VAN STRAATEN CHEMICAL COMPANY

PRIORITY TOXIC POLLUTANTS

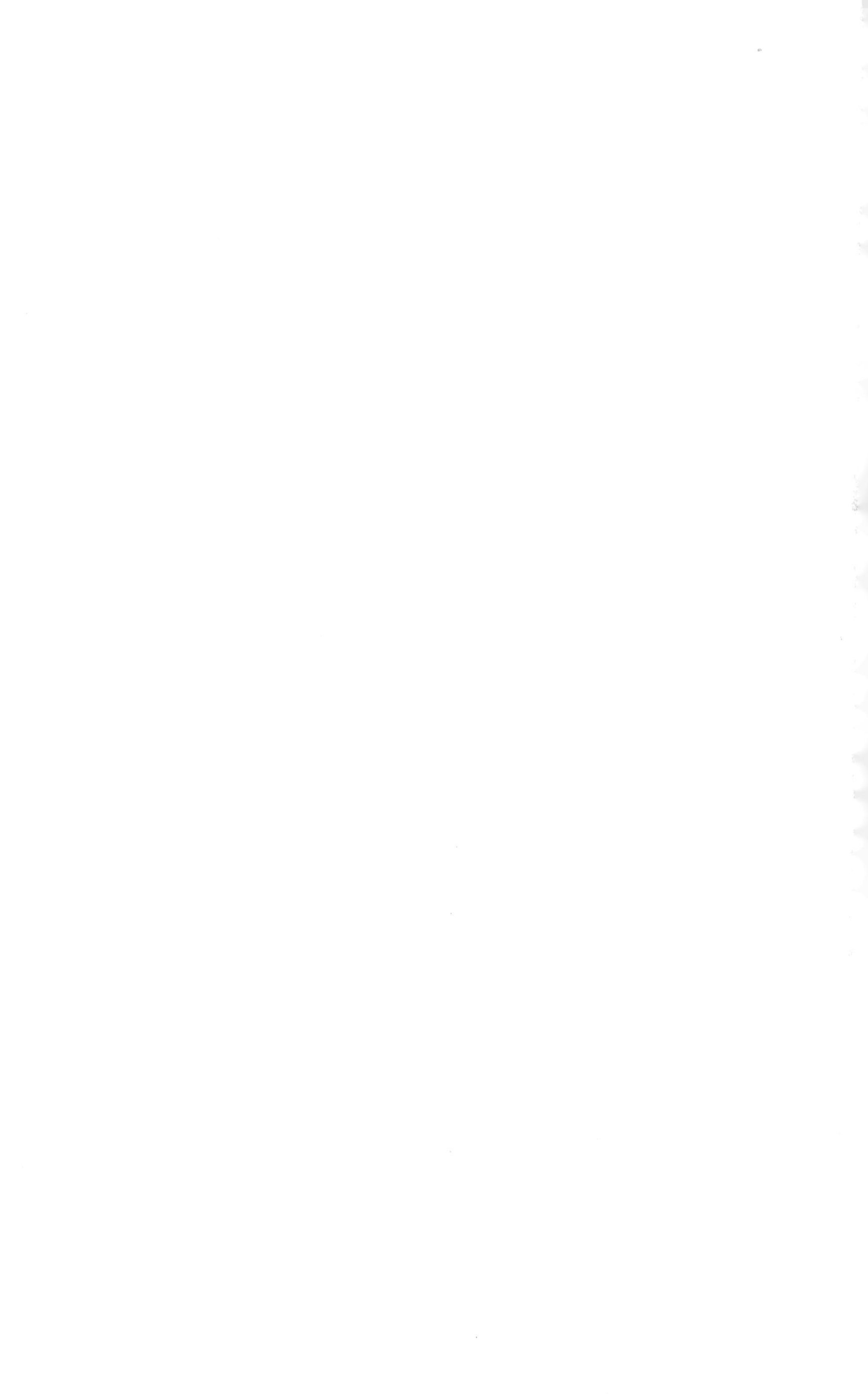

PRIORITY TOXIC POLLUTANTS

Health Impacts and Allowable Limits

Edited by Marshall Sittig

NOYES DATA CORPORATION

Park Ridge, New Jersey, U.S.A.

1980

Published in the United States of America by
Noyes Data Corporation
Noyes Building, Park Ridge, New Jersey 07656

Library of Congress Cataloging in Publication Data

Main entry under title:

Priority toxic pollutants.

  Bibliography: p.
  Includes index.
  1. Toxicology--Dictionaries. 2. Pollution--Toxi-
cology--Dictionaries. 3. Water quality--Standards--
Dictionaries. I. Sittig, Marshall. [DNLM: 1. Air
pollutants--Encyclopedia. 2. Water pollutants--Encyclo-
pedia. 3. Toxicology--Encyclopedia. WA13 P958]
RA1193.P74   363.7'394   80-311
ISBN 0-8155-0797-6

FOREWORD

This book is a practical manual of priority toxic pollutants arranged alphabetically in encyclopedic form. It is intended to provide explicit, instant information for the characterization and identification, as well as the allowable levels, of 65 priority toxic pollutants (actually reflecting 129 individual compounds), their derivatives or degradation products or intermedia transfers.

Compelled by a consent decree obtained in a federal court by public interest groups, the Environmental Protection Agency has promulgated criteria on allowable limits and profuse guidelines on how to interpret them and also how to determine further such criteria.

Here, in ready reference form, are the essentials of the criteria and guidelines which so far have been published relating to these priority toxic pollutants. Each typical pollutant is characterized with descriptions of its:

> Occurrence
> Physical Properties
> Chemical Properties
> Uses
> Toxic Effects
> Current Levels of Exposure
> Special Groups at Risk
> Existing Guidelines and Standards
> Summary of Proposed Criteria
> Bases for the Human Health Criteria
> Pertinent References

Only the basic 65 priority pollutants are assigned numbers in the text, however the toxic hazards of all of the 129 compounds are covered. It should be noted that the bibliography beginning on page 42 is discrete and separate from the references following any particular pollutant.

Advanced composition and production methods developed by Noyes Data are employed to bring this durably bound book to you in a minimum of time. Special techniques are used to close the gap between "manuscript" and "completed book." Industrial technology is progressing so rapidly that time-honored, conventional typesetting, binding and shipping methods are no longer suitable. We have bypassed the delays in the conventional book publishing cycle and provide the user with an effective and convenient means of reviewing up-to-date information in depth.

The expanded table of contents serves as a subject index and provides easy access to the information contained in this book.

CONTENTS

Contents

INTRODUCTION

A new era is at hand in industrial pollution control. Whereas the efforts of the U.S. Environmental Protection Agency in the past have been directed to the control of so-called conventional pollutants in the nation's water supply, a new set of guidelines has now been mandated.

Based on a consent decree obtained in Federal court by public interest groups, the EPA has been directed to establish standards for a list of 65 "priority" toxic pollutants (actually reflecting 129 individual compounds) to regulate discharges of such materials to the nation's waterways for the protection of both aquatic and human life.

The priority toxic pollutants are of concern to those involved in air pollution control and solid waste disposal as well because intermedia transfers of these pollutants will then directly affect water quality.

This volume then is intended to provide in ready reference form the essentials of the criteria which have been proposed (1)-(65) for the control of priority toxic pollutants.

CONVENTIONAL WATER POLLUTANTS

Section 304(a)(4) of the Clean Water Act requires that:

> The administrator shall, within 90 days after the date of enactment
> of the Clean Water Act of 1977 and from time to time thereafter,
> publish and revise as appropriate information identifying conventional
> pollutants, including but not limited to, pollutants classified as biolog-
> ical oxygen demand, suspended solids, fecal coliform, and pH. The
> thermal component of any discharge shall not be identified as a con-
> ventional pollutant under this paragraph.

On July 28, 1978 the Agency published a *Federal Register* notice designating biochemical oxygen demand (BOD), pH, fecal coliform bacteria, and total suspended solids (TSS) as conventional pollutants (43 *FR* 32857). The Agency also proposed three pollutants for addition to the list. Public comments were solicited on the addition of chemical oxygen demand (COD), oil and grease and phosphorus. In this notice the Agency identified two criteria for selection of conventional pollutants. First, conventional pollutants are generally those pollutants which are naturally occurring, biodegradable, oxygen demanding materials, and solids and which have characteristics similar to naturally occurring biodegradable substances. Second, conventional pollutants include those classes of pollutants which traditionally have been the primary focus of wastewater control. Based on these criteria, EPA concluded that conventional pollutants may include suspended solids, oxygen demanding substances and nutrients. The Agency also stated that conventional pollutants may, in some cases, be used as indicators of toxic pollutants.

EPA, as of July 30, 1979 (66), established oil and grease as a conventional pollutant and also withdrew its proposal to add COD and phosphorus to the conventional pollutant list. The following then comprises the list of conventional pollutants designated pursuant to section 304(a)(4) of the Act:

(1)   Biological oxygen demand (BOD)

(2)   Total suspended solids (nonfilterable) (TSS)

(3)   pH

(4)   Fecal coliform

(5)   Oil and grease

THE CONSENT DECREE

Actions were entered into by a number of public interest law groups to force the U.S. Environmental Protection Agency to set more definite provisions for the enforcement of the Federal Water Pollution Control Act Amendments of 1972.

The EPA was unable to promulgate many of these regulations by the dates contained in the Act. In 1976, a suit was instituted by several environmental groups including Natural Resources Defense Council, Environmental Defense Fund, and Citizens for a Better Environment. This resulted in a settlement agreement or consent decree which was approved by the Court. This original consent decree in 1976 (67) was modified by a second such decree in 1979 (68).

These agreements required EPA to develop a program and adhere to a schedule for promulgating best available technology (BAT) effluent limitations guidelines, pretreatment standards and new source performance standards for 21 major industries and for 65 "priority" pollutants and classes of pollutants which may issue from these industries.

DEFINITION OF 65 PRIORITY POLLUTANTS

Under paragraph 11 of the Consent Decree in *Natural Resources Defense Council, et al, v. Train,* (67), EPA must publish criteria for 65 specified toxic pollutants. The criteria are to state maximum recommended concentrations consistent with the protection of aquatic life and human health. They are as follows:

(1)   Acenaphthene
(2)   Acrolein
(3)   Acrylonitrile
(4)   Aldrin/Dieldrin
(5)   Antimony and compounds
(6)   Arsenic and compounds
(7)   Asbestos
(8)   Benzene
(9)   Benzidine
(10) Beryllium and compounds
(11) Cadmium and compounds
(12) Carbon tetrachloride
(13) Chlordane (technical mixture and metabolites)
(14) Chlorinated benzenes (other than dichlorobenzenes)
(15) Chlorinated ethanes (including 1,2-dichloroethane, 1,1,1-trichloroethane, and hexachloroethane)
(16) Chloroalkyl ethers (chloromethyl, chloroethyl, and mixed ethers)
(17) Chlorinated naphthalenes
(18) Chlorinated phenols (other than those listed elsewhere; includes trichlorophenols and chlorinated cresols)
(19) Chloroform
(20) 2-Chlorophenol
(21) Chromium and compounds
(22) Copper and compounds
(23) Cyanides
(24) DDT and metabolites

(25) Dichlorobenzenes (1,2-, 1,3-, and 1,4-dichlorobenzenes)
(26) Dichlorobenzidine
(27) Dichloroethylenes (1,1-, and 1,2-dichloroethylene)
(28) 2,4-Dichlorophenol
(29) Dichloropropane and dichloropropene
(30) 2,4-Dimethylphenol
(31) Dinitrotoluene
(32) Diphenylhydrazine
(33) Endosulfan and metabolites
(34) Endrin and metabolites
(35) Ethylbenzene
(36) Fluoranthene
(37) Haloethers [other than those listed elsewhere; includes chlorophenyl phenyl ethers, bromophenyl phenyl ether, bis(dichloroisopropyl) ether, bis(chloroethoxy) methane and polychlorinated diphenyl ethers]
(38) Halomethanes (other than those listed elsewhere; includes methylene chloride, methylchloride, methylbromide, bromoform, dichlorobromomethane, trichlorofluoromethane, dichlorodifluoromethane.)
(39) Heptachlor and metabolites
(40) Hexachlorobutadiene
(41) Hexachlorocyclohexane
(42) Hexachlorocyclopentadiene
(43) Isophorone
(44) Lead and compounds
(45) Mercury and compounds
(46) Naphthalene
(47) Nickel and compounds
(48) Nitrobenzene
(49) Nitrophenols (including 2,4-dinitrophenol, dinitrocresol)
(50) Nitrosamines
(51) Pentachlorophenol
(52) Phenol
(53) Phthalate esters
(54) Polychlorinated biphenyls (PCBs)
(55) Polynuclear aromatic hydrocarbons (including benzoanthracenes, benzopyrenes, benzofluoranthene, chrysenes, dibenzoanthracenes, and indenopyrenes) (PAHs)
(56) Selenium and compounds
(57) Silver and compounds
(58) 2,3,7,8-tetrachlorodibenzo-p-dioxin (TCDD)
(59) Tetrachloroethylene
(60) Thallium and compounds
(61) Toluene
(62) Toxaphene
(63) Trichloroethylene
(64) Vinyl chloride
(65) Zinc and compounds

THE DEFINITION AND USE OF INDICATOR POLLUTANTS

The difficulties of analyses for other toxic pollutants has prompted EPA to propose a new method of regulating certain toxic pollutants (69). For toxic pollutants for which historical data is limited and relatively inexpensive analytical methods are not well developed, EPA is proposing numerical limitations on indicator pollutants, including BOD_5, COD, TSS, oil and grease, TKN, ammonia, chromium (total), and phenol (total). The data available to EPA generally show that when these indicator pollutants are controlled, the concentrations of toxic pollutants are significantly lower than when indicator pollutants are present in high concentrations. While the relationships between indicator pollutants and toxic pollutants are not quantifiable on a one-to-one basis, control of an indicator will reasonably assure control of toxics with similar physical and chemical properties responsive to similar treatment mechanisms.

This method of toxics regulation obviates the difficulties, high costs, and delays of monitoring and analyses that would result from limitations solely on the toxic pollutants. When an indicator limitation is violated, a discharger may be required to monitor for some or all of the toxic pollutants or to utilize biomonitoring techniques.

RELATIONSHIP TO WATER QUALITY STANDARDS

Because EPA has raised significant issues about the relationship of section 304(a) criteria to section 303 water quality standards in an Advance Notice of Proposed Rulemaking (ANPRM) 43 FR 29588, July 10, 1978, it is appropriate to highlight certain aspects of this relationship (70).

A water quality standard is developed through State or Federal rulemaking procedures and may be directly translated into an enforceable discharge or effluent limitation in a point source discharge (NPDES) permit under section 301(b)(1)(C), or may form the basis of best management practices for nonpoint sources under section 208 of the Act. A water quality standard for a particular water body consists basically of two parts: (1) A use for which the water body is to be protected or designated (such as agriculture, recreation, or fish and wild-life); and (2) a numerical or qualitative pollutant concentration limit which will support that use. (See ANPRM, 43 *FR* at 29589, 28590).

Establishing the use component of a water quality standard for a given water body, in light of the goals of the Act and the value of the water body for various purposes, involves a de-termination of what use is attainable. In determining whether a use is attainable, considera-tion is given to environmental, technological, social, economic and institutional factors [40 *CFR* 130.17(c)(1)].

The second (concentration) component of a standard, in contrast, involves a decision about the water quality or constituent concentration that must be provided if a particular use is to be maintained. Thus this component of a water quality standard, like a section 304(a) criterion, is founded on scientific considerations.

A section 304(a) criterion is not a water quality standard and in itself has no regulatory ef-fect. Only if a section 304(a) criterion is adopted by a State through rulemaking or prom-ulgated by EPA under section 303 (or is incorporated in a standard under another statutory authority) through rulemaking or adjudication, does the section 304(a) criterion acquire regulatory significance. Moreover, that significance is restricted in two important ways. First, if a section 304(a) criterion is translated into the concentration component of a wa-ter quality standard, scientific considerations specific to a given water body may be taken into account. A criterion which has been established as generally necessary to support a specified use may not be required to maintain that use in a particular water body. For example, in some cases ecosystem adaptation may enable a viable balanced aquatic popula-tion to exist in waters with high natural background levels of certain pollutants.

Similarly, toxicity of certain compounds may be less in some waters because of differences in acidity, temperature, water hardness, and other factors. (Conversely, some natural water characteristics may increase the impact of certain pollutants.)

Second, a section 304(a) criterion adopted by a State or federally promulgated under sec-tion 303 acquires regulatory weight only when a particular water body is designated for the use which the criterion is designed to protect. A water body designated for agricultural use, for example, might not have to achieve the same concentration levels as a water body designated for the protection and propagation of fish, shellfish, and wildlife. The criteria issued on March 15, 1979 (70), which reflect levels for the protection of aquatic life and human health would not necessarily be required to protect other uses such as agricul-ture.

EPA has established regulations and policies concerning section 304(a) water quality criteria and section 303 concentrations and uses. This program was summarized in the ANPRM, and public comment was invited on a variety of questions about the direction this program should take in the future.

Issues raised in the ANPRM potentially affect the significance of the criteria issued on March 15, 1979 (70). For instance, EPA's policy for its current (1976) water quality cri-teria (the "Red Book" criteria) is that "a State may adopt a numerical concentration for a Red Book pollutant which is less stringent than the Red Book number, but only if a State provides adequate technical justification for the deviation." (43 *FR* at 29590) Fail-ure to provide adequate technical justification may result in EPA disapproval of that por-tion of the water quality standard and, subsequently, in EPA proposal and potential prom-ulgation of the more restrictive limit. The EPA is considering extending this policy con-cerning Red Book criteria to its new toxic pollutant criteria after such criteria are published as final, and solicits comments on this option.

The ANPRM also stated that it is EPA's current policy generally not to promulgate standards for pollutants which States have not addressed in their standards. As stated in that notice, EPA is contemplating altering this policy for some or all of the 65 toxic pollutants. Thus, EPA might "provide a list of pollutants for which water quality standards must be developed" either by the States or by EPA (43 *FR* at 29591). This policy will be developed in future rulemaking efforts separate from the issuance of water quality criteria for public comment today. Persons wishing to comment on this policy option will therefore be able to make their views known at that time.

RELATIONSHIP TO DRINKING WATER STANDARDS

It is not expected that health-based water quality criteria will necessarily be the same as standards or guidelines issued by EPA under other Acts since other authorities may mandate different considerations. The mandate for establishing standards for drinking water at the tap under the Safe Drinking Water Act (SDWA), for instance, expressly requires consideration of economic and technical feasibility, whereas feasibility is not a factor in developing section 304 water quality criteria.

In addition the extrapolation model used to estimate the risk associated with the Interim Primary Drinking Water Standards was somewhat different from that used in calculating water quality criteria. Thus, the criteria issued on March 15, 1979 (70) are not intended to serve as drinking water tap standards, nor are these criteria expected to be the same as recommended maximum contaminant levels (RMCL's), nonenforceable health-based goals, which are also mandated under the SDWA. While RMCL's are more like section 304 criteria than tap water standards, specific mandates of the SDWA such as the consideration of multimedia exposure, as well as the different methods for setting contaminant levels under the two Acts may result in differences between RMCL's and the criteria published for comment on March 15, 1979 (70).

In the future, a State or EPA may through rulemaking proceedings consider using the health-based section 304(a) criteria for a public water supply designated use standard under section 303. In such a case, consideration may be given to whether pollutants are more effectively removed before they reach the ambient water (i.e., at the point of discharge), or at a drinking water treatment works.

EPA PRETREATMENT STANDARDS

General pretreatment regulations were set forth by the Environmental Protection Agency in 1978 (71). These regulations were among the first implementation documents setting forth the 65 priority toxic pollutants. These general pretreatment regulations were established in accordance with the original consent decree (67) to prevent the discharge of pollutants through publicly owned treatment works (POTW's) which interfere with, pass through, or otherwise are incompatible with the treatment works. Subsequently, changes in the general pretreatment regulations have been proposed (72).

AMPLIFICATION TO 129 SPECIFIC PRIORITY POLLUTANTS

EPA concluded that it had to define specific toxic pollutants for analyses. The list of 65 pollutants and classes of pollutants potentially includes thousands of specific pollutants; and the expenditure of resources in government and private laboratories would be overwhelming if analyses were attempted for all of these pollutants. Therefore, in order to make the task more manageable, EPA selected 129 specific toxic pollutants for study in this rulemaking and other industry rulemakings. The criteria for selection of these 129 pollutants included frequency of occurrence in water, chemical stability and structure, amount of the chemical produced, availability of chemical standards for measurement, and other factors (69).

The group of pollutants and classes of pollutants, potentially including thousands of specific compounds, was thus lengthened to a list of 129 priority pollutants (Table 1) which serves as the basis for the proposed BAT, new source performance standards, and pretreatment standards for new and existing sources. The 129 toxic pollutants are divided into three major groups: organics, pesticides and PCBs and inorganics.

Table 1: Recommended List of Toxic Pollutants, Revised April 1977

(1) *acenaphthene	*dinitrotoluene
(2) *acrolein	(35) 2,4-dinitrotoluene
(3) *acrylonitrile	(36) 2,6-dinitrotoluene
(4) *benzene	(37) *1,2-diphenylhydrazine
(5) *benzidine	(38) *ethylbenzene
(6) *carbon tetrachloride (tetrachloromethane)	(39) *fluoranthene
*chlorinated benzenes (other than dichlorobenzenes)	*haloethers (other than those listed elsewhere)
(7) chlorobenzene	(40) 4-chlorophenyl phenyl ether
(8) 1,2,4-trichlorobenzene	(41) 4-bromophenyl phenyl ether
(9) hexachlorobenzene	(42) bis(2-chloroisopropyl) ether
*chlorinated ethanes (including 1,2-dichloroethane, 1,1,1-trichloroethane, and hexachloroethane)	(43) bis(2-chloroethoxy) methane
(10) 1,2-dichloroethane	*halomethanes (other than those listed elsewhere)
(11) 1,1,1-trichloroethane	(44) methylene chloride (dichloromethane)
(12) hexachloroethane	(45) methyl chloride (chloromethane)
(13) 1,1-dichloroethane	(46) methyl bromide (bromomethane)
(14) 1,1,2-trichloroethane	(47) bromoform (tribromomethane)
(15) 1,1,2,2-tetrachloroethane	(48) dichlorobromomethane
(16) chloroethane	(49) trichlorofluoromethane
*chloroalkyl ethers (chloromethyl, chloroethyl, and mixed ethers)	(50) dichlorodifluoromethane
(17) bis(chloromethyl) ether	(51) chlorodibromomethane
(18) bis(2-chloroethyl) ether	(52) *hexachlorobutadiene
(19) 2-chloroethyl vinyl ether (mixed)	(53) *hexachlorocyclopentadiene
*chlorinated naphthalenes	(54) *isophorone
(20) 2-chloronaphthalene	(55) *naphthalene
*chlorinated phenols (other than those listed elsewhere; includes trichlorophenols and chlorinated cresols)	(56) *nitrobenzene
(21) 2,4,6-trichlorophenol	*nitrophenols (including 2,4-dinitrophenol and dinitrocresol)
(22) para-chloro meta-cresol	(57) 2-nitrophenol
(23) *chloroform (trichloromethane)	(58) 4-nitrophenol
(24) *2-chlorophenol	(59) 2,4-dinitrophenol
*dichlorobenzenes	(60) 4,6-dinitro-o-cresol
(25) 1,2-dichlorobenzene	*nitrosamines
(26) 1,3-dichlorobenzene	(61) N-nitrosodimethylamine
(27) 1,4-dichlorobenzene	(62) N-nitrosodiphenylamine
*dichlorobenzidine	(63) N-nitrosodi-n-propylamine
(28) 3,3'-dichlorobenzidine	(64) *pentachlorophenol
*dichloroethylenes (1,1-dichloroethylene and 1,2-trans-dichloroethylene)	(65) *phenol
(29) 1,1-dichloroethylene	*phthalate esters
(30) 1,2-trans-dichloroethylene	(66) bis(2-ethylhexyl) phthalate
(31) *2,4-dichlorophenol	(67) butyl benzyl phthalate
*dichloropropane and dichloropropene	(68) di-n-butyl phthalate
(32) 1,2-dichloropropane	(69) di-n-octyl phthalate
(33) 1,2-dichloropropylene (1,2-dichloropropene)	(70) diethyl phthalate
(34) *2,4-dimethylphenol	(71) dimethyl phthalate
	*polynuclear aromatic hydrocarbons
	(72) benzo[a]anthracene (1,2-benzanthracene)
	(73) benzo[a]pyrene (3,4-benzopyrene)
	(74) 3,4-benzofluoranthene
	(75) benzo[k]fluoranthene (11,12-benzofluoranthene)

(continued)

Table 1: (continued)

(76) chrysene	*hexachlorocyclohexane (all isomers)
(77) acenaphthylene	(102) a-BHC-Alpha
(78) anthracene	(103) b-BHC-Beta
(79) benzo[ghi]perylene (1,12-	(104) r-BHC (lindane)-Gamma
benzoperylene)	(105) g-BHC-Delta
(80) fluorene	*polychlorinated biphenyls (PCBs)
(81) phenanthrene	(106) PCB-1242 (Aroclor 1242)
(82) dibenzo[a,h]anthracene	(107) PCB-1254 (Aroclor 1254)
(1,2,5,6-dibenzanthracene)	(108) PCB-1221 (Aroclor-1221)
(83) indeno[1,2,3-cd]pyrene	(109) PCB-1232 (Aroclor-1232)
(84) pyrene	(110) PCB-1248 (Aroclor-1248)
(85) *tetrachloroethylene	(111) PCB-1260 (Aroclor-1260)
(86) *toluene	(112) PCB-1016 (Aroclor-1016)
(87) *trichloroethylene	(113) *toxaphene
(88) *vinyl chloride (chloroethylene)	(114) *antimony (total)
*pesticides and metabolites	(115) *arsenic (total)
(89) *aldrin	(116) *asbestos (fibrous)
(90) *dieldrin	(117) *beryllium (total)
(91) *chlordane (technical mixture	(118) *cadmium (total)
and metabolites)	(119) *chromium (total)
*DDT and metabolites	(120) *copper (total)
(92) 4,4'-DDT	(121) *cyanide (total)
(93) 4,4'-DDE (p,p'-DDX)	(122) *lead (total)
(94) 4,4'-DDD (p,p'-TDE)	(123) *mercury (total)
*endosulfan and metabolites	(124) *nickel (total)
(95) a-endosulfan-Alpha	(125) *selenium (total)
(96) b-endosulfan-Beta	(126) *silver (total)
(97) endosulfan sulfate	(127) *thallium (total)
*endrin and metabolites	(128) *zinc (total)
(98) endrin	(129) **2,3,7,8-tetrachlorodibenzo-
(99) endrin aldehyde	p-dioxin
*heptachlor and metabolites	
(100) heptachlor	
(101) heptachlor epoxide	

*Specific compounds and chemical classes as listed in the consent decree.
**This compound was specifically listed in the consent decree; however, due to its
  extreme toxicity we are recommending that laboratories not acquire an analytical standard for this compound.

Source: Reference (73)

APPLICATION TO 21 INDUSTRIES

The original consent decree (67) required EPA to review 65 toxic pollutants discharged by
21 industrial categories. The 21 industrial categories and the SIC classifications pertinent
to those industries are shown in Table 2.

Table 2: Subcategories of 21 Industries

(1) Timber Products Processing

SIC 2411—Logging Camps and Logging Contractors (Camps Only)
SIC 2421—Saw Mills and Planing Mills, General
SIC 2426—Hardwood Dimension and Flooring Mills
SIC 2429—Special Purpose Sawmills, Not Elsewhere Classified
SIC 2431—Millwork
SIC 2434—Wood Kitchen Cabinets
SIC 2435—Hardwood Veneer and Plywood
SIC 2436—Softwood Veneer and Plywood

(continued)

Table 2: (continued)

SIC 2439—Structural Wood Members, Not Elsewhere Classified
SIC 2491—Wood Preserving
SIC 2499—Wood Products, Not Elsewhere Classified (Furniture Mills)
SIC 2661—Building Paper and Building Board Mills (Hardboard Only)

(2) Steam Electric Power Plants

SIC 4911—Electric Services (Limited to Steam-Electric Power Plants)

(3) Leather Tanning and Finishing

SIC 31—Leather and Leather Products

(4) Iron and Steel Manufacturing

SIC 3312—Blast Furnaces (Including Coke Ovens), Steel Works and
  Rolling Mills
SIC 3313—Electrometallurgical Products
SIC 3315—Steel Wire Drawing and Steel Nails and Spikes
SIC 3316—Cold Rolled Steel Sheet, Strip and Bars
SIC 3317—Steel Pipe and Tubes

(5) Petroleum Refining

SIC 2911—Petroleum Refining [Including (1) Topping Plants; (2) Top-
  ping and Cracking Plants; (3) Topping, Cracking and Petro-chemical
  Plants; (4) Integrated Plants; and, (5) Integrated and Petro-chemical
  Plants]

(6) Inorganic Chemicals Manufacturing

SIC 2812—Alkalies and Chlorine
SIC 2813—Industrial Glasses
SIC 2816—Inorganic Pigments
SIC 2819—Industrial Inorganic Chemicals, Not Elsewhere Classified

(7) Textile Mills

SIC 22—Textile Mill Products
SIC 23—Apparel and Other Finished Products Made from Fabrics
  and Similar Materials

(8) Organic Chemicals Manufacturing

SIC 2865—Cyclic (Coal Tar) Crudes, and Cyclic Intermediates, Dyes,
  and Organic Pigments (Lakes and Toners)
SIC 2869—Industrial Organic Chemicals, Not Elsewhere Classified

(9) Nonferrous Metals Manufacturing

SIC 2819—Industrial Inorganic Chemicals, Not Elsewhere Classified
  (Bauxite Refining Only)
SIC 3331—Primary Smelting and Refining of Copper
SIC 3332—Primary Smelting and Refining of Lead
SIC 3333—Primary Smelting and Refining of Zinc
SIC 3334—Primary Production of Aluminum
SIC 3339—Primary Smelting and Refining of Nonferrous Metals, Not
  Elsewhere Classified
SIC 3341—Secondary Smelting and Refining of Nonferrous Metals

(10) Paving and Roofing Materials (Tars and Asphalt)

SIC 2951—Paving Mixtures and Blocks
SIC 2952—Asphalt Felts and Coatings
SIC 3996—Linoleum, Asphalted-Felt-Base, and Other Hard Surface
  Floor Coverings, Not Elsewhere Classified

(11) Paint and Ink Formulation and Printing

SIC 2711—Newspapers; Publishing, Publishing and Printing
SIC 2721—Periodicals; Publishing, Publishing and Printing

(continued)

Table 2: (continued)

SIC 2731—Books; Publishing, Publishing and Printing
SIC 2732—Book Printing
SIC 2741—Miscellaneous Publishing
SIC 2751—Commercial Printing, Letterpress and Screen
SIC 2752—Commercial Printing, Letterpress and Lithographic
SIC 2753—Engraving and Plate Printing
SIC 2754—Commercial Printing, Gravure
SIC 2761—Mainfold Business Forms
SIC 2771—Greeting Card Publishing
SIC 2793—Photoengraving
SIC 2794—Electrotyping and Stereotyping
SIC 2795—Lithographic Platemaking and Related Services
SIC 2851—Paints, Varnishes, Lacquers, Enamels, and Allied Products
SIC 2893—Printing Ink
SIC 3951—Pens, Mechanical Pencils, and Parts and Stamp Pads (Inked
  Materials Only)
SIC 3952—Lead Pencils, Crayons, and Artists' Materials
SIC 3955—Carbon Paper and Inked Ribbons

(12) Soap and Detergent Manufacturing

SIC 2841—Soap and Other Detergents, Except Specialty Cleaners

(13) Auto and Other Laundries

SIC 7211—Power Laundries, Family and Commercial
SIC 7213—Linen Supply
SIC 7214—Diaper Service
SIC 7215—Coin-operated Laundries and Dry Cleaning
SIC 7216—Dry Cleaning Plants, Except Rug Cleaning
SIC 7217—Carpet and Upholstery Cleaning
SIC 7218—Industrial Laundries
SIC 7219—Laundry and Garment Services, Not Elsewhere Classified
None—Auto Wash Establishments

(14) Plastic and Synthetic Materials Manufacturing

SIC 282—Plastic Materials and Synthetic Resins, Synthetic and Other
  Manmade Fibers, Except Glass

(15) Pulp and Paperboard Mills; and Converted Paper Products

SIC 2611—Pulp Mills
SIC 2621—Paper Mills, Except Building Paper Mills
SIC 2631—Paperboard Mills
SIC 2641—Paper Coating and Glazing
SIC 2642—Envelopes
SIC 2643—Bags, Except Textile Bags
SIC 2645—Die-cut Paper and Paperboard and Cardboard
SIC 2646—Pressed and Molded Pulp Goods
SIC 2647—Sanitary Paper Products
SIC 2648—Stationery, Tablets, and Related Products
SIC 2649—Converted Paper and Paperboard Products, Not Elsewhere
  Classified
SIC 2651—Folding Paperboard Boxes
SIC 2652—Set-up Paperboard Boxes
SIC 2653—Corrugated and Solid Fiber Boxes
SIC 2654—Sanitary Food Containers
SIC 2655—Fiber Cans, Tubes, Drums, and Similar Products
SIC 2661—Building Paper and Building Board Mills
SIC 2782—Blankbooks, Looseleaf Binders and Devices

(16) Rubber Processing

SIC 2822—Synthetic Rubber (Vulcanizable Elastomers)
SIC 2891—Rubber Cement

(continued)

Table 2: (continued)

SIC 3011—Tires and Inner Tubes
SIC 3021—Rubber and Plastics Footwear (Rubber Only)
SIC 3031—Reclaimed Rubber
SIC 3041—Rubber and Plastics Hose and Belting (Rubber Only)
SIC 3069—Fabricated Rubber Products, Not Elsewhere Classified
SIC 3293—Gaskets, Packing, and Sealing Devices (Rubber Packing Only)

(17) Miscellaneous Chemicals

SIC 2831—Biological Products
SIC 2833—Medicinal Chemicals and Botanical Products
SIC 2834—Pharmaceutical Preparations
SIC 2861—Gum and Wood Chemicals
SIC 2879—Pesticides and Agricultural Chemicals, Not Elsewhere Classified
SIC 2891—Adhesive and Sealants
SIC 2892—Explosives
SIC 2895—Carbon Black
SIC 2899—Chemicals and Chemical Preparation, Not Elsewhere Classified
SIC 3861—Photographic Equipment and Supplies

(18) Machinery and Mechanical Products Manufacturing

SIC 3021—Rubber and Plastics Footwear (Balance)
SIC 3041—Rubber and Plastics Hose and Belting (Balance)
SIC 3079—Miscellaneous Plastics Products
SIC 3293—Gaskets, Packing, and Sealing Devices (Balance)
SIC 3321—Gray Iron Foundries
SIC 3322—Malleable Iron Foundries
SIC 3324—Steel Investment Foundries
SIC 3325—Steel Foundries, Not Elsewhere Classified
SIC 3351—Rolling, Drawing, and Extruding of Copper
SIC 3353—Aluminum Sheet, Plate, and Foil
SIC 3354—Aluminum Extruded Products
SIC 3355—Aluminum Rolling and Drawing, Not Elsewhere Classified
SIC 3356—Rolling, Drawing and Extruding of Nonferrous Metals, Except Copper and Aluminum
SIC 3357—Drawing and Insulating of Nonferrous Wire
SIC 3361—Aluminum Foundries (Castings)
SIC 3362—Brass, Bronze, Copper, Copper Base Alloy Foundries (Castings)
SIC 3369—Nonferrous Foundries (Castings), Not Elsewhere Classified
SIC 3398—Metal Heat Treating
SIC 3399—Primary Metal Products, Not Elsewhere Classified
SIC 3411—Metal Cans
SIC 3412—Metal Shipping Barrels, Drums, Kegs, and Pails
SIC 3421—Cutlery
SIC 3423—Hand and Edge Tools, Except Machine Tools and Hand Saws
SIC 3425—Hand Saws and Saw Blades
SIC 3429—Hardware, Not Elsewhere Classified
SIC 3431—Enameled Iron and Metal Sanitary Ware
SIC 3432—Plumbing Fixture Fittings and Trim (Brass Goods)
SIC 3433—Heating Equipment, Except Electric and Warm Air Furnaces
SIC 3441—Fabricated Structural Metal
SIC 3442—Metal Doors, Sash, Frames, Molding and Trim
SIC 3443—Fabricated Platework (Boiler Shops)
SIC 3444—Sheet Metal Work
SIC 3446—Architectural and Ornamental Metal Work
SIC 3448—Prefabricated Metal Buildings and Components
SIC 3449—Miscellaneous Metal Work
SIC 3451—Screw Machine Products
SIC 3452—Bolts, Nuts, Screws, Rivets and Washers

(continued)

Table 2: (continued)

SIC 3462—Iron and Steel Forgings
SIC 3463—Nonferrous Forgings
SIC 3465—Automotive Stampings
SIC 3466—Crowns and Closures
SIC 3469—Metal Stampings, Not Elsewhere Classified
SIC 3482—Small Arms Ammunition
SIC 3483—Ammunition, Except for Small Arms, Not Elsewhere Classified
SIC 3484—Small Arms
SIC 3489—Ordnance and Accessories, Not Elsewhere Classified
SIC 3493—Steel Springs, Except Wire
SIC 3494—Valves and Pipe Fittings, Except Plumbers' Brass Goods
SIC 3495—Wire Springs
SIC 3496—Miscellaneous Fabricated Wire Products
SIC 3497—Metal Foil and Leaf
SIC 3498—Fabricated Pipe and Fabricated Pipe Fittings
SIC 3499—Fabricated Metal Products, Not Elsewhere Classified
SIC 3511—Steam, Gas, and Hydraulic Turbines and Turbine Generator Set Units
SIC 3519—Internal Combustion Engines, Not Elsewhere Classified
SIC 3523—Farm Machinery and Equipment
SIC 3524—Garden Tractors and Lawn and Garden Equipment
SIC 3531—Construction Machinery and Equipment
SIC 3532—Mining Machinery and Equipment, Except Oil Field Machinery and Equipment
SIC 3533—Oil Field Machinery and Equipment
SIC 3534—Elevators and Moving Stairways
SIC 3535—Conveyors and Conveying Equipment
SIC 3536—Hoists, Industrial Cranes, and Monorail Systems
SIC 3537—Industrial Trucks, Tractors, Trailers, and Stackers
SIC 3541—Machine Tools, Metal Cutting Types
SIC 3542—Machine Tools, Metal Forming Types
SIC 3544—Special Dies and Tools, Die Sets, Jigs and Fixtures and Industrial Molds
SIC 3545—Machine Tool Accessories and Measuring Devices
SIC 3546—Power Driven Hand Tools
SIC 3547—Rolling Mill Machinery and Equipment
SIC 3549—Metalworking Machinery, Not Elsewhere Classified
SIC 3551—Food Products Machinery
SIC 3552—Textile Machinery
SIC 3553—Woodworking Machinery
SIC 3554—Paper Industries Machinery
SIC 3555—Printing Trades Machinery and Equipment
SIC 3559—Special Industry Machinery, Not Elsewhere Classified
SIC 3561—Pumps and Pumping Equipment
SIC 3562—Ball and Roller Bearings
SIC 3563—Air and Gas Compressors
SIC 3564—Blowers and Exhaust and Ventilation Fans
SIC 3565—Industrial Patterns
SIC 3566—Speed Changers, Industrial High Speed Drives, and Gears
SIC 3567—Industrial Process Furnaces and Ovens
SIC 3568—Mechanical Power Transmission Equipment, Not Elsewhere Classified
SIC 3569—General Industrial Machinery and Equipment, Not Elsewhere Classified
SIC 3572—Typewriters
SIC 3573—Electronic Computing Equipment
SIC 3574—Calculating and Accounting Machines, Except Electronic Computing Equipment
SIC 3576—Scales and Balances, Except Laboratory
SIC 3579—Office Machines, Not Elsewhere Classified
SIC 3581—Automatic Merchandising Machines

(continued)

Table 2: (continued)

SIC 3582—Commercial Laundry, Dry Cleaning, and Pressing Machines
SIC 3585—Air Conditioning and Warm Air Heating Equipment and Commercial and Industrial Refrigeration Equipment
SIC 3586—Measuring and Dispensing Pumps
SIC 3589—Service Industry Machines, Not Elsewhere Classified
SIC 3592—Carburetors, Pistons, Piston Rings, and Valves
SIC 3599—Machinery, Except Electrical, Not Elsewhere Classified
SIC 3612—Power, Distribution, and Specialty Transformers
SIC 3613—Switchgear and Switchboard Apparatus
SIC 3621—Motors and Generators
SIC 3622—Industrial Controls
SIC 3623—Welding Apparatus, Electric
SIC 3624—Carbon and Graphite Products
SIC 3629—Electrical Industrial Apparatus, Not Elsewhere Classified
SIC 3631—Household Cooking Equipment
SIC 3632—Household Refrigerators and Home and Farm Freezers
SIC 3633—Household Laundry Equipment
SIC 3634—Electric Housewares and Fans
SIC 3635—Household Vacuum Cleaners
SIC 3639—Household Appliances, Not Elsewhere Classified
SIC 3641—Electric Lamps
SIC 3643—Current-Carrying Wiring Devices
SIC 3644—Noncurrent-Carrying Wiring Devices
SIC 3645—Residential Electric Lighting Fixtures
SIC 3646—Commercial, Industrial, and Institutional Electric Lighting Fixtures
SIC 3647—Vehicular Lighting Equipment
SIC 3648—Lighting Equipment, Not Elsewhere Classified
SIC 3651—Radio and Television Receiving Sets, Except Communication Types
SIC 3652—Phonograph Records and Prerecorded Magnetic Tape
SIC 3661—Telephones and Telegraph Apparatus
SIC 3662—Radio and Television Transmitting, Signaling, and Detection Equipment and Apparatus
SIC 3671—Radio and Television Receiving Type Electron Tubes, Except Cathode Ray
SIC 3672—Cathode Ray Television Picture Tubes
SIC 3673—Transmitting, Industrial, and Special Purpose Electron Tubes
SIC 3674—Semiconductors and Related Devices
SIC 3675—Electronic Capacitors
SIC 3676—Resistors, for Electronic Applications
SIC 3677—Electronic Coils, Transformers and Other Inductors
SIC 3678—Connectors, for Electronic Applications
SIC 3679—Electronic Components, Not Elsewhere Classified
SIC 3691—Storage Batteries
SIC 3692—Primary Batteries, Dry and Wet
SIC 3693—Radiographic X-ray, Fluoroscopic X-ray, Therapeutic X-ray, and Other X-ray Apparatus and Tubes; Electromedical and Electrotherapeutic Apparatus
SIC 3694—Electrical Equipment for Internal Combustion Engines
SIC 3699—Electrical Machinery, Equipment, and Supplies, Not Elsewhere Classified
SIC 3711—Motor Vehicles and Passenger Car Bodies
SIC 3713—Truck and Bus Bodies
SIC 3714—Motor Vehicle Parts and Accessories
SIC 3715—Truck Trailers

(continued)

Table 2: (continued)

SIC 3721—Aircraft
SIC 3724—Aircraft Engines and Engine Parts
SIC 3728—Aircraft Parts and Auxiliary Equipment, Not Elsewhere Classified
SIC 3731—Ship Building and Repairing
SIC 3732—Boat Building and Repairing
SIC 3743—Railroad Equipment
SIC 3751—Motorcycles, Bicycles, and Parts
SIC 3761—Guided Missiles and Space Vehicles
SIC 3764—Guided Missile and Space Vehicle Propulsion Units and Propulsion Unit Parts
SIC 3769—Guided Missile and Space Vehicle Parts and Auxiliary Equipment, Not Elsewhere Classified
SIC 3792—Travel Trailers and Campers
SIC 3795—Tanks and Tank Components
SIC 3799—Transportation Equipment, Not Elsewhere Classified
SIC 3811—Engineering, Laboratory, Scientific, and Research Instruments and Associated Equipment
SIC 3822—Automatic Controls for Regulating Residential and Commercial Environments and Appliances
SIC 3823—Industrial Instruments for Measurement, Display and Control of Process Variables; and Related Products
SIC 3824—Totalizing Fluid Meters and Counting Devices
SIC 3825—Instruments for Measuring and Testing of Electricity and Electrical Signals
SIC 3829—Measuring and Controlling Devices, Not Elsewhere Classified
SIC 3832—Optical Instruments and Lenses
SIC 3841—Surgical and Medical Instruments and Apparatus
SIC 3842—Orthopedic, Prosthetic, and Surgical Appliances and Supplies
SIC 3843—Dental Equipment and Supplies
SIC 3851—Ophthalmic Goods
SIC 3873—Watches, Clocks, Clockwork Operated Devices and Parts
SIC 3911—Jewelry, Precious Metal
SIC 3914—Silverware, Plated Ware, and Stainless Steel Ware
SIC 3915—Jewelers' Findings and Materials, and Lapidary Work
SIC 3931—Musical Instruments
SIC 3942—Dolls
SIC 3944—Games, Toys, and Children's Vehicles; Except Dolls and Bicycles
SIC 3949—Sporting and Athletic Goods, Not Elsewhere Classified
SIC 3951—Pens, Mechanical Pencils, and Parts (Balance)
SIC 3961—Costume Jewelry and Costume Novelties, Except Precious Metal
SIC 3991—Brooms and Brushes
SIC 3993—Signs and Advertising Displays
SIC 3995—Burial Caskets

(19) Electroplating

SIC 347—Coating, Engraving, and Allied Services

(20) Ore Mining and Dressing

SIC 1011—Iron Ores
SIC 1021—Copper Ores
SIC 1031—Lead and Zinc Ores
SIC 1041—Gold Ores
SIC 1044—Silver Ores
SIC 1051—Bauxite and Other Aluminum Ores
SIC 1061—Ferroalloy Ores, Except Vanadium
SIC 1092—Mercury Ores

(continued)

Table 2: (continued)

> SIC 1094–Uranium-Radium-Vanadium Ores
> SIC 1099–Metal Ores, Not Elsewhere Classified

(21) Coal Mining

> SIC 1111–Anthracite
> SIC 1112–Anthracite Mining Services
> SIC 1211–Bituminous Coal and Lignite
> SIC 1213–Bituminous Coal and Lignite Mining Services

Source: Reference (71)

APPLICATION TO SPECIFIC INDUSTRY EXAMPLES

The application of the criteria set forth in brief in the *Federal Register* by EPA (70, 74, 75) and at more length in the full criteria documents (1 to 65) now require delineation as to their impact on the 21 industry categories.

Leather Tanning

The first industry to be the subject of a new Development Document (73) under the priority pollutant program was Leather Tanning and Finishing. EPA ascertained the presence and magnitude of the 129 specific toxic pollutants in leather tanning and finishing wastewaters in a two-phase sampling and analysis program involving 22 tanneries and two POTWs (69). The plants were selected primarily to be representative of the manufacturing processes, the prevalent mix of production among plants, and the current treatment technology in the industry.

One plant in each of the seven subcategories (see Industry Subcategorization in the paragraphs which follow) was sampled during the screening phase of the program. Three of these plants were direct dischargers and four were indirect dischargers. During the verification phase of the program, two POTWs and 15 plants in all of the seven subcategories were sampled. Nine of these 15 plants were direct dischargers, and six were indirect dischargers.

The primary objective of the field sampling program was to produce composite samples of wastewater from which concentrations of toxic pollutants could be ascertained. Sampling visits were made during three consecutive days of plant operation. Raw wastewater samples were taken either before treatment or after minimal preliminary treatment (e.g., screening), depending upon accessibility to the wastewater stream. Treated effluent samples were taken either following pretreatment (usually indirect dischargers) or following biological treatment as practiced by the industry (direct dischargers) where these technologies were in place. EPA also sampled intake water to determine the presence of toxic pollutants prior to contamination by tanning processes.

The subcategories of the leather tanning and finishing industry are defined as follows (69):

(1) Hair pulp, chrome tan, retan-wet finish—plants which process cured or raw cattle (or similar) hides into finished leather by chemically dissolving the hair (hair pulp), tanning with trivalent chromium, and retanning and wet finishing.

(2) Hair save, chrome tan, retan-wet finish—same as subcategory one, except hair is chemically loosened and mechanically removed rather than dissolved (pulped).

(3) Hair save, nonchrome tan, retan-wet finish—plants which process cured or raw cattle (or similar) hides into finished leather by chemically loosening and mechanically removing the hair, tanning with pri-

marily vegetable tannins, alum, syntans, oils, or other chemicals, and retanning and wet finishing.

(4)   Retan-Wet Finish—Plants which process previously unhaired and tanned hides or splits into finished leather by retanning and wet finishing, including coloring, fat-liquoring, and mechanical conditioning.

(5)   No beamhouse—Plants which process previously unhaired and pickled sheepskins or cattlehides into finished leather by tanning with trivalent chromium or other chemicals, and retanning and wet finishing.

(6)   Through-the-blue—Plants which process cured or raw cattle (or similar) hides into the blue stage only, by chemically dissolving the hair and tanning using trivalent chromium, with no retanning or wet finishing.

(7)   Shearling—Plants that process cured or raw sheep (or similar) skins into finished leather by retaining the hair on the skin, tanning with trivalent chromium or other chemicals, and retanning and wet finishing.

EPA has gone on to categorize the presence or absence of the 129 specific priority pollutants in leather tanning and finishing industry effluents as follows:

(1)   Toxic pollutants not detected in treated effluents (eighty).

(2)   Toxic pollutants detected in treated effluents at two plants or less (twenty).

(3)   Toxic pollutants detected in treated effluents at or below the nominal detection limit (twelve).

(4)   Toxic pollutants detected in treated effluents in significant concentrations (seventeen).

Control technology applicable to the leather tanning and finishing industry has then been proposed by EPA in a comprehensive document (73).

Textile Mills

In a somewhat similar manner to that by which the effluents from the leather tanning and finishing industry were categorized, the effluents from the textile industry have been divided as follows (76) with respect to the 129 priority toxic pollutants:

(1)   Toxic pollutants not detected in treated effluents (sixty-five).

(2)   Toxic pollutants detected at only one plant and at less than the nominal detection limit in the treated effluent (twenty).

(3)   Toxic pollutants detected in treated effluents at or below the nominal detection limit (fifteen).

(4)   Toxic pollutants detected in treated effluent above the nominal detection limit (twenty-nine).

Control technology applicable to the textile mills point source category and priority toxic pollutants is being developed by EPA (77).

Timber Products Processing

The application of the new priority toxic pollutants concept has been addressed to the timber product processing industry (insulation board and hardboard and wood preserving segments) in a recent publication by EPA (78).

CRITERIA DEVELOPMENT PROCEDURES IN GENERAL

Section 304(a) of the Clean Water Act [33 U.S.C. 1314(a)], requires EPA to publish and periodically update water quality criteria. These criteria are to reflect the latest scientific knowledge on the identifiable effects of pollutants on public health and welfare, aquatic life, and recreation (70).

A section 304(a) water quality criterion is a qualitative or quantitative estimate of the concentration of a water constituent or pollutant in ambient waters which, when not exceeded, will ensure a water quality sufficient to protect a specified water use. Under the Act a criterion is a scientific entity, based solely on data and scientific judgment. It does not reflect considerations of economic or technological feasibility. A criterion based on the protection and propagation of fish, shellfish and wildlife, for example, is simply the best estimate informed scientists are able to make of the maximum concentration of a given pollutant that can be tolerated while still maintaining protection of aquatic life. A criterion intended for the protection of human health, by the same reasoning, is the best estimate of the concentration which may exist and still not pose an undue risk to humans who drink water without further treatment or eat fish or shellfish from the water.

The information and scientific judgments contained in a section 304(a) criteria document could be used to develop enforceable standards under several sections of the Act such as section 302 (water quality-based-effluent limitations), section 303 (water quality standards), and section 307(a) (toxic pollutant effluent standards). It is important to observe, however, that before an enforceable standard is set under any of these statutory authorities, administrative rulemaking procedures by either the States or EPA will provide interested parties the opportunity to participate in the setting of standards. Final publication of these criteria under section 304(a) will therefore have no regulatory impact on any party.

The development of water quality criteria reflecting the latest scientific knowledge is necessarily an ongoing process. Section 304 reflects awareness of this fact in its requirement that criteria periodically be revised. As new information becomes available indicating that an existing criterion should be revised, or that criteria should be established for substances which have not yet been addressed, it is expected that new or revised criteria will be developed. The draft criteria issued for comment on March 15, 1979 (70) are part of this ongoing program. It should be recognized therefore that, when published after public comment, these criteria will not be "cast in concrete" but will be updated in future years when additional information becomes available indicating such a need.

EPA recognizes that the quality and quantity of the data in the criteria documents varies, and has undertaken a program to expand the data base dealing with bioconcentration factors and aquatic toxicity. Further data generation can be expected in the future. Comment is invited on what constitutes a sufficient data base for final criterion formulation and on how the quality of the criteria may best be expressed.

The criteria issued for comment on March 15, 1979 (70) are of two basic kinds: (1) Concentrations estimated to be protective of aquatic life and wildlife, and (2) concentrations relevant to the protection of human health. Criteria are not now being issued to protect recreation, agricultural or industrial uses, since a general lack of data precludes such an effort at this time. As data become available, however, appropriate criteria will be developed.

The criteria for protection of aquatic life and wildlife and criteria for the protection of human health were derived separately from essentially different data bases utilizing methods designed specifically to address the concerns of the two separate areas. The methods for deriving criteria in each of these areas are discussed briefly below.

Criteria Development for Carcinogens

Because methods do not now exist to establish the presence of a threshold for most, if not all, carcinogenic effects, EPA's policy is that there is no scientific basis for estimating safe levels for carcinogens.

The draft criteria for carcinogens therefore state that the recommended concentration for maximum protection of human health is zero. In addition, the documents present a range of concentrations estimated to pose various degrees of incremental cancer risk. For example, a document might indicate that exposure to a carcinogen through the lifetime daily consumption of water and edible aquatic organisms could result in one additional case of cancer in a population of 1,000,000 at a concentration of 0.1 μg/l, and of 1 additional cancer in a population of 100,000 at a level of 1.0 μg/l. Other risk-concentration pairs may be calculated by simple extrapolation.

This range of risk estimates is presented for information purposes and does not indicate any acceptable risk level, since as noted the only known exposure guaranteeing maximum protection of human health is zero. However, because in many situations the achievement of zero levels may be infeasible, it may be necessary to identify a maximum target risk level to be recommended in the interim.

The EPA is considering a level in the range of 10^{-7} to 10^{-5} as such a target. Concentrations corresponding to the target risk level would become a part of the criteria used by States and EPA for developing and reviewing water quality standards. It should be recognized that particular circumstances may call for the recommendation of risk levels of greater stringency than the target. Such circumstances might exist, for example, where significant exposure to a particular pollutant occurs through other routes, or where several potential carcinogens are present in the same water. Also, as noted above, feasibility and other considerations taken into account in applying the criteria in section 303 or other regulatory standards may result in enforceable standards which pose a less stringent level of risk. EPA invites public comment on the desirability of establishing an interim target risk level, and on the level at which such a target should be set.

Risk assessment from animal data is performed using the one-hit model recommended in the Agency's Interim Cancer Procedures and Guidelines for Health Risk and Economic Impact Assessments of Suspect Carcinogens (41 *FR* 21402, May 29, 1976). The model has been modified to account for spontaneous tumor incidence and to adjust for tumors not observed because of premature, chemical-induced death. EPA is aware that other models for risk extrapolation exist and have been used by EPA under other Acts, as well as by other Federal agencies. The one-hit model has recently been endorsed by the four agencies in the Interagency Regulatory Liaison Group. It is one of the most conservative models available, since it is less likely to underestimate risk at the low doses typical of environmental exposure.

Because of the uncertainties associated with dose and animal-to-human extrapolation and other unknown factors, because of the use of average exposure assumptions, and because of the serious public health consequences that could result if risk were underestimated, EPA believes that it is prudent to use conservative methods to estimate risk in the water quality criteria program.

It should be observed that extrapolation models provide only rough estimates of risk since a variety of assumptions are built into any model. Models using widely different assumptions may produce estimates ranging over several orders of magnitude. Since there is at present no way to demonstrate the scientific validity of any model, the use of risk extrapolation models is a subject of debate in the scientific community. However, risk extrapolation is generally recognized as the only tool available at this time for estimating health hazards associated with suspect nonthreshold toxicants and has been endorsed by EPA and other agencies as a useful means of assessing the risks associated with various chemicals.

Risk assessment based on extrapolation from epidemiological dose-response data is made by direct proportionality estimates from the levels of exposure to pollutants and the related incidence of cancer in man.

If data permit, assessments are based on data in which the tumor incidence resulted from ingestion of the particular compound. However, data from animals or humans exposed by other routes are used where ingestion data are lacking and there is no indication that the mode of toxicity is route-specific.

CRITERIA DEVELOPMENT GUIDELINES FOR AQUATIC LIFE PROTECTION

The Guidelines (70, 79) assume that water quality criteria for aquatic life should protect both the presence and uses of aquatic organisms. Since some substances may be more toxic in freshwater than in saltwater, or vice versa, separate water quality criteria are derived for freshwater and saltwater organisms for each substance. However, for some chemicals sufficient data were not available to derive one or both of the criteria using the Guidelines. The Guidelines are intended to describe an objective, consistent, and appropriate way of using the available pertinent information to derive such criteria. The Guidelines should not be interpreted as implying that the various ways of obtaining test results, such as static vs. flow-through or measured vs. estimated bioconcentration factors, are equally good.

Small letters in parentheses refer to the footnotes on page 25.

Section I. Identify needed criteria—

    (A)   Usually the substance of concern can be easily classified as either ionizable or nonionizable.

        (1)   Separate criteria should usually be derived for each individual nonionizable chemical, except possibly for a compound and one or more of its metabolites and degradation products, or structurally similar compounds that only differ in the number and location of atoms of a specific halogen, only exist as commercial mixtures of the various compounds, are difficult to measure individually, and apparently have similar chemical, biological, and toxicological properties.

        (2)   For an ionizable chemical, one criterion should usually be derived for all forms that are in chemical equilibrium. Separate criteria should usually be derived for each different form, e.g., valence state or bonding structure, that is not in chemical equilibrium with another chemical for which a criterion has been or is being derived.

    (B)   Based on information on chemical, biological and toxicological properties, determine for which substances criteria are needed.

    (C)   For each substance, determine if criteria are needed for both fresh- and saltwater. If both criteria are needed, all of the following must be completed once for freshwater and once for saltwater.

Section II. Data base—

    (A)   Collect all available data on the toxicity of the substance to fish, aquatic invertebrates, and aquatic plants and on the bioconcentration of the substance by aquatic organisms.

    (B)   Discard all data that are not either (1) published or (2) available in manuscript form and obtained using standard test procedures.

    (C)   Discard all data obtained using brine shrimp.

    (D)   Discard data that were not obtained using species resident in North America, Hawaii, or Puerto Rico. Resident North American species of fish are defined as those listed in "A List of Common and Scientific Names of Fishes from the United States and Canada," 3rd ed., Special Publication No. 6, American Fisheries Society, Washington, D.C., 1970.

    (E)   Discard questionable data. For example, discard data obtained using organisms that were previously exposed to significant concentrations of the test material. Discard data from tests for which there was no control treatment, in which control mortality was unacceptably high, or in which distilled or deionized water was used as the dilution water.

Section III. Fish acute values—

(A) Use the following kinds of data on toxicity to fish (times are ±3 hours):

    (1) 24-, 48-, 72-, and 96-hour LC_{50} values.

    (2) 24-, 48-, 72-, and 96-hour EC_{50} values based on immobilization.

(B) If values are available from one test for more than one of the specified time periods, use only the one for the longest duration. For use of comparable values for times other than those listed above, see Section XIV.

(C) Multiply all values based on unmeasured concentrations by an adjustment factor of 0.77 to simulate results based on measured concentrations (a).

(D) Multiply all 24-, 48-, and 72-hour values by adjustment factors of 0.66, 0.81, and 0.92, respectively, to simulate 96-hour values (b).

(E) Multiply all values from static and renewal tests by an adjustment factor of 0.71 to simulate values from flow-through tests (c).

Section IV. Invertebrate acute values—

(A) Use the following kinds of data on toxicity to invertebrates (times are ±3 hours):

    (1) 48-hour LC_{50} values for daphnids and other cladocerans, midge larvae, and embryos and larvae of barnacles and bivalve molluscs.

    (2) 48-hour EC_{50} values based on abnormal development of embryos and larvae of barnacles and bivalve molluscs.

    (3) 48-hour EC_{50} values based on immobilization of daphnids and midge larvae.

    (4) 96-hour EC_{50} values based on decreased shell deposition for oysters.

    (5) 24-, 48-, 72-, and 96-hour EC_{50} values based on loss of equilibrium for shrimp and crabs.

    (6) 24-, 48-, 72-, and 96-hour EC_{50} values based on immobilization for invertebrate species not named above.

(B) If values are available from one test for more than one of the specified time periods, use only the one for the longest duration. For use of comparable values for times other than those listed above, see Section XIV.

(C) Multiply all values based on unmeasured concentrations by an adjustment factor of 0.77 to simulate results based on measured concentrations (a).

(D) Multiply all 24-, 48-, and 72-hour values from steps A5 and A6 by adjustment factors of 0.26, 0.43, and 0.61, respectively, to simulate 96-hour values (h). Do not adjust the 48-hour values from steps A1, A2, and A3.

(E) Multiply all values from static and renewal tests by an adjustment factor of 1.1 to simulate values from flow-through tests (i).

Section V. Fish chronic values—

(A) Chronic values are calculated as the geometric mean of the limits on the Maximum Acceptable Toxicant Concentration (MATC) obtained from a life-cycle test or a partial life-cycle test, or one-half the geometric mean of the limits obtained from an embryo-larval test (e).

    Note: Some authors report "MATC limits" that are not MATC limits as defined in the Glossary at the end of this section.

Section VI. Invertebrate chronic values—

(A) Chronic values are calculated as the geometric mean of the MATC limits obtained from a life-cycle test or a partial life-cycle test.

    Note: Some authors report "MATC limits" that are not MATC limits as defined in the Glossary at the end of this section.

Section VII. Final values related to water quality—

(A)   If the toxicity of the substance is affected by a water quality characteristic such as hardness for freshwater organisms or salinity for saltwater organisms, the criterion for that substance in that water should be related to that water quality characteristic. Since data of the right kind may not be available to determine whether such a statistically significant relationship exists for both acute and chronic toxicity to both fish and invertebrates, extrapolations from one species to another, assumptions, and judgments may have to be used instead of statistical tests.

(B)   Deriving a relationship (do separately for fish acute values, invertebrate acute values, fish chronic values, and invertebrate chronic values).

   (1)   For each species for which comparable toxicity values are available at two or more different values of the water quality characteristic, perform a least squares regression of the natural logarithms of the toxicity values (adjusted when necessary) on the natural logarithms of the water quality characteristic values. If there are three or more values of the water quality characteristic, test the significance of the relationship using a regression F-test.

   (2)   Determine whether or not each slope is meaningful, taking into account not only the results of the regression F-test, but also the range and number of values of the water quality characteristic tested. For example, a slope from a statistically significant regression may be of limited value if it is based only on data for a narrow range of the water quality characteristic. On the other hand, even though a regression based on only two data points can not be tested for statistical significance, a slope based on a line drawn between only two data points may be meaningful if it is consistent with other information and if the two points cover a broad enough range of the water quality characteristic. If a meaningful slope is not obtained for any species, go to step B13.

   (3)   Calculate the mean slope (S) as the geometric mean of all of the meaningful slopes for individual species.

   (4)   For each species calculate the geometric mean (T) of the toxicity values (adjusted when necessary) and the geometric mean (C) of the related water quality characteristic values.

   (5)   For each species calculate a value for L, the logarithmic intercept, using the equation: $L = \ln T - S(\ln C)$.

   (6)   Calculate the average logarithmic intercept (I) as the arithmetic average of all of the logarithmic intercepts (L) for individual species.

   (7)   Select the appropriate value for the species sensitivity factor (F):

	. . . . . Fish		. . Invertebrates . .	
	Acute	Chronic	Acute	Chronic
Freshwater	3.9	6.7	21	5.1
Saltwater	3.7	6.7	49	5.1

   (8)   Calculate $J = I/F$.

   (9)   For each species calculate the geometric mean (W) of the toxicity values (adjusted when necessary) that were based on measured concentrations and obtained using flow-through procedures and the geometric mean (X) of the related water quality characteristic values.

  (10)   For each species, calculate a value for Y using the equation:
$Y = \ln W - S(\ln X)$.

  (11)   Obtain R by selecting the lower of J from step B8 and all the values of Y from step B10.

(12) Write the final value as: $e^{[R + S(\ln \text{Water Quality Characteristic})]}$
where the value of R is that obtained in step B11, and the value of
S is that obtained in step B3.

(13) If steps B1 to B12 have been completed for fish acute values, invertebrate acute values, fish chronic values, and invertebrate chronic values,
go to step C, If not, go to step B1.

(C) If, after reviewing all the data, an overall relationship cannot be established between toxicity and any water quality characteristic, go to Section VIII.

(D) If a relationship was derived for at least one, but not all, of the four kinds of
toxicity data (fish acute, invertebrate acute, fish chronic, and invertebrate
chronic), the other relationships should be derived as per steps B4 to B12 except that the slope should be obtained by extrapolation from the slopes for
the available relationships, rather than as per B3.

(E) Go to Section XII.

Section VIII. Final fish acute value—

(A) For each fish species for which acute values are available calculate the geometric mean of all the acute values (adjusted when necessary).

(B) Calculate the geometric mean of all of the geometric means for individual species.

(C) Obtain the Final Fish Acute Value by selecting the lower value obtained from
1 and 2:

(1) Divide the overall geometric mean by the species sensitivity factor of
3.9 for freshwater fish or 3.7 for saltwater fish (d).

(2) For each species calculate the geometric mean of all of the acute values (adjusted when necessary) based on measured concentrations and
obtained using flow-through procedures comparable to those in Methods for Acute Toxicity Tests with Fish, Macroinvertebrates and Amphibians (80). More than one geometric mean should be calculated
for a species if the available information indicates that substantially
different acute values are obtained under different test conditions or
with different life stages. Select the lowest of all of the means for
individual species.

Section IX. Final invertebrate acute value—

(A) For each invertebrate species for which acute values are available calculate the
geometric mean of all the acute values (adjusted when necessary).

(B) Calculate the geometric mean of all of the geometric means for individual species.

(C) Obtain the Final Invertebrate Acute Value by selecting the lower value obtained
for 1 and 2:

(1) Divide the overall geometric mean by the species sensitivity factor of
21 for freshwater invertebrates or 49 for saltwater invertebrates (j).

(2) For each species calculate the geometric mean of all of the acute values (adjusted when necessary) based on measured concentrations and
obtained using flow-through procedures comparable to those set forth
by EPA (80). More than one geometric mean should be calculated
for a species if the available information indicates that substantially
different acute values are obtained under different test conditions or
with different life stages. Select the lowest of all of the means for individual species.

Section X. Final fish chronic value—

(A) For each fish species for which chronic values are available calculate the geometric mean of all the chronic values.

(B)   Calculate the geometric mean of all of the geometric means for individual species.

(C)   Obtain the Final Fish Chronic Value by selecting the lower value obtained from 1, 2 and 3:

   (1)   Divide the overall geometric mean by the species sensitivity factor of 6.7 (f).

   (2)   For each species calculate the geometric mean of all of the chronic values. Select the lowest of all of the means for individual species.

   (3)   For each matched pair of MATC limits and 96-hour LC_{50} values from flow-through tests and obtained using measured concentrations, calculate an application factor by dividing the geometric mean of the MATC limits by the 96-hour LC_{50}. Calculate the geometric mean of all of the AF values. Obtain a calculated chronic value from $X\sqrt{YZ}$, where

   $$X = \text{geometric mean AF}$$
   $$Y = \text{geometric mean of the } LC_{50} \text{ values used in calculation of } X$$
   $$Z = \text{Final Fish Acute Value from Section VIII C (g).}$$

Section XI.   Final invertebrate chronic value—

(A)   For each invertebrate species for which chronic values are available calculate the geometric mean of all the chronic values.

(B)   Calculate the geometric mean of all of the geometric means for individual species.

(C)   Obtain the Final Invertebrate Chronic Value by selecting the lower value obtained from 1 and 2:

   (1)   Divide the overall geometric mean by the species sensitivity factor of 5.1 (k).

   (2)   For each species calculate the geometric mean of all of the chronic values. Select the lowest of all of the means for individual species.

Section XII.   Final plant value—

(A)   A plant value can be obtained from a toxicity test on algae, duckweed or other aquatic plant.

(B)   If no values are available for plants, no Final Plant Value can be derived.

(C)   Select the lowest plant value as the Final Plant Value.

Section XIII.   Residue limited toxicant concentration (RLTC)—

(A)   The RLTC is derived in order to protect (1) wildlife, including fish and birds, that eat aquatic organisms, and (2) the marketability of fish and shellfish. The diets of a variety of wildlife species consist almost entirely of aquatic life and wildlife usually eat the whole body. The marketability of fish and shellfish is determined by FDA action levels.

(B)   Use (1) an FDA action level or (2) a maximum dietary intake derived from a chronic animal study as a maximum permissible tissue concentration. To obtain a maximum dietary intake, use chronic studies on wildlife if available. Otherwise, use chronic studies on laboratory or domestic animals, such as mice, rabbits, and chickens, when available.

(C)   If no maximum permissible tissue concentration is available, no RLTC can be derived.

(D)   Discard each bioconcentration factor (BCF) that is not either (1) a steady-state value or (2) based on an exposure that lasted for 28 days or more. Use a BCF from field exposure only when enough measurements were made of the exposure concentrations. Discard bioconcentration factors obtained from exposures that caused an observable adverse effect on the test organisms. Bioconcentration factors should be corrected for the concentration in the control organisms and should be calculated using wet tissue weights. To convert values expressed on a dry weight basis to wet weight, multiply the dry weight value by 0.1 for plankton and by 0.2 for fish and other invertebrates (l).

(E) For use with the result of a chronic animal study, use only BCF values based on whole body measurements on aquatic plants and animals. Calculate the geometric mean for each species, and then the geometric mean of all of the geometric means for individual species.

(F) For use with an FDA action level for fish and shellfish, use only BCF values based on muscle (with or without skin) for fish and decapods, adductor muscle for scallops, and total living tissue for other bivalve molluscs. Calculate the geometric mean for each species, and select the highest mean.

(G) For use with an FDA action level for animal feed, use only BCF values based on whole body measurements on fish. Calculate the geometric mean for each species, and select the highest mean.

(H) For organic chemicals, if no BCF is available for aquatic organisms, a BCF can be obtained (m) from log BCF = 0.76 log P −0.23, where P is the octanol-water partition coefficient and can be either measured directly or obtained from the retention time on a calibrated reverse phase liquid chromatography system (n). As a last resort, an empirically derived partition coefficient can be used (o). A BCF obtained in this manner applies to aquatic organisms that contain about 8% lipids. If it is known that the diet of the wildlife of concern or that the organisms subject to an FDA action level contain a significantly different lipid content, an appropriate adjustment in the estimated BCF should be made.

(I) Obtain the RLTC by selecting the lowest value obtained from 1, 2, and 3:

    (1) Divide the lowest maximum permissible tissue concentration based on a chronic animal study by the BCF obtained in step E or in step H if necessary.

    (2) Divide the FDA action level for fish and shellfish by the BCF obtained in step F or in step H if necessary.

    (3) Divide the FDA action level for animal feed by the BCF obtained in step G or in step H if necessary.

Section XIV. Other data—

(A) For some substances acceptable pertinent information that cannot be used in other sections will be available concerning adverse effects on aquatic organisms and their uses.

(B) For some substances data on other obviously important adverse effects, such as flavor impairment or avoidance, may be available.

(C) Sometimes LC_{50} or EC_{50} values for durations longer than those specified in Sections III and IV for a sensitive species may be lower than the Final Chronic Value, if chronic values are only available for insensitive species.

(D) Data from behavioral, microcosm, field, and physiological studies may be available.

Section XV. Final values—

(A) The Final Acute Value is obtained from the Final Fish Acute Value and the Final Invertebrate Acute Value by selecting the lower available value, or, if toxicity is related to a water quality characteristic, by selecting the value that results in the lower concentrations in the normal range of the water quality characteristic.

(B) The Final Chronic Value is obtained from the Final Fish Chronic Value, the Final Invertebrate Chronic Value, the Final Plant Value, and the RLTC by selecting the lowest available value, unless other data (see Section XIV) exist to show that a lower value should be used, or, if toxicity is related to a water quality characteristic, by selecting the value that results in the lowest concentrations in the normal range of the water quality characteristic.

Section XVI. Criterion—

(A) No criterion can be derived using the Guidelines unless either a Final Fish Chronic Value is available from Section VII or Section X, or a Final Invertebrate Chronic Value is available from Section VII or Section XI, or a good substitute is available from Section XIV for either the final fish or final invertebrate chronic value.

(B) The criterion consists of two concentrations, one that should not be exceeded on the average in a 24-hour period and one that should not be exceeded at any time during the 24-hour period. This twofold criterion describes ambient water quality conditions necessary to protect aquatic life and its uses from acute and chronic adverse effects of both cumulative and noncumulative substances without being as restrictive as a single-number criterion would have to be to provide the same degree of protection.

(C) Obtain the 24-hour average concentration by selecting the lower value obtained from 1 and 2:

    (1) The Final Chronic Value from Section XV B.

    (2) 0.44 times the Final Acute Value (q) from Section XV A.

(D) The criterion is the 24-hour average and the concentration should not exceed the Final Acute Value at any time.

Section XVII. Review—

(A) On the basis of the data collected in Section II and other pertinent information, determine if the criterion is consistent with sound scientific evidence. If it is not, another criterion should be derived using appropriate modifications in the Guidelines. The Guidelines should be modified on a case-by-case basis only if sound scientific evidence indicates the need to do so.

Alternative procedures were used to derive aquatic life criteria for many of the pollutants for which certain values required by the Guidelines for criterion formulation were not available. The alternative procedures do not replace the Guidelines but supplement them by providing data, estimated values, or assumptions about the subject pollutants so that the Guidelines can be used.

The four alternative procedures developed for this purpose are described briefly below. The procedures are listed in order of preference, that is, the second alternative procedure was considered only if a criterion could not be derived using the first procedure, and so on.

It should be noted that these procedures will not produce a criterion for all chemicals for which the Guidelines will not produce a criterion.

    (1) Use unpublished data not yet in manuscript form and use the Guidelines to obtain a criterion.

    (2) Assume that, if the 24-hour average concentration is based on 0.44 times the Final Acute Value for a chemical, the same procedure can be used for that chemical for both freshwater and saltwater organisms and for structurally similar organic compounds. (Structurally similar organic compounds are organic chemicals that have the same carbon-oxygen-nitrogen structure and the same arrangement of single, double, and triple bonds, and differ only in the substitution of hydrogen, chlorine, and bromine for each other.)

        Estimate missing Final Fish Acute Values and Final Invertebrate Acute Values, by assuming that the ratio of the Final Fish Acute Value to the Final Invertebrate Acute Value is the same for a chemical for both freshwater and saltwater organisms and for structurally similar organic compounds.

Use the Guidelines to obtain a criterion.

(3) Assume that, if the 24-hour average concentration is based on the Final Fish Chronic Value for a chemical, the same procedure can be used for that chemical for both freshwater and saltwater organisms and for structurally similar organic compounds.

If an actual, not an estimated, Final Fish Acute Value is available, estimate a Final Fish Chronic Value by assuming that either the application factor or the ratio of the Final Fish Chronic Value to the Final Fish Acute Value is the same for a chemical for both freshwater and saltwater organisms and for structurally similar organic compounds.

Use the Guidelines to obtain a criterion.

(4) If, using the Guidelines, a criterion can be derived for a chemical in one water but not the other, set a criterion for the second water to be equal to that for the first water if data exist to indicate that the toxicity of the chemical to comparable organisms is about the same in both waters, and none of the values necessary to derive the criterion in the first water have to be estimated by procedures other than those described in the Guidelines.

Footnotes

(a)   The value of 0.77 is the geometric mean of values from 89 tests on 39 toxicants (see Table 1 in Reference 79).

(b)   The value of 0.66, 0.81, and 0.92 are geometric means of 307, 196, and 103 comparisons of 24-, 48-, and 72-hour LC_{50} values, respectively, with 96-hour LC_{50} values for fish (see Table 2 in Reference 79).

(c)   The value of 0.71 is the geometric mean of values for 24 pairs of tests on 12 toxicants (see Table 3 in Reference 79).

(d)   The value of 3.9 is the antilog of the product of 1.645 times the square root of the average of the logarithmic variances calculated from 62 sets of fish LC_{50} values (see Table 4 in Reference 79). The value of 1.645 is the t-value for $P = 0.05$ for a one-tailed test so that 95% of the distribution will be above the lower limit. The value of 3.7 is derived similarly for saltwater fish.

(e)   The value of one-half is used since in only 5 of 75 comparisons were the results of a life cycle test more than a factor of two lower than the results of a comparable embryo-larval test. See: Macek, K.J., and B.H. Sleight, III, 1977. In *Aquatic Toxicology and Hazard Evaluation,* ASTM STP 634, F.L. Mayer and J.L. Hamelink, eds. American Society for Testing and Materials, Philadelphia, PA. pp 137-146. McKim, J.M., 1977. Jour. Fish Res. Bd. Canada, 34:1148-1154. Hansen, D., Personal Communication, Environmental Research Laboratory, Sabine Island, Gulf Breeze, Florida.

(f)   The value of 6.7 is the antilog of the product of 1.645 times the square root of the average of the logarithmic variances calculated from 14 sets of freshwater fish chronic values (see Table 5 in Reference 79). No comparable data are available for saltwater fish, but 6.7 is probably reasonable since the available chronic values for saltwater fish are in the same range as those for freshwater fish.

(g)   See: Andrew, R.W., et al, Evaluation of an Application Factor Hypothesis, Manuscript.

(h)   The values of 0.26, 0.43, and 0.61 are geometric means of 400, 238, and 29 comparisons of 24-, 48-, and 72-hour LC_{50} values, respectively, with 96-hour LC_{50} values for invertebrates (see Table 6 in Reference 79).

(i)   The value of 1.1 is the geometric mean of values for 12 pairs of tests on 8 toxicants (see Table 7 in Reference 79).

(j)   The value of 21 is the antilog of the product of 1.645 times the square root of the average of the logarithmic variances calculated from 25 sets of acute values for freshwater invertebrates (see Table 8 in Reference 79). The value of 49 is derived similarly for saltwater invertebrates.

(k)   The value of 5.1 is the antilog of the product of 1.645 times the square root of the average of the logarithmic variances calculated from 9 sets of freshwater invertebrate chronic values (see Table 9 in Reference 79). No comparable data are available for saltwater invertebrates, but 5.1 is probably reasonable since the available chronic values for saltwater invertebrates are in the same range as those for freshwater invertebrates.

(l)   The values of 0.2 and 0.1 were derived from data published in: McDiffett, W.F., 1970. Ecology 51:975-988. Brocksen, R.W., et al, 1968. J. Wildlife Management 32:51-75. Cummins, K.W., et al, 1973. Ecology 54:336-345. Pesticide Analytical Manual, Volume I, Food and Drug

Administration, 1969. Love, R.M., 1957. In the Physiology of Fishes, Vol I, M.E. Brown, ed. Academic Press, New York. p 411. Ruttner, F., 1963. Fundamentals of Limnology. 3rd ed Trans by D.G. Frey and F.E.J. Fry. Univ of Toronto Press, Toronto. Some additional values can be found in: Sculthorpe, C.D., 1967. The Biology of Aquatic Vascular Plants, Arnold Publishing Ltd., London.

(m)   Veith, G.D., et al, An Evaluation of Using Partition Coefficients and Water Solubility to Estimate Bioconcentration Factors for Organic Chemicals in Fish. (Manuscript)

(n)   See Veith, G.D., and T.T. Morris, 1978. A Rapid Method for Estimating Log P for Organic Chemicals. Ecological Research Report. EPA-600/3-78-049. U.S. Environmental Protection Agency. Duluth, MN 15 pp.

(o)   See Leo, A.J., 1975. In *Symposium on Structure-Activity Correlations in Studies of Toxicity and Bioconcentration with Aquatic Organisms.* G.D. Veith and D.E. Konasewich, eds. International Joint Commission, Windsor, Ontario, pp 151-176.

(p)   Tests with copper, zinc, diazinon, simazine, TFM and 2,3-D have shown that exposures to some concentrations above the MATC for short periods of time do not adversely affect survival, growth or reproduction.

(q)   The value of 0.44 is the geometric mean of the quotients of the highest concentration that killed 0 to 10% of the organisms divided by the LC_{50} in 219 acute toxicity tests (see Table 10 in Reference 79).

Glossary

LC_{50}: The concentration of a toxicant in water which is lethal to 50% of the organisms of a particular species under a given set of conditions in a specified length of time (i.e., 24-, 48-, 96-hours).

EC_{50}: The concentration of a toxicant in water required to produce a defined effect in 50% of the organisms of a particular species in a specified length of time.

Maximum Acceptable Toxicant Concentration (MATC): The highest concentration of toxicant that has no adverse effect on survival, growth or reproduction of a species based on the results of a life-cycle or partial life-cycle toxicity test. A life-cycle or partial life-cycle test cannot produce a value for the MATC; a test can only produce limits within which the MATC must fall.

Life-Cycle Toxicity Test: Consists of exposing several groups of individuals of one species to different concentrations of a toxic agent throughout a life cycle in order to study the effect of the toxic agent on the survival, growth and reproduction of the species. To insure that all life stages and life processes are exposed, the test begins with embryos or newly hatched larvae less than 48 hours old, continues through maturation and reproduction, and with fish ends not less than 30 days (90 days for salmonids) after the hatching of the next generation.

Partial Life-Cycle Toxicity Test: Consists of exposing several groups of individuals of one species to different concentrations of a toxic agent through part of a life-cycle in order to study the effect of the toxic agent on survival, growth and reproduction. Partial life-cycle tests are conducted with fish species that require more than a year to reach sexual maturity, so that the test can be completed in less than 15 months, but still expose all major life stages to the toxicant. With fish, exposure to the toxic agent begins with immature juveniles at least 2 months prior to active gonad development, continues through maturation and reproduction, and ends not less than 30 days (90 days for salmonids) after the hatching of the next generation.

Application Factor (AF): For fish, the quotient of the maximum acceptable toxicant concentration (MATC) divided by the 96-hour LC_{50} (AF = MATC/96-hour LC_{50}).

Embryo-Larval Toxicity Test: A 28-day (60 to 90 days for salmonids) toxicity test involving exposure during the early life stages of a fish from fertilization through embryonic, larval, and early juvenile development. The biological effects measured are hatchability, survival, growth and deformities.

Bioconcentration Factor (BCF): Quotient of the concentration of a chemical in the tissue of an aquatic organism divided by the concentration in the water in which the organism resides.

Equilibrium Bioconcentration Factor: A BCF that is constant over a period of time such as one week.

Partition Coefficient: The quotient of the solubility of a compound in octanol divided by its solubility in water.

Empirically Derived Partition Coefficient: Partition coefficient that is calculated from measured partition coefficients for structures which contain the important interactive fragments of the chemicals for which partition coefficients must be calculated.

Maximum Permissible Tissue Concentration: The maximum concentration of a substance in aquatic organism tissue that causes no toxic effects when consumed by man or other animals.

FDA Action Level: The concentration of a substance in edible materials considered by FDA to be unacceptable for human or animal consumption.

Residue Limited Toxicant Concentration (RLTC): The highest toxicant concentration in water that will not produce a tissue residue in aquatic organisms that is above a maximum permissible tissue concentration.

Static Technique: In the static technique test solution and test organisms are placed in test chambers and kept there for the duration of the test.

Renewal Technique: The renewal technique is like the static technique except that the test organisms are periodically exposed to fresh test solution of the same composition, usually once every 24 hours, either by transferring the test organisms from one test chamber to another or by replacing the test solution.

Flow-Through Technique: In the flow-through technique test solutions flow into and out of the test chambers on a once through basis for the duration of the test. Two procedures can be used. In the first large volumes of the test solutions are prepared before the beginning of the test and these flow through the test chambers. In the second and more common procedure fresh test solutions are prepared continuously or every few minutes in a toxicant delivery system.

Geometric Mean: The geometric mean of N numbers is obtained by taking the Nth root of the product of the N numbers. Alternatively, the geometric mean can be calculated by adding the logarithms of the N numbers, dividing the sum by N, and taking the antilog of the quotient. The geometric mean of two numbers can also be calculated as the square root of the product of the two numbers. The geometric mean of the number is that number.

Logarithmic Variance: The logarithmic variance of a set of numbers is the variance of the logarithms of the numbers. Either natural (base e) or common (base 10) logarithms can be used to calculate geometric means and logarithmic variances as long as they are used consistently within each set of data, i.e., the antilog used must match the logarithm used.

HUMAN HEALTH ASSESSMENT OF PRIORITY POLLUTANT EFFECTS

The objective of the health effect assessments chapters of the various water criteria documents (1 to 65) is to estimate ambient water concentrations which protect public health. The assessments review all relevant information on individual chemicals or chemical classes in order to derive criteria which represent, in the case of suspect or proven carcinogens, various levels of incremental cancer risk; and, in the case of other pollutants, no observable effect levels.

Ideally, water quality criteria should represent levels for compounds in ambient water which would not pose a hazard to the human population. However, in any realistic assessment of human health hazard, a fundamental distinction must be made between absolute safety and recognition of some risk. Criteria for absolute safety would have to be based on detailed knowledge of dose/response relationships in humans including all sources of chemical exposure, the types of toxic effects elicited, the existence of thresholds for the toxic effects, the significance of toxicant interactions, and the variances of sensitivities and exposure levels within the human population. In practice, such absolute criteria cannot be established because of deficiencies in both the available information and the means of interpreting this information. Consequently, the water quality human health effects documents propose criteria which minimize or specify the potential risk of adverse human effects due to substances in ambient water. Potential social or economic costs and benefits are not considered in the formulation of the criteria.

Two types of biological endpoints have been used in developing water quality criteria, stochastic (nonthreshold) effects and nonstochastic (threshold) effects.

As defined by the International Commission on Radiological Protection (87), "stochastic effects are those for which the probability of an effect occurring, rather than its severity, is regarded as a function of the dose without threshold." For such effects, which may be regarded as "all or none" phenomena, thresholds or "no effect" levels cannot be established because even extremely small doses must be assumed to elicit a finite increase in the incidence of the response. Carcinogens, mutagens, and, in some cases, teratogens elicit stochastic effects. Consequently, safe levels, i.e., levels which will produce no adverse effects, cannot be established for carcinogens and mutagens. Instead, water quality criteria for such compounds are presented as a range of water concentrations associated with a corresponding change in incremental risk.

In contrast, nonstochastic effects are those for which the severity of the effect varies with the dose, and for which thresholds may, therefore, occur. The threshold assumption is based on the premise that in such systems a reserve capacity exists which is thought to be depleted before clinical disease ensues. Since this reserve capacity varies between individuals, it is necessary to incorporate safety factors to compensate for possible errors in the derivation of the criterion. Alternatively, it may be assumed that the rate of damage will not be significant over the life span of the organism. Thus, for chemicals which induce only nonstochastic effects, water quality criteria can be derived which will presumably correspond to a "no observable effects level."

In some instances, criteria are based on organoleptic characteristics, i.e., thresholds for taste or odor. Such criteria are established when insufficient information is available on toxicologic effects or when the criterion based on organoleptic effects is below that of the criterion based on toxicologic data. It is recognized that criteria based on organoleptic effects do not necessarily represent satisfactory approximations of low risk levels (70).

The list of Consent Decree pollutants contains both individual chemical species and classes of compounds. The health assessment chapters, likewise, review information either on broad chemical classes or on individual species as appropriate.

In some cases separate criteria for each chemical in a class are derived because at times even relatively small structural changes can significantly affect chronic toxicity. However, for some chemical classes insufficient data are available on all of the individual compounds of the class. In such instances, a criterion is derived for the entire class or criteria are derived only for certain individual chemicals in the class. The specific reasons for accepting either alternative are detailed in the appropriate health effects chapters.

Lastly, for some chemicals and chemical classes, the data are insufficient for the derivation of any criteria. In these cases, no criteria are given and deficiencies in the available information are detailed.

The human health effects chapters attempt to assess all information on the individual chemicals or classes of chemicals which might be useful in developing water quality criteria. Although primary emphasis is placed on identifying epidemiologic and toxicologic data, the assessments typically contain discussions on four topics: Existing levels of human exposure, pharmacokinetics, toxicity, and criterion formulations.

For all the EPA ambient water quality criteria documents (1 to 65), an attempt was made to include the known relevant information. Due to severe time constraints, however, an exhaustive literature review was not conducted for 15 documents (Chlordane, Chloroform, Heptachlor, Tetrachloroethylene, Arsenic, Carbon Tetrachloride, Dichlorethylenes, Hexachlorobutadiene, Selenium, Dioxin, Trichloroethylene, Benzene, Beryllium, Dichlorobenzene, Nitrosamines) and these documents were not subjected to formal peer review (70). For the remaining 50 documents, more detailed literature searches and reviews were performed. Since each of the latter 50 documents was prepared by a scientist who had either conducted original research on the compound or who had previously reviewed the toxicity of the compound, the probability of overlooking significant data is reduced.

Review articles and reports were used for data evaluation and synthesis. Scientific judgment was exercised in reviewing and evaluating the data in each document and identifying the adverse effects for which protective criteria are sought. In addition, each of these documents was reviewed by a peer committee of scientists familiar with the compound(s) under consideration. Each committee evaluated the quality of the available data, the completeness of the data summary, and the validity of the derived criterion.

In the analysis and organization of the data, an attempt is made to be consistent in both format and the application of accepted—or at least acceptable—scientific principles. The evaluation procedures used in the hazard assessment process follow the principles detailed by the National Academy of Sciences (89) and guidelines of the EPA's Carcinogenicity Assessment Group.

Exposure

The exposure section of the health effects chapters in the various criteria documents (1 to 65) reviews known information on the current levels of human exposure to the individual pollutant from all sources. Much of the data were obtained from monitoring studies of air, water, food, soil, and human or animal tissue residues. The major purpose of this section in each document is to provide background information on the contribution of exposure from water relative to all other sources. Consequently, this section is subdivided into exposure from ingestion in water, ingestion in food, inhalation, and dermal contact.

Information with regard to exposure is often valuable in developing a water quality criterion. Typically, a uniform exposure assumption is used in formulating the criteria which includes the consumption of contaminated drinking water and contaminated fish products. Exposure data, however, are useful for comparing the assumed intake to the expected contribution based upon available information. In addition knowledge of exposure from all sources, not limited to drinking water and ingesting fish, can be used to justify the formulation of criteria based upon exposure to ambient water but recognizing contributions to total body intake from additional exposure routes.

The use of fish consumption as a typical exposure factor requires the quantification of pollutant residues in the edible portion of the ingested species. Bioconcentration factors are used to relate the expected pollutant residue in aquatic organisms to the pollutant concentration in the ambient waters in which they live.

In order to estimate the average per capita intake of a pollutant due to consumption of contaminated fish and shellfish, a BCF appropriate for the average U.S. diet was developed.

The consumable fish and shellfish were divided into four categories: freshwater fishes, saltwater fishes, molluscs, and decapods (82). Three different procedures were used for estimating the BCF depending upon the availability of edible portion bioconcentration data and lipid solubility properties of the chemical. Generally speaking available BCF data are data for the whole fish rather than the edible portions and the data, at best, cover several species.

For lipid-soluble chemicals the average edible portion % lipids is derived for each of the four categories of consumable fish and shellfish products (91). Based on consumption factors (82), the average % lipids are weighted to give the % lipids for the average diet.

Since data indicate that the BCF for lipid-soluble compounds are proportional to the % lipids, factors for whole fish can be adjusted to edible portion BCF's. This is a necessary adjustment since most experimental BCF data are for whole body and not edible portion. Given a specific lipid-soluble pollutant there are, in many cases, at least one BCF and corresponding % lipid value.

With values for the % lipids in the average diet, and the whole fish BCF with corresponding lipid value, a single BCF can be calculated that estimates the weighted average bioconcentration factor.

Example:

Weighted average % lipids for average diet = 2.3%
Measured BCF of 17 for trichloroethylene with bluegills at 1% lipids
Weighted average BCF for average diet equals

$$\frac{17 \times 2.3\%}{1\%} = 39.1$$

As an estimator, 39 is used for the BCF

In those cases where a measured steady-state bioconcentration factor is not available, the equation log BCF = 0.76 log P – 0.23 can be used (95) to estimate the BCF for aquatic organisms that contain about 8% lipids from the octanol-water partition coefficient P. An adjustment for % lipids in the average diet versus 8% is made in order to derive the weighted average bioconcentration factor.

For nonlipid-soluble compounds, measured BCF's are needed in order to calculate representative BCF's for each of the four categories of consumed fish and shellfish. Usually, however, BCF information does not exist for all four categories and relative approximations are made based upon known species data. The known and estimated BCF's for each category of fish/shellfish are weighted according to fish consumption factors, and a weighted BCF representative of the average diet is derived.

Example: Given a BCF of 15 for arsenic in bay scallops and other information as shown:

	Average Diet Consumption (%)	BCF Estimate
Freshwater fishes	12	1
Saltwater fishes	61	1
Saltwater molluscs	9	15
Saltwater decapods	18	1

Note: The weighted BCF for arsenic is 2.26 for the average diet. As an estimator, 2.3 is used.

In addition to estimating current levels of human exposure, the exposure section provides, when available, information on special groups at risk based on unusual susceptibility or unusual levels of exposure.

Pharmacokinetics

This section of each criteria document (1 to 65) is intended to briefly summarize the available information on the absorption, distribution, metabolism, and elimination of the compound(s) in humans and experimental mammals. Such information can be extremely useful in species to species extrapolation, in assessing the body burdens from long-term low-level exposures, and in characterizing the mode of toxic action. Differences or similarities in pharmacokinetic data on chemicals within a class were sometimes used in evaluating the appropriateness of developing a single water quality criterion for a class of chemicals.

Toxic Effects

This section of each criteria document (1 to 65) summarizes the following types of information on both humans and experimental mammals: acute, subacute, and chronic toxicity; synergistic or antagonistic (action); teratogenicity; mutagenicity; and carcinogenicity.

The major goals of this section are to assess the suitability of data for use in establishing water quality criteria and to determine which biological endpoint, i.e., stochastic, nonstochastic, or organoleptic, should be selected for use in criterion formulation.

Because this section attempts to assess potential human health effects, data on documented human effects were actively sought. However, several problems with human epidemiological studies usually preclude the use of such data in generating water quality criteria. These problems, as summarized by the National Academy of Science (89) are presented below:

(1) Epidemiology cannot tell what effects a material will have until after humans have been exposed. One must not conduct what might be hazardous experiments on man.

(2) If exposure has been ubiquitous, it may be impossible to assess the effects of a material, because there is no unexposed control group. Statistics of morbidity obtained before use of a new material can sometimes be useful, but when latent periods are variable and times of introduction and removal of materials overlap, historical data on chronic effects are usually unsatisfactory.

(3) It is usually difficult to determine doses in human exposures.

(4) Usually, it is hard to identify small changes in common effects, which may nonetheless be important if the population is large.

(5) Interactions in a "nature-designed" experiment usually cannot be controlled.

Although these problems often prevent the use of epidemiological data in quantitative risk estimates, qualitative similarities or differences between documented effects in humans and observed effects in experimental mammals are extremely useful in assessing the validity of animal-to-man extrapolations. Therefore, in each case an attempt is made to identify and utilize both epidemiologic and animal dose response data. Criteria derived from such a confirmed data base are considered to be most reliable.

The decision to establish a criterion based on stochastic effects is made by evaluating information on carcinogenicity and mutagenicity. The first steps in the process of estimating risk are to determine whether the compound is likely to cause cancer in humans and to determine whether the data are adequate for the derivation of a water quality criterion. The criteria for the qualitative decision of carcinogenicity are outlined briefly in the EPA Interim Cancer Guidelines (93), in an article by Albert, et al (81), and in the IRLG guidelines on carcinogenic risks (86).

The assumption is made that a substance which induces a statistically significant response in animals by any route of exposure has the capability of causing cancer in humans from ingestion of this substance in water and edible aquatic organisms taken from that water. A chemical which has not induced a significant cancer response in humans or experimental animals is not identified as a possible carcinogen, even though its metabolites or close structural analogues might induce a carcinogenic response or even though they are mutagenic in in vitro systems.

It is recognized that some potential human carcinogens would not be identified by the rules above. However, the derivation of a criterion concentration cannot be justified for them. There are other compounds for which there is plausible, but weak, qualitative evidence of carcinogenicity in experimental animal systems but which cannot be given a valid criterion concentration. This occurs in cases where the only evidence of animal or human carcinogenicity is obtained in a special carcinogen bioassay system such as mouse skin painting or strain A mouse pulmonary adenoma. The derivation of a criterion concentration for human consumption from these studies is considered invalid regardless of the qualitative outcome.

In addition there are some compounds (e.g., nickel and beryllium) which are carcinogenic in humans via inhalation in one chemical form but have induced no response in animals or humans via ingestion of their soluble salts. For beryllium a criterion concentration is developed because of a finding of tumors in animals at a site removed from the injection site, but for nickel no criterion is recommended because no evidence of tumors exists from administration of nickel solutions by either ingestion or injection.

For those compounds which were not reported to induce carcinogenic effects or for those compounds on which carcinogenic effects data were lacking or insufficient, an attempt is made to define a No Observable Effect Level (NOEL). In many respects, the evaluation of these studies is similar to that of carcinogenicity bioassays. In order to more closely approximate conditions of human exposure, preference is given to chronic studies involving oral exposures (dietary or in water) over a significant proportion of the organism's life span. Greatest confidence is placed in those studies which demonstrated dose related adverse effects as well as no effect levels. Considerable variability was encountered in the biological endpoints used to define NOELs which ranged from gross effects such as mortality to more subtle changes in biochemical, physiological, or pathological parameters.

Given the variety of effects which some chemicals cause and the problems encountered in animal-to-man extrapolations, the derivation of a NOEL was obtained using chronic data if available. Teratogenicity, reproductive impairment, and behavioral effects may be significant consequences of environmental contamination. However, when such effects were seen, carcinogenic or other chronic toxic effects were usually also observed and subsequently used in deriving the criterion.

Teratogenicity studies, for the most part, involve doses near the maximum tolerated levels and administration schedules which do not reasonably approximate environmental exposures. Studies designed to determine reproductive impairment are often conducted over long periods at low doses. However, the threshold doses for reproductive effects often exceed the threshold for other biological endpoints (e.g., changes in organ weights). Information on behavioral effects, which is of considerable potential significance, is not available on most of the compounds under study. Consequently, most NOELs derived from chronic studies are based either on gross toxic effects or on effects which can be directly related to functional impairment or defined pathological lesions.

For compounds on which adequate chronic toxicity studies are not available, studies on acute and subacute toxicity assume greater significance. Acute toxicity studies usually involve single exposures at lethal or near lethal doses. Subacute studies usually involve exposures over about 10% of the life span of the test organisms, e.g., 90 days for the rat with an average life span of 30 months. Such studies are useful in establishing the nature of the toxic effects, including the target organs, metabolic behavior, physiological/biochemical effects, and patterns of retention and tissue distribution. The utility of acute and subacute studies in deriving environmentally meaningful NOEL's is uncertain although McNamara (88) has developed application factors for such derivations.

In some cases where adequate data are not available from studies using oral routes of administration, NOEL's for oral exposures are estimated from dermal or inhalation studies. Such estimates involved approximations of the total dose based on assumptions about breathing rates and/or magnitude of absorption.

Criterion Rationale

This section of each criterion document (1 to 65) reviews existing standards for the chemical(s), summarizes data on current levels of human exposure, attempts to identify special groups at risk, and defines the basis for the recommended criterion.

Information on existing standards is included primarily for comparison with the proposed water quality criteria. Some of these standards, such as those recommended by Occupational Safety and Health Administration (OSHA) or American Conference of Governmental Industrial Hygienists (ACGIH), are based on toxicological data but are intended as acceptable levels of occupational rather than environmental exposure. Other levels, such as those recommended by the National Academy of Sciences (89) or EPA (94) are more comparable to the proposed water quality criteria. Emphasis is placed on detailing the bases for the existing standards, wherever possible.

Summaries of current levels of human exposure specifically address the applicability of the data to generating water quality criteria. The identification of special groups at risk—either because of geographical or occupational differences in exposure or biological differences in susceptibility to the compound(s) focused on the impact that these groups should have on the development of water quality criteria.

In the section on the basis for the recommended criteria in each criteria document (1 to 65) all of the data used in developing the criteria were summarized and, if necessary, qualified.

CRITERIA DEVELOPMENT GUIDELINES FOR HUMAN HEALTH PROTECTION

The derivation of water quality criteria from data on laboratory animal toxicity tests is essentially a two-step procedure. First, a total daily intake for humans must be estimated which establishes either a defined level of risk for stochastic effects or NOEL for nonstochastic effects. Secondly, some assumptions must be made about the contribution of contaminated water and fish/shellfish consumption to the total daily intake of the chemical. These assumptions may then be used to calculate the water quality criterion as it relates to the tolerable daily intake.

Stochastic Effects

After the decision has been made that the compound has the potential of causing cancer in humans and that data exist which permit the development of a criterion, the water concentration which is estimated to cause a lifetime carcinogenic risk of 10^{-5} is determined. This concentration is calculated by fitting the available data to a dose-response model. A risk level of 10^{-5} was selected for the purpose of comparing the carcinogenic effects among the various compounds. The model chosen for this purpose incorporates several concepts assembled from different sources. The basic dose response model is the one-hit model.

$$(1) \qquad P = 1 - \exp\,[-BD]$$

where P is the probability of getting an observable case of cancer in a lifetime because of exposure to a daily dose D of the compound, and B is a constant determined by the data. The quantity B is the only parameter in the model and it is interpreted as a quantitative indicator of the carcinogenic effectiveness of the compound. At low doses (low enough so that $P < 0.1$), P is directly proportional to the dose D and B is the slope of the dose-response line obtained when P is plotted against D. Because the model approximates a straight line through the origin at low doses, it is sometimes called a linear, no-threshold dose-response model. It states that any exposure to a carcinogen, however small, results in some chance of cancer occurrence, and the probability (or the risk) of getting cancer from low exposure increases linearly with the dose.

This model is used for risk estimations because it is consistent with three basic concepts in chemical carcinogenesis: (a) The dose-response curve for mutagenesis in bacterial systems is linear with no threshold for both radiation- and chemical-induced damage; (b) there are both theoretical reasons, based on valid concepts of the mechanisms of chemical carcinogenesis, as well as a wealth of data, which indicate that chemicals which cause mutations are likely to induce cancer in animals and therefore presumably in people; and (c) epidemiology studies in human populations exposed to animal carcinogens (radiation, aflatoxin, cigarette smoke) show an incidence-exposure relationship that is linear down to very small doses with no evidence of a threshold.

Evidence for some chemicals suggests that extremely small doses are detoxified safely and therefore do not contribute to the induction of cancer. If this were true the risk at such low exposures would be either zero or much smaller than the one-hit model would predict. The possibility of threshold mechanisms has given support to other dose-response models (85) for extrapolation of cancer risk such as the log-probit, logit and multistage models. These models are nonlinear and result in lower risks than the one-hit model for a given low exposure.

Since the experimental tumor incidence data generally provide no clue as to which model is correct, the choice must be made on the basis of policy. The agency has chosen the one-hit model because it is consistent with the three basic facts previously mentioned and because it gives greater risk estimates than other plausible models. The entire procedure, both in the choice of the model and in the selection of which of several sets of carcinogenic data to use in the model, is designed to determine roughly how severe the carcinogenic hazard could be if the chemical does have the potential of causing cancer in humans. The hazard is not likely to be higher but could be lower if some threshold or nonlinear response exists. Therefore the water quality criterion concentrations derived from the procedure are intended to be estimates of the smallest concentrations that are likely to give rise to a 10^{-5} risk.

In analyzing animal data where the control (untreated) group has a spontaneous incidence of tumors equal to P_c and the treated group has an incidence of the same tumor type of P_t, the incidence that can be attributed to the treatment alone, P, can be found by the following argument. If the process initiating a spontaneous tumor is independent of the chemical process which initiates an induced tumor, then in the treated group where both processes are occurring simultaneously, the animals have tumors either because they are spontaneous (with probability P_c) or because they are not spontaneous (which has probability $1 - P_c$) and they are induced by the chemical (with a probability P). Therefore,

$$(2) \qquad P_t = P_c + (1 - P_c)P$$

$$P = (P_t - P_c)/(1 - P_c)$$

The quantity P, due to chemically-induced tumors, is the quantity appearing in the one-hit model, equation (1). The correction for spontaneous tumors given in equation (2) is called the Abbott's correction. Using it, the one-hit model takes the form:

$$(3) \qquad P = (P_t - P_c)/(1 - P_c) = 1 - \exp{[-BD]}$$

Another modification of the one-hit model is needed to deal with experiments that are terminated earlier than the natural lifetime of the animals because of early tumor occurrence and for cases where the data are given in terms of the time when a certain fraction (usually 50%) of the animals have tumors. It is known, from an extensive series of rat experiments by Druckrey (84) with different nitrosamine compounds, that for a certain daily dosage, d, the time when 50% of the animals get tumors, t_{50} is shorter with higher doses and the relationship between t_{50} and d is $d(t_{50})^m = K$, where K and m are constants characteristic of the compound. He found that for the compounds tested m ranged from 2.0 to 4.0 with most of them close to 3.0. This observation is consistent with the findings of Doll (83) that the age progression of human chemically-induced cancers also increases as t^3. This time dependence of the progression of tumors during a lifetime can be incorporated into the one-hit model for lifetime incidence equation (3) by expressing time as fraction of a lifetime and writing

$$(4) \qquad P = (P_t - P_c)/(1 - P_c) = 1 - \exp\left[-BDt^3\right]$$

This formulation of the dose-response model is equivalent to equation (3) for lifetime exposures. If the chemical is so potent and the doses are so large that treated animals die prematurely at times significantly less than 1.0, then the premature termination of the experiment will have the effect of increasing the value of B, the potency of the compound.

The dose-response model (4) has features of the Weibull time-to-tumor model (90), which is $P = k(t - w)^m$, where w, k and m are constants. This can be shown by noticing that, for small values of D, equation (4) is approximately $P = BDt^3$ which is the Weibull model with m = 3, w = 0 and k = BD.

Selection of Data and Use of the Extrapolation Model: After determining that a substance is carcinogenic and that the existing information is adequate for developing a water criterion, a choice must be made of which of the data sets from several studies to use in the model. For some chemicals, several studies in different animal species and strains, each run at several doses and possible different routes of exposure, are available. It is also necessary to correct for metabolism differences between species and absorption factors via different routes. The procedures used in evaluating these data are consistent with the approach of making a maximum-likely risk estimate. They are listed below:

(1) The tumor incidence data are separated according to the organ site or tumor type. For each dose group the tumor incidence in treated versus controls is tested for significance using the Fisher exact test at the $p < 0.05$ level of significance.

(2) The set of data (i.e., the dose and incidence data) used in the model is the set where the incidence is statistically significantly higher than controls at the lowest dose group. If the lowest dose group has more than one tumor site that is statistically significant, then the set used is the one which gives the highest value of the potency factor B. In case both matched and pooled controls are reported (as in the NCI bioassay program), the pooled controls are not used if their tumor incidence is significantly different from matched controls. When the two control groups are not significantly different, the one giving the highest value of B is actually used, although in this case the choice of controls usually has only a trivial effect on the value of B.

(3) Each of the available carcinogenicity reports is analyzed in a similar way. The dose units in each report are converted to mg/kg/day averaged over the time span of the study (the time until terminal sacrifice).

In calculating the mg/kg/day equivalent of a dietary dose of a certain ppm, a standard conversion factor (F), assumed to be characteristic of the species, is used as follows: mg/kg/day = ppm x F. The factor F is the percent of the adult animal weight that is consumed as food each day. For rats, F = 0.05; for mice, F = 0.13. For comparison of inhalation and ingestion experiments, the assumption is made that 100% is absorbed via each route unless experimental measurements are available.

(4) The value of B used for the criterion is the highest value obtained from any of the studies.

(5) Dose conversions between species are done on a body surface area basis. It is known that the effective dose, d, in mg per day of direct-acting drugs is proportional to the body surface area. This relationship holds for humans of various sizes from infants to adults and

for extrapolations between laboratory animals and humans. It is known to be approximately true also for oxygen and calorie consumption rates. Since a crude approximation to body surface area is the body weight, w, to the two-thirds power, one can write $d = k/w^{1/3}$, so that the ratio between the animal specific dose, $(d/w)_A$ and the equivalent human specific dose, $(d/w)_H$ is:

$$\frac{(d/w)_H}{(d/w)_A} = \left(\frac{w_A}{w_H}\right)^{1/3}$$

Therefore the specific dose (mg/kg/day) to humans required to produce an effect is smaller than the specific dose that would produce that effect in animals. It follows that, when the doses are expressed as mg/kg body weight/day, the potency in humans is higher than that in animals by the ratio $(W_H/W_A)^{1/3}$.

(6) If human epidemiology studies and associated exposure information are available for the compound they are always used in some way. If they show a carcinogenic effect, even when the route is inhalation, the data are analyzed to give an estimate of the linear dependence of cancer rates on lifetime average dose, which is equivalent to the factor B. If they show no carcinogenic effect then it is assumed that the real value of B is less than can be observed in the experiment, and an upper limit value of B is calculated assuming hypothetically that the true incidence is just below the level of detection in the cohort studied, which is determined largely by the sample sizes. Whenever possible human data are used in preference to animal bioassay data.

Calculation of the Water Quality Criterion Concentration: After the value of B has been determined the lifetime risk, P, from an average daily exposure of x mg/kg/day is found from the equation $P = Bx$. Therefore if the lifetime risk is set at $P = 10^{-5}$ for calculation purposes, the intake, I in mg/day for a 70-kg person can be found by the equation:

$$(5) \qquad I = 70 \times 10^{-5}/B$$

The exposure to ambient water is assumed to come from two sources; (a) drinking an average of 2 liters of water per day, and (b) ingesting an average of 18.7 grams of fish per day (82). Because of accumulation of residues in fish, the amount of the pollutant in fish (mg/kg of edible fish) is equal to a factor R times the water concentration (mg/kg of water). Therefore the total intake I can be written as the sum of two terms:

$$I \text{ (mg/day)} = [C \text{ (mg/l)} \times R \text{ (l/kg fish)} \times 0.0187 \text{ (kg fish/day)}] + [C \text{ (mg/l)} \times 2 \text{ (l/day)}]$$
$$= C[(0.0187 \times R) + 2]$$

where C is the water concentration in mg/l. Therefore the water concentration can be found from equation (5) as follows:

$$(6) \qquad C = 70 \times 10^{-5}/B \,[2 + (R \times 0.0187)]$$

This is the equation for calculating the water quality criterion for a pollutant. Under certain circumstances, criteria for exposure conditions other than 2 liters of water/day and 18.7 grams fish/day may be desired. Lifetime risk levels other than 10^{-5} may also be of interest. In such circumstances equation (7) is used and the desired levels substituted as follows:

$$(7) \qquad C = \frac{70 \times \text{(lifetime risk level)}}{B[(\text{Water intake}) + (R \times \text{Fish intake})]}$$

For example a criterion level for a lifetime risk of 10^{-6} at an exposure of 50 grams of fish/day and 1 l/day of water is

$$C = \frac{70 \times 10^{-6}}{B[1 + (R \times 0.050)]}$$

The interpretation of these equations is that if the lifetime average water concentration is kept lower than the calculated value, the lifetime risk is estimated to be lower than 10^{-5}. If a low dose threshold could be reliably established for the compound the risk would be lower than 10^{-5}.

The following is a summary of slope factors which can be used for calculating criteria for exposure risk levels other than those presented in the assessment documents. Note that in cases where human data are available a model different from the one-hit model is used for dose-response calculation. For these cases an equivalent slope factor is derived which is followed by an asterisk in the table below. Also included is a summary for a criterion based on a 10^{-5} lifetime risk assuming lifetime daily consumption of 2 liters of water and 0.0187 kg fish.

Chemical	Slope Factor, B $(mg/l/day)^{-1}$	Toxicant Concentration, Risk Level of 10^{-5} $(\mu g/l)$
Arsenic	14.00*	0.029
Benzene	0.02160*	15
Cadmium	1.09658*	10
Chloroform	0.14695	2.1
Beryllium	3.4308	0.087
Carbón tetrachloride	0.090996	2.6
Chlordane	5.36196	1.2×10^{-3}
1,1-Dichloroethylene	0.25292*	1.3
Heptachlor	30.3063	0.23×10^{-3}
Hexachlorobutadiene	0.04949	0.77
Dimethylnitrosamine	13.4	0.026
Diethylnitrosamine	38.2	0.0092
Dibutylnitrosamine	26.86	0.013
N-nitrosopyrrolidine	3.297	0.11
Tetrachlorodioxin	13.923	4.6×10^{-7}
Tetrachloroethylene	0.08440	2.0
Trichloroethylene	0.01200	21
Vinyl chloride	0.00066*	520

Mathematical Description of Extrapolation Method: *(1) Information from Chronic Study —*

nt = Number of animals exposed to the selected dose that developed tumors at some time in the study. See text for explanation of selection criteria for choosing the data set.

NT = Total number of animals exposed to selected dose level.

nc = Number of control animals with tumors.

NC = Total number of control animals.

Le = Actual maximum lifespan for test animals.

le = Length of exposure

d = Average dose per unit of time (mg/kg/day) during administration of the agent.

w = Average weight of test animals (kg).

(2) Information from General Literature —

70 kg = Average weight of people

L = Theoretical average length of life for test species, unless specified in article. It is 90 weeks for mice and 104 weeks for rats.

F = Average weight of fish consumed per day, assumed 0.0187 kilograms.

(3) Other Information —

R = Bioconcentration factor for edible portions of fish (supplied by Environmental Research Laboratory, Duluth).

(4)   Mathematical Model

$$Pt = Pc + (1 - Pc) \times [1 - e^{-t^3 BD}] \text{ where}$$

$Pt = nt \div NT$ = Proportion of the test animals with tumors.

$Pc = nc \div NC$ = Proportion of control animals with tumors.

$D = (d \times le)/Le$ = Lifespan weighted average dose level mg/kg/(unit of time).

$$B_A = -\ln\left[\frac{1 - Pt}{1 - Pc}\right] \div [D \times t^3]$$

$$\text{where } t = \frac{\text{lifespan for test animals}}{\text{length of life for species}} = \frac{Le}{L}$$

$$B_H = B^3\sqrt{70/w}$$

$$C = \frac{70 \times 10^{-5}}{B_H[2 + (R \times F)]} = \text{criterion level (mg/l) for man.}$$

Nonstochastic Effects

A somewhat less formalized approach is used in the derivation of water quality criteria based on nonstochastic effects. As previously described, an attempt is made to identify studies defining NOEL's in mammals. For many compounds, several effect and no effect levels are reported in the literature. The NOEL's selected for deriving the criteria is the highest NOEL that did not exceed a level reported to cause adverse effect.

The NOEL is transformed into an Acceptable Daily Intake for man (ADI) by dividing by an uncertainty factor of 10, 100, or 1,000. The guidelines for using the uncertainty factors, as given by the National Academy of Sciences (89), are outlined below:

(1)   Valid experimental results from studies on prolonged ingestion by man, with no indication of carcinogenicity. The Uncertainty Factor is 10.

(2)   Experimental results of studies of human ingestion not available or scanty (e.g., acute exposure only). Valid results of long-term feeding studies on experimental animals or in the absence of human studies, valid animal studies on one or more species. No indication of carcinogenicity. The Uncertainty Factor is 100.

(3)   No long-term or acute human data. Scanty results on experimental animals. No indication of carcinogenicity. The Uncertainty Factor is 1,000.

For a few of the chemicals or chemical classes, ADIs are estimated from threshold limit values (TLVs) or subacute/acute mammalian data. TLVs are established by the ACGIH and represent estimated levels of the compounds in the work environment which are not anticipated to result in significant adverse health effects in workers exposed 8 hours/day, 5 days/week.

The method used to derive ADIs from TLVs is essentially that recommended by Stokinger and Woodward (92) and is based on assumptions of the breathing rate and completeness of absorption.

Once an ADI is established, assumptions are made concerning the relative contribution of water to total human exposure. In some cases, criteria are developed in a manner analogous to that used in carcinogenicity studies:

$$C = ADI/[2 + (0.0187 \times R)]$$

In other cases, the bioconcentration term is omitted and an approximation is made of the proportion of the exposure attributed to water and nonwater sources. For all compounds, criteria is based on an assumed daily water consumption of 2 liters.

ANALYTICAL METHODS FOR PRIORITY POLLUTANTS

As Congress recognized in enacting the Clean Water Act of 1977, the state-of-the-art ability to monitor and detect toxic pollutants is limited. Most of the toxic pollutants were relatively unknown until only a few years ago, and only on rare occasions has EPA regulated or has industry monitored or even developed methods to monitor for these pollutants. As a result, analytical methods for many toxic pollutants, under Section 304(h) of the Act, have not yet been promulgated (69). Moreover, state-of-the-art techniques involve the use of highly expensive, sophisticated equipment, with costs ranging as high as $200,000 per unit of equipment.

When faced with these problems, EPA scientists, including staff of the Environmental Research Laboratory in Athens, Georgia and staff of the Environmental Monitoring and Support Laboratory in Cincinnati, Ohio conducted a literature search and initiated a laboratory program to develop analytical protocols. The analytical techniques used in this rulemaking were developed concurrently with the development of general sampling and analytical protocols and were incorporated into the protocols ultimately adopted for the study of other industrial categories.

A manual has been developed for analyses for priority pollutants (96) and is in the process of further revision as this volume goes to press.

Because Section 304(h) methods were available for most toxic metals, pesticides, cyanide and phenol, the analytical effort focused on developing methods for sampling and analyses of organic toxic pollutants. The three basic analytical approaches considered by EPA were infrared spectroscopy, gas chromatography (GC) with multiple detectors, and gas chromatography/mass spectrometry (GC/MS).

In selecting among these alternatives, EPA considered their sensitivity, laboratory availability, costs, applicability to diverse waste streams from numerous industries, and capability for implementation within the statutory and court-ordered time constrains of EPA's program. The Agency concluded that infrared spectroscopy was not sufficiently sensitive or specific for application in water. GC with multiple detectors was rejected because it would require multiple runs, incompatible with program time constraints. Moreover, because this method would use several detectors, each applicable to a narrow range of substances, GC with multiple detectors possibly would fail to detect certain toxic pollutants.

EPA chose GC/MS because it was the only available technique that could identify a wide variety of pollutants in many different waste streams, in the presence of interfering compounds, and within the time constraints of the program. In EPA's judgment, GC/MS and the other analytical methods for toxics used in this rulemaking represent the best state-of-the-art methods for toxic pollutant analyses available when this study was begun.

As the state-of-the-art began to mature, EPA began to refine the sampling and analytical protocols, and intends to continue this refinement to keep pace with technology advancements. Resource constraints, however, prevent EPA from reworking completed sampling and analyses to keep up with the evolution of analytical methods. As a result, the analytical techniques used in some rulemakings may differ slightly from those used in other rulemaking efforts. In each case, however, the analytical methods used represent the best state-of-the-art available for a given industry study. One of the goals of EPA's analytical proram is the promulgation of additional Section 304(h) analytical methods for toxic pollutants, scheduled to be done within calendar year 1979.

The high costs, slow pace and limited laboratory capability for toxic pollutant analyses posed difficulties unique to EPA's experience. The cost of each wastewater analysis for organic toxic pollutants ranges between $650 and $1,700, excluding sampling costs (based upon quotations recently obtained from a number of analytical laboratories). Even with unlimited resources, however, time and laboratory capability would have posed additional constraints. Although efficiency has been improving, when this study was initiated a well-trained technician using the most sophisticated equipment could perform only one complete organic analysis in an eight hour work day. Moreover, when this rulemaking study was begun there were only about 15 commercial laboratories in the United States with sufficient capability to perform these analyses. Today there are about 50 commercial laboratories known to EPA which have the capability to perform these analyses, and the number is increasing as the demand for such capability also increases.

Some attention has been given to analytical techniques in individual criteria documents but the coverage is very spotty. The only document treating this topic at any length is the one on asbestos (7).

The documents on acrolein (2), 2,4-dinitrotoluene (31), nitrobenzene (48) and phenol (52) give brief treatments of the analytical problems for these materials.

Analysis for "Indicator" Pollutants

The toxic pollutants regulated by indicator pollutants include all of the volatile (purgeable) organics, some of the acid extractable organic compounds, and the base-neutral extractable organic compounds. An "indicator" for the substituted phenolic compounds is the toxic pollutant phenol as measured by the 4-aminoantipyrine method (4AAP). This method measures simple phenol and fractions of specific substituted phenols such as 2,3,6-trichlorophenol and 2,4-dichlorophenol. While pentachlorophenol does not respond to this test, EPA concludes that when both (4AAP) phenol and other "indicator" pollutants (especially oil and grease, COD, TKN, and ammonia) are controlled, this compound and other compounds resistant to rapid biodegradation will be controlled as well. Similarly, the EPA concludes that control of zinc, lead, nickel, and copper is affected by a specific limitation on (total) chromium, and by control of TSS as an "indicator" pollutant (69).

Some of the toxic organic compounds, such as naphthalene, are readily biodegradable and are effectively controlled by BOD_5 as an "indicator." Other toxic pollutants, such as 2,4,6-trichlorophenol and dichlorobenzenes, are resistant to biological treatment and are measured more by the COD test than the BOD_5 test. COD is, therefore, an "indicator" for these toxic organic compounds, in addition to being a controlled conventional pollutant parameter. The COD test is rapidly and reliably determined by a traditional and relatively inexpensive analytical method.

Toxic pollutants such as pentachlorophenol and phthalate esters are partially treated by oil-water separation because they are immiscible in water. Thus, control of oil and grease as an "indicator" will provide control of these toxic pollutants. Other toxics such as chloroform and toluene are volatile and are air-stripped by aeration systems in activated sludge treatment. Control of BOD_5 as an "indicator" will ensure control of these volatile compounds. Many of the toxic pollutants, such as pentachlorophenol and 2,4,6-trichlorophenol, are also adsorbable on suspended solids and will be controlled by TSS as an "indicator."

Ammonia nitrogen is an oxygen-demanding non-nonconventional pollutant, and TKN is a pollutant parameter which measures the organic proteinaceous nitrogen in wastewater which ultimately contributes to ammonia nitrogen in both treatment systems and receiving streams. The conditions necessary in activated sludge systems for treating TKN and ammonia (nitrification by high solids extended aeration) are the same conditions necessary for treating many of the slowly or partially biodegradable toxic organic compounds, such as 2,4-dichlorophenol and dichlorobenzenes. Ammonia and TKN are, therefore, "indicators" for removal of these toxic pollutants (69). (TKN stands for Total Kjeldahl Nitrogen.)

In the case of the textile industry, EPA has indicated (77) that adequate control of total suspended solids will be considered evidence that such substances as pentachlorophenol are adequately controlled as well. However, phenol, chromium, copper and zinc must be monitored and controlled explicitly.

Leather Tanning and Finishing Industry

The experience in analyses of effluent from the leather tanning and finishing industry (69) is pertinent here. At both raw waste and pretreatment points, automatic samplers and flow recorders were used to take samples at 15 minute intervals. Composite samples were prepared by combining the samples on the basis of flows recorded during each 24-hour collection period. Samples for conventional and nonconventional pollutants, phenol (total) and cyanide (total) were obtained from the 24-hour composite, with the remaining sample volume combined in equal proportions for the 72-hour composite for toxic pollutants (acid and base-neutral extractable organics, pesticides, metals). Grab samples were taken in specially prepared vials for volatile (purgeable) organics. Prior to the plant visits, sample containers were carefully washed and prepared by specific methods, depending upon the type of sample to be taken. EPA took a number of other precautions to minimize potential contamination from sample components. Samples were kept on ice at 4°C prior to express shipment in insulated containers.

The analyses for toxic pollutants were performed according to groups of chemicals and associated analytical schemes. Organic toxic pollutants included volatile (purgeable), base-neutral and acid (extractable) pollutants, and pesticides. Inorganic toxic pollutants included heavy metals, cyanide, and asbestos.

The primary method used in screening and verification of the volatiles, base-neutral, and acid organics was gas chromatography with confirmation and quantification on all samples by mass spectrometry (GC/MS). Phenols (total) were analyzed by the 4-aminoantipyrine (4-AAP) method. GC was employed for analysis of pesticides with limited MS confirmation.

The EPA analyzed the toxic heavy metals by atomic absorption spectrometry (AAS), with flame or graphite furnace atomization following appropriate digestion of the sample. Samples were analyzed for cyanides by a colorimetric method, with sulfide previously removed by distillation. Analysis for asbestos was accomplished by microscopy and fiber presence reported as chrysotile fiber count. Analyses for conventional pollutants (BOD_5, TSS and pH), proposed conventionals (oil and grease and COD) and nonconventional pollutants (TKN, ammonia, and sulfide) were accomplished using "Methods for Chemical Analysis of Water and Wastes," (EPA 625/6-74-003) and amendments.

Primary Aluminum Production

The analyses of priority pollutants at a primary aluminum production facility has been discussed by Rawlings and Hoogheem (97).

THE ECONOMICS OF PRIORITY POLLUTANT CONTROL

Executive Order 12044 requires EPA and other agencies to perform Regulatory Analyses of certain regulations [43 *FR* 12661 (March 23, 1978)]. EPA's proposed regulations for implementing Executive Order 12044 require a Regulatory Analysis for major significant regulations involving annualized compliance costs of $100 million or meeting other specified criteria [43 *FR* 29891 (July 11, 1978)]. Where these criteria are met, the proposed regulations require EPA to prepare a formal Regulatory Analysis, including an economic impact analysis and an evaluation of regulatory alternatives. The proposed regulations for the leather tanning and finishing industry do not meet the proposed criteria for a formal Regulatory Analysis. Nonetheless, this proposed rulemaking satisfies the formal Regulatory Analysis requirements.

EPA's economic impact assessment for the leather industry has been published (98). This report details the investment and annualized costs for the industry as a whole and for model plants covered by the proposed leather tanning regulations. The data underlying the analysis were obtained from the Development Document, publicly available financial studies and surveys, and the EPA economic survey program described under Data Gathering Efforts. The report assesses the impact of compliance costs in terms of plant closures, production changes, price changes, employment changes, local community impacts, and balance of trade effects.

Recently economic impact documents have been prepared for the textile industry (99) and for timber products processing (100,101). It is anticipated that, as time goes on, economic impact documents will be published for the rest of the 21 affected industry categories to accompany the development documents for those industries.

RECENT DEVELOPMENTS

The story of priority pollutants is a constantly evolving one. EPA has already been petitioned by Dow Chemical Co. (102) to remove ethylbenzene, phenol, 2,4-dichlorophenol, 2,4,5-trichlorophenol and pentachlorophenol from the list of toxic pollutants.

BIBLIOGRAPHY

(The first 65 references in this Bibliography are to the Criteria Documents for the 65 Priority Toxic Pollutants. The first reference will be given in its entirety; the balance of the 65 will simply be given by PB number in the interests of saving space; all are NTIS documents and all were published in 1979.)

(1) U.S. Environmental Protection Agency, Office of Water Planning and Standards, *Acenaphthene—Ambient Water Quality Criteria*, Report No. PB-296,782, Washington, DC, Criteria and Standards Division; available from National Technical Information Service, Springfield, Virginia 22161 (1979).

(2) See above. *Acrolein—Ambient Water Quality Criteria*, Report No. PB-296,788.

(3) *Acrylonitrile—Ambient Water Quality Criteria*, Report No. PB-297,915.

(4) *Aldrin/Dieldrin—Ambient Water Quality Criteria*, Report No. PB-297,616.

(5) *Antimony—Ambient Water Quality Criteria*, Report No. PB-296,789.

(6) *Arsenic—Ambient Water Quality Criteria*, Report No. PB-292,420.

(7) *Asbestos—Ambient Water Quality Criteria*, Report No. PB-297,917.

(8) *Benzene—Ambient Water Quality Criteria*, Report No. PB-292,421.

(9) *Benzidene—Ambient Water Quality Criteria*, Report No. PB-297,918.

(10) *Beryllium—Ambient Water Quality Criteria*, Report No. PB-292,422.

(11) *Cadmium—Ambient Water Quality Criteria*, Report No. PB-292,423.

(12) *Carbon Tetrachloride—Ambient Water Quality Criteria*, Report No. PB-292,424.

(13) *Chlordane—Ambient Water Quality Criteria*, Report No. PB-292,425.

(14) *Chlorinated Benzenes—Ambient Water Quality Criteria*, Report No. PB-297,919.

(15) *Chlorinated Ethanes—Ambient Water Quality Criteria*, Report No. PB-297,920.

(16) *Chloroalkyl Ethers—Ambient Water Quality Criteria*, Report No. PB-297,921.

(17) *Chlorinated Naphthalenes—Ambient Water Quality Criteria*, Report No. PB-292,426.

(18) *Chlorinated Phenols—Ambient Water Quality Criteria*, Report No. PB-296,790.

(19) *Chloroform—Ambient Water Quality Criteria*, Report No. PB-292,427.

(20) *2-Chlorophenol—Ambient Water Quality Criteria*, Report No. PB-292,428.

(21) *Chromium—Ambient Water Quality Criteria*, Report No. PB-297,922.

(22) *Copper—Ambient Water Quality Criteria*, Report No. PB-296,791.

(23) *Cyanides—Ambient Water Quality Criteria*, Report No. PB-296,792.

(24) *DDT—Ambient Water Quality Criteria*, Report No. PB-297,923.

(25) *Dichlorobenzenes—Ambient Water Quality Criteria*, Report No. PB-292,429.

(26) *Dichlorobenzidene—Ambient Water Quality Criteria*, Report No. PB-296,793.

(27) *Dichloroethylenes—Ambient Water Quality Criteria*, Report No. PB-292,430.

(28) *2,4-Dichlorophenol—Ambient Water Quality Criteria*, Report No. PB-292,431.

(29) *Dichloropropanes/Dichloropropenes—Ambient Water Quality Criteria*, Report No. PB-296,799.

(30) *2,4-Dimethylphenol—Ambient Water Quality Criteria*, Report No. PB-292,432.

(31) *Dinitrotoluene—Ambient Water Quality Criteria*, Report No. PB-296,794.

(32) *Diphenylhydrazine—Ambient Water Quality Criteria*, Report No. PB-296,795.

(33) *Endosulfan—Ambient Water Quality Criteria*, Report No. PB-296,783.

(34) *Endrin—Ambient Water Quality Criteria*, Report No. PB-296,785.

(35) *Ethylbenzene—Ambient Water Quality Criteria,* Report No. PB-296,784.
(36) *Fluoranthene—Ambient Water Quality Criteria,* Report No. PB-292,433.
(37) *Haloethers—Ambient Water Quality Criteria,* Report No. PB-296,796.
(38) *Halomethanes—Ambient Water Quality Criteria,* Report No. PB-296,797.
(39) *Heptachlor—Ambient Water Quality Criteria,* Report No. PB-292,434.
(40) *Hexachlorobutadiene—Ambient Water Quality Criteria,* Report No. PB-292,435.
(41) *Hexachlorocyclohexane—Ambient Water Quality Criteria,* Report No. PB-297,924.
(42) *Hexachlorocyclopentadiene—Ambient Water Quality Criteria,* Report No. PB-292,436.
(43) *Isophorone—Ambient Water Quality Criteria,* Report No. PB-296,798.
(44) *Lead—Ambient Water Quality Criteria,* Report No. PB-292,437.
(45) *Mercury—Ambient Water Quality Criteria,* Report No. PB-297,925.
(46) *Naphthalene—Ambient Water Quality Criteria,* Report No. PB-296,786.
(47) *Nickel—Ambient Water Quality Criteria,* Report No. PB-296,800.
(48) *Nitrobenzene—Ambient Water Quality Criteria,* Report No. PB-296,801.
(49) *Nitrophenols—Ambient Water Quality Criteria,* Report No. PB-296,802.
(50) *Nitrosamines—Ambient Water Quality Criteria,* Report No. PB-292,438.
(51) *Pentachlorophenol—Ambient Water Quality Criteria,* Report No. PB-292,439.
(52) *Phenol—Ambient Water Quality Criteria,* Report No. PB-296,787.
(53) *Phthalate Esters—Ambient Water Quality Criteria,* Report No. PB-296,804.
(54) *Polychlorinated Biphenyls—Ambient Water Quality Criteria,* Report No. PB-296,803.
(55) *Polynuclear Aromatic Hydrocarbons—Ambient Water Quality Criteria,* Report No. PB-297,926.
(56) *Selenium—Ambient Water Quality Criteria,* Report No. PB-292,440.
(57) *Silver—Ambient Water Quality Criteria,* Report No. PB-292,441.
(58) *2,3,7,8-Tetrachlorodibenzo-p-Dioxin—Ambient Water Quality Criteria,* Report No. PB-292,442.
(59) *Tetrachloroethylene—Ambient Water Quality Criteria,* Report No. PB-292,445.
(60) *Thallium—Ambient Water Quality Criteria,* Report No. PB-292,444.
(61) *Toluene—Ambient Water Quality Criteria,* Report No. PB-296,805.
(62) *Toxaphene—Ambient Water Quality Criteria,* Report No. PB-296,806.
(63) *Trichloroethylene—Ambient Water Quality Criteria,* Report No. PB-292,443.
(64) *Vinyl Chloride—Ambient Water Quality Criteria,* Report No. PB-292,446.
(65) *Zinc—Ambient Water Quality Criteria,* Report No. PB-296,807.
(66) U.S. Environmental Protection Agency, *Federal Register* 44, No. 147, 44501-503 (July 30, 1979).
(67) Natural Resources Defense Council, et al vs Train, 8 *ERC* 2120 (D.D.C. 1976).
(68) Natural Resources Defense Council, et al vs Costle, 12 *ERC* 1833.
(69) U.S. Environmental Protection Agency, *Federal Register* 44, No. 128, 38746-38776 (July 2, 1979).
(70) U.S. Environmental Protection Agency, *Federal Register* 44, No. 52, 15926-15981 (March 15, 1979).
(71) U.S. Environmental Protection Agency, *Federal Register* 43, No. 123, 27736-27773 (June 26, 1978).
(72) U.S. Environmental Protection Agency, *Federal Register* 44, No. 210, 62260-62275 (Oct. 29, 1979).
(73) U.S. Environmental Protection Agency, *Development Document for Proposed Effluent Limitations Guidelines and Standards, Leather Tanning and Finishing Point Source Category,* Report No. EPA 440/1-79/016, Washingtion DC, Effluent Guidelines Division (July 1979).
(74) U.S. Environmental Protection Agency, *Federal Register* 44, No. 144, 43660-43697 (July 25, 1979). See also corrections in *Federal Register* 44, No. 176, 52751-52753 (Sept. 10, 1979).
(75) U.S. Environmental Protection Agency, *Federal Register* 44, No. 191, 56628-56657 (Oct. 1, 1979).
(76) U.S. Environmental Protection Agency, *Federal Register* 44, No. 210, 62204-62241 (Oct. 29, 1979).
(77) U.S. Environmental Protection Agency, *Development Document for Proposed Effluent Limitations Guidelines, New Source Performance Standards and Pretreatment Standards for the Textile Mills Point Source Category,* Washington, DC, Effluent Guidelines Division (In press, Nov. 1979).
(78) U.S. Environmental Protection Agency, *Federal Register* 44, No. 212, 62810-62846 (Oct. 31, 1979).
(79) U.S. Environmental Protection Agency, *Federal Register* 43, No. 97, 21506-21518 (May 18, 1978). See also errata listed in *Federal Register* 43, No. 129, 29028 (July 5, 1978).
(80) U.S. Environmental Protection Agency, *Methods for Acute Toxicity Tests With Fish, Macroinvertebrates and Amphibians,* Report No. EPA-660/3-75-009, Washington DC (1975).
(81) Albert, R.E., et al, "Rationale developed by the Environmental Protection Agency for the assessment of carcinogenic risks," *Jour. Natl. Cancer Institute* 58:1537-1541 (1977).
(82) Cordle, F., et al, "Human exposure to polychlorinated biphenyls and polybrominated biphenyls." *Environ. Health Perspectives* 24:157-172 (1978).
(83) Doll, R., "Weibull distribution of cancer: Implications for models of carcinogenesis," *J. Roy. Statistical Soc.* A 13:133-166 (1971).
(84) Druckrey, H., "Quantitative aspects of chemical carcinogenesis," In Rene Truhaut, ed. *Potential Carcinogenic hazards from drugs, evaluation of risks,* UICC Monograph Series, Vol. 7, Springer Verlag, New York (1967).
(85) Guess, H., et al, "Uncertainty estimates for low dose rate extrapolations of animal carcinogenicity data," *Cancer Research* 37:3475-3483 (1977).

(86)   Interagency Regulatory Liaison Group, 1979, *Scientific bases for identifying potential carcinogens and estimating their risks* (Feb. 6, 1979).

(87)   International Commission on Radiological Protection, 1977, *Recommendation of the International Commission on Radiological Protection,* Pub. No. 26, adopted Jan. 17, 1977, Pergamon Press, Oxford, England.

(88)   McNamara, B.P., "Concepts in health evaluation of commercial and industrial chemicals," In M.A. Mehlman, et al, eds., *Advances in Modern Toxicology,* Vol. 1, Part 1, Wiley and Sons, New York (1976).

(89)   National Academy of Sciences, *Drinking water and health,* National Academy of Sciences, Washington, DC (1977).

(90)   Peto, R., "Weibull distribution for continuous-carcinogenesis experiments," *Biometrics* 29:457-470 (1973).

(91)   Sidwell, V.D., et al, "Composition of the edible portion of raw crustaceans, fin-fish, and molluscs." *Marine Fisheries Review* 36:21-35 (1974).

(92)   Stokinger, M.E., and Woodward, R.L., "Toxicologic methods for establishing drinking water standards," *Jour. Am. Water Works Assoc.* 50:517 (1958).

(93)   U.S. EPA 1976, "Interim procedures and guidelines for health risk and economic impact assessments of suspected carcinogens," *Federal Register* 41 21402 (May 25, 1976).

(94)   U.S. EPA 1976, *National Interim Primary Drinking Water Regulations,* Off. of Water Supp. EPA 570/9-76-003, U.S. Environ. Prot. Agency.

(95)   Veith, G.D., et al, "An evaluation of using partition coefficients and water solubility to estimate bioconcentration factors for organic chemicals in fish," Manuscript, U.S. EPA, Duluth Laboratory, Duluth, Minnesota (1978).

(96)   U.S. Environmental Protection Agency, *Sampling and Analyses Procedures for Screening of Industrial Effluents for Priority Pollutants,* Washington, DC, Effluent Guidelines Division (published March 1977; revised April 1977; further revision in process late 1979).

(97)   Rawlings, G.D. and Hoogheem, T.J. (Monsanto Research Corp.), *Analysis of Priority Pollutants at a Primary Aluminum Production Facility,* Report No. EPA-600/2-79-087, Cincinnati, Ohio, U.S. Environmental Protection Agency (April 1979).

(98)   U.S. Environmental Protection Agency, *Economic Impact Analysis of Proposed Effluent Limitations Guidelines, New Source Performance Standards and Pretreatment Standards for the Leather Tanning and Finishing Point Sources Category,* Report No. EPA-440/2-79-019, Washington, DC, Water Economics Branch (July 1979).

(99)   U.S. Environmental Protection Agency, *Economic Impact Analysis of Proposed Effluent Limitations, Guidelines, New Source Performance Standards and Pretreatment Standards for the Textile Mills Point Source Category,* Report No. EPA 440/2-79-020, Water Economics Branch (Oct. 1979).

(100)   U.S. Environmental Protection Agency, *Economic Impact Analysis of Alternative Pollution Control Technologies: Wet Process Hardboard and Insulation Board Subcategories of the Timber Products Industry,* Report No. EPA-440/2-79-017, Washington, DC, Water Economics Branch (Aug. 1979).

(101)   U.S. Environmental Protection Agency, *Economic Impact Analysis of Alternative Pollution Control Technologies: Wood Preserving Subcategories of the Timber Products Industry,* Report No. EPA-440/2-79-018, Washington DC, Water Economics Branch (August 1979).

(102)   44 *FR* 64555-559 (Nov. 7, 1979).

It should be noted that the above bibliography is discrete and separate from the references following any particular pollutant. Unhyphenated numbers, appearing in parentheses, refer to bibliographic entries in the Introduction; hyphenated numbers pertain to the references following each of the numbered pollutants.

CRITERIA FOR SPECIFIC POLLUTANTS

In the sections which follow in the remainder of the volume, individual pollutants will be discussed using the following general outline:

- Occurrence — The manner in which the pollutant enters the environment; whether it is found in nature
- Physical Properties — The basic physical properties of the pollutant including volatility
- Chemical Properties — With special attention to reactions in the environment: oxidation and degradation
- Uses — To emphasize areas in which industrial workers and the general public may encounter the pollutant in question
- Toxic Effects — A brief account of the nature of toxic effects produced
- Current Levels of Exposure — Relating to environmental levels in general
- Special Groups at Risk — Indicating whether particular age groups, those suffering from particular diseases, or particular groups of workers are especially susceptible
- Existing Guidelines and Standards — Both domestic and international standards (if any) which have previously been established for the material in question
- Proposed EPA Water Quality Criteria
- The Basis for the Proposed EPA Criteria for human health
- A bibliography of pertinent references.

A

ACENAPHTHENE (#1)

Acenaphthene is a polynuclear aromatic hydrocarbon with a molecular weight of 154 and a formula of $C_{12}H_{10}$. It has the structural formula:

Occurrence: Acenaphthene (1,8-dihydroacenaphthylene or 1,8-ethylene naphthalene) occurs in coal tar produced during the high temperature carbonization or coking of coal. It has also been detected in cigarette smoke and gasoline exhaust condensates.

Physical Properties: The compound is a white crystalline solid at room temperature with a melting range of 95° to 97°C and a boiling range of 278° to 280°C. The vapor pressure is less than 0.02 mm Hg. Acenaphthene is soluble in water (100 mg/l), but solubility increases in organic solvents such as ethanol, toluene, and chloroform.

Chemical Properties: Acenaphthene will react with molecular oxygen in the presence of alkali-earth metal bromides to form acenaphthequinone. In the presence of alkali-earth metal hydroxides, acenaphthene reacts with ozone to produce 1,8-naphthaldehyde carboxylic acid. Acenaphthalene can be oxidized to aromatic alcohols and ketones using transition metal compounds as catalysts. Acenaphthene is stable under laboratory conditions and resists photochemical degradation in soil stability studies.

Uses: Acenaphthene is used as a dye intermediate, in the manufacture of some plastics, as an insecticide and fungicide.

Toxic Effect: Acenaphthene has been demonstrated to affect the growth of plants by causing improper nuclear division and polyploidal chromosome number. These same observations were noted in several microorganisms as well. Little information regarding aquatic toxicity was found. The freshwater acute value for bluegill was 1,700 μg/l, and the bioconcentration factor was 397. Saltwater toxicity to the sheepshead minnow was 2,230 μg/l, and no bioconcentration data were available. Data on toxicity to nonhuman mammals were few and virtually no incidences of human acenaphthene toxicity were noted. There was some information found showing organoleptic effects attributed to acenaphthene in water. A detection range of 0.02 to 0.22 mg/l was given. Laboratory experimentation points out the possibility of limited metabolism of acenaphthene to napthalic acid and naphthalic anhydride.

Current Levels of Exposure: Virtually no information is available concerning the prevalence or concentration of acenaphthene in the environment. Acenaphthene has been detected in cigarette smoke, automobile exhaust, and in urban air, and is present in coal tar and several fossil fuel oils. It has also been reported in wastewater from petrochemical, pesticide, and wood preservative industries and detected in water from a river in the Netherlands.

Special Groups at Risk: Individuals working with coal tar and/or its products face a possible risk due to increased exposure to acenaphthene, although no data are available to estimate this risk.

Existing Guidelines and Standards: No existing guidelines or standards were found.

Summary of Proposed EPA Criteria: *Freshwater Aquatic Life* — The data base for freshwater aquatic life is insufficient to allow use of the Guidelines. The following recommendation is inferred from toxicity data for saltwater organisms. For acenaphthene the criterion to protect freshwater aquatic life as derived using procedures other than the Guidelines is 110 µg/l as a 24-hour average and the concentration should not exceed 240 µg/l at any time.

Saltwater Aquatic Life — For acenaphthene the criterion to protect saltwater aquatic life as derived using the Guidelines is 7.5 µg/l as a 24-hour average and the concentration should not exceed 17 µg/l at any time.

Human Health — For the protection of human health from the toxic properties of acenaphthene, the ambient water criterion is determined to be 20 µg/l.

Basis for Proposed Human Health Criteria: So little research has been performed on acenaphthene that its mammalian and human health effects are virtually unknown. The toxicity studies available (1-1)(1-2) are inadequate for the basis of a criterion due to the experimental designs (lack of controls, small number of animals, etc.). Therefore, until more toxicological data are generated, particularly teratogenic data in view of the effects of acenaphthene on cell division, an interim criterion based upon organoleptic data is proposed. The lowest human responses were reported at 0.022 to 0.22 ppm (1-3), and thus 20 µg/l is the recommended criterion. It must be emphasized, however, that this value is not related to health effects and that the significance of odor thresholds is unknown. This value will need to be reviewed when more toxicological data are available.

References

(1-1) Knobloch, K., et al, "Acute and subacute toxicity and acenaphthene and acenaphthylene," *Med. Pracy.,* 20, 210 (1969).
(1-2) Reshetyuk, A.L., et al, "Toxicological evaluation of acenaphthene and acenaphthylene," *Gig. Tr. Prof. Zabol.,* 14, 46 (1970).
(1-3) Lillard, D.A. and Powers, J.J., *Aqueous Odor Thresholds of Organic Pollutants in Industrial Effluents,* EPA Report No. 660/4-75-002, Cowallis, Oregon, U.S.E.P.A. National Envir. Research Center (1975).

ACENAPHTHYLENE

See "Polynuclear Aromatic Hydrocarbons" (55). See also references (1-1) and (1-2) under acenaphthene.

ACROLEIN (#2)

Acrolein is the simplest unsaturated aldehyde: $CH_2{=}CH{-}CHO$.

Occurrence: Acrolein can enter the aquatic environment by its use as an aquatic herbicide, from industrial discharge, and from the chlorination of organic compounds in wastewater and drinking water treatment. It is often present in trace amounts in foods and is a component of smog, fuel combustion, wood and possibly other fires, and cigarette smoke.

An evaluation of available data indicates, that, while industrial exposure to manufactured acrolein is unlikely, acrolein is pervasive from nonmanufactured sources. Acrolein exposure will occur through food ingestion and inhalation. Exposure through the water or dermal route is less likely. However, analysis of municipal effluents of Dayton, Ohio showed the presence of acrolein in 6 of 11 samples, with concentrations ranging from 20 to 200 μg/l (2-1). The present technology for acrolein preparation employs catalytic oxidation of propene in the vapor phase. Typical reaction conditions consist of feeding propylene and air at 300° to 400°C and 30 to 45 psi over the catalyst (usually of the bismuth-molybdenum or the antimony family).

Physical Properties: Acrolein (2-propenal) is colorless, volatile liquid with a structural formula of $CH_2{=}CHCHO$ and a molecular weight of 56.07. It melts at –86.95°C, boils at 52.5 to 53.5°C, and has a density of 0.8410 g/ml at 20°C. The vapor pressure at 20°C is 215 mm Hg and its water solubility is 20.8% by weight at 30°C.

Chemical Properties: A flammable liquid with a pungent odor, acrolein is an unstable compound that undergoes polymerization to the plastic solid disacryl, especially under light or in the presence of alkali or strong acid. It is the simplest member of the class of unsaturated aldehydes, and the extreme reactivity of acrolein is due to the presence of a vinyl group ($CH_2{=}CH-$) and an aldehyde group ($-CHO$) on such a small molecule. Additions to the carbon-carbon double bond of acrolein are catalyzed by acids and bases. The addition of halogens to this carbon-carbon double bond proceeds readily.

Since it is a highly reactive organic chemical and capable of self-polymerization, the marketed product contains an inhibitor (0.1% hydroquinone) to prevent its degradation. It is extremely reactive at high pH's.

Uses: Acrolein has a wide variety of applications. It is directly used as a biocide for aquatic weed control; for algae, weed and mollusk control in recirculating process water systems; for slime control in the paper industry; and to protect liquid fuels against microorganisms. Acrolein is also used directly for crosslinking protein collagen in leather tanning and for tissue fixation in histological samples. It is widely used as an intermediate in the chemical industry. Its dimer, which is prepared by a thermal, uncatalyzed reaction, has several applications, including use as an intermediate for crosslinking agents, humectants, plasticizers, polyurethane intermediates, copolymers and homopolymers, and creaseproofing cotton. The monomer is utilized in synthesis via the Diels-Alder reaction as a dienophile or a diene.

Acrolein is widely used in copolymerization but its homopolymers do not appear commercially important. The copolymers of acrolein are used in photography, for textile treatment, in the paper industry, as builders in laundry and dishwasher detergents, as coatings for aluminum and steel panels, as well as other applications. In 1975 worldwide production was about 59 kilotons. Its largest market was for methionine manufacture. Worldwide capacity was estimated at 102 kilotons per year of which U.S. capacity was 47.6 kilotons per year.

Toxic Effects: Freshwater acute toxicity values as low as 61 μg/l have been reported. A chronic fish value of 21.8 μg/l has been demonstrated. Acrolein has been found to bioconcentrate 344 times in a freshwater fish. Saltwater acute toxicity in one fish species was found to be 240 μg/l. No bioconcentration or chronic data are available for marine species. Acrolein has been shown to produce a great variety of disorders in mammalian animals and man. However, it has not been shown to be a teratogen and only a mild to weak mutagen, if one at all, depending on the test system employed. Though it has been suspected as a carcinogen or cytotoxin, information does not definitely produce evidence of confirmation.

Current Levels of Exposure: Quantitative estimates of current levels of human exposure cannot be made based on the available data. Acrolein has not been monitored in ambient raw or finished waters. Limited data have been reported under "Occurrence" earlier in this section (2-1).

Special Groups at Risk: Since acrolein is a component of tobacco and marijuana smoke, people exposed to cigarette smoke are a group at increased risk from inhaled acrolein. In addition, acrolein is generated by the thermal decomposition of fat, so cooks are probably also at additional risk. Since acrolein has been shown to suppress pulmonary antibacterial defenses, individuals with or prone to pulmonary infections may also be at greater risk.

Existing Guidelines and Standards: The current time-weighted average TLV for acrolein established by the American Conference of Governmental Industrial Hygienists (2-2) is 0.1 ppm (0.25 mg/m^3). The same value is recommended by the Occupational Safety and Health Administration. The ACGIH standard was designed to "minimize, but not entirely prevent, irritation to all exposed individuals." Kane and Alarie (2-3) have reviewed the basis for this TLV in terms of both additional data on human irritation and their own work on the irritant effects of acrolein to mice. These investigators (2-3) concluded that "the 0.1 ppm TLV for acrolein is acceptable but is close to the highest value of the acceptable 0.02 to 0.2 ppm range predicted by this animal model."

The Food and Drug Administration permits the use of acrolein as a slime-control substance in the manufacture of paper and paperboard for use in food packaging and in the treatment of food starch at not more than 0.6% acrolein. In the Soviet Union, the maximum permissible daily concentration of acrolein in the atmosphere is 0.1 mg/m^3 (2-4). This study did not specify whether this level is intended as an occupational or ambient air quality standard.

Summary of Proposed EPA Criteria: *Freshwater Aquatic Life* — For acrolein the criterion to protect freshwater aquatic life as derived using the Guidelines is 1.2 μg/l as a 24-hour average and the concentrations should not exceed 2.7 μg/l at any time.

Saltwater Aquatic Life — The data base for saltwater aquatic life is insufficient to allow use of the Guidelines. The following recommendation is inferred from toxicity data for freshwater organisms. For acrolein the criterion to protect saltwater aquatic life as derived using procedures other than the Guidelines is 0.88 μg/l as a 24-hour average and the concentration should not exceed 2.0 μg/l at any time.

Human Health — For the protection of human health from the adverse effects of acrolein ingested through the consumption of water and fish a criterion of 6.5 μg/l is suggested.

Basis for Proposed Human Health Criteria: Although acrolein is mutagenic in some test systems and can bind to mammalian DNA, current information indicates that acrolein is not a carcinogen or cocarcinogen. Water quality criteria for acrolein could be derived from the TLV, chronic inhalation studies, and subacute oral studies using noncarcinogenic biological responses.

Stokinger and Woodward (2-5) have described a method for calculating water quality criteria from TLVs. Essentially, this method consists of deriving an acceptable daily intake (ADI) for man from the TLV by making assumptions on breathing rate and absorption. The ADI is then partitioned into permissible amounts from drinking water and other sources. However, because the TLV is based on the prevention of the irritant effects of acrolein on inhalation exposures, such a criterion would have little, if any, validity.

A criterion could also be calculated based on chronic inhalation data. Female hamsters exposed to acrolein at 9.2 mg/m^3 in the air, seven hours per day, five days per week, for 52 weeks evidenced slight hematologic changes, significant decreases in liver weight, and significant increases in lung weights (2-6).

This study cannot be used to derive a criterion by standard methods because a no observable effect level (NOEL) was not obtained. Nonetheless, by making assumptions of respiratory volume and retention, the exposure data from this study can be converted to a mg/kg dose and an equivalent water exposure level can be calculated. The average body weight for the hamsters at the end of the exposure was about 100 g. Assuming a mean minute volume of 33 ml for a 100 g hamster (2-7) and a retention of 0.75, the average daily dose is estimated at 68.3 μg/animal (9.2 mg acrolein/m^3 x 0.033 l/min x 1 m^3/1,000 liters x 60 min/hr x 7 hr/day x 5 days/7 days x 0.75) or 683 μg/kg. Using an uncertainty factor of 1,000 (2-8), an estimated unacceptable daily dose for man is 0.683 μg/kg or 47.8 μg/man, assuming a 70-kg body weight.

A criterion based on this daily dose level would be unsatisfactory for two reasons. First, as indicated above, the dose data used to derive the standard are not based on a NOEL. In this respect, the derived criterion represents an undesirably high level in water. Secondly, the criterion is based on an inhalation study. Given the probable instability of acrolein in the gastrointestinal tract, the use of inhalation data may not be suitable for deriving a criterion.

In *Drinking Water and Human Health,* the National Academy of Sciences (2-8) summarized the study by Newell (2-9) in which acrolein was added to the drinking water of rats at concentrations of 5, 13, 32, 80, and 200 mg/l for 90 days without apparent adverse effects. Because this study did not involve a chronic exposure, the National Academy of Sciences (2-8) declined to derive an acceptable daily intake for man based on this study. However, McNamara (2-10) has suggested that subacute exposures can be used to estimate chronic no-effect levels. Based on an extensive review of the literature comparing subacute and chronic toxicity tests, McNamara (2-10) noted that "for 95% of chemical compounds ... (on which data were available) ... a three-month no-effect dose (divided by a factor of 10) will produce no effects in a lifetime."

Using this approximation for acrolein, the no observable effect level for acrolein on rats can be estimated at 20 mg/l of water. Assuming a daily water consumption of 35 ml/day and a body weight of 450 g, the chronic no-effect dose for rats is estimated at 1.56 mg/kg. This value may be converted into an ADI for man by applying an uncertainty factor. Since the chronic no-effect dose is merely an estimate based on observed relationships between subacute and chronic toxicity, an uncertainty factor of 1,000 is recommended (2-8). Thus, the estimated ADI for man is 15.6 μg/kg or 109 μg/man, assuming a 70-kg body weight. Therefore, consumption of 2 liters of water daily and 18.7 g of contaminated fish having a bioconcentration factor of 790, would result in, assuming 100% gastrointestinal absorption of acrolein, a maximum permissible concentration of 6.72 μg/l for the ingested water:

$$109 \ \mu g/[2 \text{ liters} + (790 \ x \ 0.018)] \ x \ 1.0 = 6.72 \ \mu g/l$$

This criterion does not consider other significant sources of exposure to acrolein such as inhalation. In addition, this criterion may be above the organoleptic level for acrolein, which has not been determined in man.

References

(2-1) U.S. EPA *Survey of two municipal wastewater treatment plants for toxic substances,* Cincinnati, Ohio, Wastewater Res. Div. Municipal Environ. Res. Lab. (1977).

(2-2) Amer. Conference of Govt. Ind. Hygienists, *Threshold Limit Values for Chemical Substances and Physical Agents in the Workroom Environment,* Cincinnati, Ohio (1979).

(2-3) Kane, L.E. and Alarie, Y., "Sensory invitation to formaldehyde and acrolein during single and repeated exposures in mice," *J. Am. Ind. Hyg. Assoc.,* 38, 509 (1977).

(2-4) Gusev, M.Z., et al, "Substantiation of the daily average maximum permissible concentration of acrolein in the atmosphere," *Hyg. i Sanit.,* 31, 3 (1966).

(2-5) Storinger, H.E. and Woodward, R.L., "Toxicologic methods for establishing drinking water standards," *J. Amer. Water Works Assoc.,* 50, 515 (1958).

(2-6) Feron, V.J. and Kruysse, A., "Effects of exposure to acrolein vapor in hamsters simultaneously treated with benzo(2)pyrene or diethylnitrosamine," *Jour. Toxicol. Envir. Health,* 3, 379 (1977).

(2-7) Robinson, P.F., in Hoffman, R.A., et al, eds., *The Golden Hamster: Its Biology and Use in Medical Research,* Ames, Iowa State University Press (1968).

(2-8) National Academy of Sciences, *Drinking Water and Human Health,* Wash., D.C. (1977).

(2-9) Newell, G.W., *Acute and Subacute Toxicity of Acrolein,* Stanford Research Inst. Project No. 5-868-Z; summarized in Reference 2-8.

(2-10) McNamara, B.P., "Concepts in health evaluation of commercial and industrial chemicals," in Mehlman, M.A., *New Concepts in Safety Evaluation,* New York, John Wiley and Sons (1976).

ACRYLONITRILE (#3)

Acrylonitrile, $CH_2{=}CHCN$, is the commercially important organic nitrile.

Occurrence: Acrylonitrile is manufactured in the United States by the reaction of propylene with ammonia and oxygen in the presence of a catalyst. (A number of other processes are used outside the United States.) Current domestic producers of acrylonitrile are American Cyanamid Company (New Orleans, Louisiana), E.I. DuPont de Nemours Company, Inc. (Beaumont, Texas and Memphis, Tennessee), Monsanto Company (Chocolate Bayou, Texas), and The Standard Oil Company (Lima, Ohio).

Acrylonitrile is the most extensively produced aliphatic nitrile and ranks 45th on the list of high volume chemicals produced in the United States. The 1976 production of acrylonitrile was 1.6 billion pounds which is approximately seven times the 1960 production volume.

Disposal of acrylic polymers, including polyacrylonitrile, by burning results in the release of acrylonitrile monomer. Residual amounts of acrylonitrile monomer are released from fabrics such as underwear made of polyacrylonitrile fiber, and from furniture and other items made of polyacrylonitrile plastics. The public may also be exposed to acrylonitrile by ingestion of food products which have leached residual acrylonitrile monomer from polyacrylonitrile packaging materials, such as commercial plastic wraps for foods. This problem of acrylonitrile monomer leaching has led the Food and Drug Administration to ban the use of polyacrylonitrile plastic for beverage containers. Cigarette smoke has been shown by gas chromatographic analysis to contain aliphatic nitriles including acrylonitrile, propionitrile and methacrylonitrile. The presence of aliphatic nitriles in cigarette smoke may explain why higher values of thiocyanate (a known metabolic product of acrylonitrile) have been found in the blood and urine of acrylonitrile workers who were smokers compared to nonsmokers.

In brief, in addition to occupational exposure of those involved in the manufacture and processing of aliphatic nitriles, the public is exposed to acrylonitrile from the breakdown of the acrylonitrile-based polymers to monomers when the polymers are burned for disposal, by release of residual monomer from acrylic fibers and plastics, by leaching of monomer from food packaging, and from cigarette smoke.

Physical Properties: Acrylonitrile is an explosive, flammable liquid having a normal boiling point of 77°C and a vapor pressure of 80 torrs (20°C). The toxic effects of acrylonitrile are similar to cyanide poisoning although not identical. The chemical structure of acrylonitrile, $CH_2{=}CHCN$, resembles that of vinyl chloride, a material known to cause human cancer. Synonyms for acrylonitrile include cyanoethylene, 2-propenenitrile, VCN, and vinyl cyanide. Polymerization grade acrylonitrile contains a number of impurities and additives, namely, dimethylformamide, hydrogen peroxide, hydroxyanisole, methyl acrylate, phenyl ether-biphenyl mixture, sodium metabisulfite, sulfur dioxide, sulfuric acid, and titanium dioxide.

Chemical Properties: The outstanding chemical property of acrylonitrile is its ability to polymerize to high polymers and copolymers. Acrylonitrile may also be hydrodimerized to adiponitrile

Uses: The major use of acrylonitrile is in the manufacture of copolymers for the production of acrylic and modacrylic fibers by copolymerization with methyl acrylate, methyl methacrylate, vinyl acetate, vinyl chloride, or vinylidene chloride. Acrylic fibers, marketed under trade names including Acrilan, Creslan, Orlon, and Zefran, are used in the manufacture of apparel, carpeting, blankets, draperies and upholstery. Some applications of modacrylic fibers are synthetic furs and hair wigs; trade names for modacrylic fibers include Acrylan, Elura, SEF, and Verel. Acrylic and/or modacrylic fibers are manufactured from acrylonitrile by American Cyanamid Company (Milton, Florida), Dow Badishe Company (Williamsburg, Virginia), E.I. DuPont de Nemours and Company, Inc. (Camden, South Carolina and Waynesboro, Virginia), Eastman Kodak Company (Kingsport, Tennessee), and Monsanto Company (Decatur, Alabama).

Other major uses of acrylonitrile include the manufacture of acrylonitrile-butadiene-styrene (ABS) and styrene-acrylonitrile (SAN) resins (used to produce a variety of plastic products), nitrile elastomers and latexes, and other chemicals (e.g., adiponitrile, acrylamide). Acrylonitrile has been used as a fumigant; however, all U.S. registrations for this use were voluntarily withdrawn as of August 8, 1978. The U.S. Food and Drug Administration has recently banned the use of an acrylonitrile resin for soft drink bottles, but its use is still allowed in other food packaging. NIOSH estimates that 125,000 persons are potentially exposed to acrylonitrile in the workplace.

Toxic Effects: Acrylonitrile has been reported as acutely toxic to fish at concentrations as low as 10,100 μg/l and to the invertebrate, *Daphnia magna,* at 7,550 μg/l. Chronic toxic effects were not seen in *D. magna* at concentrations up to and including 3,600 μg/l. The bluegill, *Lepomis macrochirus,* concentrated acrylonitrile in its tissues by a factor of 48. The only available datum for a saltwater organism is a 96-hour LC_{50} of 24,500 μg/l for the pinfish, *Lagodon rhomboides* (3-1).

At present the body of evidence produced in both toxicity studies on laboratory animals and occupational epidemiologic studies on man suggests that acrylonitrile may be a human carcinogen. Thus, NIOSH has recently voiced its opinion that "acrylonitrile must be handled in the workplace as a suspect human carcinogen" (3-2). This judgment of NIOSH is based primarily on (1) a preliminary epidemiologic study of E.I. DuPont de Nemours and Co., Inc. on acrylonitrile polymerization workers from one particular textile fibers plant (Camden, S.C.); in this study, it was ascertained that a substantial excess risk (doubling over expected) of lung and colon cancers occurred between 1969 and 1975 in a cohort exposed between 1950 and 1955; (2) interim results from ongoing 2-year studies on laboratory rats performed by Dow Chemical Co., and reported by the Manufacturing Chemists Association (April, 1977) in which, by either drinking water or inhalation routes of acrylonitrile exposure, laboratory rats developed CNS tumors and ear canal tumors, not evident in control animals. Mammary region masses were also in excess upon exposure to 80 ppm (3-3)(3-4).

Aside from suggestive evidence of carcinogenicity in man and animals, numerous workers have reported on the other genotoxic characteristics of acrylonitrile (embryo toxicity, mutagenicity, and teratogenicity) in laboratory animals (3-5)(3-6)(3-7). Even though there is some controversy over the chronic effects of acrylonitrile (3-8), the acute toxicity of acrylonitrile is well known and the compound appears to exert part of its toxic effect through the release of inorganic cyanide (3-9)(3-10).

Current Levels of Exposure: Indices of exposure, apart from very unspecific symptoms (such as spirographic examination of the lung) in the case of chronic exposure include the determination of increased blood SCN^- level and elevated urinary SCN^- level.

It must be recognized that smoking presents a problem in ascertainment of occupational and other exposure because of the presence of nitriles in cigarette smoke. Thus, smokers

may have a blood level of approximately 3 mg % SCN⁻ in blood; the urinary SCN⁻ level
of heavy smokers may normally reach 9 mg KSCN/l in contrast to a normal urinary level
for nonsmokers of 0.2 mg/l and for occasional smokers a normal urinary level of 1.2 mg
KSCN/l. Consequently, in testing for occupational or other exposure, if it is not known
whether a person is a smoker, values of urinary KSCN of 10 mg/l cannot be considered to
result from occupational exposure. It may be advisable for the purposes of screening for
exposure to have liver function tests if urinary analysis proves to be negative. In addition,
another suggested method of screening is that of the spectrophotometric determination
of cyanomethemoglobin in blood.

The existing occupational standards are given in a section which follows shortly. These
standards are often exceeded. The production of significant amounts of acrylonitrile and
HCN from thermal decomposition of polyacrylonitrile products has already been noted.
For example, overheating of 1 kg of a polyacrylonitrile plastic about 15 g of HCN can be
formed. Thus, the amount of HCN formed in a 30 m^3 room from 100 to 200 g of polyacrylonitrile fibers corresponds to 10 to 15 times the MAC values and this underlines a
special hazard of polyacrylonitrile plants. The possible synergism of acrylonitrile and HCN
has already been alluded to.

There are few data on monitoring of ambient air and drinking water levels of acrylonitrile.
This lack of data prevents us from predicting most actual exposures of the public except
for certain groups at high risk such as occupationally exposed workers. At present, Emergency Air Standard is 2 ppm of acrylonitrile = 4.35 mg/m^3/day. Therefore, the acrylonitrile intake of a worker at threshold level = 0.90(4.35 mg/m^3)(20 m^3/day) = 78.3 mg/day,
where 0.90 is the average retention of acrylonitrile (3-22). Thus, depending on the half-life
of acrylonitrile, a substantial body burden in occupationally exposed individuals can result.

Special Groups at Risk: Shown in Table 3 below are various groups at varying degrees of
risk to acrylonitrile exposure. NIOSH has estimated that at least 125,000 individuals are
exposed occupationally.

Table 3: Groups Exposed to Acrylonitrile

```
Occupational
    (1)   Plastic
          Acrylonitrile manufacturers
          Polymer manufacturers
          Polymer molders
          Polymer combustion workers
          Furniture makers
    (2)   Fabrics
          Fiber manufacturers
          Clothing sewers
    (3)   Biological product manufacturing
          Dental polymer manufacturers
          Contact lens fabricators
          Blood filter fabricators
    (4)   Water treatment and manufacturers
    (5)   Pesticide and fumigant manufacturers
          Sprayers
          Farmers

Nonoccupational
    (1)   Accidental
          Exposure to liquid from transportational spill
          Combustion and fire (firemen and domestic personnel)
          Ingestion of contaminated water or food
          Respiration of contaminated air (environmental expos-
             ure to acrylonitrile or polyacrylonitrile plants)
    (2)   Nonaccidental
          Cigarette smokers
          Wearers of acrylic dentures
          Wearers of acrylic underwear, diapers, and sanitary
             napkins
          Ingestion of food wrapped in polyacrylonitrile wrapping
          Exposure to acrylonitrile vapors from polyacrylonitrile
             furniture
```

Source: Reference (3)

Existing Guidelines and Standards: The existing standards for acrylonitrile in various
countries and various years appear in Table 4.

**Table 4: Standards for Acrylonitrile Air Exposure Levels in Various Countries (between
1970-1974)**

Year	Country	Air (ppm)	Standard (mg/m^3)	Kind of Standard	References
1970	USSR	0.2	0.435	MAC*	(3-11)(3-12)(3-13)(3-14)
1970	Federal Republic of Germany	20.0	43.5	MAC	(3-11)(3-13)(3-15)
1970	England	20.0	43.5	MAC	(3-11)(3-13)(3-15)
1974	U.S.	20.0	43.5	TLV**	(3-11)(3-17)(3-18)(3-19)

*Hygienic goal.
**ACGIH has listed an intended change as of 1979 listing acrylonitrile as a
human carcinogen without an assigned TLV.

Source: Reference (3)

It is evident that at this time, the Russian standard was substantially less (two orders of magnitude) than the American and West European standards. Published work indicates, however, that the standard may be exceeded significantly. A study of a Yugoslavian acrylic
fiber plant indicated that their in-plant concentrations of acrylonitrile begin to approach
the TLV in the U.S.A. Other investigators (3-12)(3-13)(3-14) have noted that the air standards are often exceeded, although it is unlikely that higher concentrations occur throughout
the day.

Almost twenty years ago, it was advocated by Elkins (3-16) in the U.S.A. that the MAC
be reduced to 10 ppm (corresponding to that of HCN). According to Babanov (3-14) an
acute danger exists even from 0.85 to 6.1 mg/m³ (0.4 to 2.8 ppm) in working areas.

In January, 1978, the Occupational Safety and Health Administration (OSHA) announced
an emergency temporary standard to reduce sharply worker exposure to acrylonitrile. OSHA
director, Dr. Eula Bingham, said that, effective immediately, employee exposure to acrylonitrile must be reduced to 2 ppm averaged over an 8-hour period (TLV). Dr. Bingham
noted that the Emergency Temporary Standard was necessary because of data from studies
of workers previously exposed to acrylonitrile and laboratory tests, both of which established "exposure to acrylonitrile poses a potential carcinogenic risk to humans." While
OSHA's position is that there is no way to determine a safe level of exposure to a carcinogen,
in this case "a level was chosen to immediately minimize the hazard to the greatest extent
possible within the confines of feasibility."

The recent action of OSHA is, in fact, based upon studies done by the chemical industry
itself. In March, 1977, the Manufacturing Chemists Association (MCA) reported interim results from a study of the chronic toxicity of acrylonitrile ingestion on rats. Findings were
that ingestion of 100 and 300 ppm of acrylonitrile in drinking water produced tumors of
the CNS and ear canal. In April, 1977, there were similar tumors reported among rats ingesting 35 ppm of the substance (3-3). Confirming the laboratory results, DuPont informed
OSHA of preliminary results of an epidemiological study of workers exposed to acrylonitrile
at its textile fibers plant in Camden, S.C.

Summary of Proposed EPA Criteria: *Freshwater Aquatic Life* — For acrylonitrile the criterion to protect freshwater aquatic life as derived using the Guidelines is 130 µg/l as a 24-
hour average and the concentration should not exceed 300 µg/l at any time.

Saltwater Aquatic Life — For acrylonitrile the criterion to protect saltwater aquatic life as
derived using procedures other than the Guidelines is 130 µg/l as a 24-hour average and the
concentration should not exceed 290 µg/l at any time.

Human Health — For the maximum protection of human health from the potential carcinogenic effects of exposure to acrylonitrile through ingestion of water and contaminated aquatic organisms, the ambient water concentration is zero. The EPA is considering setting criteria at an interim target risk level in the range of 10^{-5}, 10^{-6}, or 10^{-7} with corresponding criteria of 0.08, 0.008, and 0.0008 µg/l, respectively. If water alone is consumed, the water concentration should be less than 0.084 µg/l to keep the lifetime cancer risk below 10^{-5}.

Basis for Proposed Human Health Criteria: The animal carcinogenicity studies of Norris (3-3), Quast, et al (3-4), and Maltoni, et al (3-20) and the epidemiological studies of O'Berg of DuPont (unpublished 1977) and Monson (3-21) were considered to be the most pertinent data for the determination of a water quality criterion for the protection of human health. Although the epidemiological studies showed excesses of various cancers in man, neither study had quantitative exposure data of the workers to acrylonitrile and hence could not be utilized for calculation of a safe level. The criterion was therefore developed from the animal carcinogenicity data by utilizing the linear nonthreshold model. The rat carcinogenicity studies, in general, showed a tumorigenic response to acrylonitrile whether exposure was by ingestion or inhalation. These data support the findings of the epidemiological studies.

To select data for the evaluation of an acceptable risk concentration, studies having the following attributes were chosen:

(1) There was an increase in frequency of tumors in treated rats over control rats.
(2) There was a low frequency of tumors in treated rats over control rats.
(3) Several dosage levels were tested so dose-response relationships could be interpreted.

To use the linear dose-response nonthreshold model in calculating a water concentration that results in a risk of a carcinogenicity incidence of 1/100,000, the following assumptions were made for all calculations:

(1) A maximum bioaccumulation factor of 110 for acrylonitrile, as determined for the bluegill sunfish.
(2) Consumption of water per person per day is 2 liters over a period of 70 years.
(3) Average consumption of fish per person per day is 18.7 g.
(4) Average life span for test rats is 730 days.

Specialized assumptions for converting inhalation dose to an equivalent ingestion dose were made with the Maltoni, et al (3-20) study as follows:

(1) The average rat respiration rate is 0.61 l/min-kg.
(2) The average weight for male rats is 500 g and female rats 300 g.
(3) The absorption efficiency is 90% (3-22).
(4) Since the duration of the experiment was 1,001 days, the average life span of the rat was assumed to be 1,001 days due to constraints of the equations in the linear model.
(5) The data of Young, et al (3-22) suggest that extrapolation from one dosage route to another may not be valid. Further verification of this data is needed, however, and the data of Maltoni's inhalation study was included for comparison with the water ingestion studies.

The results of the application of the linear nonthreshold model to the selected data are summarized below in Table 5.

Table 5: Analysis of Acrylonitrile Toxicity Data

Reference	Route	Location of Tumor	Sex	Dose (mg/kg)	Acceptable Risk in Water (mg/l)
Norris (3-3)	water ingestion	proliferation lesions in brain	female	12.45	1.2×10^{-4}
		mammary gland	female	4.7	1.6×10^{-4}

(continued)

Table 5: (continued)

Reference	Route	Location of Tumor	Sex	Dose (mg/kg)	Acceptable Risk in Water (mg/l)
		ear canal masses	female	12.45	9.8×10^{-4}
		ear canal masses	male	23.8	8.8×10^{-5}
Quast, et al	water ingestion	stomach	female	27.45	1.5×10^{-4}
(3-4)		stomach	male	23.8	8.8×10^{-5}
		central nervous sys.	female	11.4	8.3×10^{-5}
		central nervous sys.	male	9.6	1.9×10^{-4}
		zymbal gland	female	11.4	1.9×10^{-4}
Maltoni, et al	inhalation	gliomas	male	4.1*	18.1×10^{-4}
(3-20)		mammary gland	female	1.0*	0.6×10^{-4}
		mammary gland	male	4.1*	5.6×10^{-4}

*Calculated ingestion dose converted from inhalation.

Source: Reference (3)

In spite of the differences between the data sets, the application of linear nonthreshold model results in relatively similar calculated acceptable risk concentrations for water in each case. Due to numerous assumptions necessary for the Maltoni study as well as the potential inability to convert between dosage routes, the data from this study were not weighed as heavily as the others. Therefore, the value of 0.8×10^{-4} mg/l was selected as the recommended criterion for acrylonitrile in water. It must be emphasized that this level is based on data from a 12-month interim report and is, therefore, preliminary in nature.

Under the Consent Decree in NRDC vs Train, criteria are to state "recommended maximum permissible concentrations (including where appropriate, zero) consistent with the protection of aquatic organisms, human health, and recreational activities." Acrylonitrile is suspected of being a human carcinogen. Because there is no recognized safe concentration for a human carcinogen, the recommended concentration of acrylonitrile in water for maximum protection of human health is zero.

Because attaining a zero concentration level may be infeasible in some cases and in order to assist the Agency and States in the possible future development of water quality regulations, the concentrations of acrylonitrile corresponding to several incremental lifetime cancer risk levels have been estimated. A cancer risk level provides an estimate of the additional incidence of cancer that may be expected in an exposed population. A risk of 10^{-5}, for example, indicates a probability of one additional case of cancer for every 100,000 people exposed, a risk of 10^{-6} indicates one additional case of cancer for every million people exposed, and so forth.

In the *Federal Register* notice of availability of draft ambient water quality criteria, EPA stated that it is considering setting criteria at an interim target risk level of 10^{-5}, 10^{-6} or 10^{-7} as shown below.in Table 6. In the table the risk levels and corresponding criteria are calculated by applying a modified "one hit" extrapolation model described in the Methodology Document to the animal bioassay data. Since the extrapolation model is linear to low doses, the additional lifetime risk is directly proportional to the water concentration. Therefore, water concentrations corresponding to other risk levels can be derived by multiplying or dividing one of the risk levels and corresponding water concentrations shown in the table by factors such as 10, 100, 1,000, and so forth.

Table 6: Possible Alternative Criteria for Acrylonitrile

Exposure Assumptions	. . . . Risk Levels, ng/l			
	0	10^{-7}	10^{-6}	10^{-5}
2 liters of drinking water and consumption of 18.7 g of fish and shellfish*	—	0.008×10^{-4}	0.08×10^{-4}	0.8×10^{-4}

(continued)

Table 6: (continued)

Exposure Assumptions	0	10^{-7}	10^{-6}	10^{-5}
	. . . . Risk Levels, ng/l			
Consumption of fish and shellfish only	—	0.016×10^{-4}	0.16×10^{-4}	1.6×10^{-4}

*51% of the acrylonitrile exposure results from the consumption of aquatic organisms which exhibit an average bioconcentration potential of 110-fold. The remaining 49% of the acrylonitrile exposure results from drinking water.

Source: Reference (3)

Concentration levels were derived assuming a lifetime exposure to various amounts of acrylonitrile (1) occurring from the consumption of both drinking water and aquatic life grown in water containing the corresponding acrylonitrile concentrations and, (2) occurring solely from the consumption of aquatic life grown in the waters containing the corresponding acrylonitrile concentrations. Because data indicating other sources of exposure and the contribution to total body burden are inadequate for quantitative use, the criterion reflects the increment to risks associated with ambient water exposure only.

The water quality criterion for acrylonitrile is derived from the tumorigenic effect observed in the central nervous system of female Sprague-Dawley rats given 100 ppm acrylonitrile in drinking water. The time weighted average dose of 11.4 mg/kg/day was given for 52 weeks, and ten animals of each group were then sacrificed (interim). The incidence of brain tumors was 0/9 and 4/10 in the control and the treated groups, respectively. Assuming a fish bioconcentration of 110, the criterion is calculated from the following parameters:

$n_t = 4$	le = 368 days	L = 730 days
$N_t = 10$	Le = 368 days	w = 0.350 kg
$n_c = 0$	d = 11.4 mg/kg/day	F = 0.0187 kg/day
$N_c = 9$	R = 110	

Based on these parameters, the one-hit slope B_H is 2.0455 $(mg/kg/day)^{-1}$. The resulting water concentration of acrylonitrile calculated to keep the individual risk below 10^{-5} is 0.084 $\mu g/l$. It must be emphasized that this concentration level is based on data from a 12-month interim report and is, therefore, likely to be modified when the final report becomes available.

References

(3-1) U.S. EPA, *In-depth studies on health and environmental impacts of selected water pollutants,* U.S. Environ. Prot. Agency Report on Contract No. 68-01-4646, Wash., D.C. (1978).

(3-2) National Institute for Occupational Safety and Health, *A recommended standard for occupational exposure to acrylonitrile,* DHEW Publ. No. 78-116, Wash. D.C., U.S. Government Printing Office, (1978).

(3-3) Norris, J.M., *Status report on two-year study incorporating acrylonitrile in the drinking water of rats,* Health Environ. Res. Dow Chemical Co. (1977).

(3-4) Quast, J.F., et al, *Toxicity of drinking water containing acrylonitrile in rats: Results after 12 months,* Toxicol. Res. Lab., Health Environ. Res. Dow Chemical Co. (1977).

(3-5) Venitt, S., et al, "Mutagenicity of acrylonitrile (cyanoethylene) in *Escherichia coli,*" *Mutat. Res.,* 45, 283 (1977).

(3-6) Milvey, P., and Wolff, M., "Mutagenic studies with acrylonitrile," *Mutat. Res.,* 48, 271 (1977).

(3-7) Murray, F.J., et al, *Teratologic evaluation of acrylonitrile monomer given to rats by gavage,* Rep. Toxicol. Res. Lab. Dow Chemical Co., Midland, Mich (1976).

(3-8) Shaffer, C.B., "Toxicology of acrylonitrile," in F.A. Ayer, ed., *Environmental aspects of chemical use in rubber process operations,* Conf. Proc. (1975).

(3-9)   Fassett, D.W., "Cyanides and nitriles," *Industrial hygiene and toxicology,* Vol. II,
        New York, Interscience Publishers, (1963).
(3-10) Wilson, R.H., "Health hazards encountered in the manufacture of synthetic rubber,"
        Jour. AMA, 124, 701, (1944).
(3-11) Grahl, R., "Toxikologie und wirkungsweise von acrylonitril," *Zbl. Arbeitsmed.,* 12,
        369, (1970).
(-312) Schwaneke, R., *Zbl. Arbeitsmed,* 16, 1, (1966).
(3-13) Thiede, H. and Franzen, E., Wiss. Zschr. Martin-Luther Univ., Halle-Wittenberg,
        Meth-Naturw. Reihe, 14, 1977, (1965).
(3-14) Babanov, G.P., "Problems of industrial hygiene in the production of synthetic
        butadiene—acrylonitrile rubbers," *Gigiena Truda,* 4, 7, (1960).
(3-15) Lefaux, R., *Practical Toxicology of Plastics,* 1-43 (1966).
(3-16) Elkins, H.B., *The Chemistry of Industrial Toxicology,* 2nd Ed., London, John Wiley
        and Sons, (1959).
(3-17) Mallette, F.S., "Industrial hygiene in synthetic rubber manufacture," *Industrial Med.,*
        12, 495 (1943).
(3-18) Dudley, H.C. and Neal, P.A., "Toxicology of acrylonitrile, I, a study of the acute
        toxicity," *Jour. Ind. Hyg. Toxicol.,* 24, 27 (1942).
(3-19) Stokinger, H., et al, *Jour. Occup. Med.,* 5, 491 (1963).
(3-20) Maltoni, C., et al, "Carcinogenicity bioassays on rats of acrylonitrile administered
        by inhalation and by ingestion," *La Medicina de Lavoro,* 68, 401 (1977).
(3-21) Monson, R.R., "Mortality and cancer morbidity among B.F. Goodrich workers,"
        43, *FR,* 45762.
(3-22) Young, J.D., Slauter, R.W. and Karbowski, R.J., *The Pharmacokinetic and Metabolic
        Profile of C^{14}—Acrylonitrile Given to Rats by Three Routes,* Midland, Mich.,
        Toxicological Research Laboratory, Dow Chemical Co. (1977).

ALDRIN/DIELDRIN (#4)

Aldrin is a polychlorinated compound having the formula:

$$\begin{array}{ccccccc}
 & & CCl & & CH & & \\
ClC & & | \quad CH & & | \quad CH & & \\
 \| & & CCl_2 \quad | & & CH_2 \quad | & \| & \\
ClC & & | \quad CH & & | \quad CH & & \\
 & & CCl & & CH & &
\end{array}$$

Dieldrin is the oxy-derivative of aldrin and has the formula:

$$\begin{array}{ccccccc}
 & & CCl & & CH & & \\
ClC & & | \quad CH & & | \quad CH & & \\
 \| & & CCl_2 \quad | & & CH_2 \quad | & \rangle O \\
ClC & & | \quad CH & & | \quad CH & & \\
 & & CCl & & CH & &
\end{array}$$

Occurrence: Aldrin and dieldrin are manmade compounds belonging to the group of cyclo-
diene insecticides. They are a subgroup of the chlorinated cyclic hydrocarbon insecticides
which include DDT, BHC, etc. They were manufactured in the United States by Shell
Chemical Company until the U.S. EPA prohibited their manufacture in 1974 under the
Federal Insecticide, Fungicide and Rodenticide Act. They are currently manufactured by
Shell Chemical Company in Holland. Prior to 1974, both insecticides were available in the
United States in various formulations for broad-spectrum insect control.

The primary use of the chemicals in the past was for control of corn pests, although they
were also used by the citrus industry. Uses are restricted to those where there is no effluent discharge.

Physical Properties: Aldrin and dieldrin are white crystalline substances with aldrin melting at 104°C and dieldrin melting between 176° to 177°C. Both are soluble in organic solvents with dieldrin the less soluble of the two. The chemical name for aldrin is 1,2,3,4,10,10-hexachloro-1,4,4a,5,8,8a-hexahydro-1,4:5,8-exo-dimethanonaphthalene. The chemical name for dieldrin is 1,2,3,4,10,10-hexachloro-6,7-epoxy-1,4,4a,5,6,7,8,8a-octahydro-endo,exo-1,4:5,8-dimethanonaphthalene.

Dieldrin's persistence in the environment is due to its extremely low volatility (i.e., a vapor pressure of 1.78×10^{-7} mm mercury at 20°C) and low solubility in water (186 μg/l at 25° to 29°C). In addition, dieldrin is extremely apolar, resulting in a high affinity for fat which accounts for its retention in animal fats, plant waxes, and other such organic matter in the environment. The fat solubility of dieldrin results in the progressive accumulation in the food chain which may result in a concentration in an organism which would exceed the lethal limit for a consumer.

Chemical Properties: Aldrin is metabolically converted to dieldrin. This epoxidation has been shown to occur in several species including mammals and poultry, houseflies, locusts, soil microorganisms, a large number of *Lepidoptera* species, freshwater fish (4-1), and a number of freshwater invertebrates including protozoa, coelenterates, worms, arthropods, mollusks, and lobsters. The aldrin molecule is biologically altered in the environment to a more stable and at least equally toxic form, dieldrin. Dieldrin is known to be metabolically degraded as shown by Matsumura and Boush (4-2) and Patil, et al (4-3).

However, dieldrin is probably the most stable insecticide among the cyclodienes (i.e., isodrin-endrin; heptachlor-heptachlor epoxide). The time required for 95% of the dieldrin to disappear from soil has been estimated to vary from 5 to 25 years depending upon the microbial flora of the soil (4-4). Dieldrin applied at 100 ppm has been shown to persist in soil for more than six years (4-5), while at 25 ppm in a different soil type, a 50% loss was found at seven years (4-6). When applied to sandy soil at a rate of 100 ppm, residues could be found fifteen years later.

Uses: Aldrin use in the United States peaked at 19 million pounds in 1966 but dropped to about 10.5 million pounds in 1970. During that same period, dieldrin use decreased from 1 million pounds to about 670,000 pounds. The decreased use has been attributed primarily to increased insect resistance to the two chemicals and to development and availability of substitute materials.

Aldrin and dieldrin have been the subject of litigation bearing upon the contention that these substances cause severe aquatic environmental change and are potential carcinogens. In 1970, the U.S. Department of Agriculture cancelled all registrations of these pesticides based upon a concern to limit dispersal in or on aquatic areas. In 1972, under the authority of the Fungicide, Insecticide, Rodenticide Act as amended by the Federal Pesticide Control Act of 1972, USCS Section 135, et seq., an EPA order lifted cancellation of all registered aldrin and dieldrin for use in deep ground insertions for termite control, nursery clipping of roots and tops of nonfood plants, and mothproofing of woolen textiles and carpets where there is no effluent discharge. In 1974, cancellation proceedings disclosed the severe hazard to human health and suspension of registration of aldrin and dieldrin use was ordered; production was restricted for all pesticide products containing aldrin or dieldrin.

Toxic Effects: During the past decade, considerable information has been generated concerning the toxicity and potential carcinogenicity of the two organochlorine pesticides, aldrin and dieldrin. These two pesticides are usually considered together since aldrin is readily epoxidized to dieldrin in the environment. Both are acutely toxic to most forms of life including arthropods, mollusks, invertebrates, amphibians, reptiles, fish, birds and mammals. Dieldrin is extremely persistent in the environment. By means of bioaccumulation it is concentrated many times as it moves up the food chain.

Current Levels of Exposure: The people of the United States are exposed to aldrin and dieldrin in air, water, and food. Aldrin or dieldrin have been found in more than 85% of the air samples tested by the U.S. EPA (4-7). The levels were as high as 2.8 ng/m^3 resulting in an intake of up to 0.098 μg/day. Dieldrin can travel great distances in the air, especially when absorbed to particulate matter. Thus people can potentially be exposed to pesticide treatments from other countries.

Waters recently sampled in the United States contained aldrin or dieldrin in amounts up to 0.05 μg/l (4-8). The standard diet in the United States has been calculated to contain approximately 43 ng/g of dieldrin. Tolerances for dieldrin in cattle meat fat, milk fat, meat, and meat by-products have been petitioned for at levels of 0.3, 0.2, and 0.1 ppm respectively (4-7).

Special Groups at Risk: Children, especially infants, have a high dairy product diet that has been shown to contain dieldrin. It has also been demonstrated that human milk contains dieldrin residues and that some infants may be exposed to high concentrations of dieldrin from that source alone.

In early studies, various investigators have reported that dieldrin and several other chlorinated hydrocarbon pesticides were present in the tissues of stillborn infants. One of them also reported that dieldrin and other pesticides could be found in the blood of newborn infants.

No work has been carried out on neonatal animals with either aldrin or dieldrin; however, due to the sensitivity of neonatal animals to other carcinogens, this should be an area of great concern.

Existing Guidelines and Standards: Prior to 1974, aldrin and dieldrin were approved for use on 46 agricultural crops and for treatment of soil around fruits, grains, nuts, and vegetables (4-9). In 1974, the registration of aldrin and dieldrin was suspended on the basis of adverse health affects in rodents (39 *FR* 37251). As a result, production is restricted for all pesticide products containing aldrin or dieldrin. Aldrin and dieldrin can no longer be used for spraying and dusting, or for mothproofing in which the residues are discharged into waterways. All uses in structures occupied by humans or livestock, uses upon turf, and any use involving application to any aquatic environment are also restricted. Aldrin and dieldrin can be used for termite treatment which involves direct application to the soil and therefore little movement of the pesticides. They may also be used for treatment of some nonfood seeds and plant dipping during transplantation.

The current exposure level for both aldrin and dieldrin set by the Occupational Safety and Health Administration is an air time-weighted average (TWA) of 250 μg/m^3 for skin absorption (37 *FR* 22139). In 1969, the U.S. Public Health Service Advisory Committee recommended that the drinking water standards for both aldrin and dieldrin be 17 μg/l (4-10). Also, the U.N. Food and Agriculture Organization/World Health Organization's acceptable daily intake for aldrin and dieldrin is 0.0001 mg/kg/day (4-10).

Summary of Proposed EPA Criteria: *Freshwater Aquatic Life* — For aldrin/dieldrin, the criterion to protect freshwater aquatic life as derived using the Guidelines is 0.0019 μg/l as a 24-hour average and the concentration should not exceed 1.2 μg/l at any time.

Saltwater Aquatic Life — For aldrin/dieldrin the criterion to protect saltwater aquatic life as derived using procedures other than the Guidelines is 0.0069 μg/l as a 24-hour average and the concentration should not exceed 0.16 μg/l at any time.

Human Health — For maximum protection of human health from the potential carcinogenic effects of exposure to aldrin through ingestion of water and contaminated aquatic organisms, the ambient water concentration is zero. Concentrations of aldrin estimated to result in additional lifetime cancer risks ranging from no additional risk to an additional risk of 1 in 100,000 are presented in the Criterion document. The EPA is considering setting criteria at an interim target risk level in the range of 10^{-5}, 10^{-6}, or 10^{-7} with corresponding criteria of 4.6×10^{-2} ng/l, 4.6×10^{-3} ng/l, and 4.6×10^{-4} ng/l, respectively.

For the maximum protection of human health from the potential carcinogenic effects of exposure to dieldrin through ingestion of water and contaminated aquatic organisms, the ambient water concentration is zero. Concentrations of dieldrin estimated to result in additional lifetime cancer risks ranging from no additional risk to an additional risk of 1 in 100,000 are presented in the Criterion document ((4). The EPA is considering setting criteria at an interim target risk level in the range of 10^{-5}, 10^{-6} or 10^{-7}, with corresponding criteria of 4.4×10^{-2} ng/l, 4.4×10^{-3} ng/l, and 4.4×10^{-4} ng/l, respectively.

Basis for Proposed Human Health Criteria: The aldrin and dieldrin carcinogenicity data of Walker, et al (4-11) and the National Cancer Institute were analyzed using a linear dose-response model to calculate that concentration of dieldrin in water which is estimated to result in an excess lifetime risk of 10^{-5} in man.

It should be noted that the Walker, et al, study (4-11) used 99% pure dieldrin while the NCI study used technical grade dieldrin. Under the Consent Decree in NRDC vs Train, criteria are to state "recommended maximum permissible concentrations (including where appropriate, zero) consistent with the protection of aquatic organisms, human health, and recreational activities." Both aldrin and dieldrin are suspected of being human carcinogens. Because there is no recognized safe concentration for a human carcinogen, the recommended concentration of aldrin/dieldrin in water for maximum protection of human health is zero.

Because attaining a zero concentration level may be infeasible in some cases and in order to assist the EPA and the States in the possible future development of water quality regulations, the concentrations of aldrin and dieldrin corresponding to several incremental lifetime cancer risk levels have been estimated. A cancer risk level provides an estimate of the additional incidence of cancer that may be expected in an exposed population. A risk of 10^{-5}, for example, indicates a probability of one additional case of cancer for every 100,000 people exposed, a risk of 10^{-6} indicates one additional case of cancer for every million people exposed, and so forth.

In the *Federal Register* notice of availability of draft ambient water quality criteria, EPA stated that it is considering setting criteria at an interim target risk level of 10^{-5}, 10^{-6}, or 10^{-7} as shown in Table 7. In this table the risk levels and corresponding criteria are calculated by applying a modified "one hit" extrapolation model described in the 44 *FR* 15926, 1979. Appropriate bioassay data used in the calculation of the model are presented in the summary of pertinent data. Since the extrapolation model is linear to low doses, the additional lifetime risk is directly proportional to the water concentration. Therefore, water concentrations corresponding to other risk levels can be derived by multiplying or dividing one of the risk levels and corresponding water concentrations shown in the table by factors such as 10, 100, 1,000 and so forth.

Table 7: Possible Alternative Criteria for Aldrin/Dieldrin

Exposure Assumptions	Risk Levels, ng/l			
	0	10^{-7}	10^{-6}	10^{-5}
2 liters of drinking water and consumption of 18.7 g of fish and shellfish*				
Aldrin	0	4.6×10^{-4}	4.6×10^{-3}	4.6×10^{-2}
Dieldrin	0	4.4×10^{-4}	4.4×10^{-3}	4.4×10^{-2}
Consumption of fish and shellfish only				
Aldrin	0	4.6×10^{-4}	4.6×10^{-3}	4.6×10^{-2}
Dieldrin	0	4.5×10^{-4}	4.5×10^{-3}	4.5×10^{-2}

*99.9% of aldrin exposure results from the consumption of aquatic organisms which exhibit an average bioconcentration potential of 4,500-fold; the remaining 0.1% of aldrin exposure results from drinking water.

Source: Reference (4)

98% of dieldrin exposure results from the consumption of aquatic organisms which exhibit an average bioconcentration potential of 4,500 fold. The remaining 2% of dieldrin exposure results from drinking water.

Concentration levels were derived assuming a lifetime exposure to various amounts of aldrin/dieldrin, (1) occurring from the consumption of both drinking water and aquatic life grown in water containing the corresponding aldrin/dieldrin concentrations and, (2) occurring solely from the consumption of aquatic life grown in the waters containing the corresponding aldrin/dieldrin concentrations.

Although total exposure information for aldrin and dieldrin is discussed and an estimate of the contributions from other sources of exposure can be made, this data will not be factored into the ambient water quality criteria formulation because of the tenuous estimates. The criteria presented, therefore, assume an incremental risk from ambient water exposure only.

Summary of Pertinent Data for Aldrin — The water quality criterion for aldrin is derived from the hepatocellular carcinoma response of the B6C3F1 male mice given the low dose of aldrin in the NCI bioassay test, and on the response in the 0.1 ppm group of female CF-1 mice in the Walker, et al experiment (4-11). In the NCI study, a time-weighted average dose of 4 ppm was given in the feed for 80 weeks and the animals were observed for an additional 10 weeks before terminal sacrifice. The incidence of hepatocellular carcinoma was 3/20 and 16/49 in the control and treated groups, respectively. The slope of the one-hit dose-response curve for aldrin is calculated from the following parameters:

$$n_t = 16 \qquad\qquad Le = 90 \text{ weeks}$$
$$N_t = 49 \qquad\qquad d = 4 \text{ ppm} \times 0.13 = 0.52 \text{ mg/kg/day}$$
$$n_c = 23 \qquad\qquad L = 90 \text{ weeks}$$
$$N_c = 20 \qquad\qquad w = 0.035 \text{ kg}$$

With these parameters the slope of the one-hit dose-response curve for aldrin is 6.349 $(\text{mg/kg/day})^{-1}$.

The conversion of aldrin to dieldrin in fish results in the accumulation of dieldrin residues in fish exposed to aldrin. This makes it necessary to consider the risk resulting from intake of dieldrin stored in fish due to the presence of aldrin in water. Thus, the criterion for aldrin also depends upon the one-hit dose-response curve for dieldrin, which has a slope of 183.6 $(\text{mg/kg/day})^{-1}$ as calculated previously from the Walker, et al study (4-11).

The equation describing the risk due to aldrin in water is derived from the general relationship

$$P = B_H D$$
$$D = I/70 \text{ kg}$$
$$P = B_H \, I/70 \text{ kg}$$
$$P(70 \text{ kg}) = B_H I$$

Where:

P = individual lifetime risk (set at 10^{-5} for criterion calculation)
I = average daily human intake of the substance in question
B_H = average weight of humans.

Since aldrin in water leads to the accumulation of dieldrin residues in fish, the equation describing the risk due to aldrin is

$$P_a(70 \text{ kg}) = B_{Ha}C_a(2.0 \text{ l/day}) + B_{Ha}C_aR_{ad}(0.0187 \text{ kg/day}) +$$
$$B_{Hd}C_aR_{ad}(0.0187 \text{ kg/day})$$

Where:

P_a = risk due to aldrin (set at 10^{-5} for criterion calculation)
B_{Ha} = 6.349 $(\text{mg/kg/day})^{-1}$, the aldrin dose-response slope
B_{Hd} = 183.6 $(\text{mg/kg/day})^{-1}$, the dieldrin dose-response slope
C_a = criterion concentration for aldrin (to be calculated)

R_a = 32 l/kg, the fish bioconcentration of aldrin from aldrin
R_{ad} = 4468 l/kg, the fish bioconcentration of dieldrin from aldrin
2.0 l/day = average daily intake of water for humans
0.0187 kg/day = average daily intake of fish for humans.

The term containing R_{ad} represents intake of dieldrin resulting from the presence of aldrin in the water, and is thus multiplied by the dieldrin dose-response slope. R_{ad} is estimated by assuming that in the absence of conversion to dieldrin, aldrin would bioconcentrate 4,500 times (as dieldrin does), and that since aldrin only accumulates 32 times, the remainder of the expected aldrin residues are being stored as dieldrin.

The result is that the water concentration of aldrin should be less than 4.6×10^{-2} ng/l in order to keep the individual lifetime risk below 10^{-5}.

Summary of Pertinent Data for Dieldrin — The water quality criterion for dieldrin is based on the hepatocellular carcinoma response of the female CF-1 mice given 0.1 ppm of dieldrin continuously in the diet in the experiment of Walker, et al (4-11). In that group the incidence of type a and type b liver tumors in the 0.1 ppm group of females was 24 out of 90 animals, whereas in the controls it was 39 out of 297 animals. Assuming a fish bioconcentration factor of 4,500, the parameters of the dose-response model are:

n_t = 24	Le = 132 weeks	w = 0.025 kg
N_t = 90	le = 132 weeks	R = 4,500
n_c = 39	d = 0.1 ppm x 0.13 = 0.013 mg/kg/day	F = 0.0187 kg/day
N_c = 297	L = 132 weeks	

With these parameters the slope of the one-hit dose-response curve for dieldrin is 183.6 $(mg/kg/day)^{-1}$.

The result is that the water concentration should be less than 4.4×10^{-2} ng/l in order to keep the individual lifetime risk below 10^{-5}.

References

(4-1) Gakstatter, J.H., "Rates of accumulation of 14C-dieldrin residues in tissues of goldfish exposed to a single sublethal dose of 14C-aldrin." *Jour. Fish. Res. Board Can.*, 25, 1797 (1968).

(4-2) Matsumura, F., and Boush, G.M., "Dieldrin: Degradation by soil microorganisms," *Science,* 156, 959 (1967).

(4-3) Patil, K.C., et al, "Metabolic transformation of DDT, dieldrin, aldrin, and endrin by marine microorganisms," *Environ. Sci. Technol.,* 6, 631 (1972).

(4-4) Edwards, C.A., "Insecticide residues in soils," *Residue Rev.,* 13, 83 (1966).

(4-5) Westlake, W.E., and San Antonio, J.P., "Insecticide residues in plants, animals and soils," Page 105 in *The nature and fate of chemicals applied to soils, plants, and animals,* U.S. Dept. of Ag., 20, 9 (1960).

(4-6) Nash, R.G. and Woolson, E.A., "Persistence of chlorinated hydrocarbon insecticides in soils," *Science,* 157, 924 (1967).

(4-7) Epstein, S.S., "Case study 5: aldrin and dieldrin suspension based on experimental evidence and evaluation and societal need," *Ann. N.Y. Acad. Sci.,* 271, 187 (1976).

(4-8) Harris, R.H., et al, "Carcinogenic hazards of organic chemicals in drinking water in Hiath, H.H., et al, Eds., *Origins of Human Cancer,* New York, Cold Spring Harbor Lab. (1977).

(4-9) International Agency for Research on Cancer, "IARC monographs on the evaluation of carcinogenic risk of chemicals to man: Some organochlorine pesticides, *Aldrin,* 5, 25 (1974) and *Dieldrin,* 5, 125 (1974).

(4-10) Mrak, E.M., *Report of the Secretary's Commission on Pesticides and Their Relationship to Environmental Health,* Wash., D.C., U.S. Dept. of Health, Education and Welfare (1969).

(4-11) Walker, A.Z.T., et al, "The toxicology of dieldrin; long term oral toxicity studies in mice," *Food Cosmetic Toxicol.,* 11, 415 (1972).

ANTHRACENE

See "Polynuclear Aromatic Hydrocarbons" (55).

ANTIMONY (#5)

Antimony, symbol Sb, a silver, brittle solids, belongs to Group V-A of the Periodic Table
and lies between arsenic and bismuth. It is classified as both a metal and a metalloid. It
has an atomic number of 51 and an atomic weight of 121.8, and its principal oxidation
states are +3 and +5.

Occurrence: Antimony is a naturally occurring element which comprises between 0.2 and
0.5 ppm of the earth's crust. Environmental concentrations of antimony of 35 parts per
thousand of salinity are reported at 0.3 μg/l in seawater and at 1.1 μg/l in freshwater streams.

In the environment antimony may enter aquatic systems from natural weathering of rocks
and run-off from soils, effluents from mining and manufacturing operations, as well as
municipal and industrial discharges. Antimony concentrations are generally in the low ppm
range for uncontaminated sediments, while sediments within 1 km of a copper smelter have
shown levels of several thousand ppm.

Physical Properties: Solubilities of antimony compounds range from insolubility to fully
soluble. Most inorganic compounds of antimony are either only slightly water-soluble or
decompose in aqueous media. Antimonials in which organic ligands are bound to the element and employed therapeutically, such as potassium antimony tartrate, are water-soluble.

The brittle character of antimony metal precludes rolling, forging or drawing but accounts
for improved hardness and lowered melting point in alloys with lead, bismuth, tin, copper,
nickel, iron and cobalt.

Chemical Properties: Antimony reacts with both sulfur and chlorine to form the tri- and
pentavalent sulfides and chlorides. Oxidation to antimony trioxide, the major commercial
oxide of antimony, is achieved under controlled conditions. Stibine, antimony trihydride,
is formed by the reduction of antimony compounds in acid media using zinc or other reducing metals.

Antimony shows some definite cationic behavior but only in the trivalent state. For example, antimony(III) forms complexes with inorganic and organic acids to produce antimonial salts such as the disulfate $[Sb(SO_4)_2]^-$, the dioxalate $[Sb(C_2O_4)]^=$ and the well known
tartrate $[Sb(OH)C_4H_3O_5]^-$.

Certain antimonial complexes undergo hydrolysis or oxidation reactions and consequently
are not long-lived in the environment. Both the oxide of antimony and the trihalides are
volatile compounds, while antimony trichloride releases hydrogen chloride gas in the presence of moisture (5-1). Antimony trioxide can undergo photoreduction in the presence
of ultraviolet light in aqueous solutions.

Several metals surrounding antimony in the periodic table undergo the methylation of inorganic compounds by microorganisms to yield organometallic compounds that are stable
and mobile in water and air. Parris and Brinckman (5-2) report that although no obvious
thermodynamic or kinetic barrier prevents this reaction, biological methylation of antimony
has not been demonstrated.

Uses: The metal is heavily employed in antimonial lead, in bearings and in ammunition.
The most important antimony compound in commerce is probably antimony trioxide, a
colorless, insoluble powder, the properties of which place it in high demand as a flame-

retarding agent for many commodities. It is insoluble in water and dilute nitric or sulfuric acids but is soluble in hydrochloric and certain organic acids. It dissolves in bases to give antimonate.

A second form of antimony having commercial usefulness is antimony trisulfide, Sb_2S_3. Like the trioxide it is employed as a flame retardant in many commercial commodities. Other uses are in the manufacture of fireworks and matches. Antimony trisulfide is insoluble in water but dissolves in concentrated hydrochloric acid with the evolution of hydrogen sulfide. It is also soluble in strong alkali solution.

Consumption of antimony in the United States is of the order of 40,000 metric tons per year, of which half is obtained from recycled scrap and the balance mainly imported from countries such as Bolivia. Use in the United States is directed chiefly to the manufacture of ammunition, storage batteries and fire-proofing of textiles.

Toxic Effects: A number of biological and adverse health effects in humans and experimental animals are known to be caused by antimony in its various chemical states. Most reported effects in man arise from either occupational exposure to antimony in the course of its mining, industrial processing, and commercial use or as side effects seen with the medicinal use of antimonials as therapeutic agents in inducing emesis or for the treatment of schistosomiasis, leishmaniasis, trypanosomiasis and ulcerative granuloma. Aside from several acute poisoning episodes occurring within the context of such use, however, the toxicological threat posed by antimony to the general public appears to be quite low. This is due in large part to the very limited amounts of the element that have thus far entered into environmental media that represent potential routes of exposure for humans.

Antimony compounds have been found to be toxic to freshwater organisms at concentrations of 19,000 to 22,000 $\mu g/l$. Chronic values for freshwater organisms vary widely depending on the antimony compound. There are no bioconcentration values for antimony in freshwater organisms. Though few data exist, saltwater values for acute toxicity to marine organisms generally occur around 5,000 $\mu g/l$. No chronic data or bioconcentration values are available.

In terms of human health, pulmonary, cardiovascular, dermal, and certain effects on reproduction, development, and longevity are among the effects associated with antimony exposure. Myocardial effects are among the most serious and best characterized.

Current Levels of Exposure: It is not possible to quantitatively estimate the impact of antimony use on various compartments of the environment which are exposure sources for man. A more meaningful approach is to consider levels of antimony in those media with which human populations come in contact. Of the two major antimony production sites in the U.S. only one uses processes that entail any loss to ambient air: the installation at Laredo, Texas. Improvements in emission control have considerably reduced but not eliminated the air levels in the vicinity of the smelter. The second production operation, employing alkali leachates of Ag-Cu ore and subsequent electrowinning, recycles much of its effluent-borne antimony with apparent minor loss to the environment. Other, more general sources of airborne antimony include fossil fuel combustion and municipal incineration

Antimony in Drinking Water — Schroeder (5-3) compiled data from surveys of municipal water supplies in 94 cities and reported that levels were on average less than 0.2 $\mu g/l$ (0.2 ppb) when measured in tap water. In a related study, Schroeder and Kraemer (5-4) note that tap water levels can be increased with soft water supplies owing to the leaching of antimony from plumbing. This would mainly be reflected in "first-draw" water. The source of antimony in plumbing material would be that present in copper tubing (0.005%) and galvanized iron (0.001%).

Antimony in Food — It is far from clear what the average daily dietary intake of antimony is in the U.S. population, for wide-ranging values have been reported over the years.

The comprehensive results of the U.S. Food and Drug Administration's survey of various trace metals including antimony in various food classes, using neutron activation analysis, have recently been reported by Tanner and Friedmann (5-5). The median level and range of antimony levels for the food classes, expressed as parts per million, wet weight, are: dairy products, <0.004, <0.002 to 0.02; meat, fish and poultry, 0.008, <0.004 to 0.015; grain and cereal products, <0.01, 0.006 to 0.05; leafy vegetables, <0.006, 0.001 to 0.027; legume vegetables, 0.008, <0.002 to 0.014; garden fruits, <0.006, 0.002 to 0.011.

Based on these recent figures, Tanner and Friedmann (5-5) calculate that the daily intake for antimony is too negligible to assign a meaningful value.

Special Groups at Risk: At this time, none of the available information permits conclusive identification of populations at special risk for antimony exposure except, of course, for occupationally exposed individuals. All other types of general environmental exposures, from all media and sources, appear to represent essentially negligible antimony exposure levels for humans, as discussed earlier.

If antimony exposure levels were to reach substantially higher levels in the air or water, however, then individuals with existing chronic respiratory or cardiovascular disease problems would likely be among those at special risk in light of probable exacerbation of one or both types of health problems by antimony.

Existing Guidelines and Standards: At the present time, no standards exist regarding allowable amounts of antimony in food or water. This reflects the fact that only very small trace amounts of antimony have ever been found in food or water samples from U.S. surveys; this also reflects the general lack of any past public health problems associated with antimony exposures via food or water intake. The only present standards that exist, then, are those established for the protection of workers in occupational settings.

Existing occupational standards for exposure to antimony are reviewed in the NIOSH criteria document, *Occupational Exposure to Antimony* (5-6). These standards apply most specifically to airborne antimony, but may be useful for purposes of deriving a recommended standard for water.

As stated in the NIOSH (1978) document (5-6), the American Conference of Governmental Industrial Hygienists (ACGIH), in 1977, listed the TLV for antimony as 0.5 mg/m^3 along with a notice of intended change to a proposed TLV of 2.0 mg/m^3 for soluble antimony salts. The proposed TLV was based mainly on the reports of Taylor (5-7) and Cordasco (5-8) on accidental poisoning by antimony trichloride and pentachloride, respectively.

The NIOSH document also presented a table of exposure limits from several countries, reproduced here as Table 8; the typical standard adopted was 0.5 mg/m^3, as indicated in Table 8. The 0.5 mg/m^3 level set by ACGIH in 1968 was also recommended as the U.S. occupational exposure standard by the NIOSH (1978) criteria document, based mainly on estimated no-effect levels for cardiotoxic and pulmonary effects.

A limit of 0.5 mg/m^3 has been set by ACGIH as the TWA for antimony trioxide handling and use. The limit for antimony trioxide production was 0.5 mg/m^3 as of 1979 with a notice that this operation involves industrial substances suspect of carcinogenic potential for man.

Table 8: Hygienic Standards of Several Countries for Antimony and Compounds in the Working Environment

Country	Standard (mg/m^3)	Qualifications
Finland	0.5	not stated
Federal Republic of Germany	0.5	8-hour TWA
Democratic Republic of Germany	0.5	not stated
Rumania	0.5	not stated

(continued)

Table 8: (continued)

Country	Standard (mg/m^3)	Qualifications
USSR	0.5	for antimony dust
USSR	0.3	for fluorides and chlorides (tri- and pentavalent); obligatory control of HF and HCl
USSR	1.0	for trivalent oxides and sulfides
USSR	1.0	for pentavalent oxides and sulfides
Sweden	0.5	not stated
U.S.	0.5	8-hour TWA
Yugoslavia	0.5	not stated

Source: Reference (5-9) as quoted in Reference (5)

Summary of Proposed EPA Criteria: *Freshwater Aquatic Life* — For an antimony the criterion to protect freshwater aquatic life as derived using the Guidelines is 120 µg/l as a 24-hour average and the concentration should not exceed 1,000 µg/l at any time.

Saltwater Aquatic Life — For saltwater aquatic life, no criterion for antimony can be derived using the Guidelines, and there are insufficient data to estimate a criterion using other procedures.

Human Health — For the protection of human health from the adverse effects of antimony ingested through the consumption of contaminated water and fish a criterion of 145 µg/l is suggested.

Basis for Proposed Human Health Criteria: At the present time, there are essentially no existing community epidemiology studies that provide information on health effects associated with antimony exposure among the general population of the United States or other countries.   This is primarily due, as indicated earlier, to the lack of any recognizable public health problems having been previously associated with environmental exposures to antimony.   Rather, one is limited to extrapolating, as best as can be done, from human occupational health and animal toxicology studies.

Pulmonary, cardiovascular, dermal, and certain effects on reproduction. development, and longevity are among the health effects best associated with antimony exposure.   The pulmonary effects, however, are almost exclusively associated with inhalation exposures and have much less relevance than the other effects in considering possible bases for development of criteria for a water standard.   The pulmonary effects are, therefore, not considered here, but rather the main emphasis is placed on the latter types of effects listed.

Cardiovascular changes have been well associated with exposure to antimony and probably represent the most serious antimony-related human health effects demonstrated thus far. Specifically, in humans, various ECG changes, e.g., altered T-wave patterns, have been consistently observed following exposures to either trivalent or pentavalent antimonial compounds and have been interpreted as being indicative of at least temporary cardiotoxic effects of antimony.   Indications of even more severe, possibly permanent myocardial damage in humans have been obtained in the form of histopathological evidence of cardiac edema, myocardial fibrosis, and other signs of myocardial structural damage.

Parallel findings of functional changes in ECG patterns and of histopathological evidence of myocardial structural damage have also been obtained in animal toxicology studies using controlled exposures to antimony compounds.

As for other types of effects reasonably well associated with antimony exposures, only very limited data exist regarding such effects, and they are presently insufficient to allow definitive conclusions to be drawn regarding important exposure parameters determining their induction in humans. For example, certain skin irritation effects, e.g., rashes, have been noted to occur with high levels of occupational antimony exposure, especially under conditions of extreme heat; similar dermal effects have been reported for at least some patients undergoing therapeutic treatments with systemic injections of antimonials. There does yet exist, however, any evidence to suggest that dermal effects would result from oral ingestion of antimony compounds.

In regard to effects on reproduction, development, and longevity, the available evidence linking such effects to antimony is almost entirely derived from animal toxicology studies and consists primarily of data suggesting that (1) prenatal exposures can interfere with conception, (2) chronic oral exposure via feeding can result in postnatal retardation of growth as indexed by body weight gain, and (3) chronic oral exposure via drinking water can induce alterations in certain blood chemistry parameters and significantly shorten survival time or lifespan. Such effects, however, have not yet been well replicated in other animal studies; and only very limited analogous antimony-induced effects on reproduction have yet been demonstrated to occur in humans.

In summary, myocardial effects are among the most serious and best characterized human health effects that can presently be linked with antimony exposure; as such, setting an ambient water criterion predicated on protecting the general public from antimony-induced myocardial effects is the most desirable course of action if sufficient information on dose-effect relationships for myocardial effects exists. Failing that, then, the very limited animal toxicology literature on reproduction, development, and longevity effects would offer an alternative basis.

Dose-Effect/Dose-Response Relationships — The previous section summarized the very limited information presently available regarding a qualitative description of adverse health effects associated with antimony exposure. Ideally, the main objective of the present section would be to provide further information regarding the characterization of dose-effect/dose-response relationships that hold for the induction of the key health effects expected to provide a basis for setting a criterion for antimony.

In regard to the definition of "dose-effect" and "dose-response" relationships, Pfitzer (5-10) explains the distinction between effect and response in the following terms: "Effect" is taken to indicate the variable change due to a dose in a specific subject; and "response" is the number of individuals in a group showing that effect, i.e., the number of "reactors" showing a specific effect at a particular defined dose level. Unfortunately, it is virtually impossible to characterize key antimony-induced health effects in such quantitative terms due to the very limited data base that presently exists.

For example, data reported for the studies by Brieger, et al (5-11) suggest an inhalation no-effect level for mycardial effects as likely being around 0.5 mg/m^3. Air concentrations of antimony trisulfide ranging from 0.58 to 5.5 mg/m^3 (with most 3.0 mg/m^3) were associated with the induction of altered ECG patterns and some deaths attributed to myocardial damage among certain antimony workers (5-11). Also in parallel studies on animals, Brieger, et al (5-11) observed ECG alterations in rats and rabbits at antimony exposures of 3.1 to 5.6 mg/m^3, confirming that antimony, per se can specifically produce myocardial effects of the type observed with the occupational exposures.

Unfortunately, for present purposes, however, no adequate data exist on oral exposures to antimony compounds which would support reasonable estimates regarding likely no-effect levels for the induction of mycardial effects via antimony ingestion. Nor is there sufficient information on relative absorption rates following oral or inhalation exposures to antimony to allow for extrapolation of likely dose-effect relationships for oral exposures from the limited inhalation exposure data. Consequently, it is presently impossible to recommend a water criterion level based on projected no-effect levels for myocardial damage.

In the absence of sufficient information to develop a criterion based on known antimony mycardial effects in humans, the most viable alternative is to focus on animal toxicology studies demonstrating antimony-induced effects on reproduction, development, and longevity. From the animal studies, those pertaining to prenatal reproductive effects, e.g., Belyaeva (5-12) and Casals (5-13), employed inhalation exposures or systemic injections of antimony compounds and their result cannot presently be extrapolated very well to project the likely impact of oral exposures. Similarly, the few human studies where effects on reproduction were reported (5-12)(5-14) deal with inhalation exposures in occupational settings and cannot now be used to extrapolate likely oral exposure no-effect levels.

Turning to effects on postnatal development and longevity, a study by Gross, et al (5-15) presents evidence for growth retardation occurring when rats were chronically fed diets containing 2% antimony trioxide, but a no-effect level for growth retardation cannot be deduced from the results reported.

The studies by Schroeder and coworkers (5-16)(5-17) containing data on antimony effects on growth and longevity, on the other hand, indicate that oral exposure to 5 ppm of antimony in drinking water had no effect on the rate of growth of either rats or mice. The 5 ppm exposure level, however, was effective in producing significant, although relatively slight reductions in lifespans for animals of both species and altered blood chemistries for exposed rats. It is, therefore, recommended that the 5 ppm exposure level producing such effects be taken as a "lowest observed effect level" (LOEL) in animals that likely approximates the "no-effect" level for antimony induced effects on growth and longevity.

If one calculates acceptable daily intake for man using the value of 5 mg/l of antimony and the uncertainty factor of 100 in view of no presently available human epidemiological data regarding such effect would result in a recommended criterion of 145 μg/l.

$$\text{Dose/day} = \frac{5 \ (\text{mg/l}) \ \times \ 25 \ \text{ml/day/rat}}{0.3 \ \text{kg/rat}} = 416.67 \ (\mu\text{g/kg/day})$$

$$\frac{416}{100} = 4.16 = 4.2 \ (\mu\text{g ADI})$$

$$4.2 \times 70 = 294 \ \mu\text{g (ADI for 70 kg/man)}$$

$$2(X) + (\text{Average fish intake})(F)(X) = \text{Daily intake}$$

$$2(X) + (0.0187)(1.4)(X) = 294$$
$$99\% \quad \ldots\ldots 1\% \ldots\ldots$$

$$2.0262(X) = 294$$

$$(X) = 145 \ \mu\text{g/l}$$

In the above equations,

$$100 = \text{uncertainty factor}$$

$$2 = \text{amount of water ingested, l/day}$$

$$X = \text{antimony concentration, mg/l}$$

$$0.0187 = \text{amount of fish/shellfish products consumed, kg/day}$$

$$F = \frac{1.4 \ \text{mg Sb/kg fish}}{\text{mg Sb/l of water}} = \text{Bioconcentration Factor (BCF)}$$

Drinking water contributes 99% of the assumed exposure while eating contaminated fish products accounts for 1%. The criterion level for antimony in ambient water can alternatively can be expressed as 11 mg/l, if exposure is assumed to be from the consumption of fish and shellfish alone.

$$X \times 0.0187 \times 1.4 = 294$$

$$X \times 0.0262 = 294$$

$$X = 11.308$$

$$X = 11 \ \text{mg/l}$$

References

(5-1)   U.S. EPA *Literature study of selected potential environmental contaminants. Antimony and its compounds,* Report No. EPA-550/2-76-002, Wash., D.C., Off. Tox. Subst. U.S. Environ. Prot. Agency (1976).

(5-2) Parris, G.E., and Brinckman, F.E., "Reactions which relate to environmental mobil-
       ity of arsenic and antimony. II: Oxidation of trimethylarsine and trimethyl-
       stibine," *Environ. Sci. Technol.,* 10, 1128 (1976).
(5-3) Schroeder, H.A., "Municipal drinking water and cardiovascular death rates," *Jour.
       Am. Med. Assoc.,* 195, 81-85 (1966).
(5-4) Schroeder, H.A. and Kraemer, L.A., "Cardiovascular mortality, municipal water and
       corrosion," *Arch. Envir. Health,* 28, 303-11 (1974).
(5-5) Tanner, J.T. and Friedman, M.H., "Neutron activation analysis for trace elements
       in foods," *J. Radioanal. Chem.,* 37, 529-38 (1977).
(5-6) National Institute for Occupational Safety and Health, *Criteria for a Recommended
       Standard: Occupational Exposure to Antimony,* Wash., D.C. (Sept. 28, 1978).
(5-7) Taylor, P.J., "Acute intoxication from antimony trichloride," *Brit. Jl. Ind. Med.,*
       23, 318-21 (1966).
(5-8) Cordasco, E.M., "Newer concepts in the management of environmental pulmonary
       edema," *Angiology,* 25, 590-601 (1974).
(5-9) International Labor Office, *Occupational Exposure Limits for Airborne Toxic Sub-
       stances—A Tabular Compilation of Values from Selected Countries,* Geneva (1977).
(5-10) Pfitzer, E.A., "General concepts for dose-response and dose-effect relationship of
       toxic metals," in Nordberg, G.F., Ed., *Effects and Dose-Response Relationships
       of Heavy Metals,* Amsterdam, Elsevier (1976).
(5-11) Brieger, H., et al, "Industrial antimony poisoning," *Ind. Med. Surg.,* 23, 521-3 (1954).
(5-12) Belyaeva, A.P., "The effect of antimony on reproduction," *Gig. Truda Prof. Zabol.,*
       11, 32-37 (1967).
(5-13) Casals, J.B., "Pharmacokinetic and toxicological studies of antimony dextran glyco-
       side," *Brit. J. Pharmac.,* 46, 281-88 (1972).
(5-14) Aiello, G., "Pathology of antimony," *Folia Med.,* (Naples) 38, 100-110 (1955)
       (in Italian).
(5-15) Gross, P., et al, "Toxicological study of calcium halophosphate phosphors and anti-
       mony trioxide," *Arch. Ind. Health,* 11, 473-86 (1955).
(5-16) Kanisawa, M. and Schroeder, H.A., "Life-term studies on the effect of trace ele-
       ments on spontaneous tumors in mice and rats," *Cancer Res.,* 29, 892-95 (1969).
(5-17) Schroeder, H.A., et al, "Zirconium, niobium, antimony and lead in rats: life-term
       studies," *J. Nutr.,* 100, 59-68 (1970).

ARSENIC (#6)

Arsenic, symbol As, a member of Group V-A of the Periodic Table, is classified as a metalloid. It has an atomic number of 33 and an atomic weight of 74.92.

Occurrence: Arsenic is a naturally occurring element. The principal emission source for
arsenic in the United States is thought to be coal-fuel power plants, which emit approximately 3,000 tons of arsenic per year.

Environmental concentrations of arsenic have been reported at 5 mg/kg in the earth's crust
(6-1). Arsenic is found also in air and in all living organisms. Analysis of 1,577 U.S. surface waters showed arsenic to be present in 87 samples, with concentrations ranging from
5 to 336 μg As/l and a mean level of 64 μg As/l. Concentrations of 3.0 μg/l have been
reported in sea water.

Physical Properties: Arsenic has five electrons in its outer shell, giving rise to the oxidation states of +5, +3, 0, and –3. Arsenic as a free element (0) is rarely encountered in
natural waters. Soluble inorganic arsenate (+5) predominates under normal conditions
since it is thermodynamically more stable in water than arsenite (+3). Elemental arsenic
is a gray, crystalline material with a molecular weight of 74.92, a specific gravity of 5.727, a
melting point (at 28 atm) of 817°C, and a boiling point (sublime) of 613°C. The low toxicity
of elemental arsenic is attributed to its virtual insolubility in water or in the body fluids
(6-2).

Chemical Properties: The largest class of arsenic compounds are the organics, which are not naturally occurring. The two most common organic arsenic compounds are the arsonic acids, $RAsO(OH)_2$, and the arsinic acids, $RR'AsO(OH)$, where R and R' refer to a variety of organic (alkyl) groups (6-2).

Arsenic forms a complete series of trihalides, while arsenic(V) fluoride is the only simple pentahalide known. All of the arsenic halides are covalent compounds that hydrolyze in the presence of water. Additional information on inorganic arsenic compounds is given in Table 9.

Table 9: Properties of Some Inorganic Arsenic Compounds

Compound	Formula	Water Solubility	Specific Properties
Arsenic trioxide	As_2O_3	12×10^6 μg/l at 0°C 21×10^6 μg/l at 25°C	dissolves in water to form arsenious acid*
Arsenic pentoxide	As_2O_5	$2{,}300 \times 10^6$ μg/l at 20°C	dissolves in water to form arsenic acid**
Arsenic hydride	AsH_3	20 ml/100 g cold water	this compound and its methyl derivatives are considered to be most toxic
Arsenic(III) sulfide	As_4S_6	520 μg/l at 18°C	burns in air forming arsenic trioxide and sulfur dioxide; occurs naturally as orpiment
Arsenic sulfide	As_4S_4	–	occurs naturally as realgar
Arsenic(V) sulfide	As_4S_{10}	$1{,}400$ μg/l at 0°C	–

$^*H_3AsO_3$, $K = 8 \times 10^{-10}$ at 25°C. $^{**}H_3AsO_4$, $K_1 = 2.5 \times 10^{-4}$, $K_2 = 5.6 \times 10^{-8}$, $K_3 = 3 \times 10^{-13}$

Source: Reference (6-1)(6-2)

Uses: Arsenic and its compounds are used in the manufacturing of glass, cloth, and electrical semiconductors, as fungicides and wood preservatives, as growth stimulants for plants and animals, as well as in veterinary applications (6-2). The United States consumes half of the world production of arsenic, or about 37,500 tons/yr, and produces about 18,000 tons/yr itself.

The organic arsenic compounds considered to be of importance are those containing methyl groups, the aromatic arsenic derivatives employed as feed additives and in veterinary medicine, and others which may have importance in biological systems (6-1).

Toxic Effects: Arsenic has been shown to be toxic to both vertebrate and invertebrate freshwater aquatic organisms. Cladocerans have been reported to be more sensitive than fish to arsenic. However, certain invertebrates such as stoneflies appear to be more tolerant of arsenic than are fish.

There is a paucity of arsenic toxicity data for saltwater organisms. However, several marine studies reported LC_{50} values generally lower than those reported for comparable freshwater studies.

Arsenic has been shown to bioconcentrate in both fresh and saltwater organisms. Although no animal experiments have demonstrated carcinogenicity of arsenic, several have shown that sodium arsenate induces developmental malformations in a variety of test animals including chick embryos, hamsters, rats and mice (6-3)(6-4)(6-5)(6-6)(6-7).

Data on exposure of humans points to a causal relationship between skin cancer and high level exposures to inorganic arsenic compounds (6-8). In addition, Browning (6-9) reported the symptoms of acute arsenic poisoning by ingestion to be abdominal pain and vomiting, while acute poisoning by inhalation produces giddiness, headache, extreme general weakness and, later, nausea, vomiting, colic, diarrhea, and pains in the limbs.

Current Levels of Exposure: A broad range of arsenic levels has been found in drinking water samples.   In a U.S. Environmental Protection Agency national study of residential tap water, 66.8% of the one-time grab samples collected from 3,834 residences had arsenic levels greater than 0.1 μg/l.   The average, minimum, and maximum levels of the samples with detectable arsenic were 2.37, 0.50, and 213.6 μg/l, respectively.

In 1975 it was reported that 5 out of 566 samples collected from Interstate Carrier Water Supplies exceeded 10 μg/l and that the maximum level was 60 μg/l.   Well water samples collected during 1976 at 59 residences in a Fairbanks, Alaska suburban community had a mean arsenic content of 224 μg/l with a range from 1.0 to 2,450 μg/l.   Moderately elevated levels of arsenic, 10 to 330 μg/l, are present in potable waters of some smaller communities in Utah, Nevada, and California.   There have been a number of other reports of isolated instances of higher than usual concentration of arsenic in well waters.   The highest value reported in these studies was 21,000 μg/l in well water contaminated by arsenical grasshopper bait.

There is a wide diversity in the estimates of daily intake of arsenic in foods.   It has been estimated that the average diet provides an arsenic intake of about 1,000 μg/day.   Arsenic in a sample institutional diet amounted to about 400 μg/day.   This lower level is attributed, at least partially, to the absence of seafood, a primary source of arsenic, in the institutional diet.   In contrast to these levels, the World Health Organization reported that average arsenic intakes for Canada, the United Kingdom, the United States, and France varied from 25 to 33 μg/day; specific values ranged from 7 to 60 μg/day.   A survey of food made in Great Britain indicated that 100 μg of arsenic would be consumed daily from all sources.

The levels of atmospheric arsenic in locations where major arsenic emitting sources are absent range from below the detection limit of 1 to 83 ng/m^3 with an average of 3 ng/m^3. The annual average near major emission sources (copper, lead, and zinc smelters, cotton gins, pesticide manufacturers, and glass manufacturers) ranged from 3 to 5,900 ng/m^3 with most below 290 ng/m^3.   Assuming normal daily inhaled volumes of 21.2 and 11.1 m^3 for men and women respectively, the ranges of daily airborne arsenic exposures in uncontaminated areas are 21 to 1,760 ng and 11 to 921 ng for men and women, respectively. In areas where arsenic emitting sources are located, daily inhaled exposure levels may be as high as 6,148 to 125,080 ng and 3,219 to 65,490 ng for men and women, respectively.

No quantifiable information was found concerning present levels of exposure from drugs or dermal contact.

Special Groups at Risk: Adverse effects have been demonstrated in all age groups of both sexes.

Existing Guidelines and Standards: In 1942, the U.S. Public Health Service set a maximum allowable level of 50 μg/l for arsenic in drinking water supplied by interstate carrier water supplies.   The arsenic standard remained at that level in the 1962 revision of the Drinking Water Standards and has been continued in the U.S. Environmental Protection Agency Drinking Water Standards which became effective in June of 1977.

The American Conference of Governmental and Industrial Hygienists (1977) has set 0.5 mg/m^3 as the Threshold Limit Value-Time Weighted Average (TLV-TWA) for airborne arsenic.   This means that the time weighted average concentration of airborne arsenic for a normal 8-hour workday or 40-hour workweek should not exceed 0.5 mg/m^3.   The Conference has issued a Notice of Intended Change (as of 1979) which will reduce the TLV-TWA from 0.5 to 0.05 mg/m^3.   The ACGIH has also set limits of 0.05 ppm or 0.2 mg/m^3 for arsine and has categorized arsenic trioxide production as a human carcinogen with a notice of intended change to "suspected carcinogen."

The National Institute of Occupational Safety and Health has recommended (6-10) a ceiling level of 2 μg/m^3 for airborne inorganic arsenic for any 15-minute period of the workday.   A new OSHA standard (6-11) for airborne inorganic arsenic is 10 μg/m^3 TWA.

Summary of Proposed EPA Criteria: *Freshwater Aquatic Life* — For arsenic, the criterion to protect freshwater aquatic life, as derived using the Guidelines, is 57 µg/l as a 24-hour average and the concentration should never exceed 130 µg/l at any time.

Saltwater Aquatic Life — For arsenic, the criterion to protect saltwater aquatic life, as derived using procedures other than the Guidelines, is 29 µg/l as a 24-hour average and the concentration should never exceed 67 µg/l at any time.

Human Health — For the maximum protection of human health from the potential carcinogenic effects of exposure to arsenic through ingestion of water and contaminated aquatic organisms, the ambient water concentration is zero. Concentrations of arsenic estimated to result in additional lifetime cancer risks ranging from no additional risk to an additional risk of 1 to 100,000 are presented in the Criterion Formulation section of this document. The EPA is considering setting criteria at an interim target risk level in the range of 10^{-5}, 10^{-6}, or 10^{-7} with corresponding criteria of 0.02, 0.002, and 0.0002 µg/l, respectively.

Basis for Proposed Human Health Criteria: A number of studies have shown that arsenic is important in the etiology of human cancers. Clinical, occupational, and population studies have demonstrated that both ingestion and inhalation exposures to arsenic compounds increase the risk of cancer induction in the tissues of the lung and skin and possibly other sites. There appears to be little question that arsenic is a human carcinogen, but there has been general failure to demonstrate this effect in any animal model. Hence, it is necessary to rely totally on human data rather than supplement it with appropriate animal toxicity and carcinogenic data.

This limitation causes serious problems since animal studies are the only practical means to effectively evaluate relative toxicities, absorption rates, etc., for different compounds and routes of administration. Instead, these types of questions must be answered based on effects and observations of exposed populations recognizing the numerous unknowns (levels of arsenic and other environmental exposures, dietary patterns, genetic differences, etc.) and different routes of exposure.

A study that relates levels of arsenic ingestion to skin cancer was conducted in southwest Taiwan. A consistent dose response relationship between the exposure variables level of arsenic in drinking water and age and skin cancer prevalence was found. Questions concerning compatibility between the U.S. and Chinese populations must be raised since some areas in the U.S. have similar arsenic levels without the reported dermatological manifestations. It is very possible that major differences in dietary patterns (the Chinese diet is low in protein and fat) other environmental and/or occupational coexposures, socioeconomic status, etc., may account for the differences. However, since similar health responses have been observed in Antofagasta, Chile; Cordoba, Argentina; German vineyard workers, and those who ingest Fowler's Solution, it must be assumed that arsenic is at least one of the environmental exposures responsible for the observed effects.

Secondly, the clear dose-response relationships both by length of exposure, as indicated by age, and by level of waterborne arsenic provide additional evidence that arsenic is at least one of the agents responsible for the observed effects; it seems quite unlikely that other environmental, occupational, or socioeconomic factors which might be responsible for variations in skin tumor incidence would have a similar gradient to the waterborne arsenic gradient. Hence, it appears reasonable to use the Taiwan data as a basis for estimating a level which will not increase the lifetime risk of cancer by more than 1/100,000; it is recognized the calculated level may be quite conservative since the Taiwan experience may represent a worst case situation due to other coexposures and dietary deficiencies.

The EPA Cancer Assessment Group has developed a mathematical prediction model for estimating an acceptable level based on the published Taiwan data by Tseng (6-12).

Under the Consent Decree in NRDC vs Train, criteria are to state "recommended maximum permissible concentrations (including where appropriate, zero) consistent with the protection of aquatic organisms, human health, and recreational activities." Arsenic is suspected of being a human carcinogen. Because there is no recognized safe concentration for a human carcinogen, the recommended concentration of arsenic in water for maximum protection of human health is zero.

Because attaining a zero concentration level may be infeasible in some cases and in order to assist the EPA and states in the possible future development of water quality regulations, the concentrations of arsenic corresponding to several incremental lifetime cancer risk levels have been estimated. A cancer risk level provides an estimate of the additional incidence of cancer that may be expected in an exposed population. A risk of 10^{-5}, for example, indicates a probability of one additional case of cancer for every 100,000 people exposed, a risk of 10^{-6} indicates one additional case for every million people exposed, and so forth.

In the *Federal Register* notice of availability of draft ambient water quality criteria, EPA stated that it is considering setting criteria at an interim target risk level of 10^{-5}, 10^{-6}, or 10^{-7}, as shown in Table 10.

In Table 10 the risk levels and corresponding criteria are calculated by applying a modified "one-hit" extrapolation model to the human epidemiological data. Since the extrapolation model is linear at low doses, the additional lifetime risk is directly proportional to the water concentration. Therefore, water concentrations corresponding to other risk levels can be derived by multiplying or dividing one of the risk levels and corresponding water concentrations shown in the table by factors such as 10, 100, 1,000, and so forth.

Table 10: Possible Alternative Criteria for Arsenic

Exposure Assumptions per Day	. . . . Risk Levels, μg/l			
	0	10^{-7}	10^{-6}	10^{-5}
2 liters of drinking water and consumption of 18.7 g fish and shellfish*	0	0.0002	0.002	0.02
Consumption of fish and shellfish only	0	0.01	0.10	1.0

*Approximately 2% of the arsenic exposure results from the consumption of aquatic organisms which exhibit an average bioconcentration potential of 2.3-fold. The remaining 98% of arsenic exposure results from drinking water.

Source: Reference (6)

Due to the stable population in a rural area along the southwest coast of Taiwan, the data collected by Tseng, et al, in 1968 (6-12) may be viewed as a lifetime feeding study where measured amounts of arsenic in well water are consumed by a study population of 40,421 individuals. Thus, this data may be used to predict the lifetime probability of skin cancer caused by the ingestion of arsenic.

A model estimating the cancer rate as a function of drinking water arsenic concentration was generated using the information in its published form, which is a summary of data collected by the investigators. If the original data had been available, a more exact mathematical analysis would be possible.

It has been suggested that the relationship between the incidence of some site specific cancers, age, and exposure level of a population may be expressed as

$$(1) \qquad\qquad I(x,t) \;=\; vBx^m t^{v-1}$$

where x is the exposure level of a carcinogen, t is the age of the population, and B, m, v are unknown parameters.

However, the data collected by Tseng, et al, in 1968 (6-12) were obtained at one point in time, and since skin cancer has only a marginal effect on the death rate, the obtained rates may be viewed more accurately as the probability of having contracted skin cancer by time t. The relationship between this probability, often referred to as the cumulative probability density or prevalence, and the incidence or age specific or hazard rate may be expressed as

$$(2) \qquad F(x,t) \; = \; 1 - \exp[\textstyle\int I^t(x,s)ds]$$

The prevalence may alternatively be expressed as

$$(3) \qquad F(x,t) \; = \; 1 - \exp(-Bx^m t^v)$$

which is a Weibull distribution.

Based on information reported by Tseng, et al, in 1968 (6-12), the EPA has made estimates of F(x,t) for different age and exposure groupings for males.

To use this data, specific values for x and t had to be obtained for the intervals. Where the intervals were closed, the midpoint was utilized. For the greater than 0.6 mg/l group, the midpoint between 0.6 and the greatest recorded value 1.8 was taken resulting in 1.2 μg/l. For age 60 or greater, a value of 70 was utilized somewhat arbitrarily, being the same increase over the lower level as that in the other two age intervals.

From equation (5) it follows that

$$(4) \qquad \ln[-\ln[1 - F(x,t)]] \; - \; \ln(3) \; \div \; m\ln(x) \; \div \; v\ln(t)$$

which is multiple linear in form. Estimating the parameters by the usual least square techniques, we obtained the relationship

$$(5) \qquad \ln[-\ln[1 - F(x,t)]] \; = \; -17.548 \; \div \; 1.192\ln(x) \; \div \; 3.881\ln(t)$$

which is an excellent fit having a multiple correlation coefficient of 0.986.

Equation (5) may be expressed as

$$(6) \qquad F(x,t) \; = \; 1 - \exp[-10^{-7}(0.2429x^{1.192}t^{3.881})] \; = \; 1 - \exp[-E(t)x^{1.192}]$$

If the coefficient m = 1.192 was in fact equal to 1, then for a given value of t equation (6) would be "one-hit" in form.

To test this hypothesis, (i.e., Eo: m = 1) the student "t" test is used, giving the result

$$t_6 \; = \; \frac{1.192 - 1}{0.138} \; = \; 1.391$$

which is not significant at the 0.1 level. The value 0.138 is the standard error of m. Thus there is insufficient evidence to reject the hypothesis that the dose-response relationship is "one-hit" even at the 0.1 level even though the standard error of the regression coefficient is quite small.

Fixing m = 1 we have the relationship

$$(7) \qquad F(x,t) \; = \; 1 - \exp[g(t)x]$$

Transforming this equation to its linear form and obtaining the least square estimates of B and v, we find that

$$g(t) \; = \; \exp(-17.5393)t^{3.853}$$

where B = 2.41423 x 10^{-8} and v = 3.853.

In this case, the fit is still quite good as represented by a correlation of 0.971.

The function

$$F(x,t) = 1 - \exp[-2.41423 \times 10^{-8}(t^{3.853})]$$

is the probability of contracting skin cancer by age t given that an divividual had a lifetime exposure to x mg/l in his drinking water (and lived until age t).

In 1978 the U.S. Environmental Protection Agency calculated (6-13) the lifetime probability of cancer in the presence of competing mortality on the basis of the age-specific incidence rate. For the case where the cancer rate in the absence of exposure is near zero (as in this case where the skin cancer is of a rare form that was virtually unknown in other parts of Taiwan) the lifetime probability may be expressed as

$$Q_2(\ ) = Bx/(Bx \div p^v)$$

where $p^v = \ln 2 t_m^v$, (where t_m is the median lifetime of the population).

Assuming $t_m = 68$ and $v = 3.853$, is the same for total mortality as the appearance of skin cancer we have that

$$Q_2(\ ) = \frac{2.41423x}{2.41423x \div 6.02793}$$

The level of x that results in a lifetime probability of skin cancer equal to 10^{-5} is found by solving $Q_2(\ ) = 10^{-5}$ for x giving $x = 2.4969 \times 10^{-5}$ μg/l or 0.025 μg/l.

Under the assumption that the average consumption of water is two liters in both the U.S. and Taiwan we estimate a water criteria concentration of:

$$2(0.025) = S[2 + (0.0187 \times 2.3)] \text{ or } S = \frac{0.25}{2.0430} = 0.02447$$

Where 0.0187 is the average fish consumption in kilograms and 2.3 is the bioaccumulation factor for fish (supplied by Don Mount of U.S. EPA).

A criterion for waterborne arsenic of 0.02 μg/l would thus insure a lifetime risk of cancer of less than 10^{-5}.

It is recognized that inorganic and organic compounds differ in terms of toxicity and likely in terms of carcinogenic potential. However, since the recommended level is to be based on carcinogenic potential and no information is available concerning the relationship(s) of specific arsenic species and cancer, a single all inclusive limit must be set. Even if the data were available to permit separate standards, the level of development of the required analytical methodology is not sufficient to permit reliable and repeatable speciation measurements, a necessity before setting a standard.

For comparative purposes, the Stockinger and Woodward method was applied to the present and proposed airborne arsenic standards to compute comparable waterborne arsenic levels.

American Conference of Governmental Industrial Hygienists:

(1)   Existing Threshold Limit Value—Time Weighted Average—500 μg/m^3

$$\frac{500 \ \mu g}{m^3} \times 10m^3 \times \frac{5 \ days}{week} \times 20\% \ absorption = 5,000 \ \mu g/l$$

$$\frac{5,000 \ \mu g}{week} \times \frac{1 \ week}{7 \ days} \times \frac{1}{2 \ liters} \times \frac{Allowed}{80\% \ absorption} = 446 \ \mu g/l$$

Applying the recommended safety factor of 1/100 the comparable drinking water limit is 4.46 μg/l.

(2) Proposed Threshold Limit Value—Time Weighted Average—50 $\mu g/m^3$

$$\frac{50\ \mu g}{m^3} \times 10\ m^3 \times \frac{5\ days}{week} \times 20\%\ absorption = 500\ \mu g/wk$$

$$\frac{500\ \mu g}{week} \times \frac{1\ week}{7\ days} \times \frac{1}{2\ liters} \times \frac{Allowed}{80\%\ absorption} = 44.6\ \mu g/l$$

Applying the recommended safety factor of 1/100 the comparable drinking water limit is 0.45 $\mu g/l$.

(3) Occupational Safety and Health Administration—Eight-Hour Average—10 $\mu g/m^3$

$$\frac{10\ \mu g}{m^3} \times 10\ m^3 \times \frac{5\ days}{week} \times 20\%\ absorption = 100\ \mu g/wk$$

$$\frac{100\ \mu g}{week} \times \frac{1\ week}{7\ days} \times \frac{1}{2\ liters} \times \frac{Allowed}{80\%\ absorption} = 8.93\ \mu g/l$$

Applying the recommended safety factor of 1/100, the comparable drinking water limit is 0.08 $\mu g/l$.

Assuming that the absorption factors (20% air, 80% water) and methods recommended by Stockinger and Woodward are reasonable and that the safety of 1/100 is appropriate, it is clear that the recommended water standard is even more restrictive than the air standards. The differences are likely due at least partially to variations in extrapolation methods and levels of acceptable risk.

It is of interest to see that cancer risk would be associated with an air exposure equivalent to the recommended criterion of 0.02 $\mu g/l$. If the following assumptions are made:

(1) Total daily average absorbed arsenic from water is

$$0.8 \times 0.02[2 + (0.0267 \times 15)] = 0.0384\ \mu g$$

where 80% is the absorption rate.

(2) The breathing rate is 1 m^3/hr and 20% of the arsenic is absorbed.

Concentration levels were derived assuming a lifetime exposure to various amounts of arsenic, (1) occurring from the consumption of both drinking water and aquatic life growth in waters containing the corresponding arsenic concentrations and, (2) occurring solely from consumption of aquatic life grown in the waters containing the corresponding arsenic concentrations.

Although total exposure information for arsenic is discussed and an estimate of the contributions from other sources of exposure can be made, this data will not be factored into ambient water quality criteria formulation until additional analysis can be made. The criteria presented, therefore, assumed an incremental risk from ambient water exposure only.

Then, the air concentration, X, required to obtain the same absorbed amount of arsenic is

$$0.2 \times 24 \times X = 0.0384\ mg \quad or \quad X = 0.008\ \mu g/m^3$$

From the 1978 U.S. Environmental Protection Agency document on the risk associated with airborne arsenic, the lifetime cancer risk associated with X $\mu g/m^3$ of arsenic in the air is estimated to be

$$P = 3.418 \times 10^{-3}\ X$$

If instead of basing the risk on the most sensitive study the geometric mean of the three studies is used. The lifetime cancer risk would be

$$P = 1.95 \times 10^{-3}\ X$$

The risks associated with X = 0.008 are thus 2.73×10^{-5} and 1.56×10^{-5}. Thus if the water criterion was based on the geometric mean of the human epidemiological air studies it would be 0.013 μg/l instead of 0.02 μg/l, which is a remarkably consistent result.

References

(6-1)   U.S. EPA, *Arsenic,* Report by Subcommittee on Arsenic, Com. on Med. and Biol. Effects of Environ. Pollut. NRC/NAS, Report No. EPA 600/1-76-036, Wash., D.C., U.S. Environ. Prot. Agency (1976).

(6-2)   U.S. EPA, *Arsenic and its compounds,* Report No. EPA 560/6-76-016, Wash., D.C., U.S. Environ. Prot. Agency (1976).

(6-3)   Ancel, P., "Recherche Experimentale Sur Le Spina Bifida," *Arch. Anat. Mier. Morph. Exp.,* 36, 45 (1946).

(6-4)   Ridgeway, L.P., Karnovsky, D.A., "The effects of metals on the chick embryo: Toxicity and production of abnormalities in development," *Ann. N.Y. Acad. Sci.,* 5, 203 (1952).

(6-5)   Ferm, V.H., and Carpenter, S.J., "Malformation induced by sodium arsenate," *Jour. Reprod. Fertil,* 17, 199 (1968).

(6-6)   Hood, R.D., and Bishop, S.L., "Teratogenic effects of sodium arsenate in mice," *Arch. Environ. Health,* 24, 62 (1972).

(6-7)   Beaudoin, A.R., "Teratogenicity of sodium arsenate in rats," *Teratology,* 10, 153 (1974).

(6-8)   Tseng, W.P., et al, "Prevalence of skin cancer in an endemic area of chronic arsenicism in Taiwan," *Jour. Natl. Cancer Inst.,* 40, 453 (1968).

(6-9)   Browning, E., *Toxicity of industrial metals,* London, Buttersworth (1961).

(6-10) National Institute for Occupational Safety and Health, *Criteria for a Recommended Standard: Occupational Exposure to Inorganic Arsenic (Revised),* NIOSH Doc. No. 75-149, Wash., D.C. (1975).

(6-11) Occupational Safety and Health Administration, *Federal Register,* 43, No. 88, 19584-19631 (May 5, 1978).

(6-12) Tseng, W., "Effects and dose-response relationships of skin cancer and blackfoot disease with arsenic," *Environmental Health Perspective,* 19, 109 (1977).

(6-13) U.S. Environmental Protection Agency, *In-Depth Studies on Health and Environmental Impacts of Selected Water Pollutants,* Report on Contract 68-01-4646, Wash., D.C. (1978).

ASBESTOS (#7)

Asbestos is a broad term applied to numerous fibrous mineral silicates composed of silicon, oxygen, hydrogen, and metal cations such as sodium, magnesium, calcium, or iron. There are two major groups of asbestos, serpentine (chrysotile) and amphibole. Chrysotile is the major type of asbestos used in the manufacture of asbestos products.

Occurrence: Of the 243,527 metric tons of asbestos discharged to the environment in a recent year, 98.3% was discharged to land, 1.5% to air, and 0.2% to water. Solid waste disposal by consumers was the single largest contribution to total discharges. Although no process water is used in dry mining of asbestos ore, there is the potential for run-off from asbestos waste tailings, wet mining, and iron ore mining. Mining operations can also contribute substantially to asbestos concentrations in water via air and solid waste contamination. In addition to mining and industrial discharges of asbestos, asbestos fibers, which are believed to be the result of rock outcroppings, are found in rivers and streams.

Physical Properties: The chemical composition of different asbestos fibers varies widely and typical formulas are presented in Table 11. It should be noted that the values obtained from actual chemical analysis of the various fibers also may differ slightly from the typical formulas. Although chrysotile is considered to be a distinct mineral, the five amphibole minerals are each varieties of other minerals. These minerals differ from each other both chemically and physically with the exception that they all contain silicon and all form fibers when crushed. Good quality asbestos will form fibers with higher ratios of length to width than poorer grades.

The basic crystal form of the amphibole minerals is less complicated than for chrysotile. The basic structure consists of a double silica chain (Si_4O_{11}) that is paired back-to-back with a layer of hydrated cations between the chains (7-1).

Some typical physical properties of three different mineral forms are presented in Table 12.

Table 11: Typical Formulas for Asbestos Fibers

Serpentines	chrysotile	$Mg_3Si_2O_5(OH)_4$
Amphiboles	amosite	$(Mg,Fe)_7Si_8O_{22}(OH)_2$
	crocidolite	$Na_2(Mg,Fe)_5Si_8O_{22}(OH)_2$
	anthophyllite	$(Mg,Fe)_7Si_8O_{22}(OH)_2$
	tremolite	$Ca_2Mg_5Si_8O_{22}(OH)_2$
	actinolite	$Ca_2(Mg,Fe)_5Si_8O_{22}(OH)_2$

Source: Reference (7)

Table 12: Typical Physical Properties of Chrysotile (White Asbestos), Crocidolite (Blue Asbestos), and Amosite

Properties	Units	Chrysotile	Crocidolite	Amosite
Approximate diameter of smallest fibers	micron	0.01	0.08	0.1
Specific gravity	—	2.55	3.37	3.45
Average tensile strength	lb/in^2	3.5×10^5	5×10^5	1.75×10^5
Modulus of elasticity	lb/in^2	23.5×10^6	27.0×10^6	23.5×10^6

Source: Reference (7)

Chemical Properties: Asbestos minerals, despite a relatively high fusion temperature, are completely decomposed at temperatures of 1000°C. Both the dehydroxylation temperature and decomposition temperature increase with increased MgO content among the various amphibole species (7-1).

The solubility product constants for various chrysotile fibers range from 1.0×10^{-11} to 3×10^{-12}. Most materials have a negative surface charge in aqueous systems. However, since chrysotile has a positive (+) charge, it will attract, or be attracted to, most dispersed materials. The highly reactive surface of asbestos causes many surface reactions which are intermediate between simple absorption and a true chemical reaction. The absorption of various materials on the surface of chrysotile supports the promise that the polar surface of chrysotile has a greater affinity for polar molecules (e.g., H_2O, NH_3) than for nonpolar molecules (7-1).

Of all the asbestos minerals, chrysotile is the most susceptible to acid attack. It is almost completely destroyed within one hour in 1 N HCl at 95°C. Amphibole fibers are much more resistant to mineral acids.

The resistance of the asbestos fibers to attack by reagents other than acid is excellent up to temperatures of approximtely 100°C with rapid deterioration observed at higher temperatures. Chrysotile is completely decomposed in concentrated KOH at 200°C. In general, organic acids have a tendency to react slowly with chrysotile (7-1).

Uses: These products include asbestos cement pipe, flooring products, paper products (e.g., padding), friction materials (e.g., brake linings and clutch facings), roofing products, and coating and patching compounds. In 1975, the total consumption of asbestos in the U.S. was 550,900 thousand metric tons.

Toxic Effects: All forms of asbestos available commercially have been shown to be carcinogenic in mice, rats, rabbits, and hamsters. Occupational health studies on workers engaged in the mining, milling and manufacturing of asbestos have linked exposure of this mineral to lung carcinomas, mesotheliomas, gastrointestinal cancers, and pulmonary asbestosis.

Estimating a risk factor for ingestion of asbestos presents significant difficulties. Although gastrointestinal cancer has been linked to occupational exposures in several groups of workers, no definitive data exist on the effects of direct ingestion of asbestos, either in animals or humans. Further, only limited information exists on air exposure levels for those human studies showing excess risk of gastrointestinal cancer and peritoneal mesothelioma. Nevertheless, the most valuable data on risk are those from human inhalation exposures, and these will form the primary basis for a projected criterion.

Current Levels of Exposure: Asbestos is a ubiquitous contaminant of our air and water. Air concentrations over 24 hours in metropolitan areas usually are less than 5 ng/m^3 but range up to 20 ng/m^3. Values up to 50 ng/m^3 are found during daytime hours in locations where construction activities and traffic can be contributing sources. A significant fraction of the fibers inhaled can be brought up from the respiratory tract and swallowed. This leads to an ingestion exposure from air sources of up to 0.1 μg/day, although most of the population exposure is from 0.02 to 0.05 μg/day.

Water concentrations of asbestos are usually less than 10^6 fibers of all sizes per liter although significantly higher values (10^8 fibers per liter) have been found in circumstances where water systems have been in contact with asbestiform minerals or where contamination of the water supply exists. Fiber mass concentrations corresponding to fiber concentrations are usually less than 0.01 μg/l but could exceed 1 μg/l. Thus, direct water ingestion usually leads to exposures of less than 0.02 μg/day.

Clearly, point source pollution can cause both air and water concentrations to exceed the above values.

Special Groups at Risk: Special groups at risk may include neonates and children; however, no data exist on the relative sensitivity to asbestos of infants and children undergoing rapid growth. Concern exists because fibers deposited in the tissues of the young may have an extremely long residence time during which malignant changes could occur. In addition, risk could be influenced by differential absorption rates which have not been fully studied at this time.

Individuals on kidney dialysis machines may also be at greater risk as fluids, potentially contaminated with asbestos fibers, can enter the blood stream directly or, in selected instances, the peritoneal cavity (peritoneal dialysis).

Although no synergistic effects have been identified in the etiology of asbestos-related gastrointestinal cancer, they cannot be ruled out. Thus, people exposed to other carcinogens, initiators, or promotors could be at increased risk.

An increased risk is also associated with increased exposure to asbestos in water in municipalities such as San Francisco or Seattle where asbestos occurs naturally in water, in cities where there is an interaction between aggressive water and asbestos-cement pipe, or in cities whose water may be contaminated as a result of asbestos operations. Also, the use of asbestos cement products for the collection of water, such as in cisterns in the Virgin Islands or in roof run-offs in tropical areas, increases exposure.

Existing Guidelines and Standards: The current Occupational Safety and Health Administration (OSHA) standard for an eight-hour time-weighted average (TWA) occupational exposure to asbestos is 2 fibers longer than 5 μ in length per milliliter of air (2 fibers/ml or 2,000,000 fibers/m^3). Peak exposures of up to 10 fibers/ml are permitted for no more than ten minutes. This standard has been in effect since July 1, 1976, when it replaced an earlier one of 5 fibers/ml (TWA). In Great Britain, too, a value of 2 fibers/ml is the accepted level, below which no controls are required (7-4); the British standard, in fact, served as a guide for the OSHA standard (7-2).

The British standard was developed specifically to prevent asbestosis among working populations; data were felt to be lacking that would allow a determination of a standard for cancer (7-4).   Unfortunately, among occupational groups, cancer is the primary cause of excess death among workers. Three-fourths or more of asbestos-related deaths are from malignancy. This fact has led OSHA to propose a lower TWA standard of 0.5 fibers/ml (500,000 fibers/m^3). The National Institute for Occupational Safety and Health (NIOSH), in their criteria document for the hearings on a new standard, have proposed a value of 0.1 fiber/ml (7-3). In the discussion of the NIOSH proposal, it was stated that the value was selected on the basis of the sensitivity of analytical techniques using optical microscopy and that 0.1 fiber/ml may not necessarily protect against cancer.

Recognition that no information exists that would define a threshold for asbestos carcinogenesis was also contained in the preamble to the OSHA proposal. The existing standard in Great Britain has also been called into question by Peto (7-5), who estimates that asbestos disease may cause the death of 10% of workers exposed at 2 fibers/ml for a working lifetime.

The existing federal standard for asbestos emissions into the environment prohibits "visible emissions." No numerical value was specified because of difficulty in monitoring ambient air asbestos concentrations in the ambient air or in stack emissions. (Time-consuming and expensive electron microscopy is often required.) Some local government agencies, however, may have numerical standards (New York, 27 ng/m^3, for example).

No standards for asbestos in foods or beverages exist even though the use of filtration of such products through asbestos filters has been a common practice in past years. Asbestos filtration, however, is prohibited or limited for human drugs.

Summary of Proposed EPA Criteria: *Freshwater Aquatic Life* — For freshwater aquatic life, no criterion for asbestos can be derived using the Guidelines, and there are insufficient data to estimate a criterion using other procedures.

Saltwater Aquatic Life — For saltwater aquatic life, no criterion for asbestos can be derived using the Guidelines, and there are insufficient data to estimate a criterion using other procedures.

Human Health — For the maximum protection of human health from the potential carcinogenic effects of exposure to asbestos through ingestion of water and contaminated aquatic organisms, the ambient water concentration is zero. Concentrations of asbestos estimated to result in additional lifetime cancer risk of 1 in 100,000 are presented in the Criterion document. The EPA is considering setting criteria at an interim target risk level in the range of 10^{-5}, 10^{-6}, 10^{-7} with corresponding criteria of 300,000, 30,000, and 3,000 fibers/l, respectively.

Basis for the Proposed Human Health Criteria: A substantial body of data exists which shows increased incidence of cancer of the esophagus, stomach, colon, and rectum or peritoneal mesothelioma in humans exposed to asbestos occupationally. For several of these groups, data exist on the approximate airborne fiber concentrations to which individuals were exposed. These human data will serve as the primary basis for a standard of asbestos in water. Experimental data indicate that a major fraction of the asbestos deposited in the lungs is subsequently swallowed. In this section the dose to the gastrointestinal tract of four occupational groups will be calculated from knowledge of the air concentrations to which the workers were exposed and follow the assumption that all the asbestos inhaled subsequently passed through the gastrointestinal tract and provided the exposure that led to the observed increase in abdominal cancer. The assumption that all inhaled asbestos is ingested is an overestimate but not significantly. No account has been taken of the material that a worker may swallow directly and this quantity could be significant. However, for the purposes of a criterion, the inability to quantitate direct ingestion in the work place and to properly account for it by the present approach provides some margin of safety in the estimate of dose-response relations.

Table 13 lists the percentage of death from excess gastrointestinal cancer and peritoneal mesothelioma in four groups of asbestos workers. Calculations of this percentage were made using expected numbers of death, rather than the observed, because the latter was inflated by including other asbestos-related deaths.

Table 13: Percentage of Excess Gastrointestinal Cancers and Peritoneal Mesotheliomas in Four Groups of Asbestos Workers

| | ... Number of Excess Deaths. ... | | | Excess Deaths as Percentage of Expected Deaths in Cohort | |
Exposed Group	GI Cancer	Peritoneal Mesothelioma	Expected No. of Deaths in Cohort	GI	Peritoneal Mesothelioma
Insulation workers (chrysotile and amosite), Selikoff, et al (7-6)	39.9 (ICD 150-154)*	109	1,660.96	2.4	6.6
Insulation workers (chrysotile and amosite), Selikoff, et al (7-7)	29.4 (ICD 150-154)	22	305.20	9.6	7.2
Factory employment (amosite), Seidman, et al (7-8)	10.5 (ICD 150-154)	8	368.62	2.9	2.2
Factory employment (chrysotile, crocidolite and amosite), Newhouse and Berry (7-9)	15.8 (ICD 150-154 ex meso)	35	556.0	2.8	6.3

*Public Health Service (7-10)

Source: Reference (7)

Table 14 lists the fiber concentration estimates and an exposure index for each cohort (years of exposure x fiber concentration). This index will be used to calculate the number and mass of asbestos fibers ingested during a working lifetime. As the observed mortality is, to a large extent, after 20 years from first exposure, the intermixing of time and exposure does not present significant problems.

The average length of exposure for the insulation workers in the first group was calculated from data on employment time at entry into the cohort in 1967. Forty years was used as the working lifetime for the smaller group of New York and New Jersey insulators virtually all of whom are deceased or retired. The estimate of the person-weighted exposure index for the amosite factory is simply the average employment time multiplied by 40 fibers/ml. Data from Table 15 were used to estimate a person-weighted exposure index for the Newhouse and Berry group.

$$\text{Person-weighted exposure index} = \frac{\text{No. at risk x exposure x time}}{\text{No. at risk}} = 180$$

A detailed calculation of the daily intake of asbestos to produce a lifetime risk of 10^{-5} is given in the Criteria Document (7). Data of the occupational risk of both gastrointestinal cancer and peritoneal mesothelioma were used in Table 13. Account was taken of the fact that occupational exposures took place over a 5-day workweek and that the ingestion exposure may encompass a lifespan of 70 years. It was assumed that a worker breathes at the rate of 1 m^3/hr during work exposure for the purpose of calculating total asbestos intake per day. Using a linear dose-response relationship, and a specified risk of 10^{-5} the calculated 70-year daily intake resulting from these calculations is given in Table 16. The data from Seidman, et al, were not used because it was exclusively from amosite exposures. Assuming that two liters of water are ingested per day, this would correspond to a concentration of 300,000 fibers of all sizes per liter of water.

Table 14: Exposure Indices for Asbestos Worker Groups

Exposed Group	Air Fiber Concentration (f/ml)	Person-Weighted Exposure Average (yr)	Exposure Index (yr x f/ml)
U.S. insulators (7-6)	15	34	510
NY/NJ insulators (7-7)	15	40	600
Amosite factory workers (7-8)	40	1.9	76
British factory workers (7-9)	10-30	—	180

Source: Reference (7)

Table 15: Exposure Estimates for Workers in a British Factory

Exposure Group	Number at Risk	Exposure (f/ml)	Time of Exposure (yr)
Severe			
2 years	711	30	20
2 years	1,333	30	2
Low to moderate			
2 years	503	10	20
2 years	933	10	2

Source: Reference (7-9)

Table 16: Calculated Intake for 10^{-5} Lifetime Risk of Death from Gastrointestinal Cancer and Peritoneal Mesothelioma

Exposure Group	Estimate of Intake/Day for 10^{-5} Risk*
Selikoff, et al (7-6)	900,000
Selikoff, et al (7-7)	600,000
Newhouse and Berry (7-9)	400,000
Average	600,000

*Fibers of all lengths/day

Source: Reference (7)

A criterion for a mass concentration of asbestos can also be calculated using the conversion value of 30 μg/m^3/f/ml as derived from the data for predominantly chrysotile exposures. A value of 150 μg/m^3/f/ml for amosite appears more appropriate, based on the finding that amosite has approximately a three times greater conversion factor than chrysotile. A detailed calculation is given in the criteria document (7) and the results are summarized in Table 17. Assuming that two liters of water are ingested per day, a risk of 10^{-5} would be produced from ingesting water containing 0.05 μg/l. As mentioned in the Criteria Document, the variability in the data used to convert optical fiber counts to mass leads to a large uncertainty in the above estimate.

Considering chrysotile and depending on the source of the asbestos in water, 0.05 μg/l corresponds to from 10^6 to 20 x 10^6 fibers of all lengths per day. Such estimates are considerably higher than those derived previously and are most likely a reflection of the differences in the sizes of the fibers found in water, as compared to those found in air. Because of these uncertainties, high priority should be given to obtaining accurate size and mass distribution of typical fibers found in different circumstances (air and water) which would allow appropriate conversions to be made between fiber concentrations in air and water.

The majority of samples analyzed for the EPA to date were characterized by a concentration of all microscopic visible fibers per liter of water.

Further, techniques for the determination of fiber concentrations (as opposed to mass concentrations) have been published as interim EPA procedures. Thus, a criterion for the concentration of fibers of all sizes in water corresponding to a 10^{-5} risk will be calculated directly from the concentrations of fibers greater than 5 μm measured in the occupational circumstances that produced disease. Unfortunately, the data currently available relating to concentrations of fibers longer than 5 μm, counted by optical microscopy, determined by electron microscopy, are extremely limited. These include those by Wallingford (7-11), 15:1, Millette (7-12), 400:1; and Winer and Cossette (7-13) 1,000:1 and are only for chrysotile asbestos. Using the geometric mean of 200 for this factor from all available data, a total fiber concentration corresponding to a 10^{-5} risk can be calculated from the data of Tables 13 and 14.

Table 17: Calculated Intake for 10^{-5} Lifetime Risk of Death from Gastrointestinal Cancer and Peritoneal Mesothelioma

Exposure Group	Estimate of Intake/Day for 10^{-5} Risk (μg/l day)
Selikoff, et al (7-6)	0.14
Selikoff, et al (7-7)	0.09
Seidman, et al (7-8)	0.11
Newhouse and Berry (7-9)	0.05
Average	0.1

Source: Reference (7)

In making the calculation, one tacitly assumes the same fiber size distribution in water as in occupational air samples. Some data show that water fiber size distributions vary, and occupational air distributions have been shown to be so variable that the fraction of fibers longer than 5 μ can range over a factor of 10 depending on sampling circumstances. Although sizing of airborne and waterborne fibers have not been done using the same methods, qualitatively, water appears to have fiber distributions with more smaller fibers than in occupational air samples. Thus, an estimate assuming the same fiber size distribution in water as in air will yield a conservate criterion (from the point of view of health).

Although positive animal experiments had various experimental limitations, such data as existed were treated in the model of EPA. The data are presented in Table 18.

Considering the large number of experimental uncertainties, these values provide reasonable support for the concentration derived from human exposure data.

This document was concerned with the estimation of that concentration of asbestos in water which will produce a lifetime risk of 1 in 100,000 in a population exposed continuously. The risk estimate was made using a linear extrapolation from existing human data and would appear to constitute a conservative extrapolation. However, in the case of asbestos the risk factor of 1 in 100,000 is not conservative. If we were concerned with intermittent or localized contamination incidents of some carcinogen that, once identified, could be abated, such a value would have utility. With asbestos, however, we are concerned with an ubiquitous contaminant in the environment to which large populations are continuously exposed for decades. Further, the estimated value has a high degree of uncertainty associated with it, based upon the data from which it was derived.

Under the consent decree in NRDC vs Train, criteria are to state "recommended maximum permissible concentrations (including where appropriate, zero) consistent with the protection of aquatic organisms, human health, and recreational activities." Asbestos is suspected of being a human carcinogen. Because there is no recognized safe concentration for a human carcinogen, the recommended concentration of asbestos in water for maximum protection of human health is zero.

Table 18

Effect	Estimated 10^{-5} Dosage $(\mu g/l)$
4/42 Kidney carcinomas 0/49 control	3.2
12/42 Malignancies 2/49 control	1.1

Source: Reference (7-14)

Because attaining a zero concentration level may be infeasible in some cases and in order to assist the EPA and states in the possible future development of water quality regulations, the concentrations of asbestos corresponding to several incremental lifetime cancer risk levels have been estimated. A cancer risk level provides an estimate of the additional incidence of cancer that may be expected in an exposed population. A risk of 10^{-5}, for example, indicates a probability of one additional case of cancer for every 100,000 people exposed, a risk of 10^{-6} indicates one additional case of cancer for every million people exposed, and so forth.

In the *Federal Register* notice of availability of draft ambient water quality criteria, EPA stated that it is considering setting criteria at an interim target risk level of 10^{-5}, 10^{-6}, or 10^{-7} as shown in Table 19.

Concentration levels were derived assuming a lifetime exposure to various amounts of asbestos occurring from the consumption of drinking water only.

Although total exposure information for asbestos is discussed and an estimate of the contributions from other sources of exposure can be made, this data will not be factored into ambient water quality criteria formulation until additional analysis can be made. The criteria presented, therefore, assume an incremental risk from ambient water exposure only.

In Table 19 the risk levels and corresponding criteria are calculated by applying a modified "one-hit" extrapolation model described in the Methodology Document in the human epidemiological data presented in Criterion Document. Since the extrapolation model is linear to low doses, the additional lifetime risk is directly proportional to the water concentrations corresponding to other risk levels can be derived by multiplying or dividing one of the risk levels and corresponding water concentrations shown in the table by factors such as 10, 100, 1,000 and so forth.

Table 19: Possible Alternative Criteria for Asbestos

Exposure Assumption	. . . . Risk Levels, fibers per liter.			
	0	10^{-7}	10^{-6}	10^{-5}
2 liters of drinking water Consumption of fish and shellfish only	—	3,000	30,000	300,000
	. . . . .no criterion			

Source: Reference (7)

References

(7-1)   Speil, S., and Leineweber, J.P., "Asbestos minerals in modern technology," *Environ. Res.,* 2, 166 (1969).

(7-2)   National Institute for Occupational Safety and Health, *Criteria for a Recommended Standard: Occupational Exposure to Asbestos,* NIOSH Doc. No. 72-10267, Wash., D.C. (1972).

(7-3)   National Institute for Occupational Safety and Health, *Revised Recommended Asbestos Standard,* NIOSH Doc. No. 77-169, Wash., D.C. (Dec. 1976).

(7-4)   British Occupational Hygiene Society, "Hygiene standard for chrysotile asbestos dust," *Am. Occup. Hyg.,* 11, 47 (1968).

(7-5)   Peto, J., "The hygiene standard for asbestos," *Lancet,* No. 8062, 484 (1968).

(7-6)   Selikoff, I.J., et al, "Mortality experience of insulation workers in the U.S. and Canada, 1943-1977," *Am. New York Acad. Sci.,* (In Press-1979).

(7-7)   Selikoff, I.J., "Lung cancer and mesothelioma during prospective surveillance of 1249 asbestos insulation workers 1963-74," *Ann. New York Acad. Sci.,* 271, 448 (1976).

(7-8)   Seidman, H., et al, "Long term observation following short-term employment in an amosite asbestos factory," *Ann. New York Acad. Sci.,* (In Press-1979).

(7-9)   Newhouse, M.L. and Berry, G., "Patterns of disease among long term asbestos workers in the U.K.," *Ann. New York Acad. Sci.* (In Press-1979).

(7-10) U.S. Public Health Service, *International Classification of Diseases: Adapted for Use in the U.S.,* DHEW/PHS Publ. No. 1693, Wash., D.C. (1967-69).

(7-11) Wallingford, K.M., "Chrysotile Asbestos in Industry," Paper before Wash.-Balt. Section of Amer. Ind. Hygiene Assoc. (Feb. 1978).

(7-12) Millette, J.R., U.S. EPA Health Effects Research Lab (reported in Reference 7).

(7-13) Winer, A.A. and Cossette, M., "The Effect of Aspect Ratio," Paper before N.Y. Acad. of Sci., Conf. on Health Hazards of Asbestos Exposure, New York City (June 24-27, 1978).

(7-14) Gibel, W., et al, "Tierexperimentelle untersuchungen uber eine kanzerogene wirkung von asbestfiltematerial nach oraler aufnahme," *Arch. Geschwulstforsch.,* 46, 437 (1976).

B

BENZENE (#8)

Benzene, C_6H_6, is the simplest aromatic hydrocarbon. It has a molecular weight of 78.1.

Occurrence: Benzene is produced principally from coal tar distillation and from petroleum by catalytic reforming of light naphthas from which it is isolated by distillation or solvent extraction. It is also produced in coal processing and coal coking operations. Benzene has been detected at various concentrations in lakes and streams and finished drinking water.

Physical Properties: Benzene is a volatile, colorless, liquid hydrocarbon. Pure benzene has a boiling point of 80.1°C and a melting point of 5.5°C. Benzene has a density less than that of water (0.87865 at 20°C) and is soluble in water at concentrations which have been shown to be toxic to aquatic organisms. Benzene is also readily soluble in natural fats and fat-soluble substances. It may bioaccumulate in living organisms and appears to accumulate in animal tissues that exhibit a high lipid content or represent major metabolic sites such as liver and brain. The solubility and volatile nature of benzene indicate possible environmental mobility.

Chemical Properties: Benzene undergoes the typical reactions of aromatic hydrocarbons including: chlorination, nitration, oxidation, and sulfonation. It is volatile and reasonably stable to biodegradation in the environment.

Uses: The broad utility spectrum of benzene (commercially sometimes called "Benzol") includes its use as: an intermediate for synthesis in the chemical and pharmaceutical industries including the manufacture of styrene, cyclohexane, detergents, and pesticides, a thinner for lacquers, a degreasing and cleaning agent, a solvent in the rubber industry, an antiknock fuel additive, a general solvent in laboratories, a solvent for industrial extraction and rectification, and in the preparation and use of inks in the graphic arts industries. In the United States today, benzene is used extensively (over 4 million metric tons annually) in the chemical industry and its use is expected to increase when additional production facilities become available.

Toxic Effects: Benzene is a leukemic agent in humans. While animal studies have been negative, human case histories and epidemiological studies have provided confirmatory evidence of the causal relationship of benzene exposure to leukemia. Benzene has also been demonstrated to affect aquatic life adversely. Reproductive impairment has been observed in fish at benzene concentrations well below the lethal level. Benzene in the environment has been demonstrated to exert deleterious effects at many levels of the food chain.

Current Levels of Exposure: The major source of human exposure to benzene is through the respiratory route. The annual average exposure of an individual to ambient benzene from all air sources is 1.03 ppb (8-1). The U.S. EPA (8-2) has attempted to put into perspective the known and unknowns about total benzene exposure for its National Drinking Water Program. Based upon the assumptions utilized, air was the predominant source of benzene absorbed by the general population. This source contributed more than 80% of the total daily benzene uptake for an adult male living in an urban environment. Assumed benzene content in drinking water included levels of 0.1, 0.2, 1 and 10 μg/l, food was 250 μg/l and ambient air was 50 μg/m^3. The total daily intake at the 10 μg/l benzene level for drinking water was 1.128 mg/day of which 1.4% came from the water, 17.7% came from food and 80.9% came from ambient air exposure.

As shown by Mara and Lee (8-1) certain occupational groups have potential exposure to benzene over and above the ambient levels. The representative industry activities include chemical manufacturing, coking operations, gasoline service stations, petroleum refineries, and solvent operations.

Special Groups at Risk: There is some suggestion that there may be a genetic predisposition to benzene toxicity; this subject is reviewed by Goldstein (8-3). Although there are many more cases of benzene-induced hematotoxicity in males than in females because of occupational exposure, there is evidence to suggest that exposed females have a greater chance of developing severe disease. Age does not seem to affect hematotoxicity.

Existing Guidelines and Standards: Existing U.S. air standards for occupational exposure to benzene include 10 ppm (32 mg/m^3) set in 1974 (8-4) and an emergency temporary level of 1 ppm set by the U.S. Occupational Safety and Health Administration in 1977 (8-5), and 10 ppm (30 mg/m^3) set by the American Conference of Governmental Industrial Hygienists in 1979. This limitation by ACGIH in 1979 also bears the notation that benzene is "an industrial substance suspect of carcinogenic potential for man." The emergency level of 1 ppm for benzene proposed by OSHA is in the courts as this volume goes to press with the AFL-CIO labor union and OSHA defending the proposed standard and DuPont, Uniroyal, Exxon, U.S. Steel, The Chemical Manufacturers Association and the Chemical Specialties Manufacturers Association opposing it. The U.S. Supreme Court will rule in its 1979-1980 session.

Foreign standards include 16 ppm promulgated by Czechoslovakia in 1969, and 6 ppm (20 mg/m^3) promulgated by the Soviet Union in 1967. OSHA also prohibits repeated or prolonged skin exposure to liquid benzene. No standard for benzene in water exists, but Cleland and Kingsburg (8-6), using several assumptions and ACGIH air standards, have suggested values of 1,071 and 414 μg/l for ingested water, and a different value, 107 μg/l for ingested water based on the potential carcinogenicity of benzene.

Summary of Proposed EPA Criteria: *Freshwater Aquatic Life* — For benzene the criterion to protect freshwater aquatic life as derived using the Guidelines is 3,100 μg/l as a 24-hour average and the concentration should not exceed 7,000 μg/l at any time.

Saltwater Aquatic Life — The data base for saltwater aquatic life is insufficient to allow use of the Guidelines. The following recommendation is inferred from toxicity data for freshwater organisms. For benzene the criterion to protect saltwater aquatic life as derived using procedures other than the Guidelines is 920 μg/l as a 24-hour average and the concentration should not exceed 2,100 μg/l at any time.

Human Health — For the maximum protection of human health from the potential carcinogenic effects of exposure to benzene through ingestion of water and contaminated aquatic organisms, the ambient water concentration is zero. Concentrations of benzene estimated to result in additional lifetime cancer risks ranging from no additional risk to an additional risk of 1 in 100,000 are presented in the criterion formulation section of this document. The EPA is considering setting criteria at an interim target risk level in the range of 10^{-5}, 10^{-6}, or 10^{-7} with corresponding criteria of 15 μg/l, 1.5 μg/l, and 0.15 μg/l, respectively.

Basis for the Proposed Human Health Criteria: The Natl. Acad. Sci./Natl. Res. Coun. in its review of drinking water and health (8-7) concluded that existing animal and human data did not allow the establishment of limits for benzene in drinking water. This was because the animal results were not statistically significant and were based on nonoral administration of benzene. In addition, the occupational studies on human exposure did not contain adequate information on degree of exposure or size of the population at risk, and did not rule out exposure to other chemicals besides benzene.

Since the publication of the Natl. Acad. Sci./Natl. Res. Coun. report (8-7) epidemiological studies by Aksoy, Infante, et al and Ott, et al have appeared. These studies include information on degree of benzene exposure and size of the population at risk, and rule out exposure to solvents other than benzene. The U.S. EPA Carcinogen Assessment Group has made use of these three occupational studies to calculate a leukemia dose-response curve (8-8). The slope of this curve is 0.024074, in units of lifetime risk of leukemia per ppm exposure to benzene in air. Since 1 ppm is 3.25 mg/m^3, and assuming a respiratory rate of about 24 m^3/day, the benzene intake per individual at 1 ppm is:

$$(3.25 \text{ mg/m}^3)(24 \text{ m}^3/\text{day}) = 78 \text{ mg/day}$$

To calculate the benzene intake resulting in a lifetime risk of leukemia of 10^{-5}, one solves the following equation for x,

$$\frac{x}{10^{-5}} = \frac{78 \text{ mg/day}}{0.024074}$$

resulting in 0.032 mg/day.

The U.S. EPA total exposure analysis indicates that the total body exposure may be as high as 1.1 mg/day of benzene. This was derived using estimates which have varying degrees of support in terms of hard data. The specific use of the total exposure estimates for calculation of water criterion does not seem warranted at this particular time because of a general lack of knowledge about the accuracy of the estimates. It can be said, however, that from a general weight of evidence perspective, it appears that air exposure may contribute the majority of total exposure.

The total exposure consideration should be factored into the criterion development at a later date when additional data is available. Under the Consent Decree in *NRDC vs Train*, criteria are to state "recommended maximum permissible concentrations (including where appropriate, zero) consistent with the protection of aquatic organisms, human health, and recreational activities." Benzene is suspected of being a human carcinogen. Because there is no recognized safe concentration for a human carcinogen, the recommended concentration of benzene in water for maximum protection of human health is zero.

Because attaining a zero concentration level may be infeasible in some cases and in order to assist the Agency and States in the possible future development of water quality regulations, the concentrations of benzene corresponding to several incremental lifetime cancer risk levels have been estimated. A cancer risk level provides an estimate of the additional incidence of cancer that may be expected in an exposed population. A risk of 10^{-5}, for example, indicates a probability of one additional case of cancer for every 100,000 people exposed, a risk of 10^{-6} indicates one additional case of cancer for every million people exposed, and so forth.

In the *Federal Register* notice of availability of draft ambient water quality criteria, EPA stated that it is considering setting criteria at an interim target risk level of 10^{-5}, 10^{-6}, and 10^{-7} as shown in Table 20. In the table, the risk levels are calculated by applying a modified "one-hit" extrapolation model described in the Methodology Document to the human epidemiology data presented in the Summary of Pertinent Data. Since the extrapolation model is linear at low doses, the additional lifetime risk is directly proportional to the water concentration. Therefore, water concentration corresponding to other risk levels can be derived by multiplying or dividing one of the risk levels and corresponding water concentrations shown in the table by factors such as 10, 100, and so forth.

Concentration levels were derived assuming a lifetime exposure to various amounts of benzene, (1) occurring from the consumption of both drinking water and aquatic life grown in waters containing the corresponding benzene concentrations and, (2) occurring solely from consumption of aquatic life grown in the waters containing the corresponding benzene concentrations.

Table 20: Possible Alternative Criteria for Benzene

Exposure Assumptions (per day)	Risk Levels and Corresponding Criteria, μg/l			
	0	10^{-7}	10^{-6}	10^{-5}
2 liters of drinking water and consumption of 18.7 grams fish and shellfish*	0	0.15	1.5	15
Consumption of fish and shellfish only	0	2.5	25	250

*6% of the benzene exposure results from the consumption of aquatic organisms which exhibit an average bioconcentration potential of 6.9-fold. The remaining 94% of benzene exposure results from drinking water.

Source: Reference (8)

Although total exposure information for benzene is discussed and an estimate of the contributions from other sources of exposure can be made, this data will not be factored into ambient water quality criteria formulation until additional analysis can be made. The criteria presented, therefore, assume an incremental risk from ambient water exposure only.

Three epidemiology studies of workers exposed to benzene vapors on their jobs, performed by Infante, Ott, and Askoy, were reviewed by the CAG for the Office of Air Quality Planning and Standards (8-8). Their result was that the potency for humans breathing benzene continuously is B = 0.02407. This means that the lifetime risk of getting leukemia, R, equals 0.024074 times the lifetime average continuous exposure, X, measured as ppm of benzene by volume in air, or R = BX. Therefore, the air concentration, X, resulting in a risk of 10^{-5} is X = R/B = 10^{-5}/0.024074 = 4.1539 x 10^{-4} ppm.

Since the air concentration corresponding to 1 ppm of benzene is 3.25 x 10^{-3} μg/m^3 and since people breathe an average of 24 m^3/day of air, the daily intake that would result in a risk of 10^{-5} is: 4.154 x 10^{-4} ppm x 3.25 x 10^3 mg/m^3/ppm x 24 m^3/day = 32.4 μg/day.

It is assumed that the fraction of benzene intake reaching the target site is the same via inhalation and ingestion of water and fish, a daily benzene intake of 32.4 μg through drinking water and fish alone would also cause a leukemia risk of 10^{-5}. The water concentration giving this intake is: C = (32.4 μg/day)/[2 + (6.9 x 0.0187)] = 15.22 μg/l = 15 μg/l.

References

(8-1) Mara, S.J. and Lee, S.S., *Human Exposures to Atmospheric Benzene*, Report on Contract 68-01-4314 with Stanford Research Inst., Wash., D.C., U.S. Environmental Protection Agency (1977).

(8-2) Mitre Corp., *Environmental Sources of Benzene Exposure: Source Contribution Factors*, Report on Contract No. EPA 68-01-4635, Wash., D.C., U.S. Environmental Protection Agency (1978).

(8-3) Goldstein, G.D., "Hematotoxicity in Humans," *Jour. Toxical. Envir. Health Supp.* 2, 69 (1977).

(8-4) National Institute for Occupational Safety and Health, *Criteria for a Recommended Standard: Occupational Exposure to Benzene*, NIOSH Doc. No. 74-137, Wash., D.C. (1974).

(8-5) National Institute for Occupational Safety & Health, *Revised Recommendation for an Occupational Exposure Standard for Benzene*, Wash., D.C. (1977).

(8-6) Cleland, J.G. and Kingsbury, G.L., *Multimedia Environmental Goals for Environmental Assessment*, Report No. EPA 600/7-77-136, Wash., D.C., U.S. Environmental Protection Agency (1977).

(8-7) National Academy of Sciences/National Research Council, *Drinking Water and Health*, Wash., D.C., Nat. Acad. of Sci. (1977).

(8-8) Albert, R., Carcinogen Assessment Group's final report on the population risk to ambient benzene exposures., Wash., D.C., U.S. Environmental Protection Agency (Sept. 12, 1978).

BENZIDINE (#9)

Benzidine is an aromatic amine with a molecular weight of 184.24. It has the formula $H_2NC_6H_4C_6H_4NH_2$.

Occurrence: In general, exposure to benzidine compounds occurs in factories that synthesize benzidine and its congeners and convert them to dyes. It is also probable that some exposure occurs when the closed system used in synthesis is cleaned. Exposure also occurs from breathing contaminated air, ingesting contaminated food, and wearing contaminated clothing. Pointing of brushes by Japanese kimono painters results in the ingestion of benzidine dyes, although ingestion is not generally an important source of exposure.

Physical Properties: Benzidine is a grayish-yellow, white, or reddish-gray crystalline powder (melting point 128°C; boiling point 400°C), benzidine's solubility increases as water temperature rises. One gram of benzidine will dissolve in 2.5 liters of cold water. Solubility is greatly enhanced with dissolution into organic solvents. Benzidine is easily converted to and from its salt.

Chemical Properties: Diazotization reactions involving benzidine will result in colored compounds (color will vary with molecular structure). Because of their color, azo compounds are important as dyes for industrial use. The pKa values for the amino groups in benzidine were reported to be 4.66 and 3.57.

It has been stated that benzidine resists physical and biological degradation. Benzidine in water is oxidatively degraded by free radical, enzymatic or photochemical processes (9-3). Its half-life in water has been estimated to be 100 days. Air oxidation of benzidine in water seems to occur readily (9-1).

Humic material seems to bind 3,3'-dichlorobenzidine tightly and its degradation appears to be slower than benzidine, but the half-lives of the two compounds are the same (9-3). There is no information available on the dimethyl- and dimethoxy derivatives. This deficiency must be corrected.

Benzidine is converted to a chloramine type compound during water chlorination processes. Soil and intestinal bacteria reduce benzidine azo dyes to free benzidine, and although aquatic organisms might also cause this same transformation, no data are available to prove this point. It should be remembered that the hydrochlorides of benzidine are much more soluble in water than the free amines and are more resistant to degradation than the latter.

Uses: Benzidine is used as a chemical intermediate for the production of dyestuffs.

Toxic Effects: Benzidine (4,4'-diaminobiphenyl) is a proven human carcinogen, its primary site of tumor induction is the urinary bladder. It is also mutagenic. The incidence of bladder tumors in humans resulting from occupational exposure to aromatic amines (benzidine) was first researched in Germany in 1895. The first cases of this condition in the United States were diagnosed in 1931 and reported in 1934. Several studies implicating the high risk of bladder tumors in workers exposed to benzidine and other aromatic amines are well documented.

Adversary proceedings under section 307(a) of the Federal Water Pollution Control Act resulted in the promulgation of a toxic pollutant effluent standard for benzidine. The ambient water criterion upon which the standard was based was 0.1 μg/l (42 *FR* 2588, January 12, 1977).

Current Levels of Exposure: It is essential that consideration be given to the manner in which benzidine and its congeners and the dyes derived from them contaminate water supplies. In most cases these chemicals are a hazard only in the vicinity of dye and pigment plants where wastes escape or are discharged. A field survey of the Buffalo and Niagara river areas using the chloramine-T method, with a sensitivity of 0.2 μg/l, showed no benzidine in the samples. However, this method of analysis is photosensitive and leads to low estimates of benzidine. Moreover, the samples may have been below the level of detectability or oxidative degradation may have converted the benzidine compounds to materials not detectable by the analytical method used (9-1). A Japanese survey of the Sumida River area detected 0.082, 0.140, and 0.233 mg/l of benzidine in the water. The authors believed that the benzidine came from azo dyes by H_2S or SO_2 reduction (9-2).

Information on 3,3'-dimethylbenzidine, 3,3'-dimethoxybenzidine, and 3,3'-dichlorobenzidine and their dye derivatives as water contaminants is nonexistent and research should be instituted to correct this deficiency.

Special Groups at Risk: A potential health hazard exists in the production of benzidine and its congeners and their conversion to azo dyes. There is no maximum permissible level of contamination in the industrial environment although there are specific regulations governing the manufacture of benzidine and its congeners (39 *FR* 3756). These standards have reduced the risks to benzidine workers.

The use of benzidine and its congeners poses a potential risk to workers in biochemical, chemical, and microbiological laboratories where these chemicals are used as analytical reagents. The greatest risk occurs in laboratories working with known carcinogens when good laboratory practices are not enforced. No epidemiological evidence is available to determine the exact extent of the problem.

The risk to the general population from benzidine, its congeners, and their dyes is unknown, but contamination of water supplies, which is known to occur in Japan (9-2), poses a yet to be determined risk. There also is a potential risk for workers in the garment, leather, and homecraft industries where the benzidine dyes are used.

Existing Guidelines and Standards: In 1973 the Environmental Protection Agency proposed but did not promulgate a toxic pollutant standard for benzidine (30 *FR* 35388). The industrial standards instituted by the Occupational Safety and Health Administration in 1974 excluded from regulation any compounds containing less than 0.1% benzidine. These standards did not recognize a safe level of water contamination and provided no provisions for environmental monitoring.

New standards for benzidine discharges have been proposed (41 *FR* 27012) based upon information on the toxicological and environmental effects and the fate of benzidine. These standards, promulgated in 1977, established an ambient water criterion for benzidine of 0.1 µg/l. Effluent standards were set at 10 µg/l (daily average) with a maximum for any single day of 50 µg/l. Based on a monthly average, daily loading was limited to 0.13 kg/1,000 kg of benzidine produced. The standards set for users of benzidine-based dyes were the same except that the maximum daily effluent concentration of benzidine was limited to 25 µg/l (42 *FR* 2617).

Summary of Proposed EPA Criteria: *Freshwater Aquatic Life* — For freshwater aquatic life, no criterion for benzidine can be derived using the Guidelines, and there are insufficient data to estimate a criterion using other procedures.

Saltwater Aquatic Life — For saltwater aquatic life, no criterion for benzidine can be derived using the Guidelines, and there are insufficient data to estimate a criterion using other procedures.

Human Health — For the maximum protection of human health from the potential carcinogenic effects of exposure to benzidine through ingestion of water and contaminated aquatic organisms, the ambient water concentration is zero. Concentrations of benzidine estimated to result in additional lifetime cancer risks ranging from no additional to an additional risk of 1 in 100,000 are presented in the Criterion Formulation section of this document. The EPA is considering setting criteria at an interim target risk level in the range of 10^{-5}, 10^{-6}, or 10^{-7}, with corresponding criteria of 1.67 x 10^{-3} µg/l, 1.67 x 10^{-4} µg/l, and 1.67 x 10^{-5} µg/l, respectively.

Basis for the Proposed Human Health Criteria: The available data concerning the carcinogenicity of benzidine in experimental animals are severely limited. It is extremely difficult to extrapolate the experimental results to man because, with the possible exception of the dog and the rabbit, the target organs are different. Moreover, the metabolites produced by the various species, in general, differ significantly from those produced by man (9-4), although 3-hydroxybenzidine and its conjugation products are common to both man and animals.

Despite the limitations of the available data, a suggested criterion for benzidine was calculated using the linear nonthreshold model described in 44 *FR* 15926 March 15, 1979. The calculation assumes a risk of 1 in 100,000 of developing cancer as a result of daily consumption of 2 liters of benzidine contaminated water and the daily consumption of 18.7 g of benzidine contaminated aquatic organisms. Based on the data of Zavon, et al, (9-5), a benzidine criterion of 1.67×10^{-3} μg/l is suggested to be adequate to protect the population consuming the water and the contaminated aquatic organisms.

Epidemiological data indicate that exposure to benzidine is associated with an increase in bladder cancer in man. The possibility that benzidine may be found in wastewater may also pose a problem. In order to determine the extent of the potential problem, measurements must be made of wastewater not only for benzidine but also for its congeners. Moreover, further evaluation must be made on these chemicals and their azo dye derivatives to determine their stability to microbiological degradation. It is essential that studies of their carcinogenicity in experimental animals can be made at doses which produce a bare minimum of liver pathology. A detailed pharmacokinetic study should be undertaken to establish routes of absorption, body transport, storage and excretion of benzidine, its congeners, and the azo dyes synthesized from them. Programs covering both industrial hygienic and epidemiologic aspects of exposure to benzidine and its congeners to establish the degree of dermal and pulmonary absorption are a necessity if we are to prevent this chemically induced cancer from occurring.

Under the Consent Decree in *NRDC vs Train*, criteria are to state "recommended maximum permissible concentrations (including where appropriate, zero) consistent with the protection of aquatic organisms, human health, and recreational activities." Benzidine is suspected of being a human carcinogen. Because there is no recognized safe concentration for a human carcinogen, the recommended concentration of benzidine in water for maximum protection of human health is zero.

Because attaining a zero concentration level may be infeasible in some cases and in order to assist the EPA and States in the possible future development of water quality regulations, the concentrations of benzidine corresponding to several incremental lifetime cancer risk levels have been estimated. A cancer risk level provides an estimate of the additional incidence of cancer that may be expected in an exposed population. A risk of 10^{-5}, for example, indicates a probability of an additional case of cancer for every 100,000 people exposed, a risk of 10^{-6} indicates an additional case of cancer for every million people exposed.

In the *Federal Register* notice of availability of draft ambient water quality criteria, EPA stated that it is considering setting criteria at an interim target risk level of 10^{-5}, 10^{-6} or 10^{-7} as shown in Table 21.

Table 21: Possible Alternative Criteria for Benzidine

Exposure Assumptions	Risk Levels and Corresponding Criteria, μg/l			
	0	10^{-7}	10^{-6}	10^{-5}
2 liters of drinking water and consumption of				
18.7 grams of fish and shellfish*	0	1.67×10^{-5}	1.67×10^{-4}	1.67×10^{-3}
Consumption of fish and shellfish only	0	5.24×10^{-5}	5.24×10^{-4}	5.24×10^{-3}

*32% of benzidine exposure results from the consumption of aquatic organisms which exhibit an average bioconcentration potential of 50-fold. The remaining 68% of benzidine exposure results from drinking water.

In the table, the risk levels are calculated by applying a modified "one-hit" extrapolation model described in 44 *FR* 15926 March 15, 1979. Appropriate epidemiological data used in the calculation of the model are presented in Summary of Pertinent Data. Since the extrapolation model is linear to low doses, the additional lifetime risk is directly proportional to the water concentration. Therefore, water concentrations corresponding to other risk levels can be derived by multiplying or dividing one of the risk levels and corresponding water concentrations shown in the table by factors such as 10, 100, 1,000, etc.

Concentration levels were derived assuming a lifetime exposure to various amounts of benzidine, (1) occurring from the consumption of both drinking water and aquatic life grown in water containing the corresponding benzidine concentrations and, (2) occurring solely from the consumption of aquatic life grown in the waters containing the corresponding benzidine concentrations.

Although total exposure information for benzidine is discussed and an estimate of the contributions from other sources of exposure can be made, this data will not be factored into the ambient water quality criteria formulation because of the tenuous estimates. The criteria presented, therefore, assume an incremental risk from ambient water exposure only.

Summary of Pertinent Data — The data from the human epidemiology study of Zavon, et al (9-5) were used to estimate the concentration of benzidine in water calculated to keep the lifetime cancer risk below 10^{-5}. In this study 25 workers in a benzidine manufacturing plant were observed for the appearance of bladder tumors after a mean exposure period of 13.61 years, their average age at the end of exposure was 44 years and at the end of a 13-year observation was 57 years. The men not showing evidence of cancer had a mean exposure period of 8.91 years, their average age at the end of exposure was 43 years and at the end of observation 56 years. The estimated total accumulated dose of 200 mg/kg was estimated from average urinary levels of benzidine in these workers at the end of a workshift [see Zavon, et al (9-5)]. The criterion was calculated from the following parameters:

- Average weight of man = 70 kg;
- Observed incidence of bladder cancer = 13/25 (52%);
- Accumulated dose = 200 mg/kg;
- Bioconcentration factor of benzidine = 50;
- X = average daily exposure producing lifetime risk of 10^{-5};
- B^* = potency factor, which is an estimate of the linear dependency of cancer rates on lifetime average dose; and
- C = concentration of benzidine in water, calculated to produce a lifetime risk of 10^{-5}, assuming a daily ingestion of 2 liters of water and 0.0187 kg fish.

Workers were assumed to have received 200 mg/kg of benzidine in a lifetime. At the end of a 13-year observation period, the average age of the workers was 57 years. Therefore, benzidine exposure on an mg/day basis amounts to:

$$\frac{200 \times 70}{365 \times 57} = 0.673 \text{ mg/day}$$

This gives a response at 57 years of 52% so that:

$$0.52 = 1 - e^{-B(0.673)}$$

$$B = \frac{0.734}{0.673} = 1.091$$

$$B^* = B\left(\frac{tf}{tf}\right)^3 = 1.091\left(\frac{70}{57}\right)^3 = 2.021$$

$$(2.021)\ (X) = 10^{-5}$$
$$X = 4.9 \times 10^{-6} \text{ mg/day to obtain a rate}$$
$$\text{of } 10^{-5} \text{ or } 4.9 \times 10^{-3} \mu g/day$$

Therefore:

$$C[2 + (50 \times 0.0187)] = 4.9 \times 10^{-3}$$

$$C = 1.67 \times 10^{-3} \ \mu g/l$$

From this data the concentration of benzidine in water calculated to keep lifetime cancer risk below 10^{-5} is 1.67×10^{-3} $\mu g/l$.

References

(9-1) Howard, P.N. and Saxena, J., *Persistence and Degradability Testing of Benzidine and Other Carcinogenic Compounds*, Report EPA-560/5-76-005, Wash., D.C., U.S. Environmental Protection Agency (1976).

(9-2) Takemura, N. et al, "A survey of the pollution of the Sumida river, especially on the aromatic amines in the water," *Int. Jl. Air Water Poll.* 9, 665 (1965);

(9-3) Radding, S.B. et al, *Review of the Environmental Fate of Selected Chemicals*, Report EPA 560/5-75-001; Wash., D.C., U.S. Environmental Protection Agency (1975).

(9-4) Haley, T.J., *Benzidine Revisited: A Review of The Literature and Problems Associated With the Use of Benzidine and Its Congeners; Clin. Toxicol.* 8, 13 (1975).

(9-5) Zavon, M.R. et al, "Benzidine exposure as a cause of bladder tumors," *Arch. Environ. Health* 27, 1 (1973).

BENZO[a]ANTHRACENE

See "Polynuclear Aromatic Hydrocarbons" (55).

3,4-BENZOFLUORANTHENE

See "Polynuclear Aromatic Hydrocarbons" (55).

BENZO[k]FLUORANTHENE

See "Polynuclear Aromatic Hydrocarbons" (55).

BENZO[ghi]PERYLENE

See "Polynuclear Aromatic Hydrocarbons" (55).

BENZO[a]PYRENE

See "Polynuclear Aromatic Hydrocarbons" (55).

BERYLLIUM (#10)

Beryllium, symbol Be, is an element in Group II of the Periodic Table. It has an atomic number of 4 and an atomic weight of 9.013.

Occurrence: Beryllium has been identified in 5.4% of 1,577 U.S. surface waters at concentrations ranging from 0.01 to 1.22 μg/l, with a mean of 0.19 μg/l (10-1). The major source of beryllium in the environment is the combustion of fossil fuels (10-2). Beryllium enters the waterways through weathering of rocks and soils, through atmospheric fallout and through discharges from industrial and municipal operations.

Physical Properties: Beryllium is a dark gray metal of the alkaline earth family. It is the only stable light metal. It has a SG of 1.85 and a high melting point of about 1285°C.

Chemical Properties: Beryllium forms chemical compounds in which its valence is +2. At acid pH it behaves as a cation but forms anionic complexes at pH greater than 8. The chemical properties of beryllium have been stated to be intermediate between those of magnesium and aluminum.

Uses: Beryllium is less dense than aluminum and is used in the production of light alloys, copper and brass. World production was reported as approximately 250 tons annually.

Toxic Effects: In the aquatic environment, beryllium is acutely toxic to fish at concentrations as low as 87 μg/l and chronically toxic to *Daphnia magna* at a concentration of less than 3 μg/l (10-3). Beryllium acute toxicity to fish is greatly affected by water quality. In very soft water, beryllium is reportedly more than 100 times as toxic as in very hard water. Beryllium has been reported to bioconcentrate to levels 1,000 times those of the surrounding water. Since beryllium is an element, it may be expected to persist indefinitely in the environment in some form.

Less than 50% of ingested beryllium was absorbed from the intestine of rats. Inhaled insoluble beryllium compounds are cleared from the lungs only slowly, if at all. Injected beryllium initially concentrates preferentially in liver and bone, but liver beryllium is gradually mobilized and transferred to the skeleton. Beryllium has been shown to inhibit several enzyme systems, including alkaline phosphatase, phosphoglucomutase, and potassium activated ATPase.

Beryllium has been reported to interfere with DNA metabolism in liver and to induce chromosomal and mitotic abnormalities. It has also been shown to increase misincorporation of nucleotides during polymerization by DNA polymerase.

Intravenously administered beryllium has been found to be either excreted in urine or deposited in kidney or bone. Cows injected with beryllium excreted little of it in their milk. The half life for beryllium in several species ranged from 890 days in rats to 1,770 days in monkeys.

The LD_{50} for intravenously injected beryllium has been reported to be as low as 0.44 mg/kg in rats. Ingested beryllium is much less toxic, with an oral LD_{50} of 9.7 mg/kg (10-4). Inhaled aerosols were acutely toxic to rats at 194 μg/m^3 and caused pathologic changes within 3 months at 42 μg/m^3.

In humans short-term exposure to beryllium oxide in air at 4 mg/m^3 produced a high incidence of disease and some fatalities. Acute disease in humans has been produced by as little as 100 μg/m^3. The National Academy of Sciences reported in 1958 that human exposure to air containing 25 μg/m^3 or less did not produce acute disease.

In one form or another beryllium causes ocular inflammation and contact dermatitis, rhinitis, pharyngitis, tracheobronchitis and acute pneumonitis. In animals beryllium has caused rachitic bone changes and osteosclerotic changes.

The onset of chronic toxicity in humans may follow exposure by as long as 5 years. Symptoms include pneumonitis with cough, chest pain, and general weakness (Hardy and Stoeckle, 1959). Systemic effects include right heart enlargement with cardiac failure, enlargement of liver and spleen, cyanosis, digital clubbing and kidney stones.

Beryllium has been implicated as a teratogen in snails and has inhibited limb regeneration in the salamander, *Amblystoma punctatum*.

Lung and bone cancers are firmly associated with beryllium exposure. While beryllium is known to cause these cancers when administered by inhalation or injection, it has not been shown to cause them by ingestion, although such studies have been conducted. While early human epidemiological studies were inconclusive, the bulk of more recent work supports the hypothesis that beryllium is a human carcinogen.

Current Levels of Exposure: Concentrations of beryllium in the water supplies tend to be quite low. For example, analysis of 1,577 samples from U.S. surface waters and lakes showed beryllium present in 5.4% of the samples with concentrations ranging from 0.01 to 1.22 μg/l with a mean of 0.19 μg/l (10-1). The concentration of beryllium in seawater was reported equal to 6 x 10^{-4} μg/l.

Measurements of beryllium in air samples collected from 100 stations of the National Air Sampling Network indicated that the average 24-hour concentration was less than 0.0005 μg/m^3. The maximum value recorded at these stations during 1964 to 1965 was 0.0008 μg/m^3. Thus, the maximum reported value was only 0.4% of the threshold limit value set by the American Conference of Governmental Industrial Hygienists in 1977. An average concentration of 0.0281 μg/m^3 was reported within one-half mile of a large beryllium plant near Reading, Pa. Concentrations closer to the plant reached 0.0827 μg/m^3.

Three brands of West German cigarettes were reported to contain beryllium levels of 0.47, 0.68, and 0.74 μg per cigarette with 4.5, 1.6, and 10.0% of the beryllium content, respectively, inhaled in the smoke. It was estimated that the total beryllium intake for humans was about 100 μg/day with only a minor fraction by inhalation. Analysis of lung tissue at autopsy, from persons with no known industrial exposure to beryllium, showed maximum concentrations of 1.98 μg/100 g tissue.

Special Groups at Risk: Studies such as those of Sterner and Eisenbud (10-5) have suggested that a small percentage of the population is sensitive to extremely low concentrations of beryllium in the air, probably through the development of an immune reaction. There is no evidence at present for the development of sensitivity to concentrations of beryllium present in food or water or that sensitivity to low levels of beryllium in the air is aggravated by ingestion of beryllium. No other special groups can be identified as special risks.

Existing Guidelines and Standards: Beryllium is the subject of a Criterion Document (10-6). The present standard for occupational exposure prescribes an 8-hour time weighted average of 2.0 μg/m^3 with a ceiling concentration of 5.0 μg/m^3. In addition, the present standard allows a peak concentration above the ceiling concentration of 25 μg/m^3 for a maximum duration of 30 minutes (10-6).

OSHA has since recommended (10-7) that occupational exposure to beryllium and its compounds not exceed 1 μg/m^3 (averaged over an 8-hour work day) and a ceiling limit of 5 μg/m^3 (measured over a 15-minute sampling period).

The threshold limit value (TLV) for beryllium was set at 2μg/m^3 by the American Conference of Governmental Industrial Hygienists (1979) with the notation that beryllium is "an industrial substance suspect of carcinogenic potential for man."

EPA National Emission Standards for Hazardous Air Pollutants set the criterion as: not more than 10 g in 24 hours or emissions which result in maximum outplant concentrations of 0.01 μg/m^3, 30-day average (10-4).

The EPA proposed a water quality standard of 11 μg/l for the protection of aquatic life in soft fresh water; 1,100 μg/l for the protection of aquatic life in hard fresh water; and 100 μg/l for continuous irrigation on all soils except 500 mg/l for irrigation on neutral to alkaline lime-textured soils (10-4). The NAS/NAE *Water Quality Criteria* (10-8) recommendation for marine aquatic life is: hazard level, 1.5 μg/l; minimal risk of deleterious effects, 0.1 mg/l; and application factor, 0.01 (applied to 96-hr LC_{50}). Their recommendation for irrigation water is 0.10 mg/l for continuous use on all soils.

Summary of Proposed EPA Criteria: *Freshwater Aquatic Life* — For beryllium the criterion to protect freshwater aquatic life as derived using the Guidelines is

$$e^{[1.24 \ln (\text{hardness}) - 6.65]}$$

as the 24-hour average concentration, and the concentration at any time should not exceed

$$e^{[1.24 \ln (\text{hardness}) - 1.46]}$$

Saltwater Aquatic Life — No criterion for beryllium can be derived using the Guidelines, and there are insufficient data to estimate a criterion using other procedures.

Human Health — For the maximum protection of human health from the potential carcinogenic effects of exposure to beryllium through ingestion of water and contaminated aquatic organisms, the ambient water concentration is zero. Concentrations of beryllium estimated to result in additional lifetime cancer risks ranging from no additional risk to an additional risk of 1 in 100,000 are presented in the Criterion Formulation section of this document. The EPA is considering setting criteria at an interim target risk level in the range of 10^{-5}, 10^{-6}, or 10^{-7} with corresponding criteria of 0.087 μg/l, 0.0087 μg/l, and 0.00087 μg/l, respectively.

Basis for the Proposed Human Health Criteria: Experiments have shown cancer by beryllium can be experimentally produced in laboratory animals. Cancer has been produced by inhalation, intratracheal instillation, and intravenous injection of beryllium. Beryllium chloride has been shown to increase the error frequency of nucleotide base incorporation into DNA in an in vitro assay designed to detect potential metal mutagen/carcinogens. Finally, evidence is accumulating that inhalation of beryllium may cause lung cancer in humans.

Epidemiological studies have failed to establish an incontrovertible link between beryllium exposure and human cancer, and cancer was not produced in one experimental study by ingestion of beryllium. However, beryllium has definitely been shown to induce osteosarcomas in rabbits following intravenous administration (10-9). Therefore, it is possible that cancer would be induced in humans if a large enough amount of beryllium were ingested. The occurrence of beryllium rickets after ingestion of food supplemented with beryllium sulfate shows that toxic amounts can be absorbed. In addition, Reeves (10-12) reported data that show that 0.35% of ingested beryllium is retained in the tissue of rats after 24 weeks of feeding.

The only experiments conducted to date in which beryllium was ingested over a long period of time were those of Schroeder and Mitchener (10-10)(10-11). Five ppm beryllium was added to the food and water of rats for a lifetime. Although Schroeder and Mitchener found no statistically significant difference in tumor frequency between controls and experimental rats and mice, there was a slight excess of lymphoma leukemias in the treated group compared to the controls.

The high frequency of osteosarcomas induced in rabbits given Be intravenously, the results of mutagenicity studies, and the ingestion-uptake-retention studies of Be, comprise a strong argument that Be-laden water poses a carcinogenic risk.

Although the Schroeder and Mitchener "lymphoma leukemia" experiment showed an effect significant at the 0.09 level, this result is sufficient to calculate a criterion level as long as it is remembered: (1) that it is not the Schroeder and Mitchener, but the previously mentioned results that establish that Be poses a carcinogenic risk to man, and that (2) EPA is relying on the Schroeder and Mitchener study (10-10)(10-11) because it is the only available data for oral ingestion from which a concentration range can be calculated. To extrapolate from the Be studies where the route of administration was by injection would yield a lower, and, EPA believes, less valid number for oral ingestion.

Under the Consent Decree in *NRDC vs Train*, criteria are to state "recommended maximum permissible concentrations (including where appropriate, zero) consistent with the protection of aquatic organisms, human health, and recreational activities." Beryllium is suspected of being a human carcinogen. Because there is no recognized safe concentration for a human carcinogen, the recommended concentration of beryllium in water for maximum protection of human health is zero.

Because attaining a zero concentration level may be infeasible in some cases and in order to assist the EPA and States in the possible future development of water quality regulations, the concentrations of beryllium corresponding to several incremental lifetime cancer risk levels have been estimated. A cancer risk level provides an estimate of the additional incidence of cancer that may be expected in an exposed population. A risk of 10^{-5}, for example, indicates a probability of one additional case of cancer for every 100,000 people exposed, a risk of 10^{-6} indicates one additional case of cancer for every million people exposed.

In the *Federal Register* notice of availability of draft ambient water quality criteria, EPA stated that it is considering setting criteria at an interim target risk level of 10^{-5}, 10^{-6} or 10^{-7} as shown in Table 22 below. In the table, the risk levels are calculated by applying a modified "one-hit extrapolation model described in the Methodology Document to the animal bioassay data presented in Appendix I. Since the extrapolation model is linear at low doses, the additional lifetime risk is directly proportional to the water concentration. Therefore, water concentrations corresponding to other risk levels can be derived by multiplying or dividing one of the risk levels and corresponding water concentrations shown in the table by factors such as 10, 100, 1,000, etc.

Table 22: Possible Alternative Criteria for Beryllium

Exposure Assumptions (per day)	Risk Levels and Corresponding Criteria, μg/l			
	0	10^{-7}	10^{-6}	10^{-5}
2 liters of drinking water and consumption of 18.7 grams fish and shellfish*	0	0.00087	0.0087	0.087
Consumption of fish and shellfish only	0	0.0056	0.056	0.56

*15% of the beryllium exposure results from the consumption of aquatic organisms which exhibit an average bioconcentration potential of 19-fold. The remaining 85% of beryllium exposure results from drinking water.

Concentration levels were derived assuming a lifetime exposure to various amounts of beryllium, (1) occurring from the consumption of both drinking water and aquatic life grown in waters containing the corresponding beryllium concentrations and, (2) occurring solely from consumption of aquatic life grown in the waters containing the corresponding beryllium concentrations. Because data indicating other sources of beryllium exposure and their contributions to total body burden are inadequate for quantitative use, the figures reflect the incremental risks associated with the indicated routes only.

Summary of Pertinent Data —Although beryllium was shown to produce bone osteosarcomas at an extremely low dose via intravenous injection, the experiments of Schroeder and Mitchener (10-10) on rats and mice at 5 ppm in drinking water induced no observed carcinogenic response, except for a small statistically insignificant excess rate of "lymphoma leukemias" in female mice and in grossly observed tumors of all sites in male rats. The small absorption from the gastrointestinal tract is presumably the reason for the lack of significant effect. If beryllium is carcinogenic via ingestion it must be less potent than observed by Schroeder and Mitchener (10-10). Therefore, that experiment can be used to estimate the maximum risk that beryllium could pose, or equivalently, the lowest concentration which leads to a 10^{-5} lifetime risk.

In the male rats given 5 ppm in the drinking water, 9 out of 33 treated animals had grossly observed tumors of some type, whereas 4 out of 26 controls had tumors. With a bioaccumulation factor of 1.0, the parameters of the extrapolation model are: $n_t = 9$; $N_t = 33$; $n_c = 4$; $N_c = 26$; Le = 1,126 days; le = 1,126 days; d = 5 ppm x 0.05 = 0.25 mg/kg/day; L = 1,126 days; w = 0.385 kg; and R = 19.0.

The result is that the water concentration does not need to get any lower than 0.087 μg/l in order to keep the lifetime risk below 10^{-5}.

References

(10-1)   Kopp, J.F. and Kroner, R.C., *A five year study of trace metals in waters of the United States*, Fed. Water Pollut. Control Admin., U.S. Dep. Inter., Cincinnati, Ohio (1967).

(10-2)   Tepper, L.B., "Beryllium," *CRC Crit. Rev. Toxicol.* 1, 235 (1972).

(10-3)   U.S. Environmental Protection Agency, *In-Depth Studies on Health and Environmental Impacts of Selected Water Pollutants*, Wash., D.C. (1978).

(10-4)   U.S. EPA, *Multimedia environmental goals for environmental assessment. Vol. II MEG charts and background information*, Report No. EPA-60017-77-136b, Wash., D.C., U.S. Environ. Prot. Agency (1977).

(10-5)   Sterner, J.H. and Eisenbud, M., "Epidemiology and beryllium intoxication," *Arch. Ind. Hyg.*, Occup. Med. 4, 123 (1951).

(10-6)   National Institute for Occupational Safety and Health, *Criteria for a Recommended Standard: Occupational Exposure to Beryllium*, NIOSH Doc. No. 72-10268, Wash., D.C. (1972).

(10-7)   Occupational Safety and Health Admin., *Proposed Standard for Occupational Exposure to Beryllium*, Wash., D.C. (1977).

(10-8)   National Academy of Sciences/National Academy of Engineering, *Water Quality Criteria*, Wash., D.C. (1972).

(10-9)   Cloudman, A.M., et al, "Bone changes following intravenous injections of beryllium," *Am. Jour. Pathol.*, 25, 810 (1949).

(10-10) Schroeder, H.A. and Mitchener, M., "Life-term studies in rats: effects of aluminum, barium, beryllium and tungsten," *Jour. Nutr.* 105, 420 (1975).

(10-11) Schroeder, H.A. & Mitchener, M., "Life-term effects of mercury, methylmercury and nine other trace metals on mice," *Jour. Nutr.* 105, 452 (1975).

(10-12) Reeves, A.L., "Absorption of beryllium from the gastrointestinal tract," *AMA Arch. Envir. Health* 11, 209 (1965).

BHC

See "Hexachlorocyclohexane" (41).

BIS(2-CHLOROETHOXY)METHANE

See "Haloethers" (37).

BIS(2-CHLOROETHYL) ETHER

See "Chloroalkyl Ethers" (16).

BIS(2-CHLOROISOPROPYL) ETHER

See "Haloethers" (37).

BIS(CHLOROMETHYL) ETHER

See "Chloroalkyl Ethers" (16).

BIS(2-ETHYLHEXYL) PHTHALATE

See "Phthalate Esters" (53).

BROMOFORM

See "Halomethanes" (38).

4-BROMOPHENYL PHENYL ETHER

See "Haloethers" (37).

BUTYL BENZYL PHTHALATE

See "Phthalate Esters" (53).

C

CADMIUM (#11)

Cadmium, symbol Cd, is an element in Group II of the Periodic Table. It has an atomic number of 48 and an atomic weight of 112.41.

Occurrence: Most freshwaters in the United States contain less than 1 μg per liter of cadmium, although levels as high as 120 μg per liter have been reported. Cadmium reaches waterways as fallout from air and in effluents from pigments, plastics, alloys and other manufacturing operations as well as from municipal effluents. Cadmium is strongly adsorbed to clays, muds, humic and organic materials and some hydrous oxides, all of which tend to remove it from the water column by precipitation.

Physical Properties: Cadmium is a soft, white metal with a density of 8.65 and a melting point of 321°C. The solubility of cadmium compounds in water depends on the nature of the compounds and on water quality.

Chemical Properties: Cadmium dissolves readily in mineral acids. Cadmium is precipitated from solution by carbonate, hydroxide and sulfide ions and forms soluble complexes with other anions.

Uses: Cadmium is used in electroplating, paint and pigment manufacture and as a stabilizer in plastics manufacture. (11-1).

Toxic Effects: In the aquatic environment, cadmium is acutely toxic to fish at concentrations as low as about 1 μg per liter (11-2, 11-3). Chronic toxicity to fish has been reported at approximately the same levels (11-4). Water quality also affects cadmium toxicity independent of its effect on solubility. Tabata (11-5) and Carroll, et al (11-3), have shown that in acute tests calcium ion protects fishes against cadmium toxicity. Cadmium has been reported to bioconcentrate in fish tissues to levels 2,000 times as great as those of ambient waters (11-6). Since cadmium is an element, it will not be destroyed and may be expected to persist indefinitely in the environment in some form.

Cadmium tends to accumulate in liver and kidney of exposed organisms. In humans the threshold for kidney dysfunction is about 200 mg/kg in the renal cortex (11-7). Cadmium has been identified as a cause of Itai-Itai disease in Japan and has been implicated as a mutagen and carcinogen (11-8).

Current Levels of Exposure: Food represents the major route of human exposure, with air contributing only a negligible amount to the total intake, except in tobacco smokers. Drinking water normally would account for less than 10% of the daily total absorption for the vast majority of the population. Percutaneous absorption is inconsequential.

It is recognized that approximately 100,000 Americans have potential occupational exposure to cadmium. The spectrum of occupational exposure varies from negligible to those situations producing acute and/or chronic toxicity and even death. While efforts are being made by those in occupational health to reduce exposure to a minimum and eliminate adverse health effects, it must be recognized that no general environmental standard can prevent damage from overexposure in the occupational setting.

Special Groups at Risk: Persons with severe nutritional deficiency, i.e., calcium, zinc, protein, vitamin C and D, etc., which may be aggravated by cadmium are conceivably at special risk, although human data concerning these effects are scant. Such a risk is obviously additive since these deficiencies can in and of themselves be sufficient to cause disability and/or fatal disease. Obviously, persons in such precarious physiologic balance are particularly vulnerable to a wide variety of biologic and chemical hazards.

Some persons with diets that are adequate in terms of vital nutrients, calories, etc., but who subsist on otherwise skewed diets such as vegetarians or those eating unusual quantities of visceral meats, fish, or seafoods, which can contain rather large amounts of cadmium, may also be at increased risk. The additional risk to such population groups posed by an additional exposure increment from ambient cadmium remains to be assessed.

Existing Guidelines and Standards: Numerous domestic official agencies, foreign governments, and private parties have suggested standards or limits for cadmium in various environmental media. The more germane of these are presented in Table 23. In the following table, estimated permissible concentration of WH1 is derived from the assumption that the maximum daily safe dosage results from 24 hour exposure to air containing the estimated permissible concentration in air, assuming 100% absorption and that the same dose is therefore permissible in the volume of water consumed per day; WH2 is the estimated permissible concentration of the substance in water, based on considerations of the safe maximum body concentration and the biological half-life of the substance.

Table 23: Cadmium—Regulatory Standards, Limits, or Criteria for Human Health Protection

Regulatory Standards	. . . . Media		
	Air (Inhalation) (μg/m^3)	Water (Ingestion) (μg/l)	Food (Ingestion) (μg/ml)
OSHA (1974)	100*	—	—
NIOSH (1977)	40 (11-11)	—	—
EPA (1975)	—	10**	—
FDA (1978)	—	—	0.5***
WHO (1971)	—	10**	—
ACGIH (1977)	50†	—	—
MEG/EPC (1977)	0.12	WH1-1.9	—
	—	WH2-0.7	—
NAS/NAE (1972)	—	10	—
USSR (suggested)††	—	1	—
Canada (1968)	—	10	—
Ohio†††	—	5 (streams)	—

*For cadmium fume. Limit for cadmium dust is 200 μg/m^3.
**μg/ml.
***Based on ceramic pottery and enamelware leaching solution test.
†Cadmium oxide production is noted as "Industrial Substances Suspect of Carcinogenic Potential for Man."
††Krasovskii, G.N., et al (11-9).
†††Lykins, B.W., Jr. and Smith, J.M. (11-10).

Source: Reference (11)

Summary of Proposed EPA Criteria: *Freshwater Aquatic Life* — For cadmium the criterion to protect freshwater aquatic life as derived using the guidelines is:

$$e^{[0.87 \ln (\text{hardness}) - 4.38]}$$

as a 24 hour average. Cadmium concentration should not exceed the following at any time.

$$e^{[1.30 \ln (\text{hardness}) - 3.92]}$$

Saltwater Aquatic Life — For cadmium the criterion to protect saltwater aquatic life as derived using the guidelines is: 1.0 μg per liter as a 24 hour average and the concentration should not exceed 16 μg per liter at any time.

Human Health — For the protection of human health from the toxic properties of cadmium ingested through water and through contaminated aquatic organisms, the ambient water criterion is determined to be 10 μg per liter.

Basis for the Proposed Human Health Criteria: There is no doubt that cadmium is a teratogen in several rodent species when given in large parenteral doses. Doses of this magnitude (4 to 12 mg/kg) would surely produce severe, if not fatal toxic symptoms in man. In the human only small amounts of cadmium cross the placental barrier.

Only one report from Russia suggests any effect, i.e., low birth weight and several children with rickets or dental trouble. Details are lacking in this report and it should not be construed as implicating cadmium without further data.

The studies of whether cadmium is mutagenic are inconsistent. The reports of chromosomal aberrations in both Itai-Itai patients and cadmium workers are conflicting. Dominant lethal studies have been negative as are tests for spermatocytic chromosome aberrations in male mice and their first-generation offspring. Studies of mutagenic activity in nonmammalian life forms have given inconsistent results.

There is no question that the injection of cadmium into rodents results in injection-site sarcomas and interstitial cell tumors of the testis. Sarcoma production in rats is a common sequela to the injection of irritants and could be regarded as a nonspecific response to fibroblast injury. Interstitial tumors appear to result from the hyperplasia and metaplasia of tissue regeneration following vascular mediated testicular damage. There is no evidence that these tumors are malignant neoplasms; however, this does not refute the tumorigenic potential of cadmium.

The human evidence for the carcinogenicity of cadmium is conjectural, based on very small numbers, and confounded by exposures to other elements which are known to be human carcinogens. The reports on British battery workers and the work of Lemen, et al, (11-12) suggest an increase in prostrate and lung cancer. These men were also exposed to nickel and/or arsenic, but in amounts of approximately $\frac{1}{100}$ of cadmium exposure level.

Kolonel's work (11-13) confirmed neither of these sites, but suggested an association with renal cancer. This work is inadequate in that it assumes an exposure to cadmium based upon an occupational questionnaire. There have be no case reports of renal cancer in known cadmium-exposed workers. Cigarette smoking would appear to have a firmer association with renal neoplasia, rather than cadmium. The geographic distribution of prostate cancer (Japan, Sweden, USA) suggests that an inverse relationship exists to cadmium exposure. From the known mortality study data cited, it might be argued that cadmium exposure reduces general mortality or is a potent protective factor against cardiovascular disease. The case for cadmium as a carcinogen is not persuasive when the existing data are critically reviewed, but it has been viewed by some as suggestive from the public health perspective.

It is not recommended that cadmium be considered a suspect human carcinogen for purposes of calculating a water quality criterion. However, the weight of evidence for oncogenic potential of cadmium is sufficient to be qualitatively suggestive and is not to be ignored from a public health point of view. The EPA Carcinogen Assessment Group has reviewed cadmium and their summary is included in the appendices of the criteria document (11).

The criterion is based on established health effects. The data implicating cadmium as a cause of emphysema and renal tubular proteinuria is firmly established. Emphysema has been reported only after airborne exposures and has been documented for both man and animal. It would seem to result from a direct effect upon lung tissue of which cadmium salts are known irritants.

There is evidence from occupational studies that the kidney is more sensitive to the effects of cadmium than the lung. In exposed workers proteinuria occurs in higher incidence and in a shorter time period than emphysema. It seems entirely justified to conclude that the kidney is the critical target organ.

It is generally accepted that the critical cadmium level at which renal dysfunction occurs is approximately 200 μg/g wet weight of renal cortex. Autopsy studies indicate that the average kidney concentration in nonsmokers is approximately $\frac{1}{12}$ this level. In smokers, the concentration is about twice as high, i.e., 30 to 39 μg/g.

Friberg (11-7) has estimated that the critical level is reached at daily ingestion levels of 250 to 350 μg per day over 50 years. Since the average, nonoccupationally exposed American probably does not have an intake from all sources exceeding 25 to 50 μg, there would again seem to be a reasonable safety factor of 5 to 12 in existence. While this is not the comfortable margin of many orders of magnitude usually recommended by toxicologists, it should provide a margin of safety to the general public for the foreseeable future.

NIOSH (11-11) recommends that workers should not be exposed to airborne cadmium at a concentration greater than 40 μg/m^3 as a time weighted exposure for up to a 40 hour work week. This standard is designed to protect the health and safety of workers over an entire working lifetime. Compliance should prevent adverse effects on the health of the worker. Several studies have indicated no adverse effects at levels of 31 and 16 to 29 μg/m^3.

Effects of renal function (proteinuria) and a reduction in mean pulmonary function have been noted at levels of 66 μg/m^3, although some of these workers probably had experienced exposure, at least intermittently to cadmium fume at higher, but unknown concentrations. The limit of 40 μg/m^3 offers a greater and probably sufficient margin of safety, in comparison with the 50 μg/m^3 recommended by ACGIH and Lauwerys, et al (11-14).

From the figure 40 μg/m^3 it can be calculated that a worker might absorb about 1,000 μg during a work week, i.e., 40 μg/m^3 x 10 m^3 inhaled per day x 5 days x 0.5 (lung absorption rate). This is approximately 286 μg per day intake and 143 μg per day absorbed. To this the average daily intake from food and general environmental sources can be added, i.e., 10 to 50 μg. This suggests that an exposed worker may have an approximate intake of 300 μg/per day and still be safe. However, a healthy worker may not be representative of the American population as a whole.

From Japanese dietary intake data where Itai-Itai disease is prevalent, and studies on the age-specific incidence of proteinuria, it is possible to estimate a no-effect level for ingested cadmium. In areas where Itai-Itai disease is most common, about 85% of the daily cadmium intake is derived from rice, the locally grown grain staple.

Nogawa, et al, (11-15) have shown that the prevalence of tubular proteinuria, as measured by retinol binding protein excretion in persons under age 70, does not begin to rise above that seen in control populations until the cadmium levels in rice exceed 0.40 to 0.49 μg/g. The Japanese diet in the area of endemic Itai-Itai disease and even in the homes of patients with the disease are precisely known.

Approximately 2,100 calories are consumed daily, with carbohydrate accounting for about 1,725 calories daily, which is equivalent to the ingestion of 430 g per day. The no-effect level for Japanese can be calculated as follows:

$$\frac{430 \text{ g/day} \times 0.45 \text{ }\mu\text{g/g (rice)}}{0.85} = 228 \text{ }\mu\text{g/day}$$

This Japanese figure is slightly below the estimate of 250 μg per day given by Friberg (11-7) as an effect level. The no-effect level for a western European or American population with correspondingly larger body size would be expected to be somewhat greater, i.e., 301 μg per day.

The Working Group of Experts for the Commission of European Communities (11-16) has estimated the threshold effect level of cadmium by ingestion at around 200 μg daily, corresponding to an actual absorption of 12 μg per day. For smokers this estimate is reduced by about 1.0 to 10.1 μg, which corresponds to an oral intake of 169 μg. Using a second approach based on metabolic modeling of the above type, this same group derived a threshold effect level of 248 μg daily when pulmonary absorption is negligible.

Using the data presented in this and preceding sections of the document, it is possible to construct several exposure scenarios encompassing possible best-to-worse case exposure situations that might be domestically encountered, as shown in Table 24.

Table 24: Alternative Scenarios for Cadmium Exposure

Exposure Sources	Exposure	Cd Intake/Day (μg)	Absorption Factor*	Cd Retention/Day (μg)
Worst Case**				
Air—occupational	0.1 mg/m^3	714.0	0.5	357.0
Air—ambient	400 μg/m^3	8.0	0.5	4.0
Air—smoking (3 packs)	3.0 μg/pack	9.0	0.5	4.5
Food	–	75.0	0.1	7.5
Drinking water	10 μg/l	20.0	0.1	2.0
Total	–	826.0	–	375.0
Average Case				
Air—ambient	0.03 μg/m^3	0.60	0.25	0.150
Air—smoking (1 pack)	3.0 μg/pack	3.00	0.25	0.750
Food	–	30.00	0.05	1.500
Drinking water	1.3 μg/l	2.60	0.05	0.130
Total	–	36.20	–	2.530
Best Case***				
Air—ambient	0.001 μg/m^3	0.02	0.25	0.005
Food	–	12.00	0.05	0.600
Water	0.5 μg/l†	1.00	0.05	0.050
Total	–	13.02	–	0.655

*These absorption factors are considered to be the most realistic available.
**Maximally exposed persons.
***Minimally exposed persons.
†Average for both sexes excluding drinking water.

Source: Reference (11)

From these scenarios it can be calculated that ingested water contributes relatively little to the daily retained cadmium entering the body, i.e., 0.53, 5.1 and 7.6%, respectively for the worst, average and best cases. Water could become a significant contributor to all over cadmium intake and retention only if the scenarios are reconstructed by substituting the worst case water data for that in the average and best cases. However, even in the very unlikely event that such situations occur, the total cadmium intake and retention remain comparatively modest, i.e., 53.6 μg per day intake and 4.4 μg per day retained in the average case. The totals for the best case substitution are substantially less, i.e., 32.02 μg per day intake and 2.605 μg per day retention. Therefore, it may be concluded that there are no circumstances in which ambient waters meeting current drinking water standards pose a threat to human health.

Based on the foregoing data and discussion, it seems entirely justifiable to conclude that water constitutes only a relatively minor portion of man's daily cadmium intake. From the above analysis it is obvious (average case scenario) that drinking water contributes substantially less to human cadmium intake and/or retention than smoking a package of cigarettes daily. From this analysis, it appears that a water criterion needs to be more stringent than the existing Primary Drinking Water Standard (10 μg per liter) to provide ample protection of human health.

References:

(11-1) Fulkerson, W. and Goeller, H.E., eds., *Cadmium the dissipated element,* Oak Ridge Natl. Lab., Oak Ridge, Tenn. (1973).

(11-2) Eaton, J., et al, "Metal toxicity to embryos and larvae of seven freshwater fish species", *Bull. Environ. Contam. Toxicol.* (In Press-1979).

(11-3) Carroll, J.J., et al, "Influences of hardness constituents on the acute toxicity of cadmium to brook trout *(Salvelinus fontinalis)*", *Bull. Environ. Contam. Toxicol.* (In Press-1979).

(11-4) Sauter, et al, *Effects of exposure to heavy metals on selected freshwater fish: Toxicity of copper, cadmium, chromium and lead to eggs and fry of seven fish species,* Ecol. Res. Ser. Report No. 600/3-76-105, U.S. Environ. Prot. Agency, Washington, D.C. (1976).

(11-5) Tabata, K., "Studies on the toxicity of heavy metals to aquatic animals and factors that decrease such toxicity-II; The antagonistic action of water hardness on the toxicity of heavy metal ions", *Bull. Tokai Reg. Fish. Res. Lab.,* 58, 215 (1969).

(11-6) Spehar, R.L., "Cadmium and zinc toxicity to flagfish, *Jordanella floridae*", *Jour. Fish Res. Board Can.,* 33, 1939 (1976).

(11-7) Friberg, L., et al, *Cadmium in the environment,* 2nd ed., Cleveland, Ohio, CRC Press (1974).

(11-8) 42 *FR* 56575 (Oct. 26, 1977).

(11-9) Krasovskii, G.N., et al, "Toxic and gonadotropic effects of cadmium and boron relative to standards for these substances in drinking water", *Environ. Health Perspect.* 13, 69 (1976).

(11-10) Lykins, B.W., Jr. and Smith, J.M., *Interim report on the impact of public law 92-500 on municipal pollution control technology,* Report EPA-600/2-76-018, U.S. Environ. Prot. Agency, Washington, D.C. (1976).

(11-11) National Institute for Occupational Safety and Health, *Criteria for a recommended standard: occupational exposure to cadmium,* NIOSH Doc. No. 76-192, Washington, D.C. (1976).

(11-12) Lemen, R.A., et al, "Cancer mortality among cadmium production workers", *Ann. N.Y. Acad. Sci.* 271, 273 (1976).

(11-13) Kolonel, L.N., "Association of cadmium with renal cancer", *Cancer* 37, 1782 (1976).

(11-14) Lauwerys, R., et al, "Placental transfer of lead, mercury, cadmium and carbon monoxide in women, I, comparison of the frequency distribution of the biological indices in maternal and umbilical cord blood", *Environ. Res.* 15, 278 (1978).

(11-15) Nogawa, K., et al, "Statistical observations of the dose-response relationships of cadmium based on epidemiological studies in the Kakehashi River basin, *Envir. Res.* 15, 185 (1978).

(11-16) Commission of the European Communities, *Criteria (Dose-Effect Relationships) for Cadmium,* New York, Pergamon Press (1978).

CARBON TETRACHLORIDE (#12)

Carbon tetrachloride, CCl_4, is the simplest perchlorinated compound. For other chloromethanes, the reader is also referred to the sections of this volume on Chloroform (19) and Halomethanes (38).

Occurrence: Carbon tetrachloride has been found in many sampled waters at levels below 1 μg per liter (12-1). Data obtained from 80 municipalities show levels of CCl_4 in finished drinking waters of 2 to 3 μg per liter and levels of CCl_4 in corresponding raw waters of 2 to 4 μg per liter (12-2). These data indicate that CCl_4 is not produced in finished drinking water as a result of the chlorination process (12-3, 12-4). Accidental CCl_4 spills have occurred and as much as 63.6 metric tons were discharged into the Ohio River in February 1977 with resulting surface water concentrations as high as 340 μg per liter.

Physical Properties: Carbon tetrachloride (tetrachloromethane, perchloromethane) has a molecular weight of 153.82, a $-22.99°C$ MP, and a $76.54°C$ BP (Weast, 1972). It is a heavy (1.594 g/ml density), colorless liquid at room temperature. The compound is relatively nonpolar and miscible with alcohol, acetone and most organic solvents. The solubility in water is 800,000 μg per liter at $25°C$ and its vapor pressure is 55.65 mm Hg at $10°C$. It has an octanol/water partitioning coefficient of 2.73.

Chemical Properties: Carbon tetrachloride may be quite stable under certain environmental conditions and the hydrolytic breakdown of carbon tetrachloride in water is estimated to to require 70,000 years for 50% decomposition. This decomposition is considerably accelerated in the presence of metals such as iron.

Uses: Carbon tetrachloride (CCl_4) is a haloalkane with a wide range of industrial and chemical applications. Approximately 423,000 metric tons (932.7 million pounds) are produced at 11 plant sites in the U.S. The bulk of this production is used in the manufacture of fluorocarbons (95% in 1973) which are used primarily as aerosol propellants. However, the demand for carbon tetrachloride is expected to decrease as the use of aerosol products decreases. Other uses of carbon tetrachloride include grain fumigation, where it is being largely replaced by other registered pesticide products; a component of fire extinguisher solutions; an industrial and chemical solvent; and a degreaser in the dry cleaning industry, where it has been largely replaced by perchloroethylene. Carbon tetrachloride also has been used as a deworming agent and an anaesthetic, but because of adverse toxicity, these uses have been discontinued.

Toxic Effects: Carbon tetrachloride produces acute and chronic toxic effects on freshwater vertebrates and acute toxic effects on freshwater invertebrates. Carbon tetrachloride also produces acute toxic effects on saltwater vertebrate species. Carbon tetrachloride has induced fish tumors in trout when the fish were exposed to the toxicant via their food.

Toxicological data for nonhuman mammals are extensive and show that the halocarbon causes liver and kidney damage (12-5, 12-6), biochemical changes in liver function (12-7), neurological damage (12-8), and liver cancer (12-9, 12-10, 12-11).

Levels of carbon tetrachloride found in aquatic organisms range from 3 to 209 μg/kg (dry weight basis) (12-12), with bioconcentration factors for the whole organisms (wet weight basis) ranging from 10 to 100 (12-13). Upon depuration by placing CCl_4 contaminated bluegills in toxicant-free water, CCl_4 residues were reduced by 50% in 24 hours.

McConnell, et al (12-1) cite the total levels of CCl_4 and trichloroethane in human tissues as from less than 1 μg/kg in the brain to 24 μg/kg in adipose tissue and conclude that there is no evidence that biomagnification via the food chain to higher trophic levels occurs to any significant extent with carbon tetrachloride.

Current Levels of Exposure: Carbon tetrachloride has been found in some waters. An EPA survey of drinking water in the U.S. revealed that 10% of the supplies surveyed had 2.4 to 6.4 μg per liter CCl_4.

Carbon tetrachloride (CCl_4) has been found in a variety of foodstuffs ranging from 1 to 20 μg/kg. Residues have been found in commercially fumigated wheat, corn, and milo in amounts ranging from 2.9 to 20.4 mg/kg after storage for 1 to 3 hours. Carbon tetrachloride residues ranging from 20 to 62 mg/kg were found in sacks of wheat following fumigation with a mixture ratio of CCl_4-EDC-EDB (10.2:8:1 by weight), and then aerated for several weeks. Residues as high as 72.6 mg/kg after 1 week of aeration were detected in wheat. After 7 weeks of aeration, 3.2 mg/kg were found. Flour made from this wheat had residues of 0.20 to 0.93 mg/kg. Amounts of CCl_4 detected in bread made from this wheat ranged from 0.04 to 0.13 mg/kg for wheat aerated for 3 days and 0.01 to 0.2 mg/kg for wheat aerated for 7 weeks.

The most extensive measurements of CCl_4 have occurred in the atmosphere. Concentrations do not vary globally since CCl_4 has been released into the atmosphere for such a long time period. Virtually no variation has been found between land and ocean, urban and rural, or northern and southern hemispheres. The maximum value detected was 0.117 mg/m^3 in Bayonne, N.J.; however, normal background levels range from 0.00078 to 0.00091 mg/m^3 in the continental and marine air masses.

The National Research Council (1978) in its assessment of nonfluorinated halomethanes in the environment (12-4) estimated total human exposure to CCl_4. Using drinking water concentrations of less than 2.0 to 3.0 μg per liter and other conventional assumptions regarding human and environmental conditions, three ranges of exposure were estimated.

Minimum, typical and maximum exposure estimates of total CCl_4 uptake were 4.54, 7.70 and 629 mg per year, respectively. The percentage contribution from fluid sources (water) was 16, 23 and 0.6%, respectively. By far the highest uptake of CCl_4 was estimated to come from atmospheric sources, 62 to 98%.

Although monitoring has provided more information on CCl_4 presence in the environment than most chemicals, there remain many relative unknowns about absorption, synergism-antagonism, etc. The estimated CCl_4 exposure from food sources is based upon only limited information compared to air and fluid uptakes. At face value, the figures indicate that while none of the three routes of exposure are negligible, inhalation is most important for CCl_4.

Special Groups at Risk: Based on the studies performed on animals, it appears as though older animals are more susceptible to the toxic effects of CCl_4 than are younger animals (12-11). Also, male animals are more susceptible than females. Age and sex have been examined as factors of CCl_4 toxicity. The findings revealed that female rats are less susceptible to the ill effects of different hepatotoxic agents and fare better than males because of different hormonal and enzyme patterns and the lack of certain proteins as compared to the male liver. The sex difference noticed in adult rats was not so apparent in young rats.

The synergistic effects of alcohol and cold must also be noted. Alcoholics have a greater susceptibility to poisoning from CCl_4. The frequent occurrence of a history of alcoholism in cases of fatal CCl_4 poisoning indicates a synergistic nephrotoxic as well as hepatotoxic effect between alcohol and CCl_4.

Finally, very obese and under-nourished persons suffering from pulmonary diseases, gastric ulcers or a tendency to vomiting, liver or kidney diseases, diabetes or glandular disturbances are especially sensitive to the toxic effects of CCl_4.

Existing Guidelines and Standards: There is neither a water standard nor an air standard for CCl_4; however, a number of standards have been recommended for inhalation in the work environment. NIOSH (12-14) has summarized the history of these standards.

Permissible Levels of Toxic Substances in the Working Environment for many countries was published by the International Labor Office in 1970. The reported carbon tetrachloride standards are presented in Table 25. The USSR values (MAC) are absolute values never to be exceeded. They are set at a value which will not be expected to produce in any exposed person any disease or other detectable deviation from normal. Some other countries tend to follow this concept in setting their standards, while still others tend to follow the concepts of the ACGIH. The intent is indicated from some of the standards presented in the table.

Table 25: Carbon Tetrachloride Inhalation Standards of Ten Countries

Country	Standard (mg/m^3)	Qualifications
Czechoslovakia	50	Normal MAC
	250	Single short exposure
Finland	160	8 hours continuous exposure
Hungary	20	8-hour average
	100	30 minutes
Japan	10	—
Poland	20	—
Rumania	50	—
UAR and SAR	625	—
USSR	20	MAC
Yugoslavia	65	—

Source: Reference (12)

The Occupational Safety and Health Administration, U.S. Department of Labor, adopted the American National Standards Institute (ANSI) standard Z37.17-1967 (1967) as the Federal standard for carbon tetrachloride (29 CFR 1910.1000). This standard is 10 mg/m^3 for an 8 hour TWA exposure, with an acceptable ceiling exposure concentration of 25 mg/m^3, and an acceptable maximum peak above the acceptable ceiling concentration for an 8 hour shift of 200 mg/m^3 for 5 minutes in any 4 hours. Finally, a standard decided upon by the FAO/WHO Expert Committee is 50 μg/kg for cooked cereal products.

Summary of Proposed EPA Criteria: *Freshwater Aquatic Life* — For carbon tetrachloride, the criterion to protect freshwater aquatic life, as derived using procedures other than the guidelines, is 620 μg per liter as a 24 hour average and the concentration should never exceed 1,400 μg per liter at any time.

Saltwater Aquatic Life — For carbon tetrachloride, the criterion to protect saltwater aquatic life, as derived using procedures other than guidelines, is 2,000 μg per liter as a 24 hour average and the concentration should never exceed 4,600 μg per liter at any time.

Human Health — For the maximum protection of human health from the potential carcinogenic effects of exposure to carbon tetrachloride through ingestion of water and contaminated aquatic organisms, the ambient water concentration is zero. Concentrations of carbon tetrachloride estimated to result in additional lifetime cancer risks ranging from no additional risk to an additional risk of 1 in 100,000 are presented in the Criterion Formulation section. The EPA is considering setting criteria at an interim target risk level in the range of 10^{-5}, 10^{-6}, or 10^{-7} with corresponding criteria of 2.6, 0.26 and 0.026 μg per liter, respectively.

Basis for the Proposed Human Health Criteria

Studies indicate that CCl_4 has a full spectrum of toxic effects. Historically, industrial and accidental exposures to CCl_4 by ingestion, inhalation and dermal routes have produced acute, subacute and chronic poisoning with fatalities. Generally speaking, acute toxicity for both man and animal can be characterized as nodular hyperplasia and cirrhosis of the liver and renal dysfunction. Mutagenic effects have not been observed and teratogenic effects have not been conclusively demonstrated.

The most significant effect to consider in terms of dose/response is the cancer-causing potential of the chemical. Current knowledge leads to the conclusion that carcinogenesis is a nonthreshold, nonreversible process. The nonthreshold concept implies that many tumors will be produced at high doses, but any dose, no matter how small, will have the probability of causing cancer. Even small carcinogenic risks have a serious impact on society when the exposed population is large, because it is likely that some cancers will be caused by exposure to CCl_4. The nonreversible concept implies that once the tumor growth process has started, growth will continue and may metastasize and involve other organs until death ensues.

There is a sufficient weight of evidence to conclude that CCl_4 is a carcinogen in laboratory animals and with appropriate assumptions is interpreted to be a suspect human carcinogen.

Under the consent decree in NRDC vs Train, criteria are to state "recommended maximum permissible concentrations (including where appropriate, zero) consistent with the protection of aquatic organisms, human health, and recreational activities". Carbon tetrachloride is suspected of being a human carcinogen. Because there is no recognized safe concentration for a human carcinogen, the appropriate concentration of carbon tetrachloride in water for maximum protection of human health is zero.

Because attaining a zero concentration level may be infeasible in some cases and in order to assist the EPA and U.S. in the possible future development of water quality regulations, the concentrations of carbon tetrachloride corresponding to several incremental lifetime cancer risk levels have been estimated.

A cancer risk level provides an estimate of the additional incidence of cancer that may be expected in an exposed population. A risk of 10^{-5}, for example, indicates a probability of one additional case of cancer for every 100,000 people exposed; a risk of 10^{-6} indicates one additional case of cancer for every million people exposed, and so forth.

In the *Federal Register* notice of availability of draft ambient water quality criteria, EPA stated that it is considering setting criteria at an interim target risk level of 10^{-5}, 10^{-6}, or 10^{-7} as shown in Table 26. In the table, the risk levels and corresponding criteria were calculated by applying a modified one-hit extrapolation model described in the Methodology Document to the animal bioassay data presented in Summary of Pertinent Data. Since the extrapolation model is linear at low doses, the additional lifetime risk is directly proportional to the water concentration. Therefore, water concentrations corresponding to other risk levels can be derived by multiplying or dividing one of the risk levels and corresponding water concentrations shown in the table by factors such as 10, 100, 1,000, and so forth.

Table 26: Possible Alternative Criteria for CCl_4

Exposure Assumptions (per day)	Risk Levels and Corresponding Criteria (μg/l)			
	0	10^{-7}	10^{-6}	10^{-5}
2 liters of drinking water and consumption of 18.7 grams fish and shellfish*	0	0.026	0.26	2.6
Consumption of fish and shellfish only	0	0.067	0.67	6.7

*Approximately 39% of the carbon tetrachloride exposure results from the consumption of aquatic organisms which exhibit an average bioconcentration potential of 69-fold. The remaining 61% of carbon tetrachloride exposure results from drinking water.

Source: Reference (12)

Concentration levels were derived assuming a lifetime exposure to various amounts of carbon tetrachloride (a) occurring from consumption of both drinking water and aquatic life grown in waters containing the corresponding carbon tetrachloride concentrations and (b) occurring solely from consumption of aquatic life grown in the waters containing the corresponding carbon tetrachloride concentrations. Although total exposure information for carbon tetrachloride is discussed and an estimate of the contributions from other sources of exposure can be made, this data will not be factored into ambient water quality criteria formulation until additional analysis can be made. The criteria presented, therefore, assume an incremental risk from ambient water exposure only.

References

(12-1) McConnell, G., et al, "Chlorinated hydrocarbons and the environment", *Endeavour* 34, 13 (1975).

(12-2) U.S. EPA, *Preliminary assessment of suspected carcinogens in drinking water,* Washington, D.C., Off. of Toxic Subst., U.S. Environ. Prot. Agency (1975).

(12-3) National Research Council, *Drinking water and health,* Washington, D.C., Natl. Acad. Sci. (1977).

(12-4) National Research Council, *Nonfluorinated halomethanes in the environment,* Washington, D.C., Natl. Acad. Sci. (1978).

(12-5) Klaassen, C.D. and Plaa, G.L., "Comparison of the biochemical alterations elicited in livers from rats treated with carbon tetrachloride, chloroform, 1,1,2-trichloroethane and 1,1,1-trichloroethane" *Biochem. Pharmacol.* 18, 2019 (1969).

(12-6) Nielsen, V.K. and Larsen, J., "Acute renal failure due to carbon tetrachloride poisoning", *Acta. Med. Scand.* 178, 363 (1965).

(12-7) Recknagel, R.O., et al, "New perspectives in the study of experimental carbon tetrachloride liver injury", In E.A. Ball, ed., *Liver,* Baltimore, Md., Williams & Wilkins (1973).

(12-8) Klaassen, C.D. and Plaa, G.L., "Relative effects of various chlorinated hydrocarbons on liver and kidney function in dogs", *Toxicol. Appl. Pharmacol.* 10, 119 (1967).

(12-9) Della Porta, G, et al, "Induction with carbon tetrachloride of liver-cell carcinomas in hamsters", *Jour. Natl. Cancer Inst.* 26, 4 (1961).

(12-10) National Cancer Institute, *Carcinogenesis bioassay of trichloroethylene,* Washington, D.C., U.S. Dep. Health Educ. Welfare (1976).

(12-11) Reuber, M.D. and Glover, E.L., "Cholangiofibrosis in the liver of buffalo strain rats injected with carbon tetrachloride", *Br. Jour. Exp. Pathol.* 48,319 (1967).

(12-12) Dickson, A.G. and Riley, J.P., "The distribution of short-chain halogenated aliphatic hydrocarbons in some marine organisms", *Mar. Pollut. Bull.* 7, 9 (1976).

(12-13) Pearson, C.R. and McConnell, G., "Chlorinated C_1 and C_2 hydrocarbons in the marine environment", *Proc. Roy. Soc. London B.* 189, 305 (1975).

(12-14) National Institute for Occupational Safety and Health, *Criteria for a Recommended Standard: Occupational Exposure to Carbon Tetrachloride,* NIOSH Doc. No. 76-133 (1976).

CHLORDANE (#13)

Chlordane is a polychlorinated compound having the structural formula:

It has the molecular formula: $C_{10}H_6Cl_8$ and a molecular weight of 409.8. The chemical name for chlordane is 1,2,4,5,6,7,8,8-octachloro-2,3,3a,4,7,7a-hexahydro-4,7-methanoindene. Pure chlordane is composed of a mixture of stereoisomers, with the cis and trans forms predominating and referred to as α- and γ-isomers, respectively.

Occurrence: Chlordane is produced by the chlorination of chlordene which, in turn, is a product of hexachlorocyclopentadiene and cyclopentadiene. Chlordane has been detected at various concentrations in ambient water, finished drinking water, rainwater, and soils. Chlordane is readily soluble in natural fats and fat-soluble substances. As a result, it accumulates in the tissues of organisms, particularly in the adipose tissue or body fat. Chlordane has been found in plankton, earthworms, shellfish, fish, birds, bird eggs, and man and several other mammals.

Physical Properties: Pure chlordane is a pale, yellow liquid. Pure chlordane is soluble in water at concentrations which have been shown to be toxic to aquatic organisms. The solubility of chlordane in water has been reported to be approximately 9 μg per liter at 25°C.

Technical grade chlordane is a mixture of various chlorinated hydrocarbons with a typical composition of approximately 24% trans-chlordane (γ), 19% cis-chlordane (α), 10% heptachlor, 21.5% chlordane isomers, 7% nonachlor and 18.5% closely-related chlorinated hydrocarbon compounds. Technical chlordane is a viscous, amber-colored liquid with a cedar-like odor and is relatively nonvolatile, having a vapor pressure of 1 x 10^{-5} mm Hg at 25°C; it is soluble in water at toxic concentrations (150 to 220 μg per liter at 22°C) and has a density greater than that of water, approximately 1.65 g/ml at 16°C.

Chemical Properties: Chlordane is a persistent chlorinated hydrocarbon insecticide. It is degradable by biological organisms and by nonbiological factors. However, its overall rate of degradation is slow. Degradation is believed to result eventually in the formation of hydrophilic products such as chlorohydrins and glycols, but the exact pathways are not known.

Uses: Chlordane is a broad spectrum insecticide of the group of polycyclic chlorinated hydrocarbons called cyclodiene insecticides. Chlordane has been used extensively over the past 30 years for termite control, as an insecticide for homes and gardens, and as a control for soil insects during the production of crops such as corn. Production of chlordane in the U.S. approached 10,000 metric tons per year in 1974 (13-1). Both the uses and the production volume of chlordane have decreased extensively since the issuance of a registration suspension notice for all food crops and home and garden uses of chlordane by the U.S. Environmental Protection Agency (13-2). However, significant commercial use of chlordane for termite control continues. In addition, under the terms of a settlement which terminated chlordane registration cancellation proceedings, chlordane will be permitted for limited usage through 1980 as an agricultural insecticide (43 *FR* 12372; March 24, 1978).

Toxic Effects: Chlordane has been demonstrated to be highly toxic to aquatic organisms, to bioconcentrate in many aquatic species, and to persist for prolonged periods in the environment. It is toxic to avian and mammalian species and exhibits carcinogenic activity in mice. Thus, chlordane in water is a hazard to both aquatic and terrestrial life.

Oxychlordane, a metabolic product of chlordane, produced in both plants and animals, has been demonstrated to be more toxic than the parent compound and to persist in the adipose tissue of mammals((13-3, 13-4, 13-5 and 13-6).

Levels of Exposure and Special Groups at Risk: Nisbet (13-7) estimated total daily intake of chlordane from all possible sources by back-calculating from the level of oxychlordane stored in tissue. A value of 9 μg per day chlordane intake was obtained. Nisbet also identified highly-exposed segments of the general population: children as a result of milk consumed; fishermen and their families because of the high consumption of fish and shellfish, especially freshwater fish; persons living downwind from treated fields; and persons living in houses treated with chlordane pesticide control agents.

Existing Guidelines and Standards: The American Conference of Governmental Industrial Hygienists (1977) adopted a time-weighted average value of 0.5 mg/m^3 for chlordane based on inhalation exposure. The short-term exposure limit (15 minutes) was set at 2 mg/m^3.

An acceptable daily dose for man has been estimated by the FAO to be 0.001 mg/kg body weight. Although a limit of 3 μg per liter was originally suggested for chlordane under the proposed Interim Primary Drinking Water Standards (13-8), the final U.S. EPA regulations (13-9) did not include a limit in view of the cancellation proceedings under the Federal Insecticide, Fungicide, and Rodenticide Act. Canadian Drinking Water Standards (13-10) list a tentative maximum permissible limit for chlordane of 3 μg per liter, which is applicable to raw water supplies in Canada.

Summary of Proposed EPA Criteria: *Freshwater Aquatic Life* — For chlordane the criterion to protect freshwater aquatic life as derived using the guidelines is 0.024 μg per liter as a 24 hour average and the concentration should not exceed 0.36 μg per liter at any time.

Saltwater Aquatic Life — For chlordane the criterion to protect saltwater aquatic life as derived using the guidelines is 0.0091 μg per liter as a 24 hour average and the concentration should not exceed 0.18 μg per liter at any time.

Human Health — For the maximum protection of human health from the potential carcinogenic effects of exposure to chlordane through ingestion of water and contaminated aquatic organisms, the ambient water concentration is zero. Concentrations of chlordane estimated to result in additional lifetime cancer risks ranging from no additional risk to an additional risk of 1 in 100,000 are presented in the Criterion Formulation section of this document. The EPA is considering setting criteria at an interim target risk level in the range of 10^{-5}, 10^{-6}, or 10^{-7}, with corresponding criteria of 1.2, 0.12 and 0.012 ng per liter, respectively.

Basis for the Proposed Human Health Criteria: Several approaches are available to estimate a criterion level for chlordane in ambient water. Using the Food and Agricultural Organization/World Health Organization value (13-11) of 0.001 mg/kg of body weight as the maximum daily human intake, and assuming an average body weight of 70 kg, the allowable intake would be 70 μg per day. Further, subtracting Nisbet's value (13-7) of 9 μg as the daily intake from fish, shellfish, milk, inhalation, etc., and assuming that the contribution from drinking water is a negligible part of this value, the ambient water criterion becomes 61 μg per day. At 2 liters per day consumption, the maximum allowable concentration would be 30 μg per liter.

The proposed U.S. EPA drinking water regulations (13-8), the Canadian standards (13-10), and the National Technical Advisory Committee (13-12) all suggest a chlordane limit of 3 μg per liter for drinking water. The latter report specifically indicates that the water treatment process has little effect on chlordane.

Although there are limitations to the procedure, the industrial inhalation exposure limit of the American Conference of Governmental Industrial Hygienists may be converted to a limit for ingestion. Assuming absorption via the GI tract for chlordane is one-fifth the absorption by inhalation:

$$0.5 \, \frac{mg}{m^3} \; \times \; 10 \, \frac{m^3}{day} \, TL \; \times \; \frac{5 \text{ day work week}}{7 \text{ day week}} \; \times \; \frac{1}{5} \; = \; 0.7 \, \frac{mg}{day}$$

Consumption of 2 liters of water daily and the consumption of 18.7 g of contaminated fish which have a bioconcentration factor of 5,500 result in a maximum permissible concentration of 6.7 μg per liter for the ingested water.

The use of inhalation data assumes an 8 hour day, time-weighted average occupational exposure in the working place with workers inhaling the toxic substance throughout such a period. Exposures for the general population should be considerably less. Such worker-exposure inhalation standards are inappropriate for the general population since they presume an exposure limited to an 8 hour day, an age bracket of the population that excludes the very young and the very old, and a healthy worker prior to exposure. Ingestion data is superior to inhalation data when the risks associated with the food and water of the water environment are being considered.

Under the consent decree in NRDC vs Train, criteria are to state "recommended maximum permissible concentrations (including where appropriate, zero) consistent with the protection of aquatic organisms, human health, and recreational activities". Chlordane is suspected of being a human carcinogen. Because there is no recognized safe concentration for a human carcinogen, the recommended concentration of chlordane in water for maximum protection of human health is zero.

Because attaining a zero concentration level may be infeasible in some cases and in order to to assist the EPA and states in the possible future development of water quality regulations, the concentrations of chlordane corresponding to several incremental lifetime cancer risk levels have been estimated. A cancer risk level provides an estimate of the additional incidence of cancer that may be expected in an exposed population. A risk of 10^{-5} for example, indicates a probability of one additional case of cancer for every 100,000 exposed, a risk of 10^{-6} indicates one additional case of cancer for every 1,000,000 people exposed, and so forth.

In the *Federal Register* notice of availability of draft ambient water quality criteria, EPA stated that it is considering setting criteria at an interim target risk level of 10^{-5}, 10^{-6} or 10^{-7} as shown in Table 27.

Table 27: Possible Alternative Criteria for Chlordane

Exposure Assumptions (per day)	Risk Levels and Corresponding Criteria (ng/l)			
	0	10^{-7}	10^{-6}	10^{-5}
2 liters of drinking water and consumption of 18.7 grams fish and shellfish*	0	0.012	0.12	1.2
Consumption of fish and shellfish only	0	0.013	0.13	1.3

*98% of the chlordane exposure results from the consumption of aquatic organisms which exhibit an average bioconcentration potential of 5,500-fold. The remaining 2% of chlordane exposure results from drinking water.

Source: Reference (13)

In the above table, the risk levels and corresponding criteria were calculated by applying a modified one-hit extrapolation model described in the Methodology Document to the animal bioassay data presented in the Summary of Pertinent Data. Since the extrapolation model is linear at low doses, the additional lifetime risk is directly proportional to the water concentration. Therefore, water concentrations corresponding to other risk levels can be derived by multiplying or dividing one of the risk levels and corresponding water concentrations shown in the table by factors such as 10; 100; 1,000; and so forth.

Concentration levels were derived assuming a lifetime exposure to various amounts of chlordane (a) occurring from the consumption of both drinking water and aquatic life grown in waters containing the corresponding chlordane concentrations and (b) occurring solely from consumption of aquatic life grown in the waters containing the corresponding chlordane concentrations. Because data indicating other sources of chlordane exposure and their contributions to total body burden are inadequate for quantitative use, the figures reflect the incremental risks associated with the indicated routes only.

Summary of Pertinent Data — The NRDC lifetime study of chlordane at 25 ppm in the diet of CD-1 mice resulted in liver carcinomas in males in 41 of 52 treated mice and in 3 of 33 controls, according to a reanalysis of slides by Dr. Reuber (CAG report). Using a fish bioconcentration factor of 5,500 the water concentration estimated to result in a lifetime risk of 10^{-5} is calculated from the extrapolation model using the following parameters:

$$
\begin{aligned}
n_t &= 41 & d &= 3.25 \text{ mg/kg/day} \\
N_t &= 52 & w &= 0.041 \text{ kg} \\
n_c &= 3 & L &= 78 \text{ weeks} \\
N_c &= 33 & F &= 0.0187 \text{ kg} \\
Le &= 78 \text{ weeks} & R &= 5,500 \\
l_e &= 78 \text{ weeks}
\end{aligned}
$$

The result is that the water concentration corresponding to a lifetime risk of 10^{-5} is 1.2 nanograms per liter.

References:

(13-1) 41 *FR* 7558 (Feb. 19, 1976).

(13-2) 40 *FR* 34456 (Dec. 24, 1975).

(13-3) Street, J.E. and Blau, S.E., "Oxychlordane: accumulation in rat adipose tissue on feeding chlordane isomers or technical chlordane", *Jour. Agric. Food Chem.* 20, 395 (1972).

(13-4) Polen, P.B., et al, "Characterization of oxychlordane, animal metabolite of chlordane", *Bull. Environ. Contam. Toxicol* 5, 521 (1971).

(13-5) Dorough, H.W., et al, "Chlordane residues in milk and fat of cows fed HCS 3260 (high purity chlordane) in the diet", *Bull. Environ. Contam. Toxicol* 10, 208 (1973).

(13-6) Mastri, C., et al, unpublished data, In 1970 evaluation of some pesticide residues in food, Food Agric. Org. United Nations/World Health Org. (1969).

(13-7) Nisbet, I.C.T., *Human Exposure to Chlordane, Heptachlor and Their Metabolites,* Report on Contract WA-7-1319A, Washington, D.C., U.S. Environmental Protection Agency (1976).

(13-8) 40 *FR* 11990 (Mar. 14, 1975).

(13-9) 40 *FR* 59566 (Dec. 24, 1975).

(13-10) Dept. of National Health and Welfare, *Canadian Drinking Water Standards and Objectives,* Ottawa (1968).

(13-11) Food and Agricultural Organization of the United Nations/World Health Organization, *1967 Evaluation of Some Pesticide Residues in Food,* Geneva (1968).

(13-12) Federal Water Pollution Control Admin., *Water Quality Criteria: Report of the National Technical Advisory Committee to the Secretary of the Interior,* Washington, D.C. (1968).

CHLORINATED BENZENES (#14)

The chlorinated benzenes, excluding dichlorobenzenes [which are covered in a separate Criteria Document (25)], are monochlorobenzene, 1,2,3-trichlorobenzene, 1,2,4-trichlorobenzene, 1,3,5-trichlorobenzene, 1,2,3,4-tetrachlorobenzene, 1,2,3,5-tetrachlorobenzene, 1,2,4,5-tetrachlorobenzene, pentachlorobenzene, and hexachlorobenzene.

Occurrence: Based on annual production in the U.S., 139,105 kkg of monochlorobenzene was produced in 1975; 12,849 kkg of 1,2,4-trichlorobenzene; 8,182 kkg of 1,2,4,5-tetrachlorobenzene; and 318 kkg of hexachlorobenzene were produced in 1973 (14-1).

The remaining chlorinated benzenes are produced mainly as by-products from the production processes for the above four chemicals. Production and use of chlorinated benzenes results in 34,278 kkg of monochlorobenzene; 8,182 kkg of trichlorobenzenes; and about 1,500 kkg of tetra-, penta-, and hexachlorinated benzenes entering the aquatic environment yearly. Annual amounts on monochlorobenzene (690 kkg) and hexachlorobenzene (1,628 kkg) contaminate solid wastes. Yearly estimates of atmospheric contamination of monochlorobenzene and tetrachlorobenzenes are 362 and 909 kkg, respectively (14-1).

Physical Properties: Chlorination of benzene yields twelve different compounds: monochlorobenzene (C_6H_5Cl); three isomers of dichlorobenzene [the subject of another criterion document (25)] ; three trichlorobenzenes; three tetrachlorobenzenes; pentachlorobenzene; and hexachlorobenzene.

All are colorless liquids or solids with a pleasant aroma. The most important properties imparted by chlorine to these compounds are solvent power, viscosity, and moderate chemical reactivity. All of the chlorobenzenes are heat-stable.

Viscosity data are not available for all the chlorinated benzenes. Nevertheless, the trend is for viscosity to increase from chlorobenzene to the more highly chlorinated benzenes. The nonflammability of these compounds follows the same trend. Chlorobenzene is flammable; trichlorobenzene is nonflammable, but gives off combustible fumes; the remaining compounds are nonflammable.

Vapor pressures of the chlorinated benzenes decrease progressively from monochlorobenzene to hexachlorobenzene, i.e., at 60°C, the vapor pressures of monochlorobenzene, trichlorobenzenes and 1,2,3,5-tetrachlorobenzene are 60, 3 to 4.4 and 2 mm of mercury, respectively. Some physical properties of the chlorinated benzenes are given below in Table 28.

Table 28: Physical Properties of Chlorobenzenes (Except Dichlorobenzenes)

Compound	MW	MP(°C)	BP(°C)	Specific Gravity	Log Octanol Water Partition
Monochlorobenzene	112.56	-45.6	131-132	1.107	2.83
1,2,3-Trichlorobenzene	181.45	52.6	218-219	1.43	–
1,2,4-Trichlorobenzene	–	17	213.5	1.454	4.23
1,3,5-Trichlorobenzene	–	63.4	208	1.45	–
1,2,3,4-Tetrachlorobenzene	215.90	47.5	254	1.46	–
1,2,3,5-Tetrachlorobenzene	–	54.5	246	–	–
1,2,4,5-Tetrachlorobenzene	–	138-140	243-246	1.858	4.93
Pentachlorobenzene	250.34	86	277	1.834	5.63
Hexachlorobenzene	284.79	230	322	2.044	6.43

Source: Reference (14)

Monochlorobenzene, which is the most polar compound, is soluble in water to the extent of 488 mg per liter at 25°. Solubilities of the other chlorobenzenes in water were not available. The chlorinated benzenes are generally good solvents for fats, waxes, oils and greases. The lipid solubility of these compounds is high and are expected to accumulate in ecosystems.

Chemical Properties: Monochlorobenzene (MCB) is used industrially as a synthetic intermediate in the production of phenol, DDT and aniline.

Uses: Monochlorobenzene is used for the synthesis of o- and p-nitrochlorobenzenes (50%), solvent uses (20%), phenol manufacturing (10%), and DDT manufacturing (7.5%). 1,2,4-trichlorobenzene is used as a dye carrier (46%), herbicide intermediate (28%), a heat transfer medium, a dielectric fluid in transformers, a degreaser, a lubricant and a potential insecticide against termites. The other trichlorobenzene isomers are not used in any quantity. 1,2,4,5-tetrachlorobenzene is the only tetrachloro-isomer used in industrial quantities. 56% of the annual consumption of 1,2,4,5-tetrachlorobenzene is used in the production of the defoliant, 2,4,5-trichlorophenoxy acetic acid; 33% in the synthesis of 2,4,5-trichlorophenol; and 11% as a fungicide. Pentachlorobenzene is used in small quantities as a captive intermediate in the synthesis of specialty chemicals.

Hexachlorobenzene in 1972 was used as a fungicide (23%) to control wheat bunt and smut on seed grains. Other industrial uses (77%) included dye manufacturing, an intermediate in organic synthesis, porosity controller in the manufacturing of electrodes, a wood preservative and an additive in pyrotechnic compositions for the military.

Data derived from U.S. International Trade Commission reports show that between 1969 and 1975, the U.S. annual production of MCB decreased by 50% from approximately 600 million pounds to approximately 300 million pounds.

Toxic Effects: *Local* — Chlorinated benzenes are irritating to the skin, conjunctiva, and mucous membranes of the upper respiratory tract. Prolonged or repeated contact with liquid chlorinated benzenes may cause skin burns.

Systemic — In contrast to aliphatic halogenated hydrocarbons, the toxicity of chlorinated benzenes generally decreases as the number of substituted chlorine atoms increases. Basically, acute exposure to these compounds may cause drowsiness, incoordination, and unconsciousness. Animal exposures have produced liver damage. Chronic exposure may result in liver, kidney, and lung damage as indicated by animal experiments.

Current Levels of Exposure: *Monochlorobenzene* — MCB has been detected in water monitoring surveys of various U.S. cities (14-1, 14-2). Levels reported were: ground water, 1.0 μg per liter; raw water contaminated by various discharges, 0.1 to 5.6 μg per liter; upland water, 4.7 μg per liter; industrial discharge, 8.0 to 17.0 μg per liter; and municipal water, 27 μg per liter. These data show a gross estimate of possible human exposure to MCB through the water route.

Evidence of possible exposure from food ingestion is indirect. MCB is stable in water and thus could be bioaccumulated by edible fish species.

The only data concerning exposure to MCB via air are from the industrial working environment. Citing various investigators (14), reported industrial exposures to MCB are: 0.02 mg per liter (average value) and 0.3 mg per liter (highest value); 0.001 to 0.01 mg per liter; and 0.004 to 0.01 mg per liter.

Trichlorobenzene — Possible human exposure to trichlorobenzene (TCB) might occur from municipal and industrial wastewater and from surface runoff (14-1). Municipal and industrial discharges contained from 0.1 to 500 μg per liter. Surface runoff has been found to contain 0.006 to 0.007 μg per liter. In the National Organic Reconaissance Survey conducted by EPA in 1975, TCB was found in drinking water at a level of 1.0 μg per liter.

Tetrachlorobenzene — No data are available on current levels of exposure. However, the report by Morita, et al (14-3), gives some indication of exposure. Adipose tissue samples obtained at general hospitals and medical examiners' offices in central Tokyo were examined. Samples from 15 individuals were examined; this represented 5 males and 10 females between the ages of 13 and 78. The tissues were examined for 1,2,4,5-TeCB as well

as for 1,4-dichlorobenzene and hexachlorobenzene. The TeCB content of the fat ranged
from 0.006 to 0.039 mg/kg of tissue; the mean was 0.019 mg/kg. The mean concentrations
of 1,4-dichlorobenzene and hexachlorobenzene were 1.7 and 0.21 mg/kg, respectively.
Interestingly, neither age nor sex correlated with the level of any of the chlorinated hydrocarbons in adipose tissue.

Pentachlorobenzene — Morita, et al (14-3), examined levels of pentachlorobenzene (QCB)
in adipose tissue samples obtained from general hospitals and medical examiners' offices
in central Tokyo. The samples were from a total of 15 people. The group found by gas
chromatography a residual level of QCB to be in the range of 0.004 to 0.020 μg/g, with a
mean value of 0.09 μg/g of fat. Blood samples from workers with occupational exposure
to pentachlorobenzene have been examined by others and it was found that their blood
samples contained higher levels of this compound than a comparable group of workers not
exposed to pentachlorobenzene.

Hexachlorobenzene — Hexachlorobenzene (HCB) appears to be distributed worldwide, with
high levels of contamination found in agricultural areas devoted to wheat and related cereal
grains and in industrial areas. HCB is manufactured and formulated for application to seed
wheat to prevent bunt; however, most of the HCB in the environment comes from agricultural processes. HCB is used as a starting material for the production of pentachlorophenol
which is marketed as a wood preservative. HCB is one of the main substances in the tarry
residue which results from the production of chlorinated hydrocarbons. HCB is formed as
a by-product in the production of chlorine gas by the electrolysis of sodium chloride using
a mercury electrode.

People in the U.S. are exposed to HCB in air, water and food. HCB is disseminated in the
air as dust particles and as a result of volatilization from sites having a high HCB concentration. Airborne, HCB-laden dust particles appear to have been a major factor in producing the blood levels in the general public living near an industrial site in Louisiana. HCB
is found in river water near industrial sites in quantities of as much as 2 μg/kg and even
in finished drinking water at 5 ng/kg. HCB occurs in a wide variety of foods, in particular,
terrestrial animal products, including dairy products and eggs. The dietary intake of HCB
has been estimated to be 0.5 μg per day in Japan and 35 μg per day in Australia. Breast-
fed infants in Australia and Norway may consume 40 μg HBC per day. HCB is found in
human tissues collected throughout the world.

Special Groups at Risk: *Monochlorobenzene* — The major group at risk from monochlorobenzene (MCB) intoxication are individuals exposed to MCB in the workplace. An elderly
female exposed to a glue containing 0.07% MCB for a period of 6 years had symptoms
of headache, irritation of the eyes and the upper respiratory tract, and was diagnosed to
have medullary aplasia. Three adults developed numbness, loss of consciousness, hyperemia
of the conjunctiva and the pharynx following exposure to high levels of MCB. Information
concerning the ultimate course of these individuals is not available. 82 workers who were
exposed to benzene, chlorobenzene and vinyl chloride, were examined for certain biochemical indices and showed a decreased catalase activity in the blood and an increase in
peroxidase, indophenol oxidase and glutathione levels.

A study has been made of the occupational exposure of workers exposed to the chemicals
involved in the manufacture of chlorobenzene at limits below the allowable levels. After
three years, cardiovascular effects were noted as pain in the area of the heart, bradycardia,
irregular variations in electrocardiogram, decreased contractile function of myocardium and
disorders in adaptation to physical loading. A Russian investigator reported on the prolonged exposure of individuals involved in the production of diisocyanates to the factory
air which contained MCB as well as other chemicals. Diseases noted include asthmatic
bronchitis, sinus arrhythmia, tachycardia, arterial dystrophy and anemic tendencies. Other
Russian scientists studied the course of pregnancy and deliveries in women exposed to air
in a varnish manufacturing factory where the air contained three times the maximum permissible level of MCB, but also included toluene, ethyl chloride, butanol, ethyl bromide and
orthosilicic acid ester. The only reported significant adverse effect of this mixed exposure
was toxemia of pregnancy.

Tetrachlorobenzene — The primary groups at risk from the exposure to TeCB are those who deal with it in the workplace. Since it is a metabolite of certain insecticides, it might be expected that certain individuals exposed to those agents might experience more exposure to TeCB especially since its elimination rate might be relatively slow in man. Individuals consuming large quantities of fish may also be at risk due to the proven bioconcentration of TeCB in fish. U.S. EPA Duluth laboratory studies show that the bioconcentration factor for 1,2,4,5-TeCB is 1,000; and for 1,2,3,5-TeCB is 4,100.

Pentachlorobenzene — At-risk groups would appear to be those in the industrial setting. There might be an expected increase in body burdens of QCB in individuals on diets high in fish due to the persistence of the compound in the food chain and to those on diets high in agricultural products containing QCB as residues of PCNB spraying.

Hexachlorobenzene — Several groups appear to be at risk; these include workers engaged directly in: (a) the manufacture of HCB or in processes in which HCB is a by-product; (b) the formulation of HCB-containing products; (c) the disposal of HCB-containing wastes; and (d) the application of HCB-containing products. They also include the general public living near industrial sites, pregnant women, fetuses, and breast-fed infants and populations consuming large amounts of contaminated fish. Two lines of evidence indicate that infants may be at risk. It has been demonstrated that human milk contains HCB, and some infants may be exposed to relatively high concentrations of HCB from that source alone. Moreover, some infants of Turkish mothers who consumed HCB-contaminated bread developed a fatal disorder called pembe yara. In some Turkish villages in the region most affected by HCB poisoning, few infants survived during the period of 1955 through 1960.

Occupational exposure is associated with an increased body burden of HCB. Plant workers in Louisiana have about 200 μg HCB/kg in blood. The HCB content of body fat exceeds 1 mg/kg in many parts of the world where HCB-contamination of the environment is extensive.

The massive episode of human poisoning in Turkey resulting from the consumption of bread prepared from HCB-treated seed wheat brought to light the misuse of HCB-treated grain. In spite of warnings, regulations and attempts at public education, HCB-treated grain apparently still finds its way into the food chain, for example, in fish food. The difficulty in tracing the source of HCB contamination in a diet for laboratory animals emphasizes the difficulties encountered in tracing the source of HCB in foodstuffs for man.

As noted previously, adipose tissue acts as a reservoir for HCB. Deletion of fat depots can result in mobilization and redistribution of stored HCB. Weight loss for any reason may result in a dramatic redistribution of HCB contained in adipose tissue; if the stored levels of HCB are high, adverse effects might ensue. Many humans restrict their dietary intake voluntarily or because of illness. In these instances, the redistribution of the HCB body burden becomes a potential added health hazard.

Current evidence would indicate that food intake may be the primary source of the body burden of HCB for the general population although inhalation and dermal exposure may be more important in selected groups, e.g., industrial workers.

Existing Guidelines and Standards: *Monochlorobenzene* — The threshold limit value (TLV) for MCB as adopted by the American Conference of Governmental Industrial Hygienists in 1971 and still current in 1979 is 75 ppm (350 mg/m^3). The American Industrial Hygiene Association Guide in 1964 considered 75 ppm to be too high. The recommended maximal allowable concentrations in air in other countries are: Soviet Union, 10 ppm; Czechoslovakia, 43 ppm; Romania, 0.05 mg per liter. The latter value for Romania is equivalent to 10 ppm.

Trichlorobenzene — The ACGIH threshold limit value (TLV) standard for TCB is 5 ppm (mg/l) as a ceiling value as of 1979. Sax (14-4) recommends a maximum allowable concentration of 50 ppm in air for commercial TCB which is a mixture of isomers. Coate, et al

(14-5), citing their studies, recommends that the TLV should be set below 25 ppm, preferably 5 ppm (mg/l). In the Soviet Union the maximum allowable concentration for TCB in water is 30 μg per liter which is an organoleptic limit. In a Soviet study of 40 rats and 8 rabbits administered TCB in drinking water at a concentration of 60 μg per liter for a period of 7 to 8 months, no effects were observed. This information was obtained from an abstract and evaluation of the study could not be done (14).

Tetrachlorobenzene — The maximal permissible concentration of TeCB in water established by the Soviet Union is 0.02 mg per liter (14-1).

Pentachlorobenzene — No guidelines or standards for pentachlorobenzene were found.

Hexachlorobenzene — As far as can be determined, the Occupational Safety and Health Administration has not set a standard for occupational exposure to HCB. HCB has been approved for use as a preemergence fungicide applied to seed grain. The Federal Republic of Germany no longer allows the application of HCB-containing pesticides. The government of Turkey discontinued the use of HCB-treated seed wheat in 1959 after its link to acquired toxic porphyria cutanea tarda was reported. Commercial production of HCB in the U.S. was discontinued in 1976. The Louisiana State Department of Agriculture has set the tolerated level of HCB in meat fat at 0.3 mg/kg. The NHMRC (Australia) has used this same value for the tolerated level of HCB in cows' milk. WHO has set the tolerated level of HCB in cows' milk at 20 μg/kg in whole milk. The New South Wales Department of Health (Australia) has recommended that the concentration of HCB in eggs must not exceed 0.1 mg/kg. The value of 0.6 μg HCB/kg/day was suggested by FAO/WHO in 1974 as a reasonable upper limit for HCB residues in food for human consumption. The FAO/WHO recommendations for residues in foodstuffs were 0.5 mg/kg in fat for milk and eggs, and 1 mg/kg in fat for meat and poultry. Russia and Yugoslavia have set the maximum tolerated level of HCB in air at 0.9 mg/m^3.

Summary of Proposed EPA Criteria: *Freshwater Aquatic Life* — Chlorobenzene: For chlorobenzene the criterion to protect freshwater aquatic life as derived using procedures other than the guidelines is 1,500 μg per liter as a 24 hour average and the concentration should not exceed 3,500 μg per liter at any time.

1,2,4-Trichlorobenzene — For 1,2,4-trichlorobenzene the criterion to protect freshwater aquatic life as derived using procedures other than the guidelines is 210 μg per liter as a 24 hour average and the concentration should not exceed 470 μg per liter at any time.

1,2,3,5-Tetrachlorobenzene — For 1,2,3,5-tetrachlorobenzene the criterion to protect freshwater aquatic life as derived using procedures other than the guidelines is 170 μg per liter as a 24 hour average and the concentration should not exceed 390 μg per liter at any time.

1,2,4,5-Tetrachlorobenzene — For 1,2,4,5-tetrachlorobenzene the criterion to protect freshwater aquatic life as derived using procedures other than the guidelines is 97 μg per liter as a 24 hour average and the concentration should not exceed 220 μg per liter at any time.

Pentachlorobenzene — For pentachlorobenzene the criterion to protect freshwater aquatic life as derived using procedures other than the guidelines is 16 μg per liter as a 24 hour average and the concentration should not exceed 36 μg per liter at any time.

Saltwater Aquatic Life — Chlorobenzene: For chlorobenzene the criterion to protect saltwater aquatic life as derived using procedures other than the guidelines is 120 μg per liter as a 24 hour average and the concentration should not exceed 280 μg per liter at any time.

1,2,4-Trichlorobenzene — For 1,2,4-trichlorobenzene the criterion to protect saltwater aquatic life as derived using procedures other than the guidelines is 3.4 μg per liter as a 24 hour average and the concentration should not exceed 7.8 μg per liter at any time.

1,2,3,5-Tetrachlorobenzene — For 1,2,3,5-tetrachlorobenzene the criterion to protect saltwater aquatic life as derived using procedures other than the guidelines is 2.6 μg per liter as a 24 hour average and the concentration should not exceed 5.9 μg per liter at any time.

1,2,4,5-Tetrachlorobenzene — For 1,2,4,5-tetrachlorobenzene the criterion to protect saltwater aquatic life as derived using the guidelines is 9.6 μg per liter as a 24 hour average and the concentration should not exceed 26 μg per liter at any time.

Pentachlorobenzene — For pentachlorobenzene the criterion to protect saltwater aquatic life as derived using procedures other than the guidelines is 1.3 μg per liter as a 24 hour average and the concentration should not exceed 2.9 μg per liter at any time.

Human Health — For the prevention of adverse organoleptic or toxicological effects, the recommended criteria for chlorinated benzenes are as follows:

Substance	Criterion (μg/l)	Basis for Criterion
Monochlorobenzene*	20	organoleptic effects
Trichlorobenzene	13	organoleptic effects
Tetrachlorobenzene	17	toxicity studies
Pentachlorobenzene	0.5	toxicity studies

* A toxicological evaluation of monochlorobenzene resulted in a level of 450 μg/l; however, organoleptic effects have been reported at 20 μg/l.

For the maximum protection of human health from the potential carcinogenic effects of exposure to HCB through ingestion of water and contaminated aquatic organisms, the ambient water concentration is zero. Concentrations of HCB estimated to result in additional lifetime cancer risks ranging from no additional risk to an additional risk of 1 in 100,000 are presented in the criterion document. The EPA is considering setting criteria at an interim target risk level in the range of 10^{-5}, 10^{-6}, or 10^{-7}, with corresponding criteria of 1.25, 0.125, and 0.0125 ng per liter, respectively.

Basis for the Proposed Human Health Criteria: *Monochlorobenzene* — There is no information in the literature which indicates that monochlorobenzene is, or is not, carcinogenic. There is enough evidence to suggest that monochlorobenzene (MCB) does cause dose-related target organ toxicity, though the data still want for an acceptable chronic toxicity study. There is little, if any, usable human exposure data primarily because the exposure was not only to MCB, but to other compounds of known toxicity.

The no observable adverse effect level (NOAEL) for derivation of the water quality criterion is derived from the information in the studies by Knapp, et al (14-6) and Irish (14-7). These are 27.25 mg/kg/day for the dog (the next highest dose was 54.5 mg/kg and showed an effect), 12.5 mg/kg/rat from the Knapp study (the next highest dose was 50 mg/kg and showed an effect), and 14.4 mg/kg/rat from the Irish study (the next highest dose was 144 mg/kg and showed an effect). When toxic effects were observed at higher doses, the dog was judged to be somewhat more sensitive than the rats. The Irish study ran over a period of 6 months which was twice as long as the Knapp study of both species.

Since the Knapp and Irish studies appear to give similar results and since there are no chronic toxicities to rely on, it was decided to take the NOAEL level from the longest term study, i.e., 14.4 mg/kg for 6 months.

Considering that there is relatively little human exposure data, that there is no long-term animal data, and that some theoretical questions, at least, can be raised on the possible effects of chlorobenzene on blood-forming tissue, it was decided to use an uncertainty factor of 1,000. From this the acceptable daily intake (ADI) can be calculated as follows.

$$\text{ADI} = \frac{70 \text{ kg} \times 14.4 \text{ mg/kg}}{1,000} = 1.008 \text{ mg/day}$$

The average daily consumption of water was taken to be 2 liters and the consumption of fish to be 0.0187 kg daily. A bioconcentration factor of 13 was utilized. This is the value reported by the Duluth EPA laboratories. The following calculation results in an acceptable criterion based on the available toxicologic data:

$$\frac{1.008}{2 + (13 \times 0.0187)} = 450\ \mu g/l$$

Varshavskaya (14-8), in the only report available, has reported the threshold concentration for odor and taste of MCB in reservoir water as being 20 μg per liter. This value is about 4.5% of the possible standard calculated above. It is, however, approximately 17 times greater than the highest concentration of MCB measured in survey sites.

Since water of disagreeable taste and odor is of significant influence on the quality of life, and thus related to health, it would appear that the organoleptic level of 20 μg per liter should be the recommended criterion.

Trichlorobenzene — While the committee recognizes a need for toxicological information in order to establish a criterion, there are no reliable published toxicological data on trichlorobenzene (TCB). The studies by Smith, et al (14-9) and Coate, et al (14-5), do not give sufficient basis for establishing a toxicological criterion. Therefore, in lieu of a criterion based on toxicological information, an organoleptic level of 13 μg per liter is recommended. It should be emphasized that this is a criterion based on aesthetic rather than on health effects. Data on human health effects need to be developed as a more substantial basis for setting a criterion for the protection of human health.

Tetrachlorobenzene — The dose of 5 mg/kg/day reported for beagles [Braun (14-10)] was utilized as the NOAEL for criterion derivation. An acceptable daily intake (ADI) can be calculated from the NOAEL by using a safety factor of 1,000 based on a 70 kg/man:

$$ADI = \frac{70\ kg \times 5\ mg/kg}{1,000} = 0.35\ mg/day$$

For the sake of establishing a water quality criterion, it is assumed that on the average, a person ingests 2 liters of water and 18.7 g of fish. Since fish may biomagnify this compound, a biomagnification factor (F) is used in the calculation. The equation for calculating an acceptable amount of TeCB in water is:

$$Criterion = \frac{350\ \mu g/day}{2 + (1,000 \times 0.0187)} = 16.9\ \mu g/l\ or\ 17\ \mu g/l$$

where 2 = 2 liters of drinking water consumed; 0.0187 kg = amount of fish consumed daily; and 1,000 = biomagnification factor. Thus the recommended criterion for TeCB in water is 17 μg per liter.

Pentachlorobenzene — A survey of the pentachlorobenzene (QCB) literature revealed no acute, subchronic or chronic toxicity data with the exception of the studies by Khera and Villeneuve (14-11). These authors found an adverse effect on the fetal development of embryos exposed in utero to pentachlorobenzene. The adverse effect has not been labeled teratogenic because the abnormality was an increased incidence of extra ribs and sternal defects. The lowest level of exposure to the pregnant rat was 5 mg/kg. The criterion rationale is based on this exposure level. Since there was no NOAEL an uncertainty factor of 5,000 is used. The use of this factor has precedent in the pesticide literature. From this, the ADI can be calculated as follows.

$$ADI = \frac{70\ kg \times 5\ mg/kg}{5,000} = 0.07\ mg$$

The average daily consumption of water was taken to be 2 liters and the consumption of fish to be 0.0187 kg daily. The bioconcentration factor for QCB is 7,800; therefore,

$$\text{Recommended criterion} = \frac{0.07}{2 + (7,800 \times 0.0187)} = 0.47 \ \mu g/l \ (\text{or } 0.5 \ \mu g/l)$$

The recommended water quality criterion for pentachlorobenzene is 0.5 μg per liter.

Hexachlorobenzene — Among the studies reviewed by this document, only two appear suitable for use in the risk assessment: the mouse study of Cabral, et al (14-12) and the hamster study of Cabral, et al (14-13). These two studies are described in detail in Appendix I of the criteria document (14).

Under the consent decree in NRDC vs Train, criteria are to state "recommended maximum permissible concentrations (including where appropriate, zero) consistent with the protection of aquatic organisms, human health, and recreational activities". HCB is suspected of being a human carcinogen. Because there is no recognized safe concentration for a human carcinogen, the recommended concentration of HCB in water for maximum protection of human health is zero.

Because attaining a zero concentration level may be unfeasible in some cases, and in order to assist the EPA and states in the possible future development of water quality regulations, the concentrations of HCB corresponding to several incremental lifetime cancer risk levels have been estimated. A cancer risk level provides an estimate of the additional incidence of cancer that may be expected in an exposed population. A risk of 10^{-5}, for example, indicates a probability of one additional case of cancer for every 100,000 people exposed; a risk of 10^{-6} indicates one additional case of cancer for every 1,000,000 people exposed; and so forth.

In the *Federal Register,* notice of availability of draft ambient water quality criteria, EPA stated that it is considering setting criteria at an interim target risk level of 10^{-5}, 10^{-6}, or 10^{-7} as shown in Table 29. As shown in the table, the risk levels and corresponding criteria are calculated by applying a modified one-hit extrapolation model described in the *Federal Register,* 44 *FR* 15926, March 15, 1979. Appropriate bioassay data used in the calculation of the model is presented in Summary of Pertinent Data. Since the extrapolation model is linear at low doses, the additional lifetime risk is directly proportional to the water concentration. Therefore, water concentrations corresponding to other risk levels can be derived by multiplying or dividing one of the risk levels and corresponding water concentration shown in the table by factors such as 10; 100; 1,000; and so forth.

Table 29: Possible Alternative Criteria for Hexachlorobenzene

Exposure Assumptions (per day)	Risk Levels and Corresponding Criteria (μg/l)			
	0	10^{-7}	10^{-6}	10^{-5}
2 liters of drinking water and consumption of 18.7 grams fish and shellfish*	0	0.0125	0.125	1.25
Consumption of fish and shellfish only	0	0.0126	0.126	1.26

*99% of the HCB exposure results from the consumption of aquatic organisms which exhibit an average bioconcentration potential of 12,000-fold. The remaining 1% of HCB exposure results from drinking water.

Source: Reference (14)

Concentration levels were derived assuming a lifetime exposure to various amounts of HCB (a) occurring from the consumption of both drinking water and aquatic life grown in waters containing the corresponding HCB concentrations and (b) occurring solely from consumption of aquatic life grown in the waters containing the corresponding HCB concentrations. Because data indicating other sources of HCB exposure and their contributions to total body burden are inadequate for quantitative use, the figures reflect the incremental risks associated with the indicated routes only.

Summary of Pertinent Data on HCB — The water quality criterion for HCB is based on the induction of hepatomas and hemangioendotheliomas in male Syrian Golden hamsters given a daily oral dose of 100 ppm for 80 weeks (14-13). The hepatoma incidence was 26/30 in the treated group compared with 0/40 in the control group, and the hemangioendothelioma incidence was 6/30 in the treated group, compared with 0/40 in the control group. The criterion was calculated from the following parameters:

n_t hepatoma	= 26		Le	=	80 weeks
N_t hepatoma	= 30		le	=	80 weeks
n_c hepatoma	= 0		L	=	80 weeks
N_c hepatoma	= 40		d	=	100 ppm x 0.8 = 8 mg/kg/day
n_t hemangioendothelioma	= 6		W	=	0.100 kg
N_t hemangioendothelioma	= 30		F	=	0.0187 kg
n_c hemangioendothelioma	= 0		R	=	12,000
N_c hemangioendothelioma	= 40				

Based on these parameters, the one-hit slope (B_H) is 2.2363 $(mg/kg/day)^{-1}$ for hepatomas and 0.2477 $(mg/kg/day)^{-1}$ for hemangioendotheliomas. The resulting water concentration of HCB calculated to keep the individual lifetime cancer risk below 10^{-5} is 1.25 ng per liter.

References:

(14-1) West, W.L. and Ware, S.A., *Preliminary Report, Investigation of Selected Potential Environmental Contaminants: Halogenated Benzenes,* Washington, D.C., Environ. Prot. Agency (1977).

(14-2) U.S. EPA, *Survey of Industrial Processing Data: Task I, Hexachlorobenzene and Hexachlorobutadiene Pollution from Chlorocarbon Processes,* Prepared by Mid. Res. Inst., Washington, D.C., Off. Toxic Subs., Washington, D.C. (1975).

(14-3) Morita, M. and Oishi, S., "Clearance and tissue distribution of hexachlorobenzene in rats", *Bull. Environ. Contam. Toxicol,* 14, 313 (1975).

(14-4) Sax, N.I., *Dangerous Properties of Industrial Materials,* New York, Van Nostrand Reinhold (1975).

(14-5) Coate, W.B., et al, "Chronic inhalation exposure of rats, rabbits and monkeys to 1,2,4-trichlorobenzene", *Arch. Environ. Health* 32, 249 (1977).

(14-6) Knapp, W.K., Jr., et al, "Subacute oral toxicity of monochlorobenzene in dogs and rats, *Toxicol. Appl. Pharmacol.* 19, 393 (1971).

(14-7) Irish, D.D., "Halogenated hydrocarbons: II cyclic" in Patty, F.A., ed., *Industrial Hygiene and Toxicology,* II, 2nd Ed., New York, Interscience, (1963).

(14-8) Varshavskaya, S.P., "Comparative toxicological characteristics of chlorobenzene and dichlorobenzene (ortho and para isomers) in relation to the sanitary protection of water bodies", *Hyg. San.* 33, 10 (1968).

(14-9) Smith, C.C., et al, "Subacute toxicity of 1,2,4-trichlorobenzene (TCB) in subhuman primates". *Fed. Proc.* 31, 248 (1978).

(14-10) Braun, W.H., et al, "Pharmocokinetics and toxicological evaluation of dogs fed 1,2,4,5-tetrachlorobenzene in the diet for two years", *Jour. Environ. Pathol. Toxicol.* 2, 225 (1978).

(14-11) Khera, K.S. and Villeneuve, D.C., "Teratogenicity studies on halogenated benzenes (pentachloropentachloronitro and hexabromo) in rats", *Toxicology* 5, 117 (1975).

(14-12) Cabral, J.R.P., et al, "Carcinogenesis study in mice with hexachlorobenzene", *Toxicol. Appl. Pharmacol* 45, 323 (1978).

(14-13) Cabral, J.R.P., et al, "Carcinogenic activity of hexachlorobenzene in hamsters", *Nature* (London) 269, 510 (1977).

CHLORINATED ETHANES (#15)

The chlorinated ethanes include ethyl chloride (monochloroethane), two dichloroethanes (ethylene dichloride and 1,1-DCE), two trichloroethanes (methyl chloroform and 1,1,2-TCE), two tetrachloroethanes (1,1,1,2- and 1,1,2,2-), pentachloroethane and hexachloroethane.

Occurrence: A large number of humans are industrially exposed to chloroethanes. In addition, the general population encounters these compounds in commercial products and as environmental contaminants resulting from industrial emissions including the discharge of liquid wastes.

Physical Properties: There are nine chlorinated ethanes, the properties of which vary with the number and position of the chlorine atoms (see Table 30). Both water solubility, in most cases, and vapor pressure decrease with increasing chlorination, while density and melting point increase. Chloroethane is a gas at room temperature; hexachloroethane is a solid; the rest are liquids. All are sufficiently soluble to be of potential concern as water pollutants. The only member of the series with a specific gravity less than 1 is chloroethane. The chlorinated ethanes form azeotropes with water, a characteristic which could influence their persistence in the water column. All are very soluble in organic solvents.

Table 30: Physical and Chemical Properties of Chloroethanes

Compound	Formula Weight	BP (°C)	MP (°C)	SG*	Solubility in Water (g/l)	Vapor Pressure (mm Hg)	Vapor Density**
Monochloroethane	64.52	13.1	-138.7	0.9214	5.74	1,000***	–
1,1-Dichloroethane	98.96	57.3	-98	1.1776	5	230†	–
1,2-Dichloroethane	98.96	83.4	-35.4	1.253	8.1	85†	3.42
1,1,1-Trichloroethane	133.4	74.1	-33	1.3492	480††	96***	4.55
1,1,2-Trichloroethane	133.4	113	-37.4	1.4405	†††	–	–
1,1,1,2-Tetrachloroethane	167.9	129	-68.1	1.5532	2.85	–	–
1,1,2,2,-Tetrachloroethane	167.9	146.3	-36	1.596	2.9	16†	5.79
Pentachloroethane	202.3	162	-29	1.6796	Insoluble	–	–
Hexachloroethane	236.7	186	187	2.091	Insoluble	–	–

*At 20°C; water = 1.00 at 4°C.   ††Parts per 10^6 w/w.
**Air = 1.00.   †††Slightly soluble.
***At 20°C.
†At 25°C.

Source: Reference (15)

Chemical Properties: The chlorinated ethanes undergo the usual dehalogenation and dehydrohalogenation reactions of chlorinated aliphatic compounds in the laboratory. The microbial degradation of the chlorinated ethanes has not been demonstrated, but chemical degradation of chlorinated hydrocarbons has been reported.

Uses: Chloroethanes are widely used because of their low cost and properties which make them excellent solvents, degreasing agents, fumigants and cutting fluids. Some are used in the manufacture of plastics, textiles and in the synthesis of other chemicals. About 1955, chloroethanes began to replace more toxic industrial solvents. The chlorinated ethanes are produced in large quantities and used for production of tetraethyl lead and vinyl chloride as industrial solvents, and as intermediates in the production of other organochlorine compounds.

Toxic Effects: All of the chlorinated ethanes studies show they are at least mildly toxic, toxicity increasing with degree of chlorination. Some have been found in drinking waters, in natural waters, and in aquatic organisms and foodstuffs.

Chlorinated ethanes do not bioconcentrate significantly; however, they do exhibit a greater bioconcentrating potential with increased chlorination. Bluegill are found to bioconcentrate hexachloroethane at a factor of nearly 140, whereas they bioconcentrate dichloroethane at 2. Acute toxicity to both freshwater and marine vertebrates and invertebrates seems to be dependent on the number of chlorine atoms associated with the ethane molecule. Pentachloroethane, in several instances, is the exception to this observation, e.g., freshwater invertebrates and saltwater fishes. Aquatic chronic toxicity data are sparse.

In regard to human and mammalian health, no literature concerning the teratogenicity of the chlorinated ethanes was found. Mutagenicity data were nonexistent except for a finding that showed the mild mutagenesis of 1,2-di- and 1,1,2,2-tetrachloroethane in the Ames' *Salmonella* assay. 1,2-dichloroethane induced a higher frequency of somatic mutations in *Drosophilia*. 1,2-di-; 1,1,2-tri-; 1,1,2,2-tetra-; and hexachloroethanes have all proved to be carcinogenic in rodents.

Current Levels of Exposure: Estimates of human exposure to chloroethanes via ingestion are not available for the general population. NIOSH (15-1) estimated that of over 5 million workers exposed by inhalation and dermal routes to chloroethanes, 4.5 million are exposed to 1,2-dichloroethane or 1,1,1-trichloroethane (Table 31). In the general population there are chronic exposures to variable amounts in air and finished water. Chloroethanes are present in many commercial products, and exposure of the population depends on the tendency of individuals to read and heed instructions.

Table 31: Chloroethane Exposures and Production

Chemical	Estimated Number of Workers Exposed	Annual Production Quantities (lb)
Monochloroethane	113,000	670 million (1976)
1,1-Dichloroethane	4,600	*
1,2-Dichloroethane	1,900,000	8 billion (1976)
1,1,1-Trichloroethane	2,900,000	630 million (1976)
1,1,2-Trichloroethane	112,000	**
1,1,1,2-Tetrachloroethane	***	*
1,1,2,2-Tetrachloroethane	11,000	**
Pentachloroethane	***	*
Hexachloroethane	1,500	*,†

   *Does not appear to be commercially produced in the U.S.
  **Direct production information not available.
 ***NIOSH estimates not available.
   †730,000 kg were imported in 1976.

Source: National Institute for Occupational Safety and Health, Reference (15-1)

Special Groups at Risk: Workers who are occupationally exposed to chloroethanes by inhalation and/or dermal absorption represent a special group at risk (Table 18). Epidemiological studies have not disclosed a relationship between exposure to chloroethanes and cancer; however, four chloroethanes have proven to be carcinogenic in at least one species of rodent (15-2, 15-3, 15-4, 15-5). Those individuals who are exposed to known hepatotoxins or have liver disease may constitute a group at risk.

Existing Guidelines and Standards: OSHA standards and NIOSH recommended standards are based on exposure by inhalation (15-1). They are listed on the following page. Based on information available (15-6), the National Institute for Occupational Safety and Health recommended that occupational exposures to 1,2-dichloroethane not exceed 5 ppm (20 mg/m^3) determined as a time-weighted average for up to a 10 hour work day, 40 hour work week. Peak concentrations should not exceed 15 ppm (60 mg/m^3) as determined by a 15 minute sample. The current enforced OSHA exposure standard is 50 ppm, time-weighted average for up to a 10 hour work day, 40 hour work week.

NIOSH (15-8) issued criteria for a recommended standard of 200 ppm for occupational exposures to 1,1,1-trichloroethane. This recommendation to change the standards from 350 ppm is based on central nervous system responses to acute exposures in man, cardiovascular and respiratory effects in man and animals, and the absence of reported effects in man at concentrations below the proposed limit.

Chemical	OSHA Exposure Standard (ppm)	NIOSH Recommended Exposure Standard (ppm)
Monochloroethane	1,000	none
1,1-Dichloroethane	100	none
1,2-Dichloroethane	50*	5**
1,1,1-Trichloroethane	350***	200
1,1,2-Trichloroethane	10	none
1,1,1,2-Tetrachloroethane	none	none
1,1,2,2-Tetrachloroethane	5†	1
Pentachloroethane	none	—
Hexachloroethane	1	—

Note: NIOSH has tentative plans for a Criteria Document for a Recommended Standard
for pentachloroethane and hexachloroethane.

*Reference (15-6).
**Reference (15-7).
***Reference (15-8).
†Reference (15-9).

Summary of Proposed EPA Criteria: *Freshwater Aquatic Life* — The data base for freshwater aquatic life is insufficient to allow use of the guidelines. The following recommendation is inferred from toxicity data on pentachloroethane and saltwater organisms.

For 1,2-dichloroethane the criterion to protect freshwater aquatic life as derived using procedures other than the guidelines is 3,900 μg per liter as a 24 hour average and the concentration should not exceed 8,800 μg per liter at any time. For 1,1,1-trichloroethane the
criterion to protect freshwater aquatic life as derived using procedures other than the guidelines is 5,300 μg per liter as a 24 hour average and the concentration should not exceed
12,000 μg per liter at any time.

For 1,1,2-trichloroethane the criterion to protect freshwater aquatic life as derived using
procedures other than the guidelines is 310 μg per liter as a 24 hour average and the concentration should not exceed 710 μg per liter at any time. For 1,1,1,2-tetrachloroethane
the criterion to protect freshwater aquatic life as derived using procedures other than the
guidelines is 420 μg per liter as a 24 hour average and the concentration should not exceed
960 μg per liter at any time.

For 1,1,2,2-tetrachloroethane the criterion to protect freshwater aquatic life as derived using procedures other than the guidelines is 170 μg per liter as a 24 hour average and the
concentration should not exceed 380 μg per liter at any time. For pentachloroethane the
criterion to protect freshwater aquatic life as derived using procedures other than the guidelines is 440 μg per liter as a 24 hour average and the concentration should not exceed
1,000 μg per liter at any time.

For hexachloroethane the criterion to protect freshwater aquatic life as derived using procedures other than the guidelines is 62 μg per liter as a 24 hour average and the concentration should not exceed 140 μg per liter at any time.

Saltwater Aquatic Life — The data base for saltwater aquatic life is insufficient to allow
use of the guidelines. The following recommendation is inferred from toxicity data on
pentachloroethane and saltwater organisms.

For 1,2-dichloroethane the criterion to protect saltwater aquatic life as derived using procedures other than the guidelines is 880 μg per liter as a 24 hour average and the concentration should not exceed 2,000 μg per liter at any time. For 1,1,1-trichloroethane the
criterion to protect saltwater aquatic life as derived using procedures other than the guidelines is 240 μg per liter as a 24 hour average and the concentration should not exceed
540 μg per liter at any time.

For saltwater aquatic life, no criterion for 1,1,2-trichloroethane can be derived using the guidelines, and there are insufficient data to estimate a criterion using other procedures. For saltwater aquatic life, no criterion for 1,1,1,2-tetrachloroethane can be derived using the guidelines, and there are insufficient data to estimate a criterion using other procedures.

For 1,1,2,2-tetrachloroethane the criterion to protect saltwater aquatic life as derived using procedures other than the guidelines is 70 μg per liter as a 24 hour average and the concentration should not exceed 160 μg per liter at any time. For pentachloroethane the criterion to protect saltwater aquatic life as derived using the guidelines is 38 μg per liter as a 24 hour average and the concentration should not exceed 87 μg per liter at any time.

For hexachloroethane the criterion to protect saltwater aquatic life as derived using procedures other than the guidelines is 7.0 μg per liter as a 24 hour average and the concentration should not exceed 16 μg per liter at any time.

Human Health — For the maximum protection of human health from the potential carcinogenic effects of exposure to 1,2-dichloroethane; 1,1,2-trichloroethane; 1,1,2,2,tetrachloroethane and hexachloroethane through ingestion of water and contaminated aquatic organisms, the ambient water concentration is zero. Concentrations of these chlorinated ethanes estimated to result in additional lifetime cancer risks ranging from no additional risk to an additional risk of 1 in 100,000 are presented in the Criterion Formulation section of this document. The EPA is considering setting criteria at an interim target risk level in the range of 10^{-5}, 10^{-6}, or 10^{-7} with corresponding criteria as shown in Table 32 in the text which follows.

For the protection of human health from the toxic properties of 1,1,1-trichloroethane ingested through the consumption of water and fish, the criterion is 15.7 mg per liter. There are insufficient data to derive criteria for monochloroethane; 1,1-dichloroethane; 1,1,1,2-tetrachloroethane and pentachloroethane.

Basis for the Proposed Human Health Criteria: There is insufficient mammalian toxicological information to establish a water criterion for human health for the following chloroethanes: monochloroethane; 1,1-dichloroethane; 1,1,1,2-tetrachloroethane and pentachloroethane as noted in Table 32.

Table 32: Criteria for Chloroethanes

Compound	μg/l	Criterion	Reference
Monochloroethane	*	–	–
1,1-Dichloroethane	*	–	–
1,1-Dichloroethane	7.0	Carcinogenicity data	(15-2)
1,1,1-Trichloroethane	15.7**	Mammalian toxicity data	(15-11)
1,1,2-Trichloroethane	2.7	Carcinogenicity data	(15-3)
1,1,1,2-Tetrachloroethane	*	–	–
1,1,2,2-Tetrachloroethane	1.8	Carcinogenicity data	(15-4)
Pentachloroethane	*	–	–
Hexachloroethane	5.9	Carcinogenicity data	(15-5)

*None. **mg/l.

Source: Reference (15)

Available evidence indicates that the general population is exposed to only trace levels of 1,1-dichloroethane; 1,1,1,2-tetrachloroethane and pentachloroethane. Although inhalation exposure to monochloroethane is more widespread, it is considered one of the least toxic of the chloroethanes. Should significant levels of exposure be documented in the future, it will be necessary to conduct more extensive toxicologic studies with these chloroethanes.

The criterion for 1,1,1-trichloroethane is based on the National Cancer Institute bioassay for possible carcinogenicity (15-3). Results of the study showed that the survival of both Osborne-Mendel rats and B6C3F1 mice was significantly decreased in groups receiving oral doses of 1,1,1-trichloroethane.

Chronic murine pneumonia may have been responsible for the high incidence of natural deaths. A variety of neoplasms was observed in both species; however, the incidence of specific malignancies was not significantly different from those observed in control animals. Survival time was significantly decreased in rats receiving the high dose; therefore, the criterion for 1,1,1-trichloroethane is based on the low dose in rats (750 mg/kg body weight, 5 days per week for 78 weeks), which produced toxic effects in a number of systems. It should be recognized that the actual no-observable-adverse-effect level (NOAEL) will be lower. However, use of the lowest-minimal-effect dose as an estimate of an acceptable daily intake has been practiced by the National Academy of Sciences (15-10). Thus, assuming a 70 kg body weight and using a safety factor of 1,000 (15-10), the following calculation can be derived:

$$\frac{750 \text{ mg/kg} \times 70 \text{ kg} \times 5/7 \text{ day}}{1,000} = 37.5 \text{ mg/day}$$

Therefore, consumption of 2 liters of water daily and 18.7 g of contaminated fish having a bioconcentration factor of 21 would result in, assuming 100% gastrointestinal absorption of 1,1,1-trichloroethane, a maximum permissible concentration of 15.7 mg per liter for ingested water:

$$\frac{37.5 \text{ mg/day}}{2 \text{ liters} + (21 \times 0.0187) \times 1.0} = 15.7 \text{ mg/l}$$

Based on available literature, 1,1,2-tri-; 1,1,2,2-tetra-; and hexachloroethane are considered to be carcinogenic in at least one rodent species (15-3, 15-4, 15-5). In the case of these three chloroethanes, a statistical evaluation of the incidences of hepatocellular carcinomas revealed a significant positive association between the administration of the respective chloroethanes and tumor incidence. It can be concluded that under the conditions of the NCI bioassay, 1,1,2-tri; 1,1,2,2-tetra; and hexachloroethane are carcinogenic in B6C3F1 mice, inducing (in all cases) hepatocellular carcinomas in either male or female mice.

Estimated risk levels for these chloroethanes in water can be calculated using a linear, non-threshold model with the results from the NCI bioassays (see Summary of Pertinent Data). The model assumes a risk of 1 in 100,000 of developing cancer as a result of drinking 2 liters of water per day containing chloroethane at the concentrations used in the bioassays. Allowances are also made for consuming fish from chloroethane-contaminated waters. Based upon these assumptions, the following criteria can be calculated:

Chloroethane	Dose* (mg/kg)	Criteria (μg/l)
1,1,2-trichloroethane	279	2.7
1,1,2,2-tetrachloroethane	203	1.8
Hexachloroethane	842	4.4

* 5 days per week for 78 weeks.

Under the conditions of an NCI bioassay (15-2), 1,2-dichloroethane is carcinogenic, inducing a statistically significant number of squamous cell carcinomas of the forestomach and hemangiosarcomas of the circulatory system in male rats, mammary adenocarcinomas in female rats and mice, and endometrial tumors in female mice. The criterion for 1,2-dichloroethane is based on the high dose (107 mg/kg body weight, 5 days per week for 78 weeks), which induced mammary adenocarcinomas in female rats. Using a linear, nonthreshold model and including the consumption of fish from chloroethane-contaminated waters the criterion for 1,2-dichloroethane is 7.0 μg per liter.

It must be recognized that the NCI studies were designed to provide a "yes/no" answer to the carcinogenicity of a chemical in rats and mice. In some cases it is difficult to justify extrapolation of data from NCI studies in order to assess the risk to man of chronic exposure to low concentrations of a chemical. Those who assess risk should be aware of the following: impurities in technical grade chloroethanes were not identified; chloroethanes were administered in oil which may effect absorption and metabolism; high concentrations were used; a time-weighted average dose was reported. However, doses causing toxic responses were often administered cyclically (one week, no treatment, followed by four weeks of treatment, five days per week), during some experiments dose levels were lowered or raised, for criteria calculations, doses administered five days per week were adjusted to an average daily dose as if administered seven days per week.

Under the consent decree in NRDC vs Train, criteria are to state "recommended maximum permissible concentrations (including where appropriate, zero) consistent with the protection of aquatic organisms, human health, and recreational activities". 1,2-dichloroethane; 1,1,2-trichloroethane; 1,1,2,2-tetrachloroethane and hexachloroethane are suspected of being human carcinogens. Because there is no recognized safe concentration for a human carcinogen, the recommended concentration of these chlorinated ethanes in water for maximum protection of human health is zero.

Because attaining a zero concentration level may be infeasible in some cases and in order to assist the EPA and states in the possible future development of water quality regulations, the concentrations of these chlorinated ethanes corresponding to several incremental lifetime cancer risk levels have been estimated. A cancer risk level provides an estimate of the additional incidence of cancer that may be expected in an exposed population. A risk of 10^{-5}, for example, indicates a probability of 1 additional case of cancer for every 100,000 people exposed. A risk of 10^{-6} indicates 1 additional case of cancer for every 1,000,000 people exposed, and so forth.

In the *Federal Register*, notice of availability of draft ambient water quality criteria, EPA stated that it is considering setting criteria at an interim target risk level of 10^{-5}, 10^{-6}, or 10^{-7}, as shown in Table 33. In the table, risk levels and corresponding criteria were calculated by applying a modified one-hit extrapolation model described in the 44 *FR* 15926, March 15, 1979. Appropriate bioassay data used in the calculation of the model are presented in the Summary of Pertinent Data. Since the extrapolation model is linear to low doses, the additional lifetime risk is directly proportional to the water concentration. Therefore, water concentrations corresponding to other risk levels can be derived by multiplying or dividing one of the risk levels and corresponding water concentrations shown in the table by factors such as 10; 100; 1,000; and so forth.

Table 33: Possible Alternative Criteria for Chlorinated Ethanes

Exposure Assumptions	Risk Levels and Corresponding Criteria (μg/l)			
	0	10^{-7}	10^{-6}	10^{-5}
2 liters of drinking water and consumption of 18.7 grams of fish and shellfish*				
1-2-Dichloroethane	0	0.07	0.70	7.0
1,1,2-Trichloroethane	0	0.027	0.27	2.7
1,1,2,2-Tetrachloroethane	0	0.018	0.18	1.8
Hexachloroethane	0	0.059	0.59	5.9
Consumption of fish and shellfish only				
1,2-Dichloroethane	0	1.708	17.08	170.8
1,1,2-Trichloroethane	0	0.483	4.83	48.3
1,1,2,2-Tetrachloroethane	0	0.127	1.27	12.7
Hexachloroethane	0	0.079	0.79	7.9

*4% of 1,2-dichloroethane exposure results from the consumption of aquatic organisms which exhibit an average bioconcentration potential of 4.6-fold. The remaining 96% of 1,2-dichloroethane exposure results from drinking water.

Source: Reference (15)

6% of 1,1,2-trichloroethane exposure results from the consumption of aquatic organisms which exhibit an average bioconcentration potential of 6.3-fold. The remaining 94% of 1,1,2-trichloroethane exposure results from drinking water.

14% of 1,1,2,2-tetrachloroethane exposure results from the consumption of aquatic

organisms which exhibit an average bioconcentration potential of 18-fold. The remaining
86% of 1,1,2,2-tetrachloroethane exposure results from drinking water.

75% of hexachloroethane exposure results from the consumption of aquatic organisms
which exhibit an average bioconcentration potential of 320-fold. The remaining 25% of
hexachloroethane exposure results from drinking water.

Concentration levels were derived assuming a lifetime exposure to various amounts of these
chlorinated ethanes (a) occurring from the consumption of both drinking water and aquatic
life grown in water containing the corresponding chlorinated ethane concentrations and (b)
occurring solely from the consumption of aquatic life grown in the waters containing the
corresponding chlorinated ethane concentrations.

Although total exposure information for the above chlorinated ethanes is discussed and an
estimate of the contributions from other sources of exposure can be made, this data will
not be factored into the ambient water quality criteria formulation because of the tenuous
estimates. The criteria presented, therefore, assume an incremental risk from ambient
water exposure only.

Summary of Pertinent Data for 1,2-Dichloroethane — The water quality criterion for 1,2-
dichloroethane is based on the induction of mammary adenocarcinomas in female Osborne-
Mendel rats, given an average oral dose of 107 mg/kg/day 1,2-dichloroethane over a period
of 78 weeks (15-2). The incidences of mammary adenocarcinomas were 18/50 and 0/20 in
the treated and control groups, respectively. The criterion was calculated from the following parameters:

$$n_t = 18 \qquad\qquad L = 110 \text{ weeks}$$
$$N_t = 50 \qquad\qquad d = 76.4 \text{ mg/kg/day } (107 \text{ mg/kg/day} \times {}^5\!/_7)$$
$$n_c = 0 \qquad\qquad f = 0.0187 \text{ kg/day}$$
$$N_c = 20 \qquad\qquad R = 4.6$$
$$Le = 110 \text{ weeks} \qquad w = 0.319 \text{ kg}$$
$$le = 69 \text{ weeks}$$

Based on these parameters, the one-hit slope (B_H) is 0.04765 (mg/kg/day)$^{-1}$. The concentration of 1,2-dichloroethane in water, calculated to keep the lifetime cancer risk below
10^{-5}, is 7.0 μg per liter.

Summary of Pertinent Data for 1,1,2-Trichloroethane — The water quality criterion for
1,1,2-trichloroethane is based on the induction of hepatocellular carcinomas in female
B6C3F1 mice given an average oral dose of 390 mg/kg/day over a 78 week period (15-3).
The incidences of hepatocellular carcinomas were 40/45 and 0/20 in the treated and control
groups, respectively. The criterion was calculated from the following parameters:

$$n_t = 40 \qquad\qquad L = 91 \text{ weeks}$$
$$N_t = 45 \qquad\qquad d = 279 \text{ mg/kg/day } (390 \text{ mg/kg/day} \times {}^5\!/_7)$$
$$n_c = 0 \qquad\qquad F = 0.0187 \text{ kg/day}$$
$$N_c = 20 \qquad\qquad R = 6.3$$
$$Le = 91 \text{ weeks} \qquad w = 0.029 \text{ kg}$$
$$le = 78 \text{ weeks}$$

Based on these parameters, the one-hit slope (B_H) is 0.123 (mg/kg/day)$^{-1}$. The concentration of 1,1,2-trichloroethane in water, calculated to keep the lifetime cancer risk below
10^{-5}, is 2.7 μg per liter.

Summary of Pertinent Data for 1,1,2,2-Tetrachloroethane — The water quality criterion for
1,1,2,2-tetrachloroethane is based on the induction of hepatocellular carcinomas in male
B6C3F1 mice given average oral doses of 284 mg/kg/day over a 78 week period (15-4).
The incidences of hepatocellular carcinomas were 44/49 and 1/18 in the treated and control groups, respectively. The criterion was calculated from the following parameters.

$$n_t = 44 \qquad\qquad L = 91 \text{ weeks}$$
$$N_t = 49 \qquad\qquad d = 203 \text{ mg/kg/day } (284 \text{ mg/kg/day} \times {}^5\!/_7)$$
$$n_c = 1 \qquad\qquad F = 0.0187 \text{ kg/day}$$
$$N_c = 18 \qquad\qquad R = 18$$
$$Le = 91 \text{ weeks} \qquad w = 0.035 \text{ kg}$$
$$le = 78 \text{ weeks}$$

Based on these parameters, the one-hit slope (B_H) is 0.1638 $(\text{mg/kg/day})^{-1}$. The concentration of 1,1,2,2-tetrachloroethane in water, calculated to keep the lifetime cancer risk below 10^{-5}, is 1.8 μg per liter.

Summary of Pertinent Data for Hexachloroethane — The water quality criterion for hexachloroethane is based on the induction of hepatocellular carcinomas in male B6C3F1 mice, given an average oral dose of 1,179 mg/kg/day over a 78 week period (15-5). The incidences of hepatocellular carcinomas were 31/49 and 3/20 in the treated and control groups, respectively. The criterion was calculated from the following parameters:

$$n_t = 31 \qquad\qquad L = 91 \text{ weeks}$$
$$N_t = 49 \qquad\qquad d = 842 \text{ mg/kg/day } (1,179 \text{ mg/kg/day} \times {}^5\!/_7)$$
$$n_c = 3 \qquad\qquad F = 0.0187 \text{ kg/day}$$
$$N_c = 20 \qquad\qquad R = 320$$
$$Le = 91 \text{ weeks} \qquad w = 0.032 \text{ kg}$$
$$le = 78 \text{ weeks}$$

Based on these parameters, the one-hit slope (B_H) is 0.0149 $(\text{mg/kg/day})^{-1}$. The concentration of hexachloroethane in water, calculated to keep the lifetime cancer risk below 10^{-5}, is 5.9 μg per liter.

References:

(15-1) National Institute for Occupational Safety and Health, *Chloroethanes: Review of Toxicity,* Current Intelligence Bull. No. 27, NIOSH Publ. No. 78-181, Washington, D.C. (1978).

(15-2) National Cancer Institute, *Bioassay of 1,2-Dichloroethane for Possible Carcinogenicity,* DHEW Publ. No. (NIH) 78-1305, Washington, D.C. (1978).

(15-3) National Cancer Institute, *Bioassay of 1,1,2-Trichloroethane for Possible Carcinogenicity,* DHEW Publ. No. (NIH) 78-1324, Washington, D.C. (1978).

(15-4) National Cancer Institute, *Bioassay of 1,1,2,2-Tetrachloroethane for Possible Carcinogenicity,* DHEW Publ. No. (NIH) 78-827, Washington, D.C. (1978).

(15-5) National Cancer Institute, *Bioassay of Hexachloroethane for Possible Carcinogenicity,* DHEW Publ. No. (NIH) 78-1318, Washington, D.C. (1978).

(15-6) National Institute for Occupational Safety and Health, *Criteria Document: Recommendations for an Occupational Exposure Standard for Ethylene Dichloride,* DHEW Publ. (NIOSH) 76-139, Washington, D.C. (1976).

(15-7) National Institute for Occupational Safety and Health, *Ethylene Dichloride (1,2-Dichloroethane),* Current Intell. Bull. No. 25, DHEW (NIOSH) Publ. No. 78-149, Washington, D.C. (1978).

(15-8) National Institute for Occupational Safety and Health, *Criteria for a Recommended Standard for Exposure to 1,1,1-Trichloroethane (Methyl Chloroform),* DHEW Publ. No. (NIOSH) 76-184, Washington, D.C. (1976).

(15-9) National Institute for Occupational Safety and Health, *Criteria for a Recommended Standard: Occupational Exposure to 1,1,2,2-Tetrachloroethane,* DHEW (NIOSH) Publ. No. 77-121, Washington, D.C. (1976).

(15-10) National Academy of Sciences, *Drinking Water and Health,* Washington, D.C. (1977).

(15-11) National Cancer Institute, *Bioassay of 1,1,1-Trichloroethane for Possible Carcinogenicity,* Carcinog. Tech. Rept. Ser. NCI-CG-TR-3, Washington, D.C. (1977).

CHLOROALKYL ETHERS (#16)

The most important chloroalkyl ethers are as follows (with their abbreviations):

Chloromethyl methyl ether
    $ClCH_2OCH_3$ CMME

Bis(chloromethyl) ether
    $ClCH_2OCH_2Cl$ BCME

Bis(2-chloroethyl) ether
    $ClCH_2CH_2OCH_2CH_2Cl$ BCEE

Bis(2-chloroisopropyl) ether
    $ClCH_2CHOCHCH_2Cl$
         CH_3 CH_3 BCIE

Bis(2-chloroethoxy)methane
    $ClCH_2CH_2OCH_2OCH_2CH_2Cl$ BCEXM

Bis[1,2-(2-chloroethoxy)] ethane
    $ClCH_2CH_2OCH_2CH_2OCH_2CH_2Cl$ BCEXE

Occurrence: Concern over BCEE and BCIE has arisen mainly because of their presence in river water and the drinking water of several U.S. cities. These chemicals were found at high concentrations in wastewater from chemical plants involved in the manufacturing of glycol products, rubber and insecticides.

Physical Properties: Comprehensive reviews on the physical and chemical properties and biological effects of these chemicals have been published (16-1 through 16-7). The physical constants of the four environmentally most important chloroalkyl ethers are summarized in Table 34. The boiling points are taken at 760 mm Hg.

Table 34: Physical Constants of Four Environmentally Most Significant Chloroalkyl Ethers

Compound	MW	Appearance	MP (°C)	BP (°C)	Density	n_D^{20}	Solubility
CMME	80.5	*	–	59	$d_4^{20} = 1.0605$	1.3974	**
BCME	115.0	*	–	104	$d_4^{15} = 1.328$	1.435	**
BCEE	143.01	*	-24.5*** -51.9††	176-178	$d_4^{20} = 1.213$	1.457	†
BCIE	171.07	*	–	187-188	–	1.4474	†††

  *Colorless liquid at room temperature.
  **Immediately hydrolyze in water, miscible with ethanol, ether and other solvents.
  ***Reference (16-4).
   †Practically insoluble in water, miscible with most organic solvents (especially benzene and chloroform).
  ††Reference (16-8).
  †††Practically insoluble in water; miscible with most organic solvents.

Source: Reference (16)

Chemical Properties: The chloroalkyl ethers are compounds with the general structure $RCl_x-O-R'Cl_x$, where x may be any positive integer, including zero, and R and R' are aliphatic groups. The chemical reactivity of these compounds varies widely, depending on the placement of chlorine atoms and the nature of the aliphatic groups involved. Chloromethyl methyl ether, bis(chloromethyl) ether, 1-chloroethyl ethyl ether and 1-chloroethyl methyl ether decompose in water. A half-life of 14 seconds has been calculated for bis-(chloromethyl) ether in aqueous solution. Chloromethyl methyl ether undergoes decomposition in water to form methanol, formaldehyde and hydrochloric acid. Bis(chloromethyl) ether will form spontaneously in the presence of hydrogen chloride and formaldehyde.

Uses: The chloroalkyl ethers have been widely used in laboratories and in industrial organic synthesis, textile treatment, preparation of ion exchange resins, and pesticide manufacture. They also have been used as solvents for polymerization reactions. As an end product, BCEE is an excellent solvent for fats, waxes and greases. It can be used as a scouring agent for textiles and has also been used as an insecticide, ascaricide and soil fumigant.

Toxic Effects: Both BCME and CMME are listed as human carcinogens. Limited data are available on the effects of any of the chloroalkyl ethers on aquatic life. For this reason, no water quality criterion can be established. However, because of the demonstrated carcinogenicity of BCME and CMME, human contact with these compounds should be avoided.

Following recognition of the high potency of these chemicals as carcinogens by inhalation in animals, and various epidemiological evidence linking excessive human respiratory cancer incidence to exposure, BCME and CMME have been listed as two of the fourteen carcinogens restricted by Federal regulations, effective February 11, 1974 (16-9). Realization of the potential hazard of BCME grew dramatically when it was reported that at high concentrations, vapors of HCl and formaldehyde, two commonly used chemicals in many industries and laboratories, can combine spontaneously to form BCME.

Current Levels of Exposure: There is no information available on the levels of chloroalkyl ethers in food or in the atmosphere; hence, no estimates can be made of the extent of human exposures to these compounds via these two routes. Information on the dermal exposure is also virtually nonexistent. Only incomplete data are available for the calculation of exposure via ingestion of drinking water. Therefore, only rough estimates can be made.

The highest concentration of BCEE, BCIE and BCEXE in drinking water reported by U.S. EPA (16-10) was 0.5, 1.58 and 0.03 μg per liter, respectively. Assuming that (a) these values are representative of yearly averages, (b) the average daily intake of water is 2 liters and (c) the average body weight is 70 kg, then the maximum possible daily exposure from water to BCEE, BCIE and BCEXE would be 14.3, 45.1 and 0.86 ng/kg. These values, of course, are the upper limits and are based on the dubious assumption that the highest value is representative of the yearly average and that they only apply to specific contaminated areas. For national averages, the data of Dressman, et al (16-11) and U.S. EPA (16-12), may be used. The national average concentration of BCEE or BCIE in drinking water is calculated as the mean concentration multiplied by the percent incidence of occurrence.

Thus, the average concentration in drinking water of BCEE and BCIE was, respectively, 11.5 ng per liter (0.1 μg/l x 11.5%); and 12.1 ng per liter (0.17 μg/l x 7.1%) in phase II; and 1.7 ng per liter (0.024 μg/l x 7.27%), and 7.0 ng per liter (0.11 μg/l x 6.36%) in phase III. Using the same three assumptions mentioned above, the estimated daily exposure to BCEE and BCIE would be, respectively, 0.33 ng/kg and 0.35 ng/kg in phase II, and 0.05 ng/kg and 0.20 ng/kg in phase III.

Special Groups at Risk: Exposure to BCME and CMEE appears to be confined to occupational settings. A partial list of occupations in which exposure may occur includes: ion-exchange resin makers, specific organic chemical plant workers, laboratory workers, and polymer makers. Of these groups, workers in small noncommercial laboratories should probably be particularly cautious because of the lack of monitoring and surveillance and because of the fact that this group is more likely to be relatively more heavily exposed.

Potential exposure to BCME may also occur in workplaces where vapors of hydrochloric acid and formaldehyde may coexist. The National Institute of Occupational Safety and Health (NIOSH) has already found trace levels of BCME in the textile industry. Other such places include biological, medical and chemical laboratories, and particle board and paper manufacturing plants.

Exposure to β-chloroalkyl ethers may occur in residents in areas where the source of drinking water is from the contaminated river water and the treatment of drinking water is inadequate to remove the contaminants. Individuals consuming the water in these areas may be at a greater risk than the general population. Occupational exposure to BCEE may also occur. A partial list of occupations in which exposure may occur includes: cellulose ester plant workers, degreasers, dry cleaners, textile scourers, varnish workers, and processors or makers of ethyl cellulose, fat, gum, lacquer, oil, paint, soap and tar.

Existing Guidelines and Standards: Both BCME and CMME have been recognized as human carcinogens; all contact with them should be avoided. In 1973, these two chloroalkyl ethers were listed as two of the fourteen carcinogens restricted by Federal regulation. Emergency temporary standards were established for limiting occupational exposure. These regulations applied to all preparations containing 1% (w/w) or more of the chloroalkyl ethers.

The use, storage, or handling of these chemicals must be limited to a controlled area in which elaborate precautions were specified to minimize worker exposure. Decontamination, waste disposal, monitoring and medical surveillance programs were also required (16-13). More detailed regulations have recently been established; they apply to all preparations containing 0.1% of the chloroalkyl ethers by volume or weight (16-14). Based on the known carcinogenicity of BCME in animal inhibition studies, the American Conference of Governmental and Industrial Hygienists (1979) has recommended a TLV of 1 ppb (4.71 μg/m^3) for BCME. This value is for the time-weighted average (TWA) concentration for a normal 8 hour work day or 40 hour work week, to which nearly all workers may be repeatedly exposed, day after day, without adverse effect. The ACGIH also lists BCME as a human carcinogen.

The Federal standard for BCEE is 15 ppm (90 mg/m^3). The ACGIH has recommended a time-weighted average TLV-TWA of 5 ppm (30 mg/m^3) for BCEE. For a short term exposure limit, the tentative value (TLV-STEL) suggested is 10 ppm (60 mg/m^3). These values are based on the irritant properties of the chemical to the eye and the respiratory tract. It is also recommended that appropriate measures should be taken for the prevention of cutaneous absorption. The guideline level adopted by the Philadelphia regional office of EPA for BCEE level permitted in Philadelphia's drinking water is 0.02 μg per liter. This value is based on an evaluation of the available toxicological data for BCEE by the National Environmental Research Center; a safety factor of 500,000 has been applied in the calculation.

The TLVs for the other chloroalkyl ethers are not available. The provisional operational limit suggested for BCIE was 15 ppm (16-15). The value was based on the irritant properties of the compound to the eye and respiratory tract.

Summary of Proposed EPA Criteria: *Freshwater Aquatic Life* — For freshwater aquatic life, no criterion for any chloroalkyl ether can be derived using the guidelines and there are insufficient data to estimate a criterion using other procedures.

Saltwater Aquatic Life — For saltwater aquatic life, no criteria for any chloroalkyl ether can be derived using the guidelines and there are insufficient data to estimate a criterion using other procedures.

Human Health — For the protection of human health from the toxic properties of BCIE ingested through water and through contaminated aquatic organisms, the ambient water criterion is determined to be 175.8 μg per liter. For the maximum protection of human health from the potential carcinogenic effects of exposure to BCIE through ingestion of water and contaminated aquatic organisms, the ambient water concentration is zero.

Concentrations of BCIE estimated to result in additional lifetime cancer risks ranging from no additional risk to an additional risk of 1 in 100,000 are presented in the criterion document. The EPA is considering setting criteria at an interim target risk level in the range of 10^{-5}, 10^{-6}, or 10^{-7}, with corresponding criteria of 11.5, 1.15, and 0.115 μg per liter, respectively.

For the maximum protection of human health from the potential carcinogenic effects of exposure to BCEE through ingestion of water and contaminated aquatic organisms, the ambient water concentration is zero. Concentrations of BCEE estimated to result in additional lifetime cancer risks ranging from no additional risk to an additional risk of 1 in 100,000 are presented in the criterion document. The EPA is considering setting criteria at an interim target risk level in the range of 10^{-5}, 10^{-6}, or 10^{-7} with corresponding criteria of 0.42, 0.042, and 0.0042 μg per liter, respectively.

For maximum protection of human health from potential carcinogenic effects of exposure to BCME through ingestion of water and contaminated aquatic organisms, the ambient water concentration is zero. Concentrations of BCME estimated to result in additional lifetime cancer risks ranging from no additional risk to an additional risk of 1 in 100,000 are presented in the criterion document. The EPA is considering setting criteria at an interim target risk level in the range of 10^{-5}, 10^{-6}, or 10^{-7} with corresponding criteria of 0.02, 0.002, and 0.0002 ng per liter, respectively.

Basis for Proposed Human Health Criteria: There is no empirical evidence that BCIE is carcinogenic; however, some chronic toxic effects of the compound have been noted. One approach to estimating a safe level of BCIE in drinking water utilizes the following general equation: NOAEL x SF x BW = W x Z + R x F x Z + AD – (R x F x Z), where NOAEL is no apparent adverse effect level in mammals; SF is safety factor; BW is body weight of average human (assume 70 kg); W is daily consumption of water (assume 2 liters); Z is safe level for water; R is bioconcentration factor (in l/kg); F is daily consumption of fish (assume 0.0187 kg); A is daily amount absorbed from air; and D is daily amount from total diet (including fish).

Since valid estimates on current exposure from air and total diet cannot be made, the equation can be simplified to NOAEL x SF x BW = (W + R x F) x Z. The lowest dose tested which caused minimum adverse effects was 10 mg/kg/day for the mice. However, even at this dose, there was an increased incidence of centrilobular necrosis of the liver which was not seen in the high dose group. To be conservative, a safety factor of 1/1,000 will be applied. Assuming an average human body weight of 70 kg, acceptable daily intake calculated is 700 μg per day. Using the estimated bioconcentration factor of 106 for BCIE and assuming daily consumption of 0.0187 kg fish and 2 liters of water, the safe level calculated from these data is 175.8 μg per liter. Since this safe level is calculated on the basis of several assumptions that cannot be defended, it should be regarded as a very crude estimate. Another approach to deriving a criterion has been suggested by the Carcinogens Assessment Group, EPA.

As previously stated, BCIE has not been empirically proven to be a carcinogen; nevertheless, it is mutagenic and is in a class of compounds that are known as carcinogens. Based on these facts, credence can be lent to deriving a suggested criterion based upon unpublished NCI preliminary data as of 1978 as applied to the linear, nonthreshold model.

Therefore, a lower bound water concentration of 11.5 μg per liter has been calculated such that there is a 95% confidence that this level is lower than the actual level which would produce a 10^{-5} lifetime risk due to exposure to BCIE.

Although both approaches to calculating a criterion are somewhat tenuous, the weight of evidence for the carcinogenic potential of BCIE is sufficient to be qualitatively suggestive and must not be ignored from a public health point of view. Until further conclusive data become available, the EPA feels it is prudent to consider BCIE as a potential carcinogen.

The estimated safe level of BCEE in drinking water may be calculated using the same linear, nonthreshold model as applied to BCIE. The data on the carcinogenicity of this compound by oral administration to male mice are used in the calculation. The bio-accumulation factor used is 25. Based on this approach, the calculated water quality criterion for BCEE is 0.42 μg per liter. Compliance to this level should limit human lifetime risk of carcinogenesis from BCEE in drinking water to not more than 10^{-5} (1 case in 100,000 persons at risk), assuming water to be the only source of exposure. It should also very adequately protect against noncarcinogenic toxicity since the daily dose of contaminant that would be absorbed from water containing the criterion limit is many times less than the minimal daily oral dose required to produce a detectable toxic response in animals.

The setting of drinking water standards for BCME and CMME is of academic interest only, since these α-chloroalkyl ethers may not, under ordinary conditions, exist in water for periods of time longer than a few hours. Carcinogenicity data generated by oral administration of these compounds are not available.

In the case of CMME, no criterion was calculated due to its extremely short half-life in aqueous solution. The hydrolysis rate of CMME in aqueous isopropanol has been measured. Extrapolation of the data to pure water yielded a $t_{0.5}$ of less than 1 second. BCME has a slightly longer half-life. Therefore, as a guideline, the safe level of BCME in drinking water may be calculated using the tumor incidence data from chronic rat inhalation studies (16-16). In this study, Sprague-Dawley rats were exposed to 0.1 ppm BCME 6 hours per day, 5 days per week throughout their lifetime. Additional groups of rats were given 10, 20, 40, 80, and 100 exposures to 0.1 ppm BCME. The validity of the incidence rates for humans was established by evaluating the cancer incidence in workers after accounting for their exposure.

Therefore, using the linear, nonthreshold model and a bioconcentration factor of 31, the recommended maximum permissible concentration of BCME for the ingested water is 0.2 ng per liter. Compliance to this level should limit human lifetime risk of carcinogenesis from BCME in drinking water to not more than 10^{-5}, assuming water to be the only source of exposure.

Under the consent decree in NRDC vs Train, criteria are to state "recommended maximum permissible concentrations (including where appropriate, zero) consistent with the protection of aquatic organisms, human health, and recreational activities". BCIE, BCEE and BCME are suspected of being human carcinogens. Because there is no recognized safe concentration for a human carcinogen, the recommended concentration of these chloroalkyl ethers in water for maximum protection of human health is zero.

Because attaining a zero concentration level may be infeasible in some cases and in order to assist the EPA and states in the possible future development of water quality regulations, the concentrations of BCIE, BCEE and BCME corresponding to several incremental lifetime cancer risk levels have been estimated. A cancer risk level provides an estimate of the additional incidence of cancer that may be expected in an exposed population. A risk of 10^{-5}, for example, indicates a probability of 1 additional case of cancer for every 100,000 people exposed; a risk of 10^{-6} indicates 1 additional case of cancer for every 1,000,000 people exposed; and so forth.

In the *Federal Register* notice of availability of draft ambient water quality criteria, EPA stated that it is considering setting criteria at an interim target risk level of 10^{-5}, 10^{-6}, or 10^{-7} as shown in Table 35.

Table 35: Possible Alternative Criteria for Chloroalkyl Ethers

	Risk Levels and Corresponding Criteria (μg/l)			
Exposure Assumptions	0	10^{-7}	10^{-6}	10^{-5}
2 liters of drinking water and consumption of 18.7 grams of fish and shellfish*				
Bis(2-chloroisopropyl)ether	0	0.115	1.15	11.5
Bis(2-chloroethyl)ether	0	0.0042	0.042	0.42
Bis(chloromethyl)ether	0	0.02×10^{-5}	0.02×10^{-4}	0.02×10^{-3}

(continued)

Table 35: (continued)

Exposure Assumptions	Risk Levels and Corresponding Criteria (μg/l)			
	0	10^{-7}	10^{-6}	10^{-5}
Consumption of fish and shellfish only				
Bis(2-chloroisopropyl)ether	0	0.231	2.31	23.1
Bis(2-chloroethyl)ether	0	0.0219	0.219	2.19
Bis(chloromethyl)ether	0	0.09×10^{-5}	0.09×10^{-4}	0.09×10^{-3}

*50% of BCIE exposure results from the consumption of aquatic organisms which exhibit an average bioconcentration potential of 106-fold. The remaining 50% of BCIE exposure results from drinking water.

Source: Reference (16)

In the above table, the risk levels and corresponding criteria were calculated by applying a modified one-hit extrapolation model described in the 44 *FR* 15926. Appropriate bioassay data used in the calculation of the model are presented in the Summary of Pertinent Data. Since the extrapolation model is linear to low doses, the additional lifetime risk is directly proportional to the water concentration. Therefore, water concentrations corresponding to other risk levels can be derived by multiplying or dividing one of the risk levels and corresponding water concentrations shown in the table by factors such as 10; 100; 1,000; and so forth.

19% of BCEE exposure results from the consumption of aquatic organisms which exhibit an average bioconcentration potential of 25-fold. The remaining 81% of BCEE exposure results from drinking water. 22% of BCME exposure results from the consumption of aquatic organisms which exhibit an average bioconcentration potential of 31-fold. The remaining 78% of BCME exposure results from drinking water.

Concentration levels were derived assuming a lifetime exposure to various amounts of BCIE, BCEE and BCME (a) occurring from the consumption of both drinking water and aquatic life grown in water containing the corresponding chloroalkyl ether concentrations and (b) occurring solely from consumption of aquatic life grown in the waters containing the corresponding chloroalkyl ether concentrations.

Although total exposure information for these chloroalkyl ethers is discussed and an estimate of the contributions from other sources of exposure can be made, these data will not be factored into the ambient water quality criteria formulation because of the tenuous estimates. The criteria presented, therefore, assume an incremental risk from ambient water exposure only.

Summary of Pertinent Data — Bis(2-Chloroisopropyl) Ether: A 95% lower bound estimate of the water concentration of BCIE producing 10^{-5} cancer risk is calculated from the preliminary data of the NCI study in Osborne-Mendel rats. Since there is no statistically significant tumor incidence in any treated group compared with controls, the incidence of total malignant tumors in the male rats of the low dose group is compared with that of the respective vehicle control male group. The low dose group was given 100 mg/kg/day of BCIE by intubation 5 days per week for 2 years, so that the average lifetime exposure was 71.4 mg/kg/day. The lower bound water concentration is calculated from the values and the equation shown below. To obtain an upper 95% confidence bound on the slope, the following estimate was used.

$$B_a u \; = \; \ln \left[\frac{1 \, - \, P_c(l)}{1 \, - \, P_t(u)} \right]$$

where $P_c(l)$ is the lower 2.5% confidence limit on the control malignant tumor rate and $P_t(u)$ is the upper 97.5% confidence bound on the malignant tumor rate in the treated group. The criterion was calculated from the following parameters:

n_t	= 17		le	= 104 weeks
N_t	= 50		L	= 104 weeks
n_c	= 22		d	= 71.4 mg/kg/day
N_c	= 50		w	= 0.550 kg
Le	= 104 weeks		F	= 0.0187 kg
			R	= 106

Based on these parameters, the upper 95% confidence limit on the one-hit slope (B_Hu) is 1.53×10^{-2} $(mg/kg/day)^{-1}$. Therefore, the 95% lower bound estimate of the water concentration of BCIE producing 10^{-5} lifetime cancer risk is 11.5 μg per liter.

Bis(2-Chloroethyl) Ether — The water quality criterion for BCEE is based on the induction of hepatomas in male mice (strain C57BL/6XC3H/Anf/F$_1$) given a daily oral dose of 300 ppm for 80 weeks (16-17). The tumor incidence was 14/16 in the treated group compared with 8/79 in the control group. The criterion was calculated from the following parameters:

$$
\begin{array}{ll}
n_t = 14 & L = 80\ weeks \\
N_t = 16 & d = 300\ ppm \times 0.13 = 39\ mg/kg/day \\
n_c = 8 & w = 0.030\ kg \\
N_c = 79 & F = 0.0187\ kg \\
Le = 80\ weeks & R = 25 \\
le = 80\ weeks &
\end{array}
$$

Based on these parameters, the one-hit slope (B_H) is 6.8510×10^{-1} $(mg/kg/day)^{-1}$. The resulting water concentration of BCEE calculated to keep the individual lifetime cancer risk below 10^{-5} is 0.42 μg per liter.

Bis(Chloromethyl) Ether — The water quality criterion for BCME is based on the inducation of malignant respiratory tract tumors in male Sprague-Dawley rats given 100 exposures of 0.01 ppm by inhalation 6 hours per day, 5 days per week (16-16). The average lifetime exposure was calculated to be 3.510×10^{-4} mg/kg/day. The tumor incidence was 12/20 in the treated group and 0/240 in the control rats. The criterion was calculated from the following parameters:

$$
\begin{array}{ll}
n_t = 12 & L = 104\ weeks \\
N_t = 20 & d = 3.510 \times 10^{-4}\ mg/kg/day \\
n_c = 0 & w = 0.500\ kg \\
N_c = 240 & F = 0.0187\ kg \\
Le = 104\ weeks & R = 31 \\
le = 104\ weeks &
\end{array}
$$

Based on these parameters, the one-hit slope (B_H) is 1.3603×10^{-4} $(mg/kg/day)^{-1}$. The resulting water concentration of BCME calculated to maintain the individual lifetime cancer risk below 10^{-5} is 0.02 ng per liter.

References:

(16-1)   Summers, L., "The haloalkyl ethers", *Chem. Rev.* 55, 301 (1955).

(16-2)   VanDuuren, B.L. et al, "Carcinogenicity of haloethers", *Jour. Nat. Cancer Inst.* 43, 481 (1969).

(16-3)   International Agency for Research on Cancer, *Monograph on the Evaluation of Carcinogenic Risk of Chemicals to Man, 4, Some Aromatic Amines, Hydrazines and Related Substances, N-Nitroso Compounds and Misc. Alkylating Agents,* Lyon, France (1974).

(16-4)   International Agency for Research on Cancer, *Monograph on the Evaluation of Carcinogenic Risk of Chemicals to Man, 9, Some Aziridines, N-, S- and O-Mustards and Selenium,* Lyon, France (1975).

(16-5)   Durkin, P.R, et al, *Investigation of Selected Potential Environmental Contaminants: Haloethers,* Report EPA 560/2-75-006, Cincinnati, Ohio, U.S. Environ. Prot. Agency (1975).

(16-6)   Nelson, N. *The Chloroethers--Occupational Carcinogens: A Summary of Laboratory and Epidemiological Studies,* Ann. N.Y. Acad. Sci. 271, 81 (1976).

(16-7)   National Academy of Sciences, *Drinking Water and Health,* Washington, D.C. (1977).

(16-8)   Schrenk, H.H., et al, *Acute Response of Guinea Pigs to Vapors of Some New Commercial Organic Compounds, VII, Dichloroethyl Ether,* Pub. Health Rep. 48, 1389 (1933).

(16-9)   39 *FR* 3756.

(16-10) U.S. Environmental Protection Agency, *Preliminary Assessment of Suspected Carcinogens in Drinking Water,* Report to Congress, Washington, D.C. (1975).

(16-11) Dressman, R.C., et al, "Determinative method for analysis of aqueous sample extracts for bis(2-chloro) ethers and dichlorobenzenes", *Environ. Sci. Tech.* 11, 719 (1977).

(16-12) U.S. Environmental Protection Agency, *National Organic Monitoring Survey; General Review of Results and Methodology, Phases I-III,* Office of Water Supply (1977).

(16-13) 38 *FR* 10929.

(16-14) 39 *FR* 3756.

(16-15) Gage, J.C., "The subacute inhalation toxicity of 109 industrial chemicals", *Br. Jour. Ind. Med.* 27, 1 (1970).

(16-16) Kuschner, M,. et al, "Inhalation carcinogenicity of alpha-halo ethers, III, lifetime and limited period inhalation studies with BCME at 0.1 ppm", *Arch. Envir. Health* 30, 73 (1975).

(16-17) Innes, J.R.M., et al, "Bioassay of pesticides and industrial chemicals for tumorigenicity in mice; a preliminary note", *J. Nat. Cancer Inst.* 42, 1101 (1969).

CHLORINATED NAPHTHALENES (#17)

Chlorinated naphthalenes consist of 2 fused 6 carbon-membered aromatic rings where any or all of the 8 hydrogen atoms can be replaced with chlorine. Theoretically, 76 individual isomers are possible and may exist. The commercial products are usually mixtures with various degrees of chlorination, and are presently manufactured and marketed in the U.S. (Halowaxes).

Possible impurities of these products are chlorinated derivatives, corresponding to the impurities in coal tar, or petroleum-derived naphthalene feedstocks which may include biphenyls, fluorenes, pyrenes, anthracenes, and dibenzofurans.

Occurrence: The potential for environmental exposure may be significant when these compounds are used as oil additives, in the electroplating industry, and in the fabric dyeing industry. The extent of leaching of chlorinated naphthalenes from discarded capacitors and old cable insulation (manufactured prior to curtailment of the chemical's use in such products) has not been determined.

The synthesis of chlorinated naphthalenes generally involves the chlorination of naphthalene by chlorine in the presence of catalytic amounts of ferric or antimony chloride. This production process yields mixtures of highly chlorinated naphthalenes in varying quantities by further chlorination of the lesser substituted products. Only 1-chloronaphthalene and octachloronaphthalene are readily isolated from the products of direct chlorination.

Polychlorinated naphthalenes do not occur naturally in the environment. Potential environmental accumulation can occur around points of manufacture of polychlorinated naphthalenes or products containing them, near sites of disposal of polychlorinated naphthalene-containing wastes, and, since polychlorinated biphenyls (PCB) are to some extent contaminated by polychlorinated naphthalenes, near sites of heavy polychlorinated biphenyl contamination. Because polychlorinated naphthalenes are relatively insoluble in water, they would not be expected to migrate far from their point of disposition.

Physical Properties: The physical properties of the chlorinated naphthalenes are generally dependent on the degree of chlorination. Melting points of the pure compounds range from 17°C for 1-chloronaphthalene to 198°C for 1,2,3,4-tetrachloronaphthalene. Also, as the degree of chlorination increases, the specific gravity, boiling point, fire and flash points all increase, while the vapor pressure and water-solubility decrease. Mixtures of the mono- and dichloronaphthalenes are generally liquid at room temperature, whereas mixtures of the more highly chlorinated naphthalenes tend to be waxy solids.

Chemical Properties: Chlorinated naphthalenes, like PCBs, exhibit a high degree of chemical and thermal stability as indicated by their resistance to most acids and alkalies and to dehydrochlorination (17-1).

Uses: Mixtures of tri- and tetrachloronaphthalenes (solids) comprise the bulk of market use as the paper impregnant in automobile capacitors. Less use is made of mixtures of the mono- and dichloronaphthalenes as oil additives for engine cleaning, and in fabric dyeing. In 1956, the total U.S. production of chlorinated naphthalenes was approximately 3,175 metric tons.

By 1972 production had decreased further to approximately 2,300 metric tons per year. At the present, Halochem, Inc. in Boonton, N.J., is the only manufacturer of polychlorinated naphthalenes in the U.S. Amounts of chlorinated naphthalenes processed in 1978 were less than 22 metric tons for monochloronaphthalene, less than 45 metric tons total for di-, tri- and tetrachloronaphthalene, less than 1 metric ton for pentachloronaphthalene, and virtually zero for the more highly chlorinated naphthalenes. Projected production for 1979 totals less than 270 metric tons with 20% of this total expected to be monochloronaphthalene, less than 5% pentachloronaphthalene, and none of the more highly chlorinated naphthalenes.

Toxic Effects: Limited data exist on the toxicity of chlorinated naphthalenes toward aquatic organisms. Only two pure isomers, 1-chloronaphthalene and 1,2,3,4,5,6,7,8-octachloronaphthalene, have been tested in freshwater aquatic organisms. Results from bioassays on these compounds show that the monochloro-isomer is more acutely toxic than the octachloro-isomer for a freshwater plant, a freshwater invertebrate species, and a freshwater vertebrate species.

The same trend in acute toxicity for the mono- and octachloro-isomers exists in saltwater organisms. An embryo-larval chronic toxicity test conducted on a saltwater vertebrate species for 1-chloronaphthalene demonstrated chronic toxic effects. No other chronic data exist for any other chlorinated naphthalene for any other freshwater or saltwater species.

A considerable amount of acute toxicity data on chlorinated naphthalene mixtures (Halowaxes) for saltwater organisms has been compiled. Reported acute 96 hour LC_{50} values for invertebrate species do not suggest a trend in toxicity versus degree of mixture chlorination. Other toxicity data for saltwater organisms also do not suggest a consistent trend in toxicity with an increased degree of mixture chlorination.

Halowaxes bioconcentrate in saltwater algal and saltwater invertebrate species 25- to 2,300-fold with no consistent trend for the magnitude of the bioconcentration with respect to degree of mixture chlorination (17-2, 17-3).

Chlorinated naphthalenes demonstrate acute and chronic toxic effects for a large variety of nonhuman mammals including rats (17-4), rabbits (17-5) pigs (17-6), cattle (17-7), and sheep (17-8). Generally the mono- and dichloro-isomers are only slightly toxic; the tri- tetra-, penta- and hexa-isomers are the most toxic; and the octachloro-isomer generally the least toxic in these studies. Prevalent pathological symptoms include hyperkeratosis and damage to the liver and kidney of each species. Toxicity is caused either by ingestion, inhalation, or dermal application of the toxicant.

A similar situation for chlorinated naphthalene toxicity in humans has been demonstrated (17-5, 17-9, 17-10, 17-11, 17-12). Toxicity can be caused by dermal contact, inhalation, and presumably, ingestion. The prevalent pathological symptoms are liver injury, changes in serum enzyme levels, and dermal manifestations such as chloracne. The primary hepatotoxic isomers for man seem to be penta- and hexachloronaphthalene (17-13). The higher chlorinated naphthalenes appear to be the most toxic for dermal exposure.

In several mammalian species, the chlorinated naphthalenes are metabolized to some extent to chlorinated naphthols, and to some extent are excreted unchanged (17-14, 17-15, 17-16). These studies indicate that as the degree of isomer chlorination increases, the extent of isomer metabolism to chlorinated naphthols decreases with no metabolism of pentachloro- and higher chlorinated isomers apparent (17-14, 17-15). Howard and Durkin (17-17) report that the available data on metabolism coupled with the chemical and physical similarities to polychlorinated biphenyls indicate that the higher chlorinated naphthalenes are relatively stable and are likely to persist when released to the environment.

Current Levels of Exposure: Polychlorinated naphthalenes have not been identified in drinking water samples, market basket food samples, or at standard ambient air stations. Near point sources, concentrations in water can range as high as 7.0 μg per liter and concentrations in air as high as 2.9 $\mu g/m^3$. Near a point source one fish sample had a level of 39 $\mu g/kg$ for the whole fish and a sample of apples contained 90 $\mu g/kg$ of polychlorinated naphthalenes. Polychlorinated naphthalenes have been detected in several samples of PCBs, compounds that are known to be widely distributed in the aquatic environment. Measurements of chlorinated naphthalenes in environmental samples have not been widely performed using current sensitive measurement techniques for these compounds.

Special Groups at Risk: Because of the possible potentiation of the toxicity of higher chlorinated naphthalenes by ethanol and carbon tetrachloride, individuals who ingest enough alcohol to result in liver disfunction would be a special group at risk. Individuals, e.g., analytical and synthetic chemists, mechanics and cleaners, who are routinely exposed to carbon tetrachloride or other hepatotoxic chemicals would also be at a greater risk than a population without such an exposure. Individuals involved in the manufacture, utilization, or disposal of polychlorinated naphthalenes would be expected to have higher levels of exposure than the general population.

Existing Guidelines and Standards: The only standards that presently exist for polychlorinated naphthalenes are the Occupational Safety and Health Administration's standards which were adopted from and are identical to the ACGIH TLVs. The rigor of these standards increases as the number of chlorine atoms present increases on the assumption that vapor toxicity is proportional to the number of chlorine atoms present in each compound. The present TLVs (17-18) are: 5 mg/m^3 trichloronaphthalene, 2 mg/m^3 tetrachloronaphthalene, 0.5 mg/m^3 pentachloronaphthalene, 0.2 mg/m^3 hexachloronaphthalene, 0.1 mg/m^3 octachloronaphthalene. There are no state or federal water quality or ambient air quality standards for chlorinated naphthalenes.

Summary of Proposed EPA Criteria: *Freshwater Aquatic Life* — For 1-chloronaphthalene, the criterion to protect freshwater aquatic life as derived using procedures other than the guidelines is 29 μg per liter as a 24 hour average and the concentration should never exceed 67 μg per liter at any time.

Saltwater Aquatic Life — For 1-chloronaphthalene, the criterion to protect saltwater aquatic life as derived using the guidelines is 2.8 μg per liter as a 24 hour average and the concentration should never exceed 6.4 μg per liter at any time.

Human Health — For the protection of human health from the toxic properties of chlorinated naphthalenes ingested through water and through contaminated aquatic organisms, the ambient water criteria for the various classes of chlorinated naphthalenes are in micrograms per liter as follows: 3.9 trichloronaphthalenes, 1.5 tetrachloronaphthalenes, 0.39 pentachloronaphthalenes, 0.15 hexachloronaphthalenes, and 0.08 octachloronaphthalenes.

Basis for the Proposed Human Health Criteria: There are insufficient animal toxicity data available on which to base a criterion for polychlorinated naphthalenes. However, industrial exposure to vapors of polychlorinated naphthalenes has resulted in systemic toxicity, and this toxicity is the basis for the present ACGIH (17-18) TLVs. Such a TLV can be used as a basis for developing water criteria for polychlorinated naphthalenes. It is recognized that the ACGIH TLVs apply primarily to normal adult working males and do not incorporate safety factors for sensitive populations. In order to provide a reasonable margin of safety, calculation of an acceptable concentration of polychlorinated naphthalenes in drinking water as proposed by the Stokinger and Woodward model should include a safety factor of 100 as illustrated below.

$$\frac{TLV \ (mg/m^3) \ \times \ 50 \ m^3/week}{7 \ days/week \ \times \ 100} = acceptable \ intake \ (mg/day)$$

where 50 m^3/week is the average amount of air inhaled by a normal adult in a 40 hour work week; 7 days/week is the conversion factor for daily intake; and 100 is the safety factor for sensitive populations.

Since no pharmacokinetic data are available to compare absorption efficiency by the inhalation route versus the oral route, it is assumed that absorption efficiency is the same by either route. Using the ACGIH TLV levels, the acceptable daily intakes for polychlorinated naphthalenes would be in milligrams as follows: 0.36 trichloronaphthalenes, 0.14 tetrachloronaphthalenes, 0.036 pentachloronaphthalenes, 0.014 hexachloronaphthalenes, 0.007 octachloronaphthalenes.

Assuming an average intake of 18.7 g of fish per day with a biomagnification factor of 4,800 for edible portions of aquatic species as derived in the Exposure section, and a water intake of 2 liters per day, then criteria levels in micrograms per liter for the above polychlorinated naphthalenes in water would be as follows: 3.9 trichloronaphthalenes, 1.5 tetrachloronaphthalenes, 0.39 pentachloronaphthalenes, 0.15 hexachloronaphthalenes, and 0.08 octachloronaphthalenes.

References:

(17-1)   Kover, F.D., *Environmental hazard assessment report: chlorinated naphthalenes,* EPA Publ. No. 560/8-75-001, Washington, D.C., U.S. Environ. Prot. Agency (1975).

(17-2   Walsh, G.E., et al, "Effects and uptake of chlorinated naphthalenes in marine unicellular algae", *Bull. Environ. Contam. Toxicol* 18, 297 (1977).

(17-3)   U.S. EPA, *Semi-annual report, Environ. Res. Lab., Gulf Breeze, Fla. April-September, 1976,* Environ. Prot. Agency (1976).

(17-4)   Bennett, G.A., et al, "Morphological changes in the liver of rats resulting from exposure to certain chlorinated hydrocarbons", *Jour. Ind. Hyg. Toxicol* 20, 97 (1938).

(17-5)   Hambrick, G.W., "The effect of substituted naphthalenes on the pilosebaceous apparatus of rabbit and man", *Jour. Invest. Dermat.* 28, 89 (1957).

(17-6)   Link, R.R., et al, "Toxic effect of chlorinated naphthalenes in pigs", *Jour. Am. Vet. Med. Assoc.* 133, 83 (1958).

(17-7)   Olson, C., "Bovine hyperkeratosis (X-disease, highly chlorinated naphthalene poisoning). Historical review", in Bradley C.A. and Cornelius, C.E., eds., *Advances in veterinary science and comparative medicine,* New York, Academic Press (1969).

(17-8)   Brock, W.E., et al, "Chlorinated naphthalene intoxication in sheep", *Am. Jour. Vet. Res.* 18, 625 (1957).

(17-9)   McLetchie, N.G.R. and Robertson, D., "Chlorinated naphthalene poisoning", *Br. Med. Jour.* 1, 691 (1942).

(17-10)   Kleinfeld, M., et al, "Clinical effects of chlorinated naphthalene exposure", *Jour. Occup. Med.* 14, 377 (1972).

(17-11)   Cotter, L.H., "Pentachlorinated naphthalenes in industry", *Jour. Am. Med. Assoc.* 125, 373 (1944).

(17-12)   Greenburg, L., et al, "The systemic effects resulting from exposure to certain chlorinated hydrocarbons", *Jour. Ind. Hyg. Toxicol* 21, 29 (1939).

(17-13)   American Industrial Hygiene Association, *Chloronaphthalenes,* Hyg. Guide Ser. (Jan.-Feb. 1966).

(17-14)   Cornish, H.H. and Block W.D., "Metabolism of chlorinated naphthalenes", *Jour. Biol. Chem.* 231, 583 (1958).

(17-15)   Ruzo, L., et al, "Metabolism of chlorinated naphthalenes", *Jour. Agric. Food Chem.* 24, 581 (1976).

(17-16)   Ruzo, L., et al, "Uptake and distribution of chloronaphthalenes and their metabolites in pigs", *Bull. Environ. Contam. Toxicol* 16, 233 (1976).

(17-17)   Howard, P.H. and Durkin, P.R., *Preliminary environmental hazard assessment of chlorinated naphthalenes, silicones, fluorocarbons, benzenepolycarboxylates, and chlorophenols,* EPA Publ. No. 560/2-74-001, Washington, D.C., U.S. Environ. Prot. Agency (1973).

(17-18)   American Conference of Governmental Industrial Hygienists, *TLVs Threshold Limit Values for chemical substances and physical agents in the workroom environment with intended changes,* Cincinnati, Ohio (1979).

CHLORINATED PHENOLS (#18)

The chlorinated phenols represent a group of commercially produced, substituted phenols and cresols referred to as chlorophenols and chlorocresols.

It should be noted that 2-chlorophenol is the subject of a separate criteria document (20) and the reader is referred to that section for information on that compound. The same is true for 2,4-dichlorophenol (28) and pentachlorophenol (51).

Occurrence: A summary of the methods of synthesis and principal uses of the commercially most important chlorinated phenols is presented in Table 36. Since the hydroxyl group of the phenol molecule exerts a relatively strong ortho-, para-directing influence over the electrophilic substitution of chlorine atoms, the compounds preferentially formed during the direct chlorination of phenol are 4-chlorophenol, 2-chlorophenol, 2,4-dichlorophenol, 2,6-dichlorophenol, 2,4,6-trichlorophenol, and 2,3,4,6-tetrachlorophenol. Other positional isomers may be synthesized by the hydrolysis of higher chlorobenzenes.

It is well-known that the highly toxic polychlorinated dibenzo-p-dioxins may be formed during the chemical synthesis of some chlorophenols and that the amount of contaminant formed is dependent upon the temperature and pressure control of the reaction. The toxicity of the dioxins varies with the position and number of substituted chlorine atoms and those containing chlorine in the 2,3 and 7 positions are particularly toxic. The 2,3,7,8-tetrachlorodibenzo-p-dioxin (TCDD) is considered the most toxic of all the dioxins.

Table 36: Summary of the Synthesis and Uses of Various Chlorinated Phenols

Chlorinated Phenol	Method of Synthesis	Principal Uses
4-Chlorophenol (4-CP)	Direct chlorination of phenol	To produce 2,4-DCP, and a germicide 4-chlorophenol-o-cresol
2,4-Dichlorophenol (2,4-DCP)	Direct chlorination of phenol	To produce herbicide 2,4-D, also a mothproofing cpd, an antiseptic and a miticide
2,4,5-Trichlorophenol (2,4,5-TCP)	Hydrolysis of 1,2,4,5-tetrachlorobenzene	To produce defoliant 2,4,5-T and related products. Also used directly as a fungicide, antimildew and preservative agent, algicide, bactericide
2,4,6-Trichlorophenol (2,4,6-TCP)	Direct chlorination of phenol	To produce 2,3,4,6-TCP and PCP. Used directly as germicide, bactericide, glue and wood preservative and antimildew treatment
2,3,4,6-Tetrachlorophenol (2,3,4,6-TCP)	Direct chlorination of phenol or lower chlorophenols	Used directly as bactericide, fungicide, insecticide, wood and leather preservative
Pentachlorophenol (PCP)	Direct chlorination of phenol or lower phenols	Used directly as a wood preservative, herbicide, insecticide and molluscicide
4-Chloro-o-cresol (4-C-O-C)	Direct chlorination of o-cresol	To produce the herbicide MCPA

Source: Reference (18)

Evidence has accumulated that the various chlorophenols are formed as intermediate metabolites during the microbiological degradation of the herbicides 2,4-D and 2,4,5-T and pesticides silvex, ronnel, lindane and benzene hexachloride. In view of this, it is clear that chlorinated phenols represent important compounds with regard to potential point source and nonpoint source water contamination.

Chlorophenols may be produced inadvertently by chlorination reactions which take place during the disinfection of wastewater effluents or drinking water sources. Phenol has been reported to be highly reactive to chlorine in dilute aqueous solutions over a considerable pH range.

Limited data are available on levels of chlorinated phenols present in industrial and municipal wastes, natural waters, drinking waters, or soils and sediments. 3-chlorophenol, 4-chlorophenol, and 4-chloro-3-methylphenol (4-chloro-m-cresol) have been identified in chlorinated samples of both primary and secondary effluents and pentachlorophenol was found in domestic sewage treatment effluents.

Physical Properties: Purified chlorinated phenols exist as colorless crystalline solids, with the exception of 2-chlorophenol which is a clear liquid, while the technical grades may be light tan or slightly pink due to impurities. As a group, the chlorophenols are characterized by an odor which has been described as unpleasant, medicinal, pungent, phenolic, strong or persistent.

In general, the volatility of the compounds decreases and the melting and boiling points increase as the number of substituted chlorine atoms increases. The solubility of the chlorophenols and chlorocresols, with the exception of 2,4,6-trichloro-m-cresol, range from soluble to very soluble in relatively nonpolar solvents such as benzene and petroleum ether.

Organoleptic properties manifest themselves in two forms: the ability of a compound to impart an odor to water, and to cause tainting in fish flesh as a result of exposure to chlorophenol-contaminated water. The organoleptic properties of chlorophenols have undergone rather extensive investigation. The threshold levels of monochlorophenols causing odor in water have been reported to be as low as 0.33 to 2.0 μg per liter for 2-chlorophenol.

Chemical Properties: Although chlorophenols are considered weak acids, they are stronger acids than phenol and can be converted to the corresponding phenoxide salts by various bases including sodium carbonate. It is generally accepted that chlorinated phenols will undergo photolysis in aqueous solutions as a result of ultraviolet irradiation and that photodegradation leads to the substitution of hydroxyl groups in place of the chlorine atoms with subsequent polymer formation. Microbial degradation of chlorophenols has also been reported by numerous investigators.

Uses: Chlorinated phenols are used as intermediates in the synthesis of dyes, pigments, phenolic resins, pesticides, and herbicides. Certain chlorophenols also are used directly as flea repellents, fungicides, wood preservatives, mold inhibitors, antiseptics, disinfectants, and antigumming agents for gasoline. See separate criteria documents for compounds 2-chlorophenol (20), 2,4-dichlorophenol (28), and pentachlorophenol (51)].

Toxic Effects: Virtually no data are available on the bioconcentration or bioaccumulation of the lower chlorophenols and limited data are available regarding pentachlorophenol bioconcentration. Studies using ^{14}C-labeled 2,4-dichlorophenol (DCP) demonstrated that oats and soybean seedlings concentrated DCP from dilute solutions (0.2 mg per liter) by factors of 9.2- and 0.65-fold, respectively. Bioconcentration data on pentachlorophenol may be found in the pentachlorophenol criterion document (51).

Chlorophenols, their sodium salts, and certain chlorocresols have been shown to be toxic to aquatic life, mammals, and man. In aquatic organisms it appears that the acute toxicity increases directly with the degree of chlorination. In addition, the production of odors in water and the tainting of fish flesh by the lower chlorophenols and chlorocresols has been reported to occur at extremely low concentrations. These findings, in conjunction with the potential pollution of chlorinated phenols from waste sources, inadvertent chlorination of phenols during disinfection, waste treatment degradation of herbicides and pesticides, and direct industrial and agricultural applications lead to the conclusion that chlorinated phenols represent a potential hazard to aquatic and terrestrial life.

Current Levels of Exposure: There are no available data for any of the chlorophenols on exposure levels.

Special Groups at Risk: There are no special groups at risk for the monochlorophenols, dichlorophenols, trichlorophenols or chlorocresols. Special groups at risk for the tetrachlorophenols include manufacturers, users in wood sawmills and wood treaters.

Existing Guidelines and Standards: No standards have been established for monochlorophenols, dichlorophenols, tetrachlorophenols or chlorocresols. No existing standards were
found for trichlorophenols; however, the National Academy of Sciences (18-1) calculated
a no-adverse-effect level of 0.7 mg 2,4,5-trichlorophenol per liter based on the toxicity studies
with that compound showing no-observable-effect levels (NOEL) of 10 mg/kg in dogs and
mice and 30 mg/kg in rats. These levels were used to determine an ADI of 0.1 mg/kg.

Summary of Proposed EPA Criteria: *Freshwater Aquatic Life* — For 4-chlorophenol the
criterion to protect freshwater aquatic life as derived using the guidelines is 45 μg per liter
as a 24 hour average and the concentration should not exceed 180 μg per liter at any time.
For 2,4,6-trichlorophenol the criterion to protect freshwater aquatic life as derived using
the guidelines is 52 μg per liter as a 24 hour average and the concentration should not exceed 150 μg per liter at any time.

Saltwater Aquatic Life — For saltwater aquatic life, no criterion for any chlorinated phenol
can be derived using the guidelines, and there are insufficient data to estimate a criterion
using other procedures.

Human Health — For the protection of human health from the adverse effects of chlorinated
phenols in water, the following criteria are recommended:

	Micrograms per Liter
Monochlorophenols	
3-chlorophenol	50
4-chlorophenol	30
Dichlorophenol	
2,5-dichlorophenol	3.0
2,6-dichlorophenol	3.0
Trichlorophenol	
2,4,5-trichlorophenol	10
2,4,6-trichlorophenol	100
Tetrachlorophenol *	
2,3,4,6-tetrachlorophenol	263

*This criterion is based on toxicological effects; all other criterion
are based on organoleptic effects.

Basis for the Proposed Human Health Criteria: The chlorinated phenols which are the subject of this section are the monochlorophenols (3- and 4-chlorophenol); the dichlorophenols
(2,5-; 2,6-; 2,3-; 4,6-; and 3,4-dichlorophenols); the trichlorophenols (2,4,5-; 3,4,5-; 2,4,6-;
2,3,4-; 2,3,5-; and 2,3,6-trichlorophenol) and the tetrachlorophenols (2,3,4,5; 2,3,4,6; and
2,3,5,6-tetrachlorophenols). In addition, the monochlorocresols are discussed.

Three chlorinated phenols have been the subject of separate criteria documents: 2-chloro-
phenol (20); 2,4-dichlorophenol (28); and pentachlorophenol (51). There are very little
data on most of these compounds on chronic mammalian effects. However, the organoleptic effects of these compounds have been well documented. (See Table 37.)

Table 37: Comparison of Odor Thresholds for Chlorophenols in Water

	Threshold (ppb)	Temperature (°C)	Reference
2-Chlorophenol	0.33	30	(18-4)
	2	25	(18-5)
	6	*	(18-6)
3-Chlorophenol	200	30	(18-4)
4-Chlorophenol	33	30	(18-4)
	250	25	(18-5)
	900-1,350	—	(18-6)

(continued)

Table 37: (continued)

	Threshold (ppb)	Temperature (°C)	Reference
2,4-Dichlorophenol	0.65	30	(18-4)
	2	25	(18-5)
2,5-Dichlorophenol	3.3	30	(18-4)
2,6-Dichlorophenol	3	25	(18-5)
2,4,5-Trichlorophenol	11	25	(18-4)
2,4,6-Trichlorophenol	100	30	(18-4)
	1,000	25	(18-5)
2,3,4,6-Tetrachlorophenol	915	30	(18-4)

*Temperature not specified.

There are toxicity data on 2,4,5-trichlorophenol. McCollister, et al (18-2), in a 98 day feeding study on rats, demonstrated the NOEL for 2,4,5-trichlorophenol to be 100 mg/kg. Using the National Academy of Sciences' recommended uncertainty factor of 1,000 (18-1), the ADI is calculated to be 0.1 mg/kg of body weight, or 7 mg for a 70 kg person.

For the sake of establishing water quality criteria, it is assumed that on the average a person ingests 2 liters of water and 18.7 g of fish. Since fish may bioaccumulate substances, a bioconcentration factor (BCF) is used in the calculation. The BCF for 2,4,5-trichlorophenol is 130 and was derived by U.S. EPA ecological laboratories in Duluth, Minnesota. The equation for calculating an acceptable amount of 2,4,5-trichlorophenol in water based on the ingestion of 2 liters of drinking water and 18.7 g of fish is:

$$(2\ l)X + (0.0187 \times F)X = ADI$$

where 2 l is 2 liters of drinking water; 0.0187 kg is the amount of fish consumed daily; F is bioconcentration factor (130 for 2,4,5-trichlorophenol); (2 l)X + (0.0187 x 130)X is 7.0 mg; 2X + 2.43X is 7.0; 4.43X is 7.0; and X is 1.6 mg/l.

There are no toxicity data for tetrachlorophenol, but because of the similarities between tetra- and pentachlorophenol and the lower acute toxicity of tetrachlorophenol, it is reasonable to set the water criterion on the basis of the more extensive toxicologic data base for pentachlorophenol.

The criterion is established as follows: The NOEL for pentachlorophenol is 3 mg/kg. Since the chlorophenols are rapidly excreted by mammals, an uncertainty factor of 100 is used to establish the acceptable human exposure of 0.03 mg/kg per day. A water intake of 2 liters per day and an average body weight of 70 kg are assumed. The acceptable whole body exposure is then 70 kg x 0.03 mg/kg/day, which equals 2.1 mg per day. Assuming that the total exposure is from ingesting 2 liters of drinking water and 18.7 g of fish, the following calculation has been established:

$$(2\ l)X + (0.0187 \times BCF)X = ADI$$

where 2 l is the amount of drinking water consumed; 0.0187 kg is the amount of fish consumed; BCF is the bioconcentration factor (320 for tetrachlorophenol); and ADI is the acceptable daily intake (2.1 mg).

In tetrachlorophenol, which is based on the use of chronic toxicologic data and an uncertainty factor of 100, the recommended criterion level is 263 μg per liter. Drinking water contributes 25% of the assumed exposure while eating contaminated fish products accounts for 75%. The criterion level can alternatively be expressed as 351 if exposure is assumed to be from the consumption of fish and shellfish products alone.

The organoleptic properties of the chlorinated phenols are well-known. These compounds have been reported to impart a medicinal-like odor and taste to water and to the flesh of aquatic organisms raised in contaminated water. Summaries of the reported taste/odor threshold levels of various chlorophenols in water or in aquatic organisms are presented in Table 37 and 38, respectively.

Table 38: Summary of Threshold Concentrations of Chlorinated Phenols in Water that Cause Tainting of the Flesh of Aquatic Organisms

Compound	Threshold (μg/l)	Reference
2-Chlorophenol	15.0	(18-7)
	15.0	(18-8)
3-Chlorophenol	60.0	(18-7)
4-Chlorophenol	60.0	(18-7)
	50.0	(18-8)
2,4-Dichlorophenol	5.0	(18-8)
	10.0	(18-9)

Water quality criteria for 2-chlorophenol and 2,4-dichlorophenol based on organoleptic effects were published (18-3). These criteria of 0.3 and 0.5 μg per liter, respectively, were derived from the data reported by Hoak (18-4) and are based on the odor threshold of these compounds in water.

The criteria for various other mono-, di- and trichlorophenols have been derived and are based on the lower of the odor threshold in water or the tainting threshold in aquatic organisms (18). (See Table 39.)

Table 39: Recommended Water Quality Criteria

Compound	........Criterion from........	
	Organoleptic Effects (μg/l)	Toxicological Data (μg/l)
Monochlorophenols		
3-Chlorophenol	50	none
4-Chlorophenol	30	none
Dichlorophenols		
2,5-Dichlorophenol	3.0	none
2,6-Dichlorophenol	3.0	none
Trichlorophenols		
2,4,5-Trichlorophenol	10	1,600
2,4,6-Trichlorophenol	100	–
Tetrachlorophenol*		
2,3,4,6-Tetrachlorophenol	900	263

*The criterion will be based on toxicological effects.

Since the criterion derived for tetrachlorophenol based on its toxic effects is lower than that derived as a result of its organoleptic properties, the former criterion is recommended. There are no available data on monochlorocresols upon which to base a criterion.

References:

(18-1) National Academy of Sciences, *Drinking Water and Health,* Washington, D.C. (1977).

(18-2) McCollister, D.D., et al, "Toxicologic information on 2,4,5-trichlorophenol", *Toxicol. Appl. Pharmacol* 3, 63 (1961).

(18-3) *FR* 15946 (1979).

(18-4) Hoak, R.D., "The causes of tastes and odors in drinking water", *Proc. 11th Ind. Waste Conf., Purdue Univ. Eng. Bull.* 41, 229 (1957).

(18-5) Burttschell, R.H., et al, "Chlorine derivatives of phenol causing taste and odor", *Jour. Am. Water Works Assoc.* 51, 205 (1959).

(18-6) Campbell, C.L., et al, "Effect of certain chemicals in water on the flavor of brewed coffee", *Food Res.* 23, 575 (1959).

(18-7) Schulze, E., "The effect of phenol-containing waste on the taste of fish", *Int. Revne. Ges. Hydrobiol.* 46, No. 1, 81 (1961).

(18-8) Teal, J.L., "The control of waste through fish taste", presented to American Chemical Society, national meeting (1959).

(18-9) Shumway, D.L., *Effect of effluents on flavor of salmon,* Dept. Fisheries and Wildlife Agri. Exper. Sta. Oregon State U. (1966).

CHLOROBENZENE

See "Chlorinated Benzenes" (14).

p-CHLORO-m-CRESOL

See "Chlorinated Phenols" (18).

CHLORODIBROMOMETHANE

See "Halomethanes" (38).

CHLOROETHANE

See "Chlorinated Ethanes" (15).

2-CHLOROETHYL VINYL ETHER

See "Chloroalkyl Ethers" (16).

CHLOROFORM (#19)

Chloroform, $CHCl_3$, is a chlorinated methane and the reader is also referred to criteria for Carbon Tetrachloride (12) and Halomethanes (38).

Occurrence: Chloroform appears to be ubiquitous in the environment in trace amounts and discharges into the environment result largely from chlorination of water and wastewater (19-1). Major transport routes are both waterborne and atmospheric.

Physical Properties: At ordinary temperatures and pressures, chloroform is a clear, colorless, volatile liquid with a pleasant, etheric, nonirritating odor and sweet taste. It has a boiling point range of 61° to 62°C, a melting point of –63.5°C and is nonflammable. There is no flash point. Chloroform is slightly soluble in water (7.42×10^6 μg per liter of water at 25°C). It is miscible with alcohol, benzene, ether, petroleum, ether, carbon tetrachloride, carbon disulfide and oils. Chloroform is highly refractive and has a vapor pressure of 200 mm Hg at 25°C.

Chemical Properties: At ambient environmental temperatures, chloroform is thermostable and resists decomposition. However, slow decomposition is observed following prolonged exposure to sunlight in the presence or absence of air, and in the dark when air is present. Chloroform has the potential to react with, and thereby deplete, the ozone layer since studies have shown that phosgene is a decomposition product of ozone and chloroform. There is no appreciable decomposition of chloroform at ambient temperatures in water even in the presence of sunlight. Aqueous degradation of chloroform is accelerated in the presence of aerated waters and metals such as iron with hydrogen peroxide representing the degradation product.

Uses: Chloroform has become obsolete as a widely used anesthetic in favor of other agents with more desirable properties; its uses today are mainly as a chemical solvent and as an intermediate in the production of refrigerants, plastics, and pharmaceuticals (19-1). Current annual production of chloroform approaches 120,000 metric tons.

Toxic Effects: In controlled laboratory tests, chloroform has been shown to be toxic to aquatic organisms. In mammalian species, chloroform has been demonstrated to be carcinogenic and exhibits both temporary and lasting toxic effects.

Human exposure may be incidental or occupational, or deliberate because of the prenarcosis euphoria associated with the inhalation of chloroform. Humans are exposed to chloroform by routes other than water ingestion, including food ingestion, inhalation and skin contact. Long range exposures have caused both physical and neurological disorders in humans, with liver and kidney toxic responses representing the most prevalent physical pathology. Epidemiological studies hint that there may be a relationship between cancer incidence and ingestion of water containing chloroform. The studies are inconclusive, however, and only add to the weight of evidence suggesting that chloroform exposure may be deleterious.

The chemical apparently does not significantly bioconcentrate in aquatic species (19-3) or significantly biomagnify along the food chain to higher trophic levels (19-4, 19-5) and evidence suggests that it is metabolized in humans by the liver and kidney to carbon dioxide or it is eliminated unchanged as chloroform through the lungs (19-5, 19-6).

Current Levels of Exposure: The National Academy of Science (19-7) assembled data based on human exposure to chloroform. Their calculations of human uptake are based on fluid intake, respiratory volume and food consumption data for reference man as compiled by the International Commission for Radiological Protection. Table 40 presents the data on relative human uptake from the three sources.

The uptake of chloroform from the atmosphere at minimum levels of exposure is about 10 times greater than from fluids. At maximum exposure levels, the chloroform uptake from fluids is slightly less than that from the atmosphere. At typical exposure levels, however, the human uptake from fluids is two to three times greater than from the atmosphere with slight variation by sex and age noted.

In its Statement of Basis and Purpose for an Amendment to the National Interim Primary Drinking Water Regulations on Trihalomethanes, the U.S. EPA (19-8) estimated the total human exposure to chloroform. The estimates have basic assumptions that are roughly comparable, but not exactly the same as those used by the NAS (19-7). They use newer values for chloroform content in drinking water from NOMS data, and provide estimates for human adults only. See Table 41 for the exposure estimates.

Table 40: Relative Human Uptake of Carbon Tetrachloride and Chloroform from Environmental Sources (mg/year)

Source	Adult Man CCl_4	Adult Man $CHCl_3$	Adult Woman CCl_4	Adult Woman $CHCl_3$	Child CCl_4	Child $CHCl_3$
	. . . . At Minimum Exposure Levels*.					
Fluid intake	0.73	0.037	0.73	0.037	0.73	0.036
Atmosphere	3.60	0.41	3.30	0.37	2.40	0.27
Food supply	0.21	0.21	0.21	0.21	0.21	0.21
Total	4.54	0.66	4.24	0.62	3.34	0.52

(continued)

Table 40: (continued)

Source	Adult Man		Adult Woman		Child	
	CCl$_4$	CHCl$_3$	CCl$_4$	CHCl$_3$	CCl$_4$	CHCl$_3$
	. . . . .At Typical Exposure Levels**.					
Fluid intake	1.78	14.90	1.28	10.70	1.28	10.70
Atmosphere	4.80	5.20	4.40	4.70	3.20	3.40
Food Supply	1.12	2.17	1.12	2.17	1.12	2.17
Total	7.70	22.27	6.80	17.57	5.60	16.27
	. . . . At Maximum Exposure Levels***.					
Fluid intake	4.05	321	4.05	321	1.83	223
Atmosphere	618	474	567	434	405	310
Food supply	7.33	16.4	7.33	16.4	7.33	16.4
Total	629	811	578	771	414	549

*Minimum conditions of all variables assumed: Minimum exposure-minimum intake for
fluids; minimum exposure-minimum absorption for atmosphere; and minimum exposure-minimum intake for food supplies.

**Typical conditions of all variables assumed. For CCl$_4$: 0.0025 mg/l-reference man intake
for fluids; average of typical minimum and maximum absorption for atmosphere; and
average exposure and intake for food supplies. For CHCl$_3$: median exposure-reference
man intake for fluids; average of typical minimum and maximum absorption for atmosphere; and average exposure and intake for food supplies.

***Maximum conditions of all variables assumed: maximum exposure intake for fluids; maxi-
mum exposure-maximum absorption for atmosphere; and maximum exposure-maximum
intake for food supplies.

Source: Reference (19-7)

Table 41: Uptake of Chloroform for the Adult Human from Air, Water, and Food

Source	Adult (mg/year)	Uptake (%)
	. . . . . Maximum Conditions	
Atmosphere	204	36
Water	343	61
Food supply	16	3
Total	563	100
	. . . . . Minimum Conditions.	
Atmosphere	0.41	13
Water	0.73	23
Food Supply	2.00	64
Total	3.14	100
	. . . . . . Mean Conditions	
Atmosphere	20.0	22
Water	64.04	68
Food supply	9.00	10
Total	93	100

Source: Reference (19-8)

The two exposure estimates, NAS (19-7) and the U.S. EPA (19-8) demonstrate that chloroform intake from ingesting water is likely to range from a modest to predominant percentage of total exposure with a simple minimum, mean, and maximum exposure scenario.

	Total Exposure from Water (%)	
	U.S. EPA	NAS
Minimum exposure	23	6
Mean exposure	69	67
Maximum exposure	61	40

Special Groups at Risk: A partial list of occupations in which exposure may occur includes chemists, drug makers, fluorocarbon makers, lacquer workers, polish makers, silk synthesizers and solvent workers. NIOSH estimates that 40,000 people in the U.S. may be exposed to chloroform in their working environment.

Existing Guidelines and Standards: The Occupational Safety and Health Administration's limit for chloroform in workplace air is 50 ppm or 244 mg/m^3. This is a ceiling value for a maximum 10 minute exposure that at no time shall be exceeded. NIOSH promulgated a criterion of 10 ppm (48.9 mg/m^3) in 1974 (19-9). This criterion was applied to a time-weighted exposure for as high as 10 hours per day and a 40 hour work week. Following the National Cancer Institute's (NCI) study of chloroform, NIOSH on June 9, 1976 (19-10) reduced this allowable time-weighted average exposure criterion to 2 ppm (9.8 mg/m^3).

Based on available health information, a safe level of airborne exposure to halogenated agents could not be defined. Since a safe level of occupational exposure to halogenated anesthetic agents could not be established by either animal or human investigations, NIOSH recommended that airborne exposure be limited to levels no greater than the lowest level detectable using the sampling and analysis techniques recommended (19-11). Although chloroform is not usually used as an anesthetic, it is included in the criteria and is limited to 2 ppm or 9.8 mg/m^3.

If a procedure that converts this air limit to a water limit is used, the equivalent exposure in water would be 34.9 mg per liter (19-12). In this method, complete absorption from inhalation and ingestion is assumed. The inhalation absorption may be closer to 50% and the equivalent water exposure would then be 17.4 mg per liter. The occupational limits apply to the healthy working-age population and even then if exposure level is half the limit, comprehensive medical surveillance is required. To use the occupational limit as a guide for the general population, an application factor of 100 can be used. Thus, an equivalent level in water would be 174 µg per liter. It must be remembered that the occupational limit for chloroform is based on the lowest level detectable in air using NIOSH's recommended analytical techniques and does not necessarily represent a level adequate to protect man.

In general, the use of inhalation data assumes an 8 hour day, time-weighted average, occupational exposure in the working place with workers inhaling the toxic substance throughout such a period. Exposures for the general population should be considerably less. Such worker-exposure inhalation standards are inappropriate for the general population since they presume an exposure limited to an 8 hour day, an age bracket of the population that excludes the very young and the very old, and a healthy worker prior to exposure. Ingestion data are far superior to inhalation data when the risks associated with the food and water of the aquatic environment are being considered.

Following the NCI study of chloroform (19-13), the Food and Drug Administration took action to halt the use of chloroform in drug products, cosmetic products, and food contact materials (19-14). The EPA has issued a notice of rebuttable presumption against continued registration of chloroform-containing pesticides (19-15).

The EPA has also proposed an amendment which would add to the National Interim Primary Drinking Water Regulations a section on the control of organic halogenated chemical contaminants in drinking water (19-16). The proposed limit for total trihalomethanes, which includes chloroform, is 100 µg per liter. This limit was set largely on the basis of technological and economic feasibility. Originally the limit will apply only to water supplies serving greater than 75,000 consumers; this is intended to provide an orderly upgrading of drinking water treatment in the country. The basis and purpose of the regulation are discussed in a paper by the Office of Drinking Water issued in January 1978 (19-8). This document contains a number of estimates of cancer risk attributable to the presence of chloroform in drinking water. One of these, performed by the National Academy of Sciences, using a linear nonthreshold extrapolation from animal data, estimated that the lifetime risk would fall between 1.5×10^{-7} and 17×10^{-7} per microgram of chloroform per liter of water consumed daily depending upon the data set used. The upper 95% confidence estimates would range between 3×10^{-7} and 22×10^{-7} per microgram per liter per day.

Summary of Proposed EPA Criteria: *Freshwater Aquatic Life* — For chloroform, the criterion to protect freshwater aquatic life, as derived using the guidelines, is 500 μg per liter as a 24 hour average and the concentration should never exceed 1,200 μg per liter at any time.

Saltwater Aquatic Life — For chloroform, the criterion to protect saltwater aquatic life, as derived using procedures other than the guidelines, is 620 μg per liter as a 24 hour average and the concentration should never exceed 1,400 μg per liter at any time.

Human Health — For the maximum protection of human health from the potential carcinogenic effects of exposure to chloroform through ingestion of water and contaminated aquatic organisms, the ambient water concentration is zero. Concentrations of chloroform estimated to result in additional lifetime cancer risks ranging from no additional risk to an additional risk of 1 in 100,000 are presented in the criterion formulation section of this document. The EPA is considering setting criteria at an interim target risk level in the range of 10^{-5}, 10^{-6}, or 10^{-7} with corresponding criteria of 2.1, 0.21 and 0.021 μg per liter, respectively.

Basis for the Proposed Human Health Criteria: Chloroform has several adverse effects on the human body. Safe levels of chloroform in water necessary to avoid some of these effects would be difficult to establish because adequate studies have not been conducted. The most serious effect to consider is the cancer-causing potential of the chemical. Current knowledge leads to the conclusion that carcinogenesis is a nonthreshold, nonreversible process. The nonthreshold concept implies that many tumors will be produced at high doses, but any dose no matter how small, will have the probability of causing cancer. Even small carcinogenic risks have a serious impact on society when the exposed population is large, because it is likely that some cancers will be caused by chloroform. The nonreversible concept implies that once the tumor growth process has started, growth will continue and may metastasize and involve other organs until death ensues.

Chloroform has been shown to induce cancer in two species of experimental animals. This conclusion is neither confirmed nor denied by the results of numerous epidemiology studies available, although from a public health point of view, a suspicion of a qualitative weight of evidence for confirmation probably exists.

The available information on total human exposure to chloroform from air, water and food sources suggests that drinking water contributes from 6 to 69% of the total exposure. Considering that chloroform levels in drinking water are enhanced by water treatment processes on the one hand and that chloroform levels in waste discharges may be similarly enhanced by waste treatment processes, it is difficult to utilize the total exposure information in formulating an ambient water quality criterion, except to say that exposure through water is likely to be more significant than other exposure routes.

It is therefore proposed that the total risk for carcinogenic response be allocated to the ambient water exposure conditions of ingesting 2 liters per day of water and consuming 18.7 g of potentially contaminated fish products.

Under the consent decree in NRDC vs Train, criteria are to state "recommended maximum permissible concentrations (including where appropriate, zero) consistent with the protection of aquatic organisms, human health, and recreational activities". Chloroform is suspected of being a human carcinogen. Because there is no recognized safe concentration for a human carcinogen, the recommended concentration of chloroform in water for maximum protection of human health is zero.

Because attaining a zero concentration level may be infeasible in some cases and in order to assist the EPA and states in the possible future development of water quality regulations, the concentrations of chloroform corresponding to several incremental lifetime cancer risk levels have been estimated. A cancer risk level provides an estimate of the additional incidence of cancer that may be expected in an exposed population. A risk of 10^{-5}, for example, indicates a probability of 1 additional case of cancer for every 100,000 people exposed; a risk of 10^{-6} indicates 1 additional case of cancer for every 1,000,000 people exposed; and so forth.

In the *Federal Register* notice of availability of draft ambient water quality criteria, EPA stated that it is considering setting criteria at an interim target risk level of 10^{-5}, 10^{-6}, or 10^{-7} as shown in Table 42.

Table 42: Possible Alternative Criteria for Chloroform

Exposure Assumptions (per day)	Risk Levels and Corresponding Criteria (μg/l)			
	0	10^{-7}	10^{-6}	10^{-5}
2 liters of drinking water and consumption of 18.7 grams fish and shellfish*	0	0.021	0.21	2.1
Consumption of fish and shellfish only	0	0.175	1.75	17.5

*~12% of the chloroform exposure results from the consumption of aquatic organisms which exhibit an average bioconcentration of 14-fold. The remaining 88% of chloroform exposure results from drinking water.

Source: Reference (19)

In the above table risk levels and corresponding criteria were calculated by applying a modified one-hit extrapolation model described in the methodology document to the animal bioassay data presented in Summary of Pertinent Data. Since the extrapolation model is linear at low doses, the additional lifetime risk is directly proportional to the water concentration. Therefore, water concentrations corresponding to other risk levels can be derived by multiplying or dividing one of the risk levels and corresponding water concentrations shown in the table by factors such as 10; 100; 1,000; and so forth.

Concentration levels were derived assuming a lifetime exposure to various amounts of chloroform (a) occurring from the consumption of both drinking water and aquatic life grown in waters containing the corresponding chloroform concentrations and (b) occurring solely from consumption of aquatic life grown in the waters containing the corresponding chloroform concentrations. Although total exposure information for chloroform is discussed and an estimate of the contributions from other sources of exposure can be made, this data will not be factored into ambient water quality criteria formulation until additional analysis can be made. The criteria presented, therefore, assume an incremental risk from ambient water exposure only.

Summary of Pertinent Data — The NCI bioassay (19-13) with female mice given a time-weighted average dose of 238 mg/kg of chloroform by stomach tube 5 times per week for 78 weeks is used for the water quality criterion. The treatment induced hepatocellular carcinomas in 36 of 45 animals examined, whereas the pooled control group had 1 animal with hepatocellular carcinoma out of 80 animals examined. Assuming a fish bioaccumulation factor of 14, the parameters of the extrapolation model are:

$$n_t = 36 \qquad\qquad le = 78 \text{ weeks}$$
$$N_t = 45 \qquad\qquad d = 238 \times {}^5\!/_7 = \text{mg/kg/day}$$
$$n_c = 1 \qquad\qquad w = 0.030 \text{ kg}$$
$$N_c = 80 \qquad\qquad L = 92 \text{ weeks}$$
$$Le = 92 \text{ weeks} \qquad R = 14$$
$$F = 0.0187 \text{ kg}$$

The result is that the water concentration should be less than 2.1 μg per liter in order to keep the individual lifetime risk below 10^{-5}.

References:

(19-1)   U.S. EPA, *Development document for interim final effluent limitations guidelines and new source performance standards for the significant organic products segment of the organic chemical manufacturing point source category,* Report No. EPA-440/1-75/045, Washington D.C., Environ. Prot. Agency, (1975).

(19-2)   Eschenbrenner, A.B. and Miller, E., "Induction of hepatomas in mice by repeated oral administration of chloroform, with observations of sex differences", *Jour. Nat. Cancer Inst.* 5, 251 (1945).

(19-3)   U.S. EPA, *In-depth studies on health and environmental impacts of selected water pollutants,* EPA Contract No. 68-01-4646, Washington, D.C., U.S. Environ. Prot. Agency (1978).

(19-4)   Pearson, C.R. and McConnell, G., "Chlorinated C_1 and C_2 hydrocarbons in the marine environment", *Proc. Roy. Soc. London Bull.,* 189, 305 (1975).

(19-5)   McConnell, G., et al, "Chlorinated hydrocarbons and the environment", *Endeavor* 34, 13 (1975).

(19-6)   Taylor, D.C., et al, "Metabolism of chloroform. II. A sex difference in the metabolism of (^{14}C)-chloroform in mice", *Xenobiotica* 4, 165 (1974).

(19-7)   National Academy of Sciences, *Nonfluorinated Halomethanes in the Environment,* Washington, D.C. (1978).

(19-8)   U.S. Environmental Protection Agency, *Statement of Basis for an Amendment to the National Interim Primary Drinking Water Regulations on Trihalomethanes,* Washington, D.C., Office of Water Supply (1978).

(19-9)   National Institute for Occupational Safety and Health, *Criteria for a Recommended Standard: Occupational Exposure to Chloroform,* NIOSH Doc. No. 75-114, Washington, D.C. (1975).

(19-10) National Institute for Occupational Safety and Health, *Current Intelligence Bulletin No. 9-Chloroform,* Washington, D.C. (1976).

(19-11) National Institute for Occupational Safety and Health, *Criteria for a Recommended Standard: Occupational Exposure to Waste Anesthetic Gases and Vapors,* NIOSH Doc. No. 77-140, Washington, D.C. (1977).

(19-12) Stokinger, H.E. and Woodward, R.L., "Toxicological methods for establishing drinking water standards", *Jour. Am. Water Works Assoc.* 50, 515 (1958).

(19-13) National Cancer Institute, *Report on carcinogenesis bioassay of chloroform,* Washington, D.C. (1976).

(19-14) 41 *FR* 15026, 15029 (Apr. 9, 1976).

(19-15) 41 *FR* 14588 (Apr. 6, 1976).

(19-16) 43 *FR* 5756 (Feb. 9, 1978).

CHLOROMETHYL METHYL ETHER

See "Chloroalkyl Ethers" (16).

2-CHLORONAPHTHALENE

See "Chlorinated Naphthalenes" (17).

2-CHLOROPHENOL (#20)

2-Chlorophenol (o-chlorophenol) has the structural formula

the molecular formula HOC_6H_4Cl and a molecular weight of 128.36.

Occurrence: Information concerning the presence and fate of 2-chlorophenol is incomplete or nonexistent. However, the generation of waste sources from the commercial production of 2-chlorophenol, its chemically derived products and the inadvertent synthesis of 2-chlorophenol due to chlorination of phenol in effluents and drinking water sources, may clearly indicate its importance in potential point source and nonpoint source water contamination.

The chlorination of phenol from dilute aqueous solutions and from sewage effluents has been demonstrated. However, no data regarding 2-chlorophenol concentrations in finished drinking water are available.

Physical Properties: 2-Chlorophenol has a density of 1.2573 at 25°C, a vapor pressure of 1 mm Hg at 12.1°C, melts at 8.7°C and exhibits a boiling point range of 175° to 176°C.

Chemical Properties: Microbial degradation of 2-chlorophenol under laboratory conditions has been reported. Studies on the metabolism of the herbicide, 2,4-dichlorophenoxyacetate (2,4-D), have demonstrated the dechlorination and aromatic ring degradation of 2-chlorophenol by an *Arthrobacter* species (20-1). Nachtigall and Butler (20-2) reported the complete oxidation of 2-chlorophenol by *Pseudomonas* species isolated from activated sludge. Although these laboratory studies suggested microbial oxidation as an important degradation route for 2-chlorophenol, sufficient data are not available to reach conclusions regarding the persistence of this compound in the environment.

Uses: 2-Chlorophenol is a commercially produced chemical used entirely as an intermediate in the production of other chemicals. It represents a basic chemical feedstock for the manufacture of higher chlorophenols for such uses as fungicides, slimicides, bactericides, antiseptics, disinfectants, and wood and glue preservatives. 2-Chlorophenol is also used to form intermediates in the production of phenolic resins and has been utilized in a process for extracting sulfur and nitrogen compounds from coal.

Direct chlorination leads to the formation of both 2- and 4-chlorophenols and the isomers are separated by fractional distillation since the difference in boiling points is greater than 40°C. Most of the 2-chlorophenol used commercially in the U.S. is recovered as a by-product from the manufacture of 4-chlorophenol by direct chlorination of phenol.

Toxic Effects: Although 2-chlorophenol has been reported to be less toxic than the higher chlorophenols, its low odor threshold in water and its tainting properties are considered a potential threat to certain beneficial uses of water and the utilization of aquatic life as a food source.

Current Levels of Exposure: Overall, exposure of the general population to 2-chlorophenol would be most likely in the form of consumption of phenolic-containing chlorinated drinking water. This would limit exposure primarily to water supplies contaminated by a point source of 2-chlorophenol. Such sources should be relatively easy to identify and monitor since analytical techniques for 2-chlorophenol are available. Apparently, such monitoring is not generally being done.

Since 2-chlorophenol is not a universally reported metabolite of 2,4-D, exposure of the general population via use of 2,4-D is only speculative. If small amounts of 2-chlorophenol are formed and gain access to ground water or the soil, it is not expected to persist in view of its ready susceptibility to microbial attack.

Inhalation or dermal exposure to the general population is not expected to be a significant part of any total 2-chlorophenol exposure. For industrial workers manufacturing or handling 2-chlorophenol, inhalation exposure could be the greatest threat and the hardest to control. Dermal exposure in such instances should be negligible if sensible and accepted industrial hygiene practices are followed.

Due to the lack of monitoring data or human body burden values, human exposure cannot be determined.

Special Groups at Risk: The only special group expected to be at risk for high exposure to 2-chlorophenol are industrial workers involved in the manufacturing or handling of 2-chlorophenol. No data were found to relate exposure or body burden to conditions of contact with 2-chlorophenol.

Existing Guidelines and Standards: As far as can be determined, no standards or guidelines exist for 2-chlorophenol.

Summary of Proposed EPA Criteria: *Freshwater Aquatic Life* — For 2-chlorophenol the criterion to protect freshwater aquatic life as derived using the guidelines is 60 μg per liter as a 24 hour average and the concentration should not exceed 180 μg per liter at any time.

Saltwater Aquatic Life — For saltwater aquatic life, no criterion for 2-chlorophenol can be derived using the guidelines, and there are insufficient data to estimate a criterion using other procedures.

Human Health — For the prevention of adverse effects due to the organoleptic properties of 2-chlorophenol in water, the criteria is 0.3 μg per liter.

Basis for the Proposed Human Health Criteria: Insufficient data exists to indicate that 2-chlorophenol is a carcinogenic agent. Only one study was designed to detect the promoting activity of 2-chlorophenol with dimethylbenzanthracene-initiated tumors. Although carcinogenic promoters may pose a possible carcinogenic risk to man, there are no dose/response data on which to base a qualitative risk extrapolation.

(Under certain environmental conditions, 2-chlorophenol may produce a small amount of dibenzo-p-dioxin, which is an unsubstituted analog of chlorinated dibenzo-p-dioxins. The recent NCI bioassay report of possible carcinogenicity of dibenzo-p-dioxin has concluded that dibenzo-p-dioxin was not carcinogenic for Osborne-Mendel rats or B6C3F1 mice.) In fact, insufficient health effects data exist on any chronic or acute effect of 2-chlorophenol. In view of this, the recommended criterion is based on organoleptic effects.

The data of investigations evaluating the odor of 2-chlorophenol in drinking water indicate that a low concentration is capable of causing discernable odor. None of these studies indicate if the threshold odor concentration made the water unacceptable for consumption. These studies, coupled with flavor impairment studies, suggest that the selection of 0.3 μg per liter of 2-chlorophenol would be sufficient for the prevention of adverse organoleptic effects in water.

It should be emphasized that this is a criterion based on aesthetic rather than health effects. Data on human health effects needs to be developed as a more substantial basis for setting a criterion for the protection of human health.

Thus, based on the prevention of adverse organoleptic effects, the interim criterion recommended for 2-chlorophenol is 0.3 μg per liter.

References:

(20-1)   Loos, M.A., et al, "Formation of 2,4-dichlorophenol and 2,4-dichlorophenoxyacetate by *Arthrobacter* Sp.", *Can. Jour. Microbiol.* 13, 691 (1966).

(20-2)   Nachtigall, M.H. and Butler, R.G., "Metabolism of phenols and chlorophenols by activated sludge microorganisms", *Abstr. Ann. Meet. Am. Soc. Microbiol.* 74, 184 (1974).

4-CHLOROPHENYL PHENYL ETHER

See "Haloethers" (37).

CHROMIUM (#21)

Chromium, symbol Cr, is an element in Group VI of the Periodic Table. It has an atomic weight of 52.01.

Occurrence: Chromium is a common element, present in low concentrations throughout nature. Sources of chromium in the environment have been recently reviewed (21-1). Although Cr is widely distributed, with an average concentration in the continental crust of 125 mg/kg, it is rarely found in significant concentrations in natural waters. Air levels in nonurban areas usually fall below detection limits and may be as low as 5 pg/m^3. Much of the detectable Cr in air and water is presumably derived from industrial processes, which in 1972 consumed 320,000 metric tons of the metal in the U.S. alone. A significant fraction of this amount entered the environment; additional amounts are contributed by combustion of coal and other industrial processes (21-2).

As a result, levels of Cr in air exceeding 0.010 μg/m^3 have been reported from 59 of 186 urban areas examined. Mean concentration of Cr in 1,577 samples of surface water were reported as 9.7 μg per liter (Kopp, 1969). The significance of 9.7 μg per liter as a mean value is questionable because only 25% of the samples tested contained any detectable Cr. Occasional values of total Cr [Cr(III) and Cr(IV)] exceeded 50 μg per liter, a fact which must be noted in relation to the recommended standard for domestic water supplies.

Physical Properties: The metallic element Cr belongs to the first series of transition elements, and occurs in nature primarily as compounds of its trivalent Cr(III) or hexavalent Cr(VI) forms. Generally speaking, the hexavalent compounds are relatively water-soluble and readily reduced to the more insoluble and stable forms of Cr(III) by reaction with organic reducing matter.

Chemical Properties: Chromium is a metallic element which can exist in several valence states. However, in the aquatic environment it virtually is always found in valence states +3 or +6. Hexavalent chromium is a strong oxidizing agent which reacts readily with reducing agents such as sulfur dioxide to give trivalent chromium. Cr(III) oxidizes slowly to Cr(VI), the rate increasing with temperature. Oxidation progresses rapidly when Cr(III) adsorbs to MnO, but is interfered with by Ca(II) and Mg(II) ions. Thus accumulation would probably occur in sediments where chemical equilibria favor the formation of Cr(III), while Cr(VI), if favored, would presumably dissipate in soluble forms. Hexavalent chromium exists in solution as a component of an anion, rather than a cation, and, therefore, does not precipitate from alkaline solution.

The three important anions are hydrochromate, chromate and dichromate. The proportion of hexavalent chromium present in each of these forms depends on pH. In strongly basic and neutral solutions, the chromate form predominates. As pH is lowered, the hydrochromate concentration increases. At very low pH the dichromate species predominates. In pH ranges encountered in natural waters, the proportion of dichromate ions is relatively low. In the acid portion of the environmental range, the predominant form is hydrochromate ion (63.6% at pH 6.0 to 6.2). In the alkaline portion of the range, the predominant form is chromate ion (95.7% at pH 8.5 to 7.8). The anionic form of chromium can affect its toxicity.

Trivalent chromium in solution forms numerous types of hexacoordinate complexes. Trivalent Cr forms stable hexacoordinate complexes with many molecules of biochemical interest. Interaction of Cr(III) with such compounds may involve binding to carboxy groups of proteins or smaller metabolites, coordination with certain amino acids, and binding to nucleic acids and nucleoproteins. This last reaction is of special significance in the consideration of the carcinogenic potential of Cr compounds. The field was reviewed by Mertz (21-3) and it suffices here to emphasize the stability of these Cr complexes, and the fact that the element is found combined with both RNA and DNA; an effect of Cr on the tertiary structure of nucleic acids is clearly indicated. In general, it may be concluded that reduction of Cr(VI) to Cr(III) and its subsequent coordination to organic molecules of biochemical interest explain in large measure the biological reactivity of Cr compounds. Thus, the well-known reaction of Cr with skin proteins, i.e., the tanning process, involves coordination sites of Cr(III). For reasons of solubility, however, uptake of compounds of Cr(VI) by the living organism generally exceeds that of Cr(III) compounds.

Thus, one may invoke as a likely explanation for the greater toxicity of Cr(VI) than of Cr(III) compounds their more rapid uptake by tissues due to their solubility and to the facilitation of their translocation across biological membranes. Once within cells, the Cr(VI) is likely to be reduced to the trivalent state before reacting with cell constituents such as proteins and nucleic acids.

Uses: Chromium salts are used extensively in the metal finishing industry as electroplating, cleaning and passivating agents, and as mordants in the textile industry. They also are used in cooling waters, in the leather tanning industry, in catalyst manufacture, in pigments and primer paints, and in fungicides and wood preservatives.

Toxic Effects: The toxicity of chromium has long been recognized, but detailed analysis of toxic effects is complicated by the occurrence of many different compounds of the metal; these may contain Cr in different valence states and are distinguished by their chemical, physical and toxicological properties.

In the freshwater environment, hexavalent chromium has been shown acutely toxic to invertebrates at concentrations as low as 22 μg per liter (21-4) and 17,600 μg per liter for vertebrates (21-5). For marine waters the figures are 2,000 μg per liter for invertebrates (21-6) and 30,000 μg per liter for vertebrates (21-7). Trivalent chromium is recognized as an essential trace element for humans. Hexavalent chromium in the workplace is suspected of being carcinogenic.

The general area of environmental effects of chromium compounds was recently reviewed by the U.S. EPA (21-1); a valuable discussion of the medical and biological effects of Cr in the environment is found also in a volume published by the National Academy of Sciences (21-8). Occupational hazards of chromium were assessed in a criteria document prepared by NIOSH in 1976 (21-9). Mertz (21-3) provided a valuable survey of the biochemical properties of Cr compounds.

Current Levels of Exposure: Although lower Cr limits have been prescribed for air than for water, the standard for noncarcinogenic Cr(VI) in air permits significantly greater uptake of Cr than does that for Cr(VI) in drinking water designed for human consumption. Thus, if we assume a daily consumption of 2 liters, with a fractional gastrointestinal absorption of 5%, total uptake from that source would amount to 10 μg per day.

In contrast, an alveolar ventilation of 10 m^3 per 24 hours with 50% alveolar retention of inhaled Cr, would lead to Cr uptake through the lungs of around 40 μg during an 8 hour exposure to levels of 25 μg/m^3. The upper limit for carcinogenic Cr(VI) would, similarly, cause retention of 1 to 2 μg Cr under these conditions.

Special Groups at Risk: No such groups have been identified outside the occupational environment.

Existing Guidelines and Standards: A variety of standards have been recommended for permissible Cr(VI) levels in water and air. Table 43 provides information on standards presently established in the U.S., as formulated by various agencies.

The high acceptable level of Cr in livestock water is based on the poor absorption of Cr compounds in general from the gut ("Ingestion" section). Because of this low fractional absorption, and in view of the fact that the sensitivity of the lungs to Cr appears to exceed that of other tissues, standards for Cr in air are much lower than those for water.

Table 43: Recommended or Established Standards for Cr in the U.S.

Medium	Chemical Species	Reference	Standard
Total drinking water	Cr(VI)	(21-10)	50 μg/l
Ambient water	Cr(VI)	(21-11)	50 μg/l
Total fresh water (aquatic life)	Total chromium	(21-11)	100 μg/l
Livestock water	Cr(VI)	(21-12)	1 mg/l
Work place air	Carcinogenic*	(21-9)	1 μg/m^3
	Noncarcinogenic*	(21-9)	25 μg/m^3 **
	Cr(VI)	(21-9)	50 μg/m^3 **

*Carcinogenic compounds here include all forms of
  Cr(VI) other than CrO_3 and mono- or dichromates
  of H, Li, Na, K, Rb, Cs and NH_4.
**Time-weighted average (TWA).

Source: Reference (21)

Summary of Proposed EPA Criteria: *Freshwater Aquatic Life* — For trivalent chromium
the criterion to protect freshwater aquatic life as derived using the guidelines is

$$e^{[0.83 \ln (\text{hardness}) + 2.94]}$$

as a 24 hour average and the concentration should not exceed $e^{[0.83 \ln (\text{hardness}) + 3.72]}$
at any time. For hexavalent chromium the criterion to protect freshwater aquatic life as
derived using the guidelines is 10 μg per liter as a 24 hour average concentration and the
concentration should not exceed 110 μg per liter at any time.

Saltwater Aquatic Life — For saltwater aquatic life, no criterion for trivalent chromium can
be derived using the guidelines, and there are insufficient data to estimate a criterion using
other procedures. For hexavalent chromium, the criterion to protect saltwater aquatic life
as derived using the guidelines is 25 μg per liter as a 24 hour average and the concentration
should not exceed 230 μg per liter at any time.

Human Health — For the protection of human health from the toxic properties of chromium
(except hexavalent chromium) ingested through water and contaminated aquatic organisms,
the recommended water quality criterion is 50 μg per liter.

For the maximum protection of human health from the potential carcinogenic effects of
exposure to hexavalent chromium through ingestion of water and contaminated aquatic
organisms, the ambient water concentration is zero. Concentrations of hexavalent chromium
estimated to result in additional lifetime cancer risks ranging from no additional risk to
an additional risk of 1 in 100,000 are presented in the Criterion Formulation section of
this document. The EPA is considering setting criteria at an interim target risk level in the
range of 10^{-5}, 10^{-6}, or 10^{-7} with corresponding criteria of 8, 0.8 and 0.08 ng per liter,
respectively.

Basis for Proposed Human Health Criteria: There is evidence which suggests that hexavalent chromium, Cr(VI), is a carcinogen. Based on exposure of chromium workers to
Cr(VI), Mancuso and Hueper (21-13) and Taylor (21-14), the U.S. EPA Carcinogen Assessment Group has developed a water quality criterion for Cr(VI) to keep the lifetime risk
level below 1 in 100,000.

Under the consent decree in NRDC vs Train, criteria are to state "recommended maximum permissible concentrations (including where appropriate, zero) consistent with the protection of aquatic organisms, human health, and recreational activities". Chromium(VI) is suspected of being a human carcinogen. Because there is no recognized safe concentration for a human carcinogen, the recommended concentration of Cr(VI) in water for maximum protection of human health is zero.

Because attaining a zero concentration level may be infeasible in some cases and in order to assist the EPA and states in the possible future development of water quality regulations, the concentrations of Cr(VI) corresponding to several incremental lifetime cancer risk levels have been estimated. A cancer risk level provides an estimate of the additional incidence of cancer that may be expected in an exposed population. A risk of 10^{-5}, for example, indicates a probability of 1 additional case of cancer for every 100,000 people exposed; a risk of 10^{-6} indicates 1 additional case of cancer for every 1,000,000 people exposed; and so forth.

In the *Federal Register* notice of availability of draft ambient water quality criteria, EPA stated that it is considering setting criteria at an interim target risk level of 10^{-5}, 10^{-6}, or 10^{-7} as shown in Table 44. In the table, risk levels and corresponding criteria are calculated by applying a modified one-hit extrapolation model described in the *FR* 15926, 1979 to the animal bio-assay data presented in the Summary of Pertinent Data. Since the extrapolation model is linear to low doses, the additional lifetime risk is directly proportional to the water concentration. Therefore, water concentrations corresponding to other risk levels can be derived by multiplying or dividing one of the risk levels and corresponding water concentrations shown in the table by factors such as 10; 100; 1,000; and so forth.

Table 44: Possible Alternative Criteria for Chromium

	Risk Levels and Corresponding Criteria			
Exposure Assumptions	0	10^{-7}	10^{-6}	10^{-5}
	. . . . (ng/l)			
2 liters of drinking water and consumption of 18.7 grams of fish and shellfish*	—	0.08	0.8	8
Consumption of fish and shellfish only	—	8.63	86.3	863

*~1% of the Cr(VI) exposure results from the consumption of aquatic organisms which exhibit an average bioconcentration potential of 1.0-fold. The remaining 99% of Cr(VI) exposure results from drinking water.

Source: Reference (21)

Concentration levels were derived assuming a lifetime exposure to various amounts of Cr(VI) (a) occurring from the consumption of both drinking water and aquatic life grown in water containing the corresponding Cr(VI) concentrations and (b) occurring solely from the consumption of aquatic life grown in the waters containing the corresponding Cr(VI) concentrations. Although total exposure information for Cr(VI) is discussed and an estimate of the contributions from other sources of exposure can be made, this data will not be factored into the ambient water quality criteria. The criteria presented, therefore, assume an incremental risk from ambient water exposure only. Therefore, the criterion for hexavalent chromium should be at a level of no greater than 8 ng per liter to keep the lifetime risk of cancer below 1 in 100,000.

A water quality criterion can be set for other Cr species on the basis of reasonable safety margins applied to the lowest exposure observed to produce effects. The level of 0.05 mg per liter of chromium quoted in Table 43 appears to be an acceptable risk level. This level is 500 times lower than a concentration which remained without overt toxicological effects in rats over a period of one year and over 200 times lower than a level reported not to affect dogs over four years. With the exception of hexavalent chromium, there is no reason to believe that the level of 0.05 mg per liter (50 μg per liter) permitted for ambient water poses a significant threat to human health. As a standard, this level was set in 1962 and has in the meantime been confirmed by several reviewing groups. Therefore, the recommended water quality criterion for chromium, except hexavalent chromium, is 50 μg per liter. For practical purposes, it should be noted that it is difficult to analytically distinguish between trivalent and hexavalent chromium.

Because of the low bioconcentration of chromium, consideration of the consumption of fish and shellfish does not change the recommended criterion; if 2 liters of drinking water are ingested per day, then a level of 50 μg per liter would correspond to an intake of 100 μg from water. To apportion this daily intake to both drinking water and fish and shellfish consumed, the following calculation can be used: $2X + (0.0187)(F)(X) = 100$ μg, where 2 is the amount of water ingested in liters per day; X is the chromium concentration in water (mg/l); 0.0187 is the amount of fish consumed per day (kg/day); and F is the bioconcentration factor, milligrams chromium per kilogram fish per milligram chromium in water (F = 11 for chromium); $2X + 0.2X = 100$ μg; $2.2X = 100$ μg; and $X = 45$ μg per liter (or ~50 μg per liter).

Summary of Pertinent Data — In order to calculate a water quality criterion for Cr(VI), it was necessary to assume that the population's exposure to Cr(VI) in the Mancuso and Hueper study (21-13) was the same as the exposure to Taylor's paper (21-14). Taylor's is the only study in which the cohort is large enough (1,212 people were studied) to see the effects of Cr exposure in areas other than the lungs, which are directly affected by inhaled Cr. The lung cancer risk was very high in this study. The risk of digestive cancer from Cr exposure is statistically significant in Taylor's cohort (as shown in 1974 Enterline); however, the amount of Cr to which the workers were exposed is not available for Taylor's study. Mancuso and Hueper closely studied 97 chromium workers in which they saw a high incidence of lung cancer (however, less than Taylor's study). The data on exposure in the Mancuso and Hueper study is very detailed, giving information on first exposure date, years of exposure, latent period, amount of Cr exposure in milligrams Cr per cubic meter for Cr(III) and Cr(VI) separately, and date of death.

In order to calculate a water quality criterion for Cr, it is necessary to know the exposure levels producing the digestive cancer response in Taylor's study, as the direct lung effects may not be relevant to water exposure.

The following is an account of the calculations used in estimating the water concentration of Cr(VI) which would result in a lifetime risk of dying from digestive cancer of 10^{-5}. Assuming that the average exposure in Mancuso and Heuper's study is 0.1 mg Cr/m^3 [this is the mean exposure to water-soluble chromium which is Cr(VI)], then the concentration in Taylor's study is also assumed to be 0.15 mg Cr/m^3. The total exposure in 4.146 years (the mean exposure time in Taylor's study) is

0.15 mg Cr/m^3 x 10 m^3/working day x 240 working days/year x 4.146 years = 1,492.56 mg.

If 50% of this is swallowed from the respiratory tract, then

2.018 liters/day x 365 days/year x 70 years x C mg/l = 1,492.56 x 0.5.

(The bioconcentration factor in fish is 1.0.) C is 14.47 μg per liter of Cr(VI); C is the estimated concentration in water necessary to produce the observed digestive cancer indidence in the Taylor study. The relative risk in the Taylor study is 1.533, which is statistically significant. The excessive risk corresponding to a concentration of C = 14.40 μg per liter is 0.533 p, where p is the expected population risk of digestive tract cancer. The slope of the excessive risk curve is

$$B = \frac{0.533\ p}{0.014} = 37.01\ p\ (mg/l)^{-1}$$

The water quality criterion corresponding to a risk of 10^{-5} is given by

$$X = \frac{10^{-5}}{37.01\ p}\ mg/l = \frac{10^{-2}}{37.01\ p}\ \mu g/l$$

Based on the HEW Vital Statistics of the United States (1973), the lifetime risk of dying from digestive cancer (p) is estimated by an actuarial method to be 3.5%. (Thus, from this data, p = 0.035). Therefore, the water concentration of Cr(VI) should be less than 8.0 ng per liter in order to keep the lifetime risk below 10^{-5}. Using the water concentration of 8 mg per liter, the one-hit slope (B_H) may be calculated as follows:

$$B_H = \frac{70 \times 10^{-5}}{C(2 + R \times F)}$$

where R is 1.0; F is 0.0187 kg per day; C is 8×10^{-5} mg per liter; B_H is 43.345 (mg per kg/day)$^{-1}$.

References:

(21-1) U.S. Environmental Protection Agency, *Reviews of the Environmental Effects of Pollutants: Chromium,* Report No. 600/1-78-023, Washington, D.C. (1978).

(21-2) U.S. Environmental Protection Agency, *National Emissions Inventory of Sources and Emissions of Chromium,* Report No. EPA 450/3-74-012, Washington, D.C. (1974).

(21-3) Mertz, W., "Chromium occurrence and function in biological systems", *Physiol. Rev.* 49, 163 (1969).

(21-4) Baudouin, M.F. and Scoppa, P., "Acute toxicity of various metals to freshwater zooplankton", *Bull. Environment. Contam. Toxicol* 12, 745 (1974).

(21-5) Pickering, Q.H. and Henderson, C., "The acute toxicity of some heavy metals to different species of warm water fishes", *Int. Jour. Air-Water Pollut.* 10, 453 (1966).

(21-6) Eisler, R. and Hennekey, R.J., "Acute toxicities of Cd, Cr, Hg, Ni and Zn to estuarine macro-fauna", *Arch. Environ. Contam. Toxicol* 6, 315 (1977).

(21-7) Mearns, A.J., et al, "Chromium effects on coastal organisms", *Jour. Water Pollut. Control Fed.* 48, 1929 (1976).

(21-8) National Academy of Sciences, *Chromium,* Washington, D.C. (1974).

(21-9) National Institute for Occupational Safety and Health, *Criteria for a recommended standard: occupational exposure to chromium (VI),* NIOSH Doc. No. 76-129 (1976).

(21-10) U.S. Public Health Source, Publ, No. 956, Washington, D.C. (1962).

(21-11) U.S. Environmental Protection Agency, *Quality criteria for water,* Doc. No. 440/9-76-023, Washington, D.C., Office of Planning and Standards (1976).

(21-12) National Academy of Sciences and National Academy of Eng., *Water Quality Criteria,* Washington, D.C. (1972).

(21-13) Mancuso, T.F. and Hueper, W.C., "Occupational cancer and other health hazards in a chromate plant: a medical appraisal: I, lung cancer in chromate workers", *Ind. Med. Surg.* 20, 358 (1951).

(21-14) Taylor, F.H., "The relationship of mortality and duration of employment as reflected by a cohort of chromate workers", *Am. Jour. Publ. Health* 56, 218 (1966).

CHRYSENE

See "Polynuclear Aromatic Hydrocarbons" (55).

COPPER (#22)

Copper, symbol Cu, is in Group I of the Periodic Table. Its atomic number is 29 and its atomic weight is 63.54.

Occurrence: Copper is ubiquitous in the rocks and minerals of the earth's crust. In nature, copper occurs usually as sulfides and oxides and occasionally as metallic copper. Weathering and solution of these natural copper minerals results in background levels of copper in natural surface waters at concentrations generally well below 20 μg per liter. Higher concentrations of copper are usually from anthropogenic sources. These sources include corrosion of brass and copper pipe by acidic waters, industrial effluents and fallout, sewage treatment plant effluents, and the use of copper compounds as aquatic algicides. Potential industrial copper pollution sources number in the tens of thousands in the U.S. However, the major industrial sources include the smelting and refining industries, copper wire mills, coal-burning industries, and iron- and steel-producing industries. Copper may enter natural waters directly from these sources or by atmospheric fallout of air pollutants produced by these industries. Precipitation to atmospheric fallout may be a significant source of copper to the aquatic environment in industrial and mining areas. Human exposure to copper can occur from water, food and air, and through direct contact of tissues with items that contain copper.

Physical Properties: Copper is a soft, heavy metal with a melting point of 1083°C, a boiling point of 2595°C, and a density in elemental form at 20° of 8.9 g/cc.

Chemical Properties: Elemental copper is readily attacked by organic and mineral acids that contain an oxidizing agent and is slowly soluble in ammonia water. The halogens attack copper slowly at room temperature to yield the corresponding copper halide. Oxides and sulfides are also reactive with copper.

Copper has two oxidation states: Cu(I) (cuprous) and and Cu(II) (cupric). Cuprous copper is unstable in aerated water over the pH range of most natural waters (6 to 8) and will oxidize to the cupric state. Bivalent copper chloride, nitrate, and sulfate are highly soluble in water, whereas basic copper carbonate, cupric hydroxide, oxide and sulfide will precipitate out of solution or form colloidal suspensions in the presence of excess cupric ion. Cupric ions are also adsorbed by clays, sediments, and organic particulates and form complexes with several inorganic and organic compounds. Due to the complex interactions of copper with numerous other chemical species normally found in natural waters, the amounts of the various copper compounds and complexes that actually exist in solution will depend on the pH, temperature, alkalinity, and the concentrations of bicarbonate, sulfide and organic ligands.

Uses: The extensive use of copper and its compounds by man since prehistoric times has added copper to the environment and the ecosystem in wide ranges of concentration. From 1955 to 1958, the annual U.S. production of recoverable copper was about 900,000 metric tons. By 1975, the production had risen to 1,260,000 metric tons. The world trade in refined copper amounted to 2,271,150 metric tons in 1973.

Toxic Effects: Although copper poisoning in humans is rare, ingestion of milligram quantities of ionic copper (usually from acidic waters or foods exposed to copper) can cause acute symptoms of nausea, vomiting and diarrhea. Many aquatic organisms are more sensitive than man to copper and significant changes in the aquatic community may occur at copper concentrations significantly lower than those hazardous to human health. Copper occurs at higher concentrations in freshwater than in sea water and is more toxic to aquatic life in soft acidic waters than in hard alkaline waters.

Copper is an essential trace element for humans as well as for many other life forms. In humans most of this copper requirement is obtained from food. Abnormal levels of copper intake can range from levels so low as to induce a nutritional deficiency to levels so high as to be acutely toxic.

Current Levels of Exposure: As has been mentioned earlier, principal concern has been for conditions of copper deficiency rather than copper toxicity. It has been suggested earlier that copper intakes from food and water may range from 6 to 8 mg per day, and that the percentage absorbed varies with the nutritional status. On the other hand, because of changes in food processing and, perhaps, because of better methods of analysis, copper intakes may not reach the 2 mg per day considered an adequate nutritional intake. The average concentration of copper in the U.S. water systems is approximately 134 μg per liter with a little over 1% of the samples taken exceeding the drinking water standard of 1 mg per liter. When the U.S. Public Health Service studied urban water supply systems, they found that only 11 of 969 systems had copper concentrations greater than 1 mg per liter. In 1966, the National Air Sampling Network found airborne copper concentrations ranging from 0.01 to 0.257 μg/m^3 in rural and in urban communities, respectively. Levels of copper as high as 1 to 2 μg/m^3 were found near copper smelters, but this was not considered hazardous.

Special Groups at Risk: Increased copper exposure, with associated health effects, has occasionally occurred in young children subjected to unusually high concentrations of copper in soft or treated water that has been held in copper pipes or stored in copper vessels. Discarding the first water coming from the tap can reduce this hazard. Similar problems have developed in vending machines with copper-containing conduits where acid materials in contact with the copper for periods of time have dissolved copper into the vended liquids. Other groups that may be at risk are medical patients suffering from Wilson's disease, and those patients who are being treated with copper-contaminated fluids in dialysis or by means of parenteral alimentation. These are medical instances in which the copper content of the materials used should be carefully controlled. A final group that may be subject to risk of copper toxicity consists of those people occupationally exposed to copper, e.g., industrial or farm workers.

In reviewing the medical and biologic effects of environmental pollutants, the National Research Council (22-1) pointed out that use of livers from animals fed high levels of copper in the diet could produce a baby food product that was excessively high in copper. The committee also raised the question of exposure to copper from intrauterine contraceptive devices (IUDs), but subsequent reports have failed to demonstrate any abnormal accumulation of copper because of the use of these devices.

Existing Guidelines and Standards: Far more attention has been given to the problems of copper deficiency than to the problems of excess copper in the environment. The 1 mg per liter standard which has been established for copper levels in water for human consumption has been adopted more for organoleptic reasons rather than because of any evidence of toxic levels.

The ACGIH has adopted standards for exposure to airborne copper at work. The time-weighted average for 8 hour daily exposure to copper dust is limited to 1 mg/m^3 of air. The standard for copper fume was changed in 1975 to 0.2 mg/m^3 (22-2). There are no standards for copper in medical practice such as the treatment of burns or dialysis or for parenteral feeding.

Summary of Proposed EPA Criteria: *Freshwater Aquatic Life* — For copper, the criterion to protect freshwater aquatic life as derived using the guidelines is

$$e^{[0.65 \ln (\text{hardness}) - 1.94]}$$

as a 24 hour average and the concentration should not exceed

$$e^{[0.88 \ln (\text{hardness}) - 1.03]}$$

at any time.

Saltwater Aquatic Life — For copper, the criterion to protect saltwater aquatic life as derived using the guidelines is 0.79 μg per liter as a 24 hour average and the concentration should not exceed 18 μg per liter at any time.

Human Health — For copper, the criterion to protect human health is 1 mg per liter.

Basis for the Proposed Human Health Criterion: Copper is an essential dietary element for humans and animals. A level of 2 mg per day will maintain adults in balance and has been considered adequate, although because of interactions with other dietary constituents which limit absorption and utilization, a requirement level must be considered in conjunction with such constituents as zinc, iron, fiber and ascorbic acid. The minimum level meeting requirements for copper intake in intravenous feeding was 22 μg copper per kilogram body weight.

The short biological half-life of copper and the homeostasis that exists in humans prevents copper from accumulating, even with dietary intakes considerably in excess of 2 mg per day. In the opinion of many investigators, there is much more likelihood of a copper deficiency occurring than of a toxicity developing with current dietary and environmental situations.

Although acute and chronic levels of intake may occur, there are no good data which define these levels. It has been suggested that chronic intakes of 15 mg of copper per day may produce observable effects, but if zinc and iron intakes are also increased, much higher levels may be consumed without adverse reactions. The data for acute toxicity are even more uncertain, since practically all human information stems from cases of attempted suicide.

The available literature leads to the conclusion that copper does not produce teratogenic, mutagenic or carcinogenic effects. The limited information available indicates that where such action has occurred, e.g., with mixtures of copper sulfate and lime, arsenic or enediols, the copper should be considered as interacting with the other materials and not as the active material.

The current drinking water standard of 1 mg per liter is considered to be well below any minimum hazard level, even for special groups at risk such as very young children and, therefore, it is recommended that this standard be maintained.

References:

(22-1)   National Academy of Sciences, *Copper,* Committee on Medical and Biological Effects of Environmental Pollutants, Washington, D.C. (1977).

(22-2)   Cohen, S.R., "A review of the health hazards of copper exposure", *Jour. Occup. Med.* 16, 621 (1974).

CYANIDES (#23)

The cyanide ion, CN^-, is present in metallic cyanides and in hydrogen cyanide.

Occurrence: Industrial cyanide wastes include discharges from electroplating (the largest source), as well as paint sludges and paint residues, and from the manufacture and disposal of inorganic cyanides. In addition to discharges from these industries, cyanide wastes are discharged into the environment from the pyrolysis of a number of synthetic and natural materials and from chemical, biological, and clinical laboratories. Although wool, silk, polyacrylonitrile, nylon, polyurethane, and paper are all said to liberate HCN on combustion, the amounts vary widely with the conditions.

Despite numerous potential sources of pollution, cyanide is relatively uncommon in most U.S. water supplies. A survey of 969 U.S. public water supply systems in 1970 revealed no cyanide concentrations above the mandatory limit. In 2,595 water samples, the highest cyanide concentration found was 8 ppb and the average concentration was 0.09 ppb. In part, this must be ascribed to the volatility of undissociated hydrogen cyanide which would be the predominant form in all but highly alkaline waters. Also, in part, cyanide ion would have a decided tendency to be fixed in the form of insoluble or undissociable complexes by trace metals.

Physical Properties: Because of the volatility of HCN, it tends to escape from the water column. In addition, it is readily degraded by microorganisms and by animal metabolism. For these reasons, it is not expected to bioconcentrate in aquatic organisms.

Chemical Properties: Cyanide exists in water in the free form (CN^- and HCN) which is extremely toxic or bound to organic or inorganic moieties in which it is less toxic. Free and complex forms of cyanide can be converted one to the other under conditions found in the aquatic environment. The criterion is based on free cyanide, since that is the principal toxic moiety.

Uses: Cyanide production in the U.S. is over 700,000,000 lb per year and it appears to be increasing steadily (23-1). The sources and industrial uses of cyanide compounds in the U.S. have recently been reviewed exhaustively (23-1, 23-2). Briefly, the major industrial users of cyanide in the U.S. are the producers of steel, plastics, synthetic fibers and chemicals, and the electroplating and metallurgical industries.

Toxic Effects: Cyanide is lethal to freshwater fishes at concentrations as low as about 50 μg per liter and has been shown to adversely affect invertebrates and fishes at concentrations of about 10 μg per liter. Very few saltwater data have been generated. The toxicological effects of cyanides are based upon their potential for rapid conversion by mammals to HCN. Cyanides are known to be degraded by human liver to the less toxic thiocyanate and despite their high levels of acute toxicity, are not known to be chronically toxic to humans.

Current Levels of Exposure: Since cyanide is encountered only infrequently in water supplies or in the atmosphere and since long-term and large-scale monitoring has not been carried out, insufficient data exist to estimate current levels of exposure of the general population. A number of factors contribute to the rapid disappearance of cyanide from water. Bacteria and protozoa may degrade cyanide by converting it to carbon dioxide and ammonia. Cyanide is converted to cyanate during chlorination of water supplies. An alkaline pH favors the oxidation by chlorine, whereas an acid pH favors volatilization of HCN into the atmosphere. As cited, cyanide concentrations above 8 ppb were not found in a survey of 2,595 water samples collected throughout the U.S. (23-1). Thus, these concentrations were well below the objective levels established by the PHS.

Special Groups at Risk: Although it was speculated that the elderly and the debilitated individuals in our population may be at special risk with respect to cyanide, no experimental or epidemiological studies can be cited to prove the point.

Existing Guidelines and Standards: The U.S. Public Health Service Drinking Water Standards of 1962 established 0.2 mg CN⁻ per liter as the acceptability criterion for water supplies. In addition to defining the 0.2 mg per liter criterion for cyanide, the PHS set forth an objective to achieve concentrations below 0.01 mg CN⁻ per liter in water because proper treatment will reduce cyanide levels to 0.01 mg per liter or less (23-3). The Canadian government has recently adopted criterion and objective concentrations of 0.2 and 0.02 mg CN⁻ per liter, respectively. The latter figure represents the lower limit of detection by colorimetric methods (23-4).

The U.S. PHS criterion was based on cyanide toxicity to fish and not to man. Obviously, a disparity exists between the exposure condition for man and for fish. The human experience cited involved discrete single doses by mouth, whereas the fish data are derived from continuous total body exposure. The latter conditions are not a very realistic model from which to assess the human hazard. Even chronic occupational exposures of men to hydrogen cyanide gas allows for respite at the end of each working day. No data were encountered which compared single acute oral LD_{50} doses in fish to ambient concentrations in their water which produced death within a specified interval.

Summary of Proposed EPA Criteria: *Freshwater Aquatic Life* — For free cyanide (expressed as CN), the criterion to protect freshwater aquatic life as derived using the guidelines is 1.4 μg per liter as a 24 hour average and the concentration should not exceed 38 μg per liter at any time.

Saltwater Aquatic Life — For saltwater aquatic life, no criterion for free cyanide can be derived using the guidelines, and there are insufficient data to estimate a criterion using other procedures.

Human Health — For cyanide, the criterion to protect human health from the toxic properties of cyanide ingested through water and through contaminated aquatic organisms is 0.2 mg CN⁻ per liter.

Basis for Proposed Human Health Criteria: As shown in Table 45, the criterion of 0.2 mg CN⁻ per liter allows for safety factors ranging from 41 to 2,100.

Table 45: Basis and Derivation of Cyanide Criterion

Exposure Levels*	Route	Species	Calculated Daily Exposure (mg)	Margin of Safety†	Reference
9.2 mg/m^3	Inhalation	Man	60.8**	152	(23-5)
2.5 mg/m^3	Inhalation	Man	16.5**	41	(23-2)
12 mg/kg	Oral	Rat	840***	20.8	(23-6)

*NOAEL.
**Based on 100% retention and on alveolar exchange of 6.6 m^3 for 8 hours.
***Rat data converted to human equivalent assuming food consumption of 60 g/kg for rats and 70 kg human.
†Daily exposure compared with 0.4 mg/day exposure from the consumption of 2 liters water containing 0.2 mg/l.

El Ghawabi, et al (23-5) studied the effects of chronic cyanide exposure in the electroplating sections of three Egyptian factories. A total of 36 male employees with exposures up to 15 years were studied and compared with a control group of 20 normal, nonsmoking males. Only minimal differences with respect to thyroid gland size and function were found. The El Ghawabi study was given considerable weight in formulating the NIOSH (23-2) recommendations for occupational exposure which gives a safety factor of 41 when applied to drinking water by the usual extrapolations (Table 45).

Finally, a safety factor of 2,100 is obtained using the results of a two year chronic feeding study in rats. When fed at the rate of 12 mg/kg per day over the equivalent of a lifetime, these rats showed no overt signs of cyanide poisoning and hematological values were normal. Gross and microscopic examinations of tissues revealed no abnormalities. The only abnormality found was an elevation of thiocyanate levels in the liver and kidneys.

Consequently, the ADI for man is derived by taking the no-observable-adverse-effect-level (NOAEL) in mammals (12 mg/kg per day) multiplied by the weight of the average man (70 kg) and dividing by a safety factor of 100. Thus,

$$\text{ADI} = 12 \text{ mg/kg/day} \times 70 \text{ kg} \div 100 = 8.4 \text{ mg/day.}$$

The equation for calculating the criterion for the cyanide content of water given an ADI is $2X + [(0.0187)(F)(X)] = \text{ADI}$, where 2 is the amount of drinking water per liter per day; X is the cyanide concentration in water in milligrams per liter; 0.0187 is the amount of fish consumed per kilogram per day; F is the bioconcentration factor in milligrams of cyanide per kilogram of fish per milligram of cyanide per liter of water; ADI is the limit of daily exposure for a 70 kg person (8.4 mg/day); $2X + (0.0187)(2.3)X = 8.4$; and X is 4.11 mg per liter.

Thus, the current and recommended criteria (0.2 mg per liter) has a margin of safety of 20.5 (4.11 ÷ 0.2).

No new additional evidence was encountered to suggest that the 1962 PHS Drinking Water Standard for cyanide should be lowered. The concentration of 0.2 mg per liter or less is easily achieved by proper treatment and concentrations in excess of that amount have been encountered only on rare occasions in U.S. water supplies. The experience since 1962 suggests that 0.2 mg CN⁻ per liter is a safe criterion not only for man, but for most species of fish as well. Although cyanide has been implicated in fish kills, these represent isolated, accidental and localized cases of pollution where the cyanide concentrations must have been greatly in excess of the PHS limit.

Cyanide is unlikely to become a widespread environmental pollutant because of its low degree of persistence in the biosphere. It is not accumulated or stored in mammals and there is no evidence for its biomagnification in food chains. Well-controlled attempts to show cumulative toxic effects have not been successful. No data exist to suggest that cyanide produces such irreversible effects as mutagenesis, teratogenesis or cancer.

References:

(23-1) Towill, L.E., et al, *Reviews of the Environmental Effects of Pollutants: V. Cyanide,* Oak Ridge, Tenn., Information Div., Oak Ridge National Lab. (1978).

(23-2) National Institute for Occupational Safety and Health, *Criteria for a Recommended Standard: Occupational Exposure to Hydrogen Cyanide and Cyanide Salts,* NIOSH Publ. No. 77-108, Washington, D.C. (1976).

(23-3) U.S. Public Health Service, *Drinking Water Standards,* PHS Publ. No. 956, Washington, D.C. (1962).

(23-4) Health and Welfare Canada, *Cyanide—Drinking Water Criteria Review,* Ottawa, (1977).

(23-5) El Ghawabi, S.H., et al, "Chronic cyanide exposure: a clinical, radioisotope and laboratory study", *Brit. Jl. Ind. Med.,* 32, 215 (1975).

(23-6) Howard, J.W. and Hanzal, R.F., "Chronic toxicity for rats of food treated with hydrogen cyanide", *J. Agr. Food Chem.* 3, 325 (1955).

D

DDT (#24)

DDT refers to technical DDT, which is usually composed of:

77.1% p,p'-DDT
14.9% o,p'-DDT
0.3% p,p'-DDD
0.1% o,p'-DDD
4.0% p,p'-DDE
0.1% o,p'-DDE
3.5% unidentified compounds

		R	R'	R''
DDT	1,1'-(2,2,2-trichloroethylidene)-bis(4-chlorobenzene)	$-Cl$	$-H$	$-CCl_3$
DDE	1,1'-(2,2-dichloroethenylidene)-bis(4-chlorobenzene)	$-Cl$	none	$=CCl_2$
DDD	1,1'-(2,2-dichloroethylidene)-bis(4-chlorobenzene)	$-Cl$	$-H$	$-CHCl_2$
DDMU	1,1'-(2-chloroethenylidene)bis(4-chlorobenzene)	$-Cl$	none	$=CHCl$
DDMS	1,1'-(2-chloroethylidene)-bis(4-chlorobenzene)	$-Cl$	$-H$	$-CH_2Cl$
DDNU	1,1-bis(4-chlorophenyl)ethylene	$-Cl$	none	$=CH_2$
DDOH	2,2-bis(4-chlorophenyl)ethanol	$-Cl$	$-H$	$-CH_2OH$
DDA	2,2-bis(4-chlorophenyl)acetic acid	$-Cl$	$-H$	$-COOH$

Occurrence: Human exposure to DDT is primarily by ingestion of contaminated food. Air and water intake is negligible and amounts to probably less than 0.01 mg/yr. Therefore, by EPA estimate (24) total intake of DDT per year for the average U.S. resident will be less than 3 mg/yr.

Physical Properties: The p,p'-isomer forms colorless crystals, MP 108.5°C, vp 1.9×10^{-7} torr at 20°C. It is practically insoluble in water, moderately soluble in hydroxylic and polar solvents and in petroleum oils and readily soluble in most aromatic and chlorinated solvents. The technical product is a waxy solid of indefinite MP and of similar solubility to the p,p'-isomer.

Chemical Properties: p,p'-DDT is dehydrochlorinated at temperatures above its MP to the noninsecticidal ethylene, a reaction catalyzed by ferric and aluminum chlorides and by UV light. In solution it is readily dehydrochlorinated by alkalies or organic bases. Otherwise it is stable, being unattacked by acid and alkaline permanganate or by aqueous acids and alkalies. With DDT, dehydrochlorination may proceed at temperatures as low as 50°C.

Uses: DDT, first synthesized in Germany in 1874, has been used extensively worldwide for public health and agricultural programs. Its efficacy as a broad spectrum insecticide and its low cost continue to make it the insecticide of choice for those measures for most of the world.

Following an extensive review of health and environmental hazards of the use of DDT, U.S. EPA decided to ban further use of DDT (24-2). This decision was based on several properties of DDT that had been well evidenced: (1) DDT and its metabolites are toxicants with long-term persistence in soil and water; (2) it is widely dispersed by erosion, runoff and volatilization; and (3) the low-water solubility and high lipophilicity of DDT result in concentrated accumulation of DDT in the fat of wildlife and humans which may be hazardous.

Agricultural use of DDT was canceled by the U.S. EPA in December, 1972. Prior to this, DDT had been widely used in the U.S. with a peak usage in 1959 of 80 million pounds. This amount decreased steadily to less than 12 million pounds by 1972. Since the 1972 ban, the use of DDT in the U.S. has been effectively discontinued.

Toxic Effects: DDT is acutely toxic to freshwater fishes at concentrations as low as 0.8 μg/l (24-3) and to invertebrates at 0.18 μg/l (24-4). It is chronically toxic to the fathead minnow in the range of 0.37 to 1.48 μg/l (24-5). An average bioconcentration factor of 640,000 was calculated using data on 26 species of fish. For saltwater fishes concentrations of DDT as low as 0.2 μg/l have been reported to be acutely toxic (24-6). For invertebrates the figure is 0.14 μg/l (24-7). Chronic toxicity data for saltwater organisms were not available. The average marine fish bioconcentration factor was found to be 22,467. Criteria for both freshwater and marine organisms are based on bioconcentration.

Current Levels of Exposure: Most of the reported DDT concentrations in air are associated with high usage of DDT prior to 1972. Stanley, et al (24-8) analyzed air samples from nine localities. DDT levels ranged from 0.1 ng/m^3 to 20 ng/m^3. Air samples collected in July 1970 had 0.00007 ng/m^3 (24-9) over the Atlantic Ocean. The actual levels of DDT in the ambient air at the present time are difficult to estimate but are probably at the lowest ranges of Stanley's estimates. The significance of pesticide levels in the air has been carefully reviewed and the consensus is that the levels of DDT found in the ambient air are far below levels that might add significantly to the total human intake (24-10).

Kenaga (24-11) gave the following relative values for residues of DDT and its metabolites found in various types of waters: rain water, 0.2 μg/l; fresh water, 0.02 μg/l; and seawater, 0.001 μg/l. Assuming average daily intake of water to be 2 liters in any given year, maximal DDT intake from water should be 0.007 mg. This figure is equivalent to the estimated dietary intake of DDT in a single day for a 19-year-old male (24-2). Therefore, it is concluded that DDT intake from potable water does not contribute significantly to the overall exposure.

Duggan and Corneliussen (24-12) calculated the average daily intake of total DDT residues in 1965 as 0.0009 mg/kg and decreasing to 0.0004 mg/kg in 1970. Market basket studies have shown significant declines between 1970 and 1973 of DDT and DDD residues of 86 and 89%, respectively. DDE decreased by 25% over this period of time. Dairy, meat, fish and poultry constitute 95% of the total ingested DDT sources with dairy products contributing 30% of this amount. Average human fat storage for the time period of 1970 to 1973 has decreased from approximately 8 ppm to 6 ppm in the U.S. population. Based on these declines and the most current figures of 1973 for intakes it is estimated that current levels of dietary intake are approximately 0.0001 mg/kg/day with DDE comprising over 80% of this amount. Assuming the average male weighs 70 kg the average daily intake would be 0.007 mg/day or 2.56 mg/yr.

Special Groups at Risk: The entire population of the U.S. has some low level exposure to dietary contaminants. Minimal exposure from air and water sources, however, may be more important in previously heavily sprayed agricultural areas, where large amounts of residues may still be present.

In 1975, estimated DDT production was 30 to 49 million pounds (24-13). The primary producer of DDT in the U.S. is the Montrose Chemical Co. It is assumed that there are other companies involved in the formulation of their products with DDT, but no data are available.

Groups at special risk are workmen in manufacturing plants and formulating plants and applicators, handlers and sprayers.

During such times as exceptions are granted by the U.S. EPA for crop usage or during use for public health measures, those involved in handling or applying DDT may have considerable exposure.

Estimating the number of individuals at high risk due to occupational exposure is difficult. It is estimated that 8,700 workers are involved in formulating or manufacturing all pesticides. Since DDT constitutes much less than 10% of the total, the maximal number of exposed workers would be approximately 500. Since usage of DDT is severely limited, persons exposed by application would probably be fewer.

Existing Guidelines and Standards: In 1958, U.S. Department of Agriculture began to phase out the use of DDT in insect control programs. Spraying was reduced from 4.9 million acres in 1957 to just over 100,000 acres in 1967, and DDT was used as a persistent pesticide thereafter only in the absence of an effective alternative. In 1964, the Secretary of Interior issued a directive that use of chlorinated hydrocarbons should be avoided in Department of Interior lands.

This was extended in 1970, when 16 pesticides, including DDT, were completely banned for use on Department of Interior lands. By 1969, DDT registration and usage was curtailed by the USDA in various areas of the cooperative Federal-State pest control program. In November 1969, the USDA announced its intention to discontinue all uses of DDT nonessential to human health and for which there were safe and effective substitutes. In 1970, a major cancellation of Federal registrations of DDT products by the USDA for use on 50 food crops, domestic animals, finished wood and lumber products, and use around commercial, institutional, and industrial establishments was completed.

Major responsibility for Federal regulation of pesticides under the Federal Insecticide, Fungicide and Rodenticide Act (1947) was transferred to the U.S. EPA. In January, 1971, U.S. EPA issued notices of intent to cancel all remaining Federal registrations of products containing DDT. A hearing on the cancellation of Federal registration of products containing DDT was held beginning in August, 1971 and concluding in March, 1972. The principal parties to the hearing were 31 DDT formulating companies, the USDA, the Environmental Defense Fund, and the U.S. EPA. This hearing and other evidence from four government reports including the December 1969 Mrak Commission Report were instrumental in the final cancellation of all remaining crop usages of DDT in the U.S., effective December 31, 1972.

During the same period (October 1972), a Federal Environmental Pesticide Control Act (FEPCA) was enacted which provided EPA with more effective pesticide regulation mechanisms. The cancellation order was appealed by the pesticides industry in several U.S. courts. On December 13, 1973, the U.S. Court of Appeals for the District of Columbia ruled there was substantial evidence in the record to support the U.S. EPA ban on DDT. In April 1973 the U.S. EPA, in accordance with authority granted by FEPCA, required that all products containing DDT be registered with the Agency by June 10, 1973. Since that time, the U.S. EPA has granted requests to the states of Washington and Idaho and to the Forest Services to use DDT on the basis of economic emergency and no effective alternative to DDT being available.

Authority to regulate hazards arising from the manufacturing and formulation of pesticides and other chemicals resides with the Occupational Safety and Health Administration (OSHA). Under the terms of the Occupational Safety and Health Act of 1970, the National Institute of Occupational Safety and Health has been responsible for setting guidelines, criteria, and standards for occupational exposure. The OSHA exposure limit for DDT on skin has been set a 1.0 mg/m^2. Further, DDT has been classified as a suspected occupational carcinogen that should be cautiously handled in the workplace.

The decision to ban DDT was extensively reviewed relative to scientific and economic aspects in 1975 (24-2). No new evidence was found contradicting the original finding of the Administrator in 1972. The chronology of DDT regulation is reviewed in Table 46.

Table 46: The Chronology of DDT Regulation

Year	Agency	Standard	Remarks
1971	WHO	0.005 mg/kg body weight	maximum acceptable daily intake in food
1976	U.S. EPA	0.001 µg/l	quality criteria for water
1977	Natl. Acad. Sci., Natl. Res. Counc.	—	in light of carcinogenic risk projection, suggested strict criteria for DDT and DDE in drinking water
1978	OSHA	1 mg/m^2	skin exposure
1978	U.S. EPA	0.41 µg/l 0.00023 µg/l	final acute and chronic values for water quality criteria for protection of aquatic life (freshwater)

Source: Reference (24)

Summary of Proposed EPA Criteria: *Freshwater Aquatic Life* — For DDT and metabolites the criterion to protect freshwater aquatic life as derived using the Guidelines is 0.00023 µg/l as a 24-hour average and the concentration should not exceed 0.41 µg/l at any time.

Saltwater Aquatic Life — The data base for saltwater aquatic life is insufficient to allow use of the Guidelines. The following recommendation is inferred from toxicity data for freshwater organisms.

For DDT and metabolites the criterion to protect saltwater aquatic life as derived using procedures other than the Guidelines is 0.0067 µg/l as a 24-hour average and the concentration should not exceed 0.021 µg/l at any time.

Human Health — For the maximum protection of human health from the potential carcinogenic effects of exposure to DDT through ingestion of water and contaminated aquatic organisms, the ambient water concentration is zero. Concentrations of DDT estimated to result in additional lifetime cancer risks ranging from no additional risk to an additional risk of 1 in 100,000 are presented in the Criteria document. The Agency is considering setting criteria at an interim target risk level in the range of 10^{-5}, 10^{-6}, or 10^{-7} with corresponding criteria of 0.98 ng/l, 0.098 ng/l, and 0.0098 ng/l, respectively. If water alone is consumed, the water concentration should be less than 0.36 µg/l to keep the lifetime cancer risk below 10^{-5}.

Basis for the Proposed Human Health Criteria: Since no epidemiological evidence for the carcinogenicity of DDT in man has been reported, the results of animal carcinogenicity studies conducted by feeding DDT or its metabolites over the life span of the animal are regarded as the most pertinent data. Although a number of studies have been reported for various species, the major evidence for the tumorigenicity of DDT is its ability to induce liver tumors in mice.

Under the Consent Decree in *NRDC vs Train*, criteria are to state "recommended maximum permissible concentrations (including where appropriate, zero) consistent with the protection of aquatic organisms, human health, and recreational activities." DDT is suspected of being a human carcinogen. Because there is no recognized safe concentration for a human carcinogen, the recommended concentration of DDT in water for maximum protection of human health is zero.

Because attaining a zero concentration level may be infeasible in some cases and in order to assist the Agency and States in the possible future development of water quality regulations, the concentrations of DDT corresponding to several incremental lifetime cancer risk levels have been estimated. A cancer risk level provides an estimate of the additional incidence of cancer that may be expected in an exposed population. A risk of 10^{-5}, e.g., indicates a probability of one additional case of cancer for every 100,000 people exposed, a risk of 10^{-6} indicates one additional case of cancer for every million people exposed, etc.

In the *Federal Register* notice of availability of draft ambient water quality criteria, EPA stated that it is considering setting criteria at an interim target risk level of 10^{-5}, 10^{-6} or 10^{-7} as shown in Table 47.

Table 47: Possible Alternative Criteria for DDT

Exposure Assumptions (per day)	. . .Risk Levels and Corresponding Criteria . . .			
	0	10^{-7}	10^{-6}	10^{-5}
		. . . . (ng/l).			
2 liters of drinking water and consumption of 18.7 g of fish and shellfish*	—	0.0098	0.098	0.98
Consumption of fish and shellfish only	—	0.0098	0.098	0.98

*Greater than 99% of the DDT exposure results from the consumption of aquatic organisms which exhibit an average bioconcentration potential of 39,000 fold. The remaining less than 1% of DDT exposure results from drinking water.

Source: Reference (24)

In the table risk levels are calculated by applying a modified "one-hit" extrapolation model described in the *FR* 15926, 1979, to the animal bioassay data presented in the summary of pertinent data. Since the extrapolation model is linear at low doses, the additional lifetime risk is directly proportional to the water concentration. Therefore, water concentrations corresponding to other risk levels can be derived by multiplying or dividing one of the risk levels and corresponding water concentrations shown in the table by factors such as 10, 100, 1,000, etc.

Concentration levels were derived assuming a lifetime exposure to various amounts of DDT (1) occurring from the consumption of both drinking water and aquatic life grown in water containing the corresponding DDT concentrations and, (2) occurring solely from the consumption of aquatic life grown in the waters containing the corresponding DDT concentrations. Although total exposure information for DDT is discussed and an estimate of the contributions from other sources of exposure can be made, this data will not be factored into the ambient water quality criteria formulation because of the tenuous estimates. The criteria presented, therefore, assume an incremental risk from ambient water exposure only.

The case of DDT and its possible role as a human carcinogen is complicated by several factors. Despite widespread use and exposure over thirty years, no positive associations with human cancer have been found to date, although the number of individuals studied is not statistically large. It is a chemical with high efficacy and has been extremely effective all over the world for public health measures. However, its slow biodegradability and propensity to accumulate in nontarget species have made it particularly hazardous for many fish and bird species. For mammals, however, it has a low acute toxicity as compared to other alternate pesticides.

DDT has not been shown to produce point mutations or teratogenic effects in a wide battery of tests. Some evidence for its clastogenic properties, however, make is suspect. The primary evidence for the carcinogenicity of DDT and metabolites to date has been the induction of liver tumors in mice. Studies in other species have consistently shown little or no effect and in the mice only liver tumors have shown an increase. The evidence for the carcinogenicity of DDT would be much more convincing if other species or sites of tumorigenic action could be conclusively demonstrated. This is in light of the fact that DDT has been probably the most extensively studied compound in modern science.

Current levels of exposure would seem to pose extremely small risk to persons in the U.S. DDT and DDE are preferentially stored in fatty compartments that are not actively dividing and subject to carcinogenic changes.

The use of DDT has been restricted in several countries because of its impact on the environment and its tumorigenic effect in mice. This is a reasonable proposition based on numerous reports. Therefore, the levels proposed in this document should ensure the health of wildlife and the coexisting human population.

Summary of Pertinent Data — The water quality criterion for DDT can be derived on the basis of two independent sets of data, neither of which is completely satisfactory. The first method is based on the most sensitive animal chronic bioassay available, which is the six-generation study by Turusov, et al (24-14) in CF-1 mice. The second method is based on a comparison of the lifetime incidence of nervous system cancer cases between residents of New York State (except New York City) and residents of Israel who were born in Europe or America (24-15).

The first method results in water quality concentrations so low that over 95% of surface water in the U.S. would fail to meet the criteria. This method also implies that the lifetime risk from current ambient concentrations is approximately 3%, which seems unrealistically high for DDT exposure alone in view of the absence of reported carcinogenic effects in heavily exposed populations. The second method is based on extremely tenuous assumptions, but it does use human data to put an upper limit on the carcinogenic effectiveness of DDT.

Method 1 — In the Turusov mouse study, the six generations of the lowest dose group (2 ppm) of males had 179 animals with hepatomas out of 354 animals analyzed, whereas in controls 97 out of 328 animals had hepatomas. The data used for the criterion are: n_t = 179; N_t = 354; n_c = 97; N_c = 328; Le = 104 weeks; le = 104 weeks; d = 2 x 0.13 = 0.26 mg/kg/day; w = 0.030 kg; L = 104 weeks; R = 39,000; and F = 0.0187 kg/day.

With these values the slope parameter is B_H = 18.055 $(mg/kg/day)^{-1}$. The result of the calculation is that if fish and water are consumed the water concentration should be less than 0.053 ng/l in order to keep the individual lifetime risk below 10^{-5}. If only water were consumed (F = 0) the corresponding concentration is 20 ng/l.

Method 2 — There is strong evidence that Method 1 overstates the DDT risk, either because the animal experiments overstate the human risk or because most people do not eat fish contaminated to the extent assumed in the model. The basis for stating this is that countries like Israel where the levels of DDT exposure have been high and widespread have experienced no excess cancer incidence as compared to the United States.

As an upper limit estimate of cancer risk from DDT exposure, we can make the unsupported assumption that DDT does cause human cancer with some probability which is proportional to the lifetime exposure and we can make the reductio ad absurdum argument that cancer incidence in the organ site where the largest excess in incidence occurs in Israel is due solely to DDT, which of course is not true.

Taking the nervous system as a reasonable candidate site for the action of DDT, we can make the following estimate which is intended only to put upper bounds on the carcinogenic effectiveness of DDT. The high exposure in Israel is reflected in the higher fat levels measured by Wasserman, et al (24–15). According to their data the average level in Israel is 16.33 ppm (based on three studies), whereas in the United States it is 9.04 ppm (based on ten studies).

Using the following relationship, developed by Hayes, et al and Durham, et al between the daily dose I(mg/day), and the concentration C(ppm) in body fat: log I = (1/0.7)(log C − 1.3), the difference in the average daily doses in Israel and the United States was calculated to be 0.751 − 0.323 = 0.428 mg/day.

The lifetime incidence of cancer for Israel and New York State is tabulated in the table shown on the following page.

| | . . . . . Lifetime Incidence (%) . . . . . | |
Population (males)	Nervous System	All Sites
New York State	0.5	28.8
Israel		
All Jews	1.1	24.9
Born Israel	1.3	21.4
Born Europe or America	1.1	24.1
Born Africa or Asia	0.7	18.6
Non-Jews	0.5	15.3

Relative to New York, the excess lifetime risk of nervous system cancer in migrants to Israel from Europe and America is 1.1 − 0.5 = 0.6%. This is caused by an excess intake of 0.428 mg/day. Therefore, the intake I resulting in 10^{-5} risk is: $I = (10^{-5}/0.006) \times 0.428 = 7.13 \times 10^{-4}$ mg/day. If this intake comes from fish and water, the concentration of water would be: $C = 7.13 \times 10^{-4}/[2 + (39{,}000 \times 0.0187)] = 0.98$ ng/l. If the intake comes from water alone, the concentration would be: $C = (7.13 \times 10^{-4})/2 = 0.357$ ng/l. Therefore, according to Method 2, if fish and water are consumed, the water concentration should be <0.98 ng/l in order to keep the individual lifetime risk below 10^{-5}. If only water is consumed, the corresponding concentration is 0.36 ng/l. The equivalent slope factor for Method 2 is:

$$B_H \; = \; \frac{70 \times 10^{-5}}{2 \times 3.57 \times 10^{-4}} \; = \; 0.98 \; (mg/kg/day)^{-1}$$

Method 2 is recommended because it gives some basis for avoiding the unrealistically low concentrations imposed by considering only the animal data.

References

(24-1) Archer, T.E., *Residue Reviews*, 61, 29 (1976).

(24-2) U.S. Environmental Protection Agency, *DDT–A Review of Scientific and Economic Aspects of the Decision to Ban Its Use as a Pesticide*, Report EPA 520/1-75-022, Wash., D.C. (1975).

(24-3) Marking, L.L., Evaluation of p,p'-DDT as a reference toxicant in bioassays," in *Investigations in Fish Control*, Wash., D.C., U.S. Fish Wildl. Serv. Resour. Publ. 14, 10 (1966).

(24-4) Sanders, H.O., *Toxicity of some insecticides to four species of malacostracan crustaceans*, Bur. Sport Fish. Wildl. Tech. Paper 66, 19 (1972).

(24-5) Jarvinen, A.W., et al, "Long-term toxic effects of DDT food and water exposure on fathead minnows, *Pimephales promelas*," *Jour. Fish. Res. Board Can.* 34, 2089 (1977).

(24-6) Eisler, R., *Acute toxicities of organochlorine and organophosphorus insecticides to estuarine fishes*, Tech. Paper Bur. Sport Fish. Wildl. U.S. Dept. Interior No. 46 (1970).

(24-7) Schimmel, S.C. and Patrick, J.M., *Acute Bioassays*, Semi-Annual Report, U.S. Environmental Protection Agency, Environmental Research Laboratory, Gulf Breeze, Florida (1975).

(24-8) Stanley, C.W., et al, "Measurement of atmospheric levels of pesticides," *Envir. Sci. Tech.* 5, 430 (1971).

(24-9) Prospero, J.M. & Seba, D.B., "Some additional measurements of pesticides in the lower atmosphere of the northern equatorial Atlantic Ocean," *Atmos. Environ.* 6, 363 (1975).

(24-10) Spencer, W.F., "Movement of DDT and its derivatives into the atmosphere," *Residue Rev.* 59, 91 (1975).

(24-11) Kenaga, E.E., "Factors related to bioconcentration of pesticides," in Matsumura, F., et al, *Environmental Toxicology of Pesticides*, New York, Academic Press (1972).

(24-12) Duggan, R.E. and Corneliussen, P.E., "Dietary intake of pesticide chemicals in the U.S. (III) for June 1968-April 1970," *Pesticide Monitor Jl.* 5, 331 (1972).

(24-13) National Institute for Occup. Safety and Health, *Criteria for a Recommended Standard: Occupational Exposure During the Manufacture and Formulation of Pesticides*, NIOSH Pub. No. 78-174 (July 1978).

(24-14) Turusov, V.S., et al, "Tumors in CF-1 mice exposed for six consecutive generations to DDT," *Jour. Natl. Cancer Inst.*, 51, 983 (1973).

(24-15) Wasserman, M., et al, "Storage map of organochlorine compounds in humans," *Proc. Intl. Symposium on Recent Advances in the Assessment of the Health Effects of Environmental Pollution*, 2, 1053 (1974).

DIBENZO[a,h]ANTHRACENE

See "Polynuclear Aromatic Hydrocarbons" (55).

DI-n-BUTYL PHTHALATE

See "Phthalate Esters" (53).

DICHLOROBENZENES (#25)

The dichlorobenzenes are a class of halogenated aromatic compounds represented by three structurally similar isomers: 1,2-dichloro-, 1,3-dichloro-, and 1,4-dichlorobenzene. Dichlorobenzenes have the molecular formula $C_6H_4Cl_2$ and a molecular weight of 147.01. For other chlorinated benzenes, the reader is referred to another criterion document on "Chlorinated Benzenes" (14).

Occurrence: Dichlorobenzenes have been detected at various concentrations in ambient water, groundwater, and finished drinking water. They have been found to bioconcentrate in fish tissues.

Physical Properties: 1,2-Dichloro- (1,2-DCB) and 1,3-dichlorobenzene (1,3-DCB) are liquids at normal environmental temperatures while 1,4-dichlorobenzene (1,4-DCB) is a solid. Melting points (MP), boiling points (BP) and densities for the three isomers are presented below:

Compound	MP, °C	BP, °C	Density g/ml (°C)
1,2-Dichlorobenzene	−17.6	179	1.30 (20)
1,3-Dichlorobenzene	−24.2	172	1.29 (20)
1,4-Dichlorobenzene	53.0	174	1.25 (20)

The dichlorobenzenes are soluble in water at concentrations which are toxic to aquatic organisms. The solubilities in water of the 1,2-, 1,3-, and 1,4-dichlorobenzene isomers at 25°C are 145,000 μg/l, 123,000 μg/l, and 80,000 μg/l, respectively. The dichlorobenzenes also are readily soluble in natural fats or fat-soluble substances. The logs of the octanol/water partition coefficients for 1,3-dichloro-, and 1,4-dichlorobenzene are 3.44 and 3.37, respectively (25-1). All three dichlorobenzene isomers are relatively volatile. The vapor pressure of 1,2-dichlorobenzene at 20°C is 1 mm Hg; the vapor pressure of 1,3-dichlorobenzene at 39°C is 5 mm Hg; and the vapor pressure of 1,4-dichlorobenzene at 25°C is 0.4 mm Hg.

Chemical Properties: The dichlorobenzenes are less resistant to biodegradation and less persistent than the more highly chlorinated benzenes. However, even the dichlorobenzenes appear to be reasonably stable in view of their widespread detection in water, air, soil and animals.

Uses: The major uses of 1,2-DCB are as a process solvent in the manufacturing of toluene diisocyanate and as an intermediate in the synthesis of dyestuffs, herbicides, and degreasers (25-2). 1,4-Dichlorobenzene is used primarily as an air deodorant and an insecticide, which account for 90% of the total production of this isomer. Information is not available concerning the production and use of 1,3-DCB. However, it may occur as a contaminant of 1,2- or 1,4-DCB formulations. Both 1,2-dichloro- and 1,4-dichlorobenzene are produced almost entirely as by-products during the production of monochlorobenzene. Combined annual production of these two isomers in the United States approaches 50,000 metric tons.

Toxic Effects: Human exposure to dichlorobenzene is reported to cause hemolytic anemia and liver necrosis, and 1,4-dichlorobenzene has been found in human adipose tissue. In addition, the dichlorobenzenes are toxic to nonhuman mammals, birds, and aquatic organisms and impart an offensive taste and odor to water. The dichlorobenzenes are metabolized by mammals, including humans, to various dichlorophenols, some of which are as toxic as the dichlorobenzenes.

Current Levels of Exposure: In the few samples of relatively uncontaminated groundwater and of drinking water the reported DCB levels ranged on the order of less than 0.001 to 0.003 mg/l. In the NCMS survey, median concentrations and frequency of positive samples in drinking water were low, compared to halomethanes. This data would suggest a relatively low exposure level for the general public from drinking municipally treated water. An attempt to estimate human DCB exposure doses by using available survey contaminant-level data and certain assumptions for water consumption and absorption efficiency is shown in Table 48.

Table 48: Estimated Dichlorobenzene Exposure from Drinking Water*

| | Exposure, mg | | | |
| | Daily Uptake | | Annual Uptake | |
Exposure Level	per Person	per Kilogram	per Person	per Kilogram
Minimal case				
Median level in drinking water of 0.000005 mg/l (assume 3)	6×10^{-6}	0.086×10^{-6}	2.2×10^{-3}	0.031×10^{-3}
Moderate case				
Assume level of 10^{-4} mg/l (33 x minimal, 1/33 x maximal)	200×10^{-6}	2.86×10^{-3}	73×10^{-3}	1.04×10^{-3}
Maximal case				
Maximal reported level in drinking water of 0.003 mg/l	$6{,}000 \times 10^{-6}$	860×10^{-6}	$2{,}190 \times 10^{-3}$	31.3×10^{-3}

*Assuming human water consumption of 2 l/day, absorption efficiency of 100%, and body weight of 70 kg. Values probably about equally applicable to any single isomer, but not total of all. See exposure section for data base.

A spread of about 1,000 times between "minimal" and "maximal" case exposures resulted. Even so, less than "minimal" exposures may apply for some of the population (e.g., very pure water supply) and more than "maximal" exposure for others (highly contaminated supplies). Specific data on ambient air contamination by DCBs was meager. Based on the data of Morita and Ohi (1975) an attempt is made to estimate levels of human exposure via air contamination (see Table 49).

Table 49: Estimated Dichlorobenzene Exposure from Air Contamination

| | Estimated Exposure, mg* | | | |
| | Daily Uptake | | Annual Uptake | |
Exposure Level**	per Person	per Kilogram	per Person	per Kilogram
Minimal case				
1.5×10^{-3} mg/m^3 (lowest suburban concentration reported)	0.01725	0.000246	0.63	0.09
Moderate case				
0.24 mg/m^3 (mean of all values reported from urban, suburban and indoor air)	2.76	0.0394	1,007	14
Maximal case				
1.7 mg/m^3 (reported in wardrobe air due to use of 1,4-DCB)	19.55	0.28	7,136	102

*Based on assumptions as follows: daily inspired volume for reference adult male, 23 m^3 (Natl. Acad. Sci. 1978 citing: Int. Comm. Radiol. Prot. 1975); human body weight, 70 kg (NAS, 1978); absorption efficiency by inhalation, 50%.
**Based on data of Morita and Ohi (25-13) for 1,4-DCB.

The extent of the population that may be represented by the table values is simply un-known. Some segment may be subject to less exposure (e.g., remote rural dwelling), and some to more (e.g., highly contaminated urban or industrial area air, especially contami-nated air associated with some occupations or perhaps indoor air where DCB products are used). Comparison of Tables 48 and 49 suggest greater intake doses via air than via water.

No data are available by which specific exposure to DCBs by consumption of food could be estimated. Reports of detectable, even significant levels in fish, meat, eggs, and grains representing direct contamination residues or products of degradation of other chemicals would suggest the likelihood of at least some intake by ingestion of food (probably mostly from food of lipid nature because of food-chain lipophilic bioaccumulation processes).

Data indicate the possibility of dermal absorption from unusually high-level exposure to vapors or perhaps liquids, but this would likely be significant only in special individual cir-cumstances. There are no data on the level or importance of dermal exposure for the gen-eral public, but it seems reasonable to speculate that it would be insignificant in relation to other exposure modes.

Special Groups at Risk: Persons with preexisting pathology (hepatic, renal, central nervous system, blood) or metabolic disorders, who are taking certain drugs (hormones or other-wise metabolically active), or who are otherwise exposed to DCBs or related (chemically or biologically) chemicals by such means as occupation, or domestic use or abuse (e.g., pica or "sniffing") of DCB products, might well be considered at increased risk from exposure to DCBs.

Existing Guidelines and Standards: The known current standards, guidelines, and goals for DCBs in air and water are summarized in Table 50.

Table 50: Standards, Criteria, or Goal Limits of Contamination for Dichlorobenzenes*

Medium	Standard, Criterion, Goal, etc.	1,2-DCB	1,4-DCB	Reference
Air	OSHA standard for worker exposure	50 ppm (300 mg/m^3) (ceiling)	75 ppm (450 mg/m^3) (TWA)** (car)***	(25-4) (25-5)
Air	ACGIH recommended TLV	50 ppm (300 mg/m^3) (ceiling)	75 ppm (450 mg/m^3) (limit)	(25-6)
Air	EPA, MEG: EPC-AH1†	0.12 ppm (0.714 mg/m^3)	0.18 ppm (2.07 mg/m^3)	(25-7)
Air	Russian MAC (maximal allowable concentration)	3.3 ppm	3.3 ppm (20 mg/m^3)	(25-8)
Water	EPA, MEG: EPC-WH1††	10.7 mg/l	16.1 mg/l	(25-7)
	WH2†††	4.4 mg/1	6.21 mg/l	(25-7)
Water	Russian MPC§	0.002 mg/l	0.002 mg/l	(25-9)

*Current, based on available information. Note: No known regulatory standards exist in US for any DCB isomers (1,2-, 1,3-, or 1,4-DCB) in ambient air or water.

**Time weighted average, 8 hours.

***Carcinogenicity notation in reference (25-5); carcinogenicity determination indefinite in (25-4).

†Estimated permissible concentration in air based on a model utilizing TLV.

††Estimated permissible concentration in water derived from EPC-ALL extrapolated to water intake.

†††Estimated permissible concentration in water based on maximal safe body concentration and biological half-life considerations.

§Maximum permissible concentration recognizing organoleptic effect.

For air the only officially Federally regulated limits are by the Occupational Safety and Health Administration (25-3) for 1,2-DCB and 1,4-DCB in workroom air at 300 mg/m³ and 450 mg/m³, respectively. The threshold limit value (TLV) guidelines of the American Con-ference of Governmental Industrial Hygienists (1979) are virtually the same as the OSHA stan-dards. These may need downward revision in view of human sensory responses in unacclimated persons. The Russian maximal allowable concentration (MAC) value for both 1,2-DCB and 1,4-DCB is 20 mg/m³, much lower than U.S. standards. The U.S. EPA has published multimedia environmental goals (MEGs) for health related estimated permissible concentrations in air: 1,2-DCB, 0.714 mg/m^3 (0.12 ppm) and 1,4-DCB, 1.07 mg/m^3 (0.18 ppm). The Russian and MEG limits appear to recognize the following detection limits more closely than the OSHA and ACGIH values: 1,2-DCB, 12 to 24 mg/m^3 (odor threshold), 60 to 90 mg/m^3 (very noticeable odor), 150 to 180 mg/m^3 (unpleasant odor and eye irritation); 360 to 600 mg/m^3 (painful mucosal irritation); and 960 mg/m^3 (painful irritation).

1,4-DCB is listed for inclusion among chemicals to be monitored by EPA under the Safe Drinking Water Act.

The U.S. EPA (25-7) has published MEGs for health-related EPCs in water based on different approaches (see Table 33): (1) derived from the air-health EPC extrapolated to water intake assuming daily intake and absorption efficiency values: EPA-WHI, 10.7 mg 1,2-DCB/l and 16.1 mg 1,4-DCB/l. (2) based on considerations of maximum safe body concentration and biological half-life data: EPC-WH2, 4.4 mg 1,2-DCB/l and 6.21 mg 1,4-DCB/l. The reported maximum permissible concentrations (MPCs) in Russia, recognizing organoleptic factors (odor, taste) are much more conservative: 0.002 mg/l for both 1,2-DCB and 1,4-DCB (25-9)(25-10).

Apparently, 1,3-DCB has been omitted from regulations or guidelines for media contamination, undoubtedly reflecting its insignificant environmental contamination level and potential at this time. Practically speaking, it would seem reasonable to assume that efforts to control the 1,2- and 1,4-isomers of DCB would also effectively control the 1,3-DCB as well, since it generally would accompany its isomers in total DCB contamination and would not have a significant contamination mode of its own.

Under the Federal Food, Drug and Cosmetic Act certain uses of both monochlorobenzene (MCB) and 1,4-DCB are regulated. MCB is a solvent in the manufacture of resins for food contact articles; residues in such resin products must not exceed 500 mg/kg. 1,4-DCB is an intermediate in the manufacture of other resins for coating products in food contact use; in such products 1,4-DCB residues are limited to 0.8 mg/kg. No information on regulation of residues or levels in food commodities was available.

The U.S. EPA has regulatory authority over some uses of DCBs under the Federal Environmental Pesticide Control Act of 1972. Registered under this act are 43 uses of 1,2-DCB and 304 uses of 1,4-DCB. The chlorinated benzene pesticides are categorized as Class III toxins (oral LD_{50} values ranging from 500 to 5,000 mg/kg and LC_{50} values ranging from 200 to 20,000 mg/m^3) and as such have a hazard signal "caution" and precautionary labeling requirement: "Harmful if swallowed (inhaled or absorbed through skin). Avoid breathing vapors (dust or spray mist). Avoid contact with skin (eyes or clothing). In case of contact immediately flush eyes or skin with plenty of water. Get medical attention if irritation persists."

The Department of Transportation (DOT) regulated interstate transport, and there are specific requirements in regard to handling DCBs as combustible materials (for which they are classified due to their toxic and flashpoint properties). The Coast Guard has regulatory authority for overseas transportation and has recognized toxic, aquatic life hazard, and combustible properties in requiring notification of health, pollution and fire authorities in the event of spills. DCBs have been determined to be hazardous to aquatic life in very low concentrations.

Several states have or intend legislation regulating manufacture, use, disposal, handling, and/or registration and inventory of toxic/hazardous chemicals, often mirroring Federal legislation and promulgations (25-2).

Summary of Proposed EPA Criteria: *Freshwater Aquatic Life* — For 1,2-dichlorobenzene the criterion to protect freshwater aquatic life as derived using the Guidelines is 44 μg/l as a 24-hour average and the concentration should not exceed 99 μg/l at any time.

For 1,3-dichlorobenzene the criterion to protect freshwater aquatic life as derived using procedures other than the Guidelines is 310 μg/l as a 24-hour average and the concentration should not exceed 700 μg/l at any time.

For 1,4-dichlorobenzene the criterion to protect freshwater aquatic life as derived using procedures other than the Guidelines is 190 μg/l as a 24-hour average and the concentration should not exceed 440 μg/l at any time.

Saltwater Aquatic Life — For 1,2-dichlorobenzene the criterion to protect saltwater aquatic life as derived using procedures other than the Guidelines is 15 μg/l as a 24-hour average and the concentration should not exceed 34 μg/l at any time.

For 1,3-dichlorobenzene the criterion to protect saltwater aquatic life as derived using procedures other than the Guidelines is 22 μg/l as a 24-hour average and the concentration should not exceed 49 μg/l at any time.

For 1,4-dichlorobenzene the criterion to protect saltwater aquatic life as derived using procedures other than the Guidelines is 15 μg/l as a 24-hour average and the concentration should not exceed 34 μg/l at any time.

Human Health — For the protection of human health from the toxic properties of dichlorobenzene ingested through water and through contaminated aquatic organisms, the ambient water criterion is determined to be 230 μg/l total dichlorobenzene (all isomers combined).

Basis for the Proposed Human Health Criteria: There was not a sufficient weight of evidence from human or animal tests to qualitatively suggest that DCBs are carcinogenic or mutagenic in mammals or to derive a quantitative estimate of acceptable daily intake using cancer risk extrapolation methods. In addition, there were no human data to allow an estimation of the maximum daily oral dose producing no detected adverse effect.

The most usable controlled experimental data on chronic enteric exposure in multiple animal species is that of Hollingsworth, et al (25-11)(25-12).

The maximum tested dose level producing no detectable adverse effects in these tests was 18.8 mg/kg/day over a period of 6 to 7 months, for both 1,2-DCB and 1,4-DCB. Assuming the average weight of adult humans to be 70 kg, the average daily intake of water for man to be two liters, the ingestion of 18.7 g of fish, a fish bioconcentration factor of 200, and applying an uncertainty factor of 1,000, the acceptable daily intake (ADI) of 1,2- or 1,4-DCB in man is calculated to be 1.316 mg/day.

$$ADI = \frac{18.8 \times 70}{1,000} = 1.316 \text{ mg/day}$$

The corresponding no adverse effect ambient level in water (x) would be 0.23 mg/l based on 1.316 = x[2+200 (0.0187)]. The similarity of toxicities among the DCB isomers indicates the applicability of this value to 1,3-DCB as well.

The calculation assumes that 100% of man's exposure is assigned to the ambient water pathway. The only environmental monitoring data available on the DCBs inadequate as they are, suggest that man's exposure by inhalation of the material in air may be 3,000 to 15,000 times his exposure from water. Although it is desirable to arrive at a criterion level for water based on total exposure analysis, the data base for exposure pathways other than water is not sufficient to support a factoring of the ADI level calculated from ambient water assumptions.

The calculated level of 0.23 mg/l for any DCB isomer should be considered a total, i.e., total contamination by DCB isomers whether occurring singly or in combination should not exceed the criterion level. Pending the availability of better data on relative exposure by various routes and on carcinogenic risk, this level should be adequate to prevent adverse health effects from long-term ambient water exposures.

In summary, based on the use of chronic toxicologic test data in animals, and an uncertainty factor of 1,000, the criterion level of DCBs (total) corresponding to the calculated total acceptable daily intake of 18.8 mg/kg, is 0.23 mg/l. Drinking water contributes 35% of the assumed exposure while eating contaminated fish products accounts for 65%. The criterion level for DCB can alternatively be expressed as 0.35 mg/l if exposure is assumed to be from the consumption of fish and shellfish products alone.

References

(25-1) U.S. EPA, *In depth studies on health and environmental impacts of selected water pollutants*, Report on EPA Contract No. 68-01-4646, Wash., D.C., Environ. Prot. Agency, (1978).

(25-2) West, W.L. and Ware, S.A., *Investigation of selected potential environmental contaminants: halogenated benzenes*, Washington, D.C., U.S. Environ. Prot. Agency (1977).

(25-3) 29 *CFR* 1910 (Jan. 16, 1976).

(25-4) Occupational Safety and Health Admin., *General Industry Standards*, Wash., D.C. (1976).

(25-5) Christensen, H.E. and Luginbyhl, T.T., Eds., *Suspected Carcinogens, A Subfile of the NIOSH Toxic Substances List*, Rockville, Md., NIOSH (1975).

(25-6) Amer. Conf. of Govt. Ind. Hygienists, *Threshold Limit Values for Chemical Substances in Workroom Air*, Cincinnati, Ohio (1979).

(25-7) U.S. Environmental Protection Agency, *Multimedia Environmental Goals for Environmental Assessment*, Wash., D.C., Office of Res. and Dev. (1977).

(25-8) International Agency for Research on Cancer, *Information Bulletin on the Survey of Chemicals Being Tested for Carcinogenicity*, No. 7, Lyon, France (1974).

(25-9) Stofen, D., "Tolerance Levels for Toxic Substances in Drinking Water," *Stadthyg*, 24, 109 (1973) (Translation, Oak Ridge Natl. Lab. ORNL-Tr-2975).

(25-10) Varshavskaya, S.P., "The comparative sanitary and toxicological characteristics of chlorobenzene and dichlorobenzene (ortho and para isomers) from the point of view of sanitation of water reservoirs," *Gig. Sanit.* (Russian), 33, 15 (1968).

(25-11) Hollingsworth, R.L., et al, "Toxicity of para-dichlorobenzene. Determinations on experimental animals and human subjects," *AMA Arch. Ind. Health*, 14, 138 (1956).

(25-12) Hollingsworth, R.L., et al, "Toxicity of ortho-dichlorobenzene. Studies on animals and industrial experience," *AMA Arch. Ind. Health*, 17, 180 (1958).

25-13) Morita, M. and Ohi, G., "para-Dichlorobenzene in human tissues and atmospheres in the Tokyo metropolitan area," *Environ. Pollut.*, 8, 269 (1975).

3,3'-DICHLOROBENZIDINE (#26)

The molecular formula of 3,3'-dichlorobenzidine (4,4'-diamino-3,3'-dichlorobiphenyl) is $C_{12}H_{10}Cl_2N_2$. Its molecular weight is 253.13 and its structural formula is

Occurrence: Dichlorobenzidine involves only industrial exposure. It does not occur in nature and therefore it is found only in plant environment and plant effluents.

Physical Properties: 3,3'-DCB forms brownish needles with a melting point of 132° to 133°C. It is readily soluble in alcohol, benzene, and glacial acetic acid, slightly soluble in HCl, and sparingly soluble in water (0.7 g/l at 15°C). When combined with ferric chloride or bleaching powder, a green color is produced.

Chemical Properties: 3,3'-DCB's affinity for water-suspended particulate matter and soils is uncertain; the fact that it is an organic base suggests that it may be strongly bound to soil materials.

Pyrolysis of 3,3'-DCB will most likely lead to the release of HCl. Because of the halogen substitution, 3,3'-DCB compounds probably biodegrade at a slower rate than benzidine alone. The photochemistry of 3,3'-DCB is unknown.

Assuming the clean air concentrations of ozone (2×10^{-9}M) and an average atmospheric concentration of hydroxyl radicals (3×10^{-15}M), the half-life for oxidation of 3,3'-DCBs by either of these chemical species is on the order of one and one to ten days, respectively. Furthermore, assuming a representative concentration of 10^{-10}M for peroxy radicals in sunlit oxygenated water, the half-life for oxidation by these species is approximately 100 days, given the variability of environmental, atmospheric, and aqueous conditions.

Uses: 3,3'-Dichlorobenzidine is used in the production of dyes and pigments and as a curing agent for polyurethanes.

Toxic Effects: There are few data available on the bioconcentration, bioaccumulation, and biomagnification of 3,3'-DCB in the aquatic environment. It has been shown to be experimentally bioconcentrated by fish to a significant degree, approximately 1,150-fold. However, no 3,3'-DCB was detected in fish sampled from the vicinity of a 3,3'-DCB-contaminated waste lagoon using analytical methods with sensitivities of 10 to 100 $\mu g/kg$.

3,3'-DCB has been shown to be a carcinogen in nonhuman mammals under controlled laboratory conditions. Exposure to DCB results in various types of sarcomas and adenocarcinomas. Tumors have been induced both locally (at the site of injection) and remotely (multisystem involvement after feeding) (26-1). Experiments show 3,3'-DCB to be a much less potent carcinogen in animals than the unsubstituted base (benzidine) (26-1).

No definitive evidence exists to demonstrate 3,3'-DCB as a carcinogen in man. Unlike benzidine, 3,3'-DCB exposure to humans produced no increases in urinary bladder carcinomas (26-2)(26-3). Because of the dichloro substitution, this compound may be metabolized differently from benzidine, which is carcinogenic by virtue of metabolic activation.

Current Levels of Exposure: Given the stringent precautions which must be taken in the manufacture and use of 3,3'-DCB, the level of exposure may be minimal at present, although no data are available. However, past exposure of individuals working without benefit of protective measures must present a cause for concern. In addition, the general population may receive exposure through contaminated drinking water or food (fish), although there is no significant evidence for this at the present.

Special Groups at Risk: It is estimated that between 250 and 2,500 workers receive exposure to DCB in the U.S., compared to 62 for benzidine (26-4).

Additional groups that may be at risk include workers in the printing or graphic arts professions handling the 3,3'-DCB-based azo pigments. 3,3'-DCB may be present as an impurity in the pigments, and there is some evidence that 3,3'-DCB may be metabolically liberated from the azo pigment. More information on the level of exposure to the pigments is needed.

Existing Guidelines and Standards: The American Conference of Governmental Industrial Hygienists recommended in 1977 that no exposure to 3,3'-DCB by any route should be permitted, because of a demonstrated high carcinogenic response in animals. Strict regulations have recently been promulgated by the Occupational Safety and Health Administration to minimize or eliminate occupational exposure to DCB (26-5). To date, no standards have been placed on permissible levels of 3,3'-DCB in the environment or in food.

Summary of Proposed EPA Criteria: *Freshwater Aquatic Life* — For freshwater aquatic life, no criterion for any dichlorobenzidine can be derived using the Guidelines, and there are insufficient data to estimate a criterion using other procedures.

Saltwater Aquatic Life — For saltwater aquatic life, no criterion for any dichlorobenzidine can be derived using the Guidelines, and there are insufficient data to estimate a criterion using other procedures.

Human Health — For the maximum protection of human health from the potential carcinogenic effects of exposure to dichlorobenzidine through ingestion of water and contaminated aquatic organisms, the ambient water concentration is zero. Concentrations of dichlorobenzidine estimated to result in additional lifetime cancer risks ranging from no additional risk to an additional risk of 1 in 100,000 are presented in the Criterion Formulation section of this document. The EPA is considering setting criteria at an interim target risk level in the range of 10^{-5}, 10^{-6}, or 10^{-7} with corresponding criteria of 1.69×10^{-2} $\mu g/l$, 1.69×10^{-3} and 1.69×10^{-4} $\mu g/l$, respectively.

Basis for the Proposed Human Health Criteria: The water quality criterion for 3,3'-dichlorobenzidine is based on the induction of papillary transitional cell carcinomas of the urinary bladder and hepatic carcinomas in female beagle dogs, given an oral dose of 100 mg 3,3'-dichlorobenzidine, three times per week for six weeks, then five times per week continuously for up to 7.1 years (26-6). Dose-response data for dogs were selected because dogs developed urinary bladder tumors, as do humans, when exposed to certain aromatic amines. The concentration of 3,3'-DCB in water, calculated to keep the lifetime cancer risk below 10^{-5} is 0.10 $\mu g/l$.

Under the Consent Decree in *NRDC vs Train*, criteria are to state "recommended maximum permissible concentrations (including where appropriate, zero) consistent with the protection of aquatic organisms, human health, and recreational activities." 3,3'-DCB is suspected of being a human carcinogen. Because there is no recognized safe concentration for a human carcinogen, the recommended concentration of 3,3'-DCB in water for maximum protection of human health is zero.

Because attaining a zero concentration level may be infeasible in some cases and in order to assist the EPA and States in the possible future development of water quality regulations, the concentrations of 3,3'-DCB corresponding to several incremental lifetime cancer risk levels have been estimated. A cancer risk level provides an estimate of the additional incidence of cancer that may be expected in an exposed population. A risk of 10^{-5}, e.g., indicates a probability of one additional case of cancer for every 100,000 people exposed, a risk of 10^{-6} indicates one additional case of cancer for every million people exposed, etc.

In the *Federal Register* notice of availability of draft ambient water quality criteria, EPA stated that it is considering setting criteria at an interim target risk level of 10^{-5}, 10^{-6} or 10^{-7} as shown in Table 51.

Table 51: Possible Alternate Criteria for Dichlorobenzidine

Exposure Assumptions (per day)	Risk Levels and Corresponding Criteria			
	0	10^{-7}	10^{-6}	10^{-5}
	. . . .(ng/l)			
2 liters of drinking water and consumption of 18.7 g of fish and shellfish*	0	0.169	1.69	16.9
Consumption of fish and shellfish only	0	0.185	1.85	18.5

*48% of DCB exposure results from the consumption of aquatic organisms which exhibit an average bioconcentration potential of 100-fold. The remaining 52% of DCB exposure results from drinking water.

Source: Reference (26)

The risk levels are calculated by applying a modified "one-hit" extrapolation model described in the *FR* 15926, 1979. Since the extrapolation model is linear to low doses, the additional lifetime risk is directly proportional to the water concentration. Therefore, water concentrations corresponding to other risk levels can be derived by multiplying or dividing one of the risk levels and corresponding water concentration shown in the table by factors such as 10, 100, 1,000, etc.

Concentration levels were derived assuming a lifetime exposure to various amounts of 3,3'-DCB, (1) occurring from the consumption of both drinking water and aquatic life grown in water containing the corresponding 3,3'-DCB concentrations and, (2) occurring solely from consumption of aquatic life grown in the waters containing the corresponding 3,3'-DCB concentrations.

Although total exposure information for 3,3'-DCB is discussed and an estimate of the contributions from other sources of exposure can be made, this data will not be factored into the ambient water quality criteria formulation because of the tenuous estimates. The criteria presented, therefore, assume an incremental risk from ambient water exposure only.

Summary of Pertinent Data — The water quality criterion for 3,3'-DCB is based on the induction of papillary transitional cell carcinomas of the urinary bladder and hepatic carcinomas in female beagle dogs, given an oral dose of 100 mg 3,3'-DCB, three times per week for six weeks, then five times per week continuously for periods up to 7.1 years (26-6). The incidence of urinary bladder carcinomas observed in 3,3'-DCB-treated dogs was 5/5 as compared to 0/6 in the control group. The incidences of hepatic carcinomas were 4:5 and 0/6 in 3,3'-DCB-treated and control groups, respectively.

The criterion was calculated from the following parameters: n_{tu} = 4.5 (urinary bladder carcinomas); N_{tu} = 5; n_{th} = 4 (hepatic carcinoma); N_{th} = 5; n_c = 0; N_c = 6; Le = 7.1 years; le = 7.1 years; L = 8.65 years; d (timeweighted average concentration) = 7.36 mg per kg per day; F = 0.0187 kg; R = 1,150; and W = 11.391 kg.

Based on these parameters, the one-hit slope (B_H) is 1.036 $(mg/kg/day)^{-1}$ for urinary bladder carcinomas and 0.724 $(mg/kg/day)^{-1}$ for hepatic carcinomas. The resulting water concentration for 3,3'-DCB, calculated to keep the individual lifetime cancer risk below 10^{-5}, is 1.69 x 10^{-2} $\mu g/l$. In n_{tu} = 4.5 above, the underestimate of the true number, based on Burkson's correction factor, was chosen in order to obtain a finite mathematical estimate.

References

(26-1) Rye, W.A., et al, "Facts and myths concerning aromatic diamine curing agents," *Jour. Occup. Med.*, 12, 211 (1970).

(26-2) Gerarde, H.W. and Gerarde, D.F., "Industrial experience with 3,3'-dichlorobenzidine. Epidemiological study of a chemical manufacturing plant." *Jour. Occup. Med.*, 16, 322 (1974).

(26-3) MacIntyre, D.I., "Experience of tumors in a British plant handling 3,3'-dichlorobenzidine," *Jour. Occup. Med.*, 17, 23 (1975).

(26-4) Haley, T.J., "Benzidine revisited: A review of the literature and problems associated with the use of benzidine and its congeners," *Clin. Toxicol.*, 8, 13-42 (1975).

(26-5) *Code of Federal Regulations*, Title 29, Part 10 (1977).

(26-6) Stula, E.F., Barnes, J.R., Sherman, H., Reinhardt, C.F., and Zapp, Jr., J.A., *J. Environmental Pathology and Toxicology*, 1:475-490 (1976).

DICHLOROBROMOMETHANE

See "Halomethanes" (38).

DICHLORODIFLUOROMETHANE

See "Halomethanes" (38).

1,1-DICHLOROETHANE

See "Chlorinated Ethanes" (15).

1,2-DICHLOROETHANE

See "Chlorinated Ethanes" (15).

DICHLOROETHYLENES (#27)

The dichloroethylenes consist of the three isomers: 1,1-dichloroethylene (1,1-DCE) (also commonly known as vinylidene chloride), cis-1,2-dichloroethylene (cis-1,2-DCE) and trans-1,2-dichloroethylene (trans-1,2-DCE).

Occurrence: 1,1-DCE is not shown to occur in nature and ambient levels have not been determined. This chemical is expected to be short-lived in water because of its volatilization to the atmosphere. The 1,2-DCEs have been measured in a limited number of U.S. drinking water supplies.

Physical Properties: Dichloroethylenes are clear colorless liquids with the molecular formula $C_2H_2Cl_2$ and a molecular weight of 96.95. 1,1-DCE has a water solubility of 2,500 μg/ml, a vapor pressure of 591 mm Hg, and a melting point of -122.1°C. The cis-isomer of 1,2-dichloroethylene has a water solubility of 3,500 μg/ml, a vapor pressure of 208 mm Hg, and a melting point of -80.5°C; trans-1,2-dichloroethylene has a water solubility of 6,300 μg/ml, a vapor pressure of 324 mm Hg and a melting point of -50°C. The octanol/water partition coefficient for 1,1-DCE was reported as 5.37 (log P = 0.73), indicating it should not accumulate significantly in animals.

Chemical Properties: Vinylidene chloride, 1,1-dichloroethylene, polymerizes readily and also adds chlorine to give methyl chloroform.

Uses: As of the early 1960s, neither of the 1,2-dichloroethylenes (1,2-DCEs) had wide industrial usage (27-1). However, annual production of 1,1-DCE now approximates 120,000 metric tons. It is used as a chemical intermediate in the synthesis of methylchloroform and in the production of polyvinylidene chloride copolymers (PVDCs). Among the monomers used with 1,1-DCE in copolymer production are vinyl chloride, acrylonitrile, and alkyl acrylates. The impermeability of PVDCs make them useful primarily as barrier coatings in the packaging industry. Polymers with high vinylidene chloride (1,1-DCE) content such as Saran are widely used in the food packaging industry. The heat-seal characteristics of saran coatings make them useful in the manufacture of nonflammable synthetic fiber. 1,1-DCE polymers have also been used extensively as interior coatings for ship tanks, railroad cars, and fuel storage tanks, and for coating of steel pipes and structures.

Toxic Effects: Under laboratory conditions, the dichloroethylenes have shown to be toxic to fish (27-2)(27-3). The primary effect of acute toxicity of the dichloroethylenes is depression of the central nervous system. There is concern over the toxicity of 1,1-DCE because it is toxic to the liver of experimental animals (27-4) and has a structure similar to vinyl chloride monomer, a known liver carcinogen in several species including humans (27-5)(27-6).

Current Levels of Exposure: No information was found on current levels of exposure. The reader is referred to accounts of manufacturing practice; see the section which follows.

Special Groups at Risk: The population most exposed to 1,1-DCE consists of workers in industries manufacturing or using 1,1-DCE (27-7)(27-8). 1,1-DCE was identified as a co-contaminant with vinyl chloride monomer in the working environment of polyvinylchloride production plants (27-9).

Existing Guidelines and Standards: Standards that have been established for the DCEs are applicable primarily to occupational exposures. The threshold limit values (TLV) for these compounds presently established by the American Conference of Governmental Industrial Hygienists (ACGIH) are 40 mg/m^3 (1,1-DCE) and 790 mg/m^3 (1,2-DCE). These values allow daily exposures of 286 mg 1,1-DCE per day and 5,643 mg 1,2-DCE per day. These calculations are based on the assumption of 50 m^3/work week of inhaled air averaged over a 7 day period (27-10). A separate standard has been established for 1,1-DCE, but the TLV does not distinguish between the two isomers of 1,2-DCE.

The standard for 1,2-DCE was established on the basis of no measurable effects on growth, mortality, organ and body weights, hematology, clinical chemistry, and gross and microscopic pathology at doses of up to 4,000 mg/m^3 for 6 months in rats, rabbits, guinea pigs and dogs. However, more recent data (27-12) indicate that 16 weeks' exposure at the TLV of 790 mg/m^3 of trans-1,2-DCE produces histological evidence of fatty degeneration of the liver in rats.

In the case of 1,1-DCE, the standard was established primarily on the basis of the work of Prendergast, et al (27-12) who observed increased mortality as a result of continuous exposures of guinea pigs and monkeys to 61 mg/m^3 and above for 90 days. Liver and kidney pathology were consistently only observed at 189 mg/m^3. As can be seen these industrial TLVs allow very little safety factor for sensitive populations. Recent data suggesting that 1,1-DCE is carcinogenic in mice (27-13) have not yet been taken into account.

Summary of Proposed EPA Criteria: *Freshwater Aquatic Life* — For 1,1-dichloroethylene, the criterion to protect freshwater aquatic life, (as derived using procedures other than the Guidelines), is 530 µg/l as a 24-hour average and the concentration should not exceed 1,200 µg/l at any time.

For 1,2-dichloroethylene, the criterion to protect freshwater aquatic life, (as derived using procedures other than the Guidelines), is 620 µg/l as a 24-hour average and the concentration should not exceed 1,400 µg/l at any time.

Saltwater Aquatic Life — For 1,1-dichloroethylene, the criterion to protect saltwater aquatic life, (as derived using procedures other than the Guidelines), is 1,700 µg/l as a 24-hour average and the concentration should not exceed 3,900 µg/l at any time.

For saltwater aquatic life, no criterion for 1,2-dichloroethylene can be derived using the Guidelines, and there are insufficient data to estimate a criterion using other procedures.

Human Health — For the maximum protection of human health from the potential carcinogenic effects of exposure to 1,1-dichloroethylene through ingestion of water and contaminated aquatic organisms, the ambient water concentration is zero. Concentrations of 1,1-dichloroethylene estimated to result in additional lifetime cancer risks ranging from no additional risk to 1 in 100,000 are presented in the Criterion Formulation section of this document. The EPA is considering setting criteria at an interim target risk level in the range of 10^{-5}, 10^{-6}, or 10^{-7} with corresponding criteria of 1.3 µg/l, 0.13 µg/l, and 0.013 µg/l, respectively.

Basis for the Proposed Human Health Criteria: Under the Consent Decree in *NRDC vs Train*, criteria are to state "recommended maximum permissible concentrations (including where appropriate, zero) consistent with the protection of aquatic organisms, human health, and recreational activities." 1,1-Dichloroethylene is suspected of being a human carcinogen. Because there is no recognized safe concentration for a human carcinogen, the recommended concentration of 1,1-dichloroethylene in water for maximum protection of human health is zero.

Because attaining a zero concentration level may be infeasible in cases and in order to assist the EPA and States in the possible future development of water quality regulations, the concentrations of 1,1-dichloroethylene corresponding to several incremental lifetime cancer risk levels have been estimated. A cancer risk level provides an estimate of the additional incidence of cancer that may be expected in an exposed population. A risk of 10^{-5}, e.g., indicates a probability of one additional case of cancer for every 100,000 people exposed, a risk of 10^{-6} indicates one additional case of cancer for every million people exposed, etc.

In the *Federal Register* notice of availability of draft ambient water quality criteria, EPA stated that it is considering setting criteria for 1,1-dichloroethylene at an interim target risk level of 10^{-5}, 10^{-6} or 10^{-7} as shown in Table 52.

Table 52: Possible Alternative Criteria for 1,1-Dichloroethylene (Vinylidene Chloride)

Exposure Assumptions (per day)	Risk Levels and Corresponding Criteria			
	0	10^{-7}	10^{-6}	10^{-5}
	. . . . (μg/l)			
2 liters of drinking water and consumption of 18.7 g of fish and shellfish*	0	0.013	0.13	1.3
Consumption of fish and shellfish only	0	0.214	2.14	21.4

*Approximately 7% of the 1,1-dichloroethylene exposure results from the consumption of aquatic organisms which exhibit an average bioconcentration potential of 8-fold. The remaining 93% of 1,1-dichloroethylene exposure results from drinking water.

Source: Reference (27)

The risk levels are calculated by applying a modified "one-hit" extrapolation model described in the Methodology Document to the animal bioassay data presented in Summary of Pertinent Data. Since the extrapolation model is linear at low doses, the additional lifetime risk is directly proportional to the water concentration. Therefore, water concentrations corresponding to other risk levels can be derived by multiplying or dividing one of the risk levels and corresponding water concentrations shown in the table by factors such as 10, 100, 1,000, etc.

Concentration levels were derived assuming a lifetime exposure to various amounts of 1,1-dichloroethylene (1) occurring from the consumption of both drinking water and aquatic life grown in waters containing the corresponding 1,1-dichloroethylene concentrations and (2) occurring solely from assumption of aquatic life grown in the waters containing the corresponding 1,1-dichloroethylene concentrations. Because data including other sources of 1,1-dichloroethylene exposure and their contributions to total body burden are inadequate for quantitative use, the figures reflect the incremental risks associated with the indicated routes only.

Summary of Pertinent Data — Maltoni (27-13) exposed mice to 25 ppm via inhalation for 4 hr/day, 4.5 days/week for 1 year. The interim report summarized the results after 82 weeks or 1.64 years. The control males had a kidney adenocarcinoma incidence of 0/126 and the treated males had an incidence of 16/98. The fish bioaccumulation factor is 6.9.

The parameters of the extrapolation model are: n_t = 16; N_t = 98; n_c = 0; N_c = 126; Le = 82 weeks; le = 52 weeks; d = 25 x 4/24 x 4.5/7 x 0.4 = 1.0714 ppm; w = 0.025 kg (not exceeded); L = 90 weeks; R = 6.9; D = 1.0714 x 52/82 = 0.67944 ppm; t = 82/90 = 0.91111; t^3 = 0.75633; Dt^3 = 0.51388 ppm; and B = 1/0.51388 in [(1–0/126)/(1–16/98)] = = 0.34686 (in terms of risk per ppm).

For air exposures in units of ppm, no species conversion factor is necessary. Therefore, for humans the concentration, X, giving a risk, R, of 10^{-5} is X = R/B = 10^{-5}/0.34686 = 2.8830 x 10^{-5} ppm.

Since the air concentration corresponding to 1 ppm of DCE is 4×10^{-3} $\mu g/m^3$ and since people breathe an average of 24 m^3/day of air, the daily intake of DCE that would result in a lifetime risk of 10^{-5} is:

$$2.8830 \times 10^{-5} \text{ ppm} \times 4 \times 10^3 \ \mu g/m^3/\text{ppm} \times 24 \ m^3/\text{day} = 2.7677 \ \mu g/\text{day}$$

If it is assumed that the fraction of the DCE intake reaching the target site is the same whether it is administered via limitation or ingestion of water and fish, a daily DCE intake of 2.768 μg through water and fish alone would also cause a cancer risk of 10^{-5}. The water concentration giving this intake is

$$C = \frac{2.7677 \ \mu g/\text{day}}{[2 + (6.9 \times 0.0187)] \ \text{liters/day}} = 1.2999 \ \mu g/l \cong 1.3 \ \mu g/l$$

References

(27-1) Patty, F.A., "Aliphatic halogenated hydrocarbons," *Ind. Hyg. Tox.*, 2, 1307 (1963).

(27-2) Dawson, G.W., et al, "The acute toxicity of 47 industrial chemicals to fresh and saltwater fishes," *Jour. Hazard. Mater.*, 1, 303 (1977).

(27-3) U.S. EPA, *In-depth studies on health and environmental impact of selected water pollutants*, Report on Contract No. 68-01-4646, Wash., D.C., Environ. Prot. Agency (1978).

(27-4) Jaeger, et al, "Biochemical toxicology of unsaturated halogenated monomers," *Environ. Health Perspect.*, 11, 121 (1975).

(27-5) Maltoni, C., "Predictive values of carcinogenesis bioassays," *Annu. N.Y. Acad. Sci.*, 271, 431 (1976).

(27-6) Spirtas, R., and Kaminski, R., "Angiosarcoma of the liver in vinyl chloride-polyvinyl chloride workers. Update of the NIOSH Register," *Jour. Occup. Med.*, 20, 427 (1978).

(27-7) Hushon, J. and Kornreich, M., *Air pollution assessment of vinylidene chloride*, Report on EPA Contract 68-02-1495, Wash., D.C. (1976).

(27-8) Arthur D. Little, Inc., *Vinylidene chloride monomer emissions from the monomer, polymer, and polymer processing industries*, Report for the U.S. Environ. Prot. Agency, Research Triangle Park, N.C. (Apr. 1976).

(27-9) Kramer, C. and Mutchler, J., "The correlation of clinical and environmental measurements for workers exposed to vinyl chloride," *Am. Ind. Hyg. Assoc. Jour.*, 33, 19 (1972).

(27-10) Stokinger, H.E. and Woodward, H.L., "Toxicologic methods for establishing drinking water standards," *Jour. Am. Water Works Assoc.*, 50, 515 (1958).

(27-11) Freundt, K.J., et al, "Toxicity studies on trans-1,2-dichloroethylene," *Toxicology*, 7, 141 (1977).

(27-12) Prendergast, J.A., et al, "Effects on experimental animals of long-term inhalation of trichloroethylene, carbon tetrachloride, 1,1,1-trichloroethane, dichlorodifluoromethane and 1,1-dichloroethylene," *Toxicol. Appl. Pharmacol.*, 10, 270 (1967).

(27-13) Maltoni, C., "Recent findings on the carcinogenicity of chlorinated olefins," *Environ. Health Perspect.*, 21, 1 (1977).

DICHLOROMETHYL BROMIDE

See "Halomethanes" (38).

2,4-DICHLOROPHENOL (#28)

The compound, 2,4-dichlorophenol, has the empirical formula $C_6H_4Cl_2O$, the following structural formula, and a molecular weight of 163.0.

OH

Cl

Cl

Occurrence: Little information is available on the 2,4-DCP levels present in industrial or municipal effluents, natural waters, or drinking water. A report by Sidwell (28-1) found 2,4-DCP levels in industrial plant effluents ranging from 11.4 to 73.6 mg/l and has estimated a resulting drinking water level of 1.25 mg/l.

Few data exist regarding the persistence of 2,4-DCP in the environment. 2,4-DCP is slightly soluble in water while its alkaline salts are readily soluble in aqueous solutions. Its low vapor pressure and nonvolatility from alkaline solutions would cause it to be only slowly removed from surface water via volatilization. Studies have indicated low sorption of 2,4-DCP from natural surface waters by various clays.

Physical Properties: 2,4-Dichlorophenol is a colorless, crystalline solid with a density of 1.383 g/ml at 60°F/25°C and a vapor pressure of 1.0 mm Hg at 53.0°C. The melting point of 2,4-DCP is 45°C and the boiling point is 210°C at 760 mm Hg.

2,4-DCP is slightly soluble in water at neutral pH and dissolves readily in ethanol and benzene. 2,4-DCP behaves as a weak acid and is highly soluble in alkaline solutions, since it readily forms the corresponding alkaline salt. The dissociation constant (pKa) for 2,4-DCP has been reported to be 7.48. Unlike the monochlorophenols, 2,4-DCP is not volatile from aqueous alkaline solutions.

Chemical Properties: Numerous studies on the microbial degradation of 1,4-DCP have been conducted, revealing degradation to yield succinic acid. Additionally, oxidative degradation of 2,4-DCP in natural lake waters under laboratory conditions has also been reported.

Uses: 2,4-Dichlorophenol is a commercially produced substituted phenol used entirely in the manufacture of industrial and agricultural products. As an intermediate in the chemical industry, 2,4-DCP is utilized principally as the feedstock for the manufacture of the herbicide, 2,4-dichlorophenoxyacetic acid (2,4-D), and 2,4-D derivatives (germicides, soil sterilants, etc.) and certain methyl compounds used in mothproofing, antiseptics and seed disinfectants. 2,4-DCP is also reacted with benzene sulfonyl chloride to produce miticides or further chlorinated to pentachlorophenol, a wood preservative.

Toxic Effects: Although a paucity of aquatic toxicity data exists, 2,4-DCP appears to be less toxic than the higher chlorinated phenols. 2,4-DCP's toxicity to certain microorganisms and plant life has been demonstrated and its tumor promoting potential in mice (28-2) has been reported. In addition, it has been demonstrated that 2,4-DCP can produce objectionable odors when present in water at extremely low levels (28-3). These findings, in conjunction with potential 2,4-DCP pollution by waste sources from commercial processes or the inadvertent production of 2,4-DCP due to chlorination of waters containing phenol, lead to the conclusion that 2,4-DCP represents a potential threat to aquatic and terrestrial life, including man.

Little or no information on the bioconcentration, metabolism, or excretion of 2,4-DCP appears to exist. However, an octanol/water partition coefficient of 1,200 has been reported.

Current Levels of Exposure: Human exposure to 2,4-DCP has not been monitored, but a worst-case estimate of 0.04 mg 2,4-DCP/kg body weight/day of exposure has been encountered.

Special Groups at Risk: The only group expected to be at risk for high exposure to 2,4-DCP is industrial workers involved in the manufacturing or handling of 2,4-DCP and 2,4-D. No data were found to relate exposure or body burden to conditions of contact with 2,4-DCP.

Existing Guidelines and Standards: Presently no standard for exposure to 2,4-DCP in drinking or ambient water has been set, although a standard of 0.1 mg/l for 2,4-D, a related compound, has been set (28-4).

Summary of Proposed EPA Criteria: *Freshwater Aquatic Life* — For 2,4-dichlorophenol the criterion to protect freshwater aquatic life as derived using the Guidelines is 0.4 μg/l as a 24-hour average and the concentration should not exceed 110 μg/l at any time.

Saltwater Aquatic Life — For saltwater aquatic life, no criterion for 2,4-dichlorophenol can be derived using the Guidelines, and there are insufficient data to estimate a criterion using other procedures.

Human Health — For the prevention of adverse effects due to the organoleptic properties of 2,4-dichlorophenol in water, the criterion is 0.5 μg/l.

Basis for the Proposed Human Health Criteria: Insufficient data exists to indicate that 2,4-DCP is a carcinogenic agent. One study was designed to detect promoting activity, and the effect of 2,4-DCP as a primary carcinogen could not be evaluated. In fact, only minimal health effects data exist on the acute and chronic effects of 2,4-DCP. Only one chronic study was found in which a chronic (6-month) no-effect level for 2,4-DCP of 1,000 μg/l of diet for mice, which is equivalent to 100 mg/kg body weight per day was determined. For water, a concentration of approximately one-half the dietary intake will result in equivalent dosage on a body weight basis, assuming a fluid intake two times the dry matter intake.

If food sources are not included, the maximum no-effect level of 2,4-DCP in water for mice would be 500 μg/l. Applying an uncertainty factor of 10^{-3} x maximum no-effect level as suggested by the National Academy of Sciences Safe Drinking Water Committee would result in a criterion for human health of 500 μg/l, which is approximately 250 times greater than the threshold odor concentration.

However, in addition to exposure through drinking water, additional exposure to 2,4-DCP through the daily ingestion of 18.7 g of fish and shellfish products exists. Therefore, based on the assumption of an intake of two liters of drinking water per day at a level of 500 μg/l, and a fish bioconcentrating value of 37, the total amount of 2,4-DCP exposure through both routes is 371 μg/day:

$$\frac{2 \times 500 \ \mu g/day}{2 + (37 \times 0.0187)} = 371 \ \mu g/day$$

Human health is a subject measurement in many respects. The organoleptic effect of 2,4-DCP could conceivably alter human health by causing a decrease in water consumption. This might be of particular importance to individuals with certain renal diseases or in instances where dehydration occurs as a result of vigorous exercise, manual labor, or hot weather. Although two investigators reported that low concentrations of 2,4-DCP caused discernible odor, neither indicated if the threshold odor concentration made water unacceptable for consumption. In view of the wide disparity between odor threshold concentrations and available toxicity information, the criterion recommended is based on organoleptic effects. It is suggested that a 2,4-DCP water concentration of 0.5 μg/l would be low enough to prevent objectionable organoleptic effects for most people and still be far below minimal no-effect concentrations determined in laboratory animals.

In conclusion, two criteria can be proposed. Based on the prevention of adverse organoleptic effects, the interim criterion recommended for 2,4-dichlorophenol is 0.5 μg/l in water. Based on human health effects alone, the interim criterion recommended is 371 μg/l.

References

(28-1) Sidwell, A.E., *Biological treatment of chlorophenolic wastes*, Water Pollut. Control Res. Ser. 12130 EGK, Wash., D.C., U.S. Environ. Prot. Agency (1971).

(28-2) Boutwell, R.K. and Bosch, D.K., "The tumor-promoting action of phenol and related compounds for mouse skin," *Cancer Res.*, 19, 413 (1959).

(28-3) Burttschell, R.H., et al, "Chlorine derivatives of phenol causing taste and odor," *Jour. Am. Water Works Assoc.*, 5, 205 (1959).

(28-4) National Academy of Sciences, *Drinking Water and Health*, Wash., D.C. (1977).

DICHLOROPROPANES/DICHLOROPROPENES (#29)

For purposes of discussion, dichloropropane refers to 1,2-dichloropropane and will be abbreviated "PDC" (for propylene dichloride); dichloropropene refers to 1,3-dichloropropene and will be abbreviated "DCP." In the case of the latter, the cis- or trans-isomer will be designated when known. Lack of such designation will indicate lack of further information on speciation or that a mixture of the two isomers is involved.

Occurrence: Dichloropropanes and dichloropropenes can enter the aquatic environment as discharges from industrial effluents, by runoff from agricultural land, and from municipal effluents. These compounds have been detected in New Orleans drinking water, although they were not quantified. Most data on persistence, degradation and distribution of dichloropropanes and dichloropropenes deal with their presence in soils.

Physical Properties: Dichloropropanes and dichloropropenes are liquids at environmental temperatures and have molecular weights of 112.99 and 110.97, respectively. Compositions of specific compounds are shown in Table 53.

Table 53: Properties of Dichloropropanes/Dichloropropenes

	Boiling Point (°C)	Density g/ml
Dichloropropanes		
1,1-PDC	88.1	1.132
1,2-PDC	96.4	1.156
1,3-PDC	120.4	1.188
2,2-PDC	69.3	1.112
Dichloropropenes		
1,1-DCP	76–77	1.186
1,2-DCP	77	1.182
cis-1,3-DCP	104.3	1.224
trans-1,3-DCP	112	1.217

Source: Reference (29)

Lange (1952) reports a water solubility of 270 mg/100 ml at 20°C for 1,2-dichloropropane. The vapor pressure of 1,2-dichloropropane is 40 mm Hg at 19.4°C. The water solubility at 20°C is 0.27% for cis-1,3-dichloropropene and 0.28% for trans-1,3-dichloropropene.

Chemical Properties: When heated to decomposition, 1,2-dichloropropane emits highly toxic fumes of phosgene, while 1,3-dichloropropene gives off toxic fumes of chlorides.

Dichloropropenes have been shown to undergo photochemical formation of free radicals. The cis- and trans-isomers of 1,3-dichloropropene have undergone biodehalogenation by a *Pseudomonas* species isolated from the soil. 1,3-Dichloropropene has been shown to react with biological materials (cow's milk, potatoes, humus-rich soil) to produce 3-chloroallyl methyl sulfide.

Degradation of certain of these compounds can occur in the soil. Cis- and trans-1,3-dichloropropene can be chemically hydrolyzed in moist soils to the corresponding 3-chloroalkyl alcohols, which are capable of metabolism to carbon dioxide and water by a bacterium (*Pseudomonas* sp.). Although field applications of 1,3-dichloropropene have shown between 15 and 80% decomposition, the large amount that can be absorbed (80 to 90%) can result in considerable residues existing months after application is completed. 1,2-Dichloropropane, however, appears to undergo minimal degradation in the soil, with the major route of dissipation appearing to be volatilization. The persistence and degradation of both compounds depend on susceptibility to hydrolysis, soil types and temperature.

Uses: Principal uses of dichloropropanes and dichloropropenes are as soil fumigants for the control of nematodes, in oil and fat solvents, and in dry cleaning and degreasing processes.

Stanford Research Institute in a study for the National Science Foundation in 1975, reported that 60 million pounds per year of a mixture of DCP/PDC were produced for use as a soil fumigant.

Toxic Effects:　The actions of dichloropropanes and dichloropropenes on living organisms seem to depend upon the isomer (volatility, solubility, etc.) and the individual organisms. Additionally, judging by the rapid excretion of dichloropropanes and dichloropropenes in rats, it is unlikely that these compounds will remain and accumulate in mammals.

Dichloropropanes and dichloropropenes were both shown to be mutagenic but differed in degree. However, both were shown to have a low tumor-causing potential if any at all.

Data on the toxicology of dichloropropanes have been published by Heppel and coworkers (29-2) and on dichloropropenes by Torkelson and Oyen (29-3).

Current Levels of Exposure:　Very little information is available on current levels of exposure.

Special Groups at Risk:　A partial list of occupations in which exposure to propylene dichloride may occur includes:　cellulose plastic makers; dry cleaners; fat processors; fumigant workers; gum processors; metal degreasers; oil processors; organic chemical synthesizers; rubber makers; scouring compound makers; solvent workers; stain removers; and wax makers.

Existing Guidelines and Standards:　The Am. Conf. of Govt. Ind. Hygienists (ACGIH), as of 1979 (29-1), has set a TWA standard for propylene dichloride of 75 ppm (350 mg/m^3) and a tentative STEL value of 110 ppm (510 mg/m^3).

The ACGIH has given notice of intending to set a limit as of 1979 for dichloropropene as follows:　TWA, 1 ppm (5 mg/m^3) and STEL, 10 ppm (50 mg/m^3).

Summary of Proposed EPA Criteria:　*Freshwater Aquatic Life* — For 1,1-dichloropropane the criterion to protect freshwater aquatic life as derived using procedures other than the Guidelines is 410 μg/l as a 24-hour average and the concentration should not exceed 930 μg/l at any time.

For 1,2-dichloropropane the criterion to protect freshwater aquatic life as derived using procedures other than the Guidelines is 920 μg/l as a 24-hour average and the concentration should not exceed 2,100 μg/l at any time.

For 1,3-dichloropropane the criterion to protect freshwater aquatic life as derived using procedures other than the Guidelines is 4,800 μg/l as a 24-hour average and the concentration should not exceed 11,000 μg/l at any time.

For 1,3-dichloropropene the criterion to protect freshwater aquatic life as derived using the Guidelines is 18 μg/l as a 24-hour average and the concentration should not exceed 250 μg/l at any time.

Saltwater Aquatic Life —For saltwater aquatic life, no criterion for 1,1-dichloropropane can be derived using the Guidelines, and there are insufficient data to estimate a criterion using other procedures.

For 1,2-dichloropropane the criterion to protect saltwater aquatic life as derived using procedures other than the Guidelines is 400 μg/l as a 24-hour average and the concentration should not exceed 910 μg/l at any time.

For 1,3-dichloropropane the criterion to protect saltwater aquatic life as derived using the Guidelines is 79 μg/l as a 24-hour average and the concentration should not exceed 180 μg/l at any time.

For 1,3-dichloropropene the criterion to protect saltwater aquatic life as derived using procedures other than the Guidelines is 5.5 μg/l as a 24-hour average and the concentration should not exceed 14 μg/l at any time.

Human Health — For the protection of human health from the adverse effects of dichloropropanes and dichloropropenes ingested through the consumption of contaminated fish and water, the following criteria are suggested: dichloropropanes, 200 μg/l and dichloropropenes, 0.63 μg/l.

Basis for the Proposed Human Health Criteria

The Ostwald coefficient O is defined as the ratio of the concentration of a gas in a liquid to the concentration of the gas in an equivalent volume of gas above that liquid. By definition, the Ostwald coefficient of a gas and water at any particular temperature could be expressed as

$$\frac{\text{water solubility (g/l)}}{\substack{\text{conc. of vapor (g/l) at a partial pressure} \\ \text{equal to vapor pressure}}}$$

In the criteria formulation, the Ostwald coefficient for water is used as that for blood. A review of data on volatile anesthetic agents indicated this approach was acceptable. The applicability of this procedure can be used to estimate X_b.

The determined blood concentrations of PDC in rabbits and dogs after a 7-hour exposure period are from exposure data, blood levels that are calculated based on the Ostwald coefficient determined here (see below) and a hematocrit of 0.50. The data are shown in Table 54.

Table 54: Blood Concentration vs Exposure Levels for PDC

Animal	Exposure Concentration	Blood Concentration Found	Blood Concentration Calculated
	. . . . (mg/l).		
Rabbits	10.3	15–29	28.6
Rabbits	6.9	6–11	16.7
Dogs	4.7	13–16	13.0

Source: Reference (29)

Dichloropropane —It was determined that vapor pressure P (20°C) = 40 mm Hg and P (38°C) = 90 mm Hg. Unfortunately the only solubility data available was that for 20°C. However, data available on trichloroethylene and chloroform indicated that

$$\frac{P_{38°C}}{P_{20°C}} = 0.512$$

A similar relationship was found for ether. This factor was utilized for PDC:

$$\text{Solubility in water} = 2.7 \text{ g/l}$$

$$\text{Concentration in air} = \frac{n}{V} = \frac{P}{RT} = \frac{40}{62 \times 293} =$$

$$0.0022 \text{ mol/l} = 0.25 \text{ g/l}$$

$$\text{at } 20°C = \frac{2.7}{0.25} = 10.8$$

$$\text{at } 38°C = 10.8 \times 0.512 = 5.5$$

Dichloropropene — A valid vapor pressure value for DCP could not be identified as such. Therefore, the vapor in air density of DCP (cis- and trans-) of 1.4 at 37.8°C is used. Vapor air density (D) can be expressed as:

$$D = \frac{PD}{P'} + \frac{P'-P}{P'}$$

where

P = vapor pressure (at 37.8°)
P' = ambient pressure (760 mm Hg)
D = vapor density (3.8 for DCP)

Therefore

$$P = \frac{P'D-P}{D-1} = 109 \text{ mm Hg}$$

This is a feasible relationship to the vapor pressure of 90 mm Hg at 38°C reported for PDC. An assumption of parallelism for plots of log vapor pressure vs 1/T for PDC and DCP is reasonable. Thus, the vapor pressure of DCP at 20°C can be assumed to be 59 mm Hg. This conversion is necessary since the only available solubility data for DCP is at 20°C. Thus,

$$\frac{n}{V} = \frac{P}{RT} = \frac{59}{62 \times 293} = 0.0032 \text{ mol/l}$$

$$= 0.36 \text{ g/l}$$

solubility of DCP in water at 20°C = 1.0 g/l

$$\text{at } 20°C = \frac{1.0 \text{ g/l}}{0.36 \text{ g/l}} = 2.8$$

$$\text{at } 38°C = 2.8 \times 0.512 = 1.4$$

D-D^R in one study was found to have a vapor pressure of 35 mm Hg at 20°C; in another it was found to have a vapor pressure of 31.3 mm Hg at 20°C.

If these values are accurate, then the mixture of PDC and DCP can be assumed to be a negative deviation from Raoult's law. Measurements of partial pressure of binary solutions show that most of them can be classified as deviating from Raoult's law, either positively or negatively. The implication of this behavior of mixtures of PDC and DCP has been discussed in this document as regards the interpretation of mutagenicity data.

The derivation of k is the most speculative portion of the model. From the data presented earlier, it can be assumed that the rat excretes 80% of a dose in 24 hours. It is likely, however, that PDC and DCP fit a two-compartment pharmacokinetic model, at the least. Only the first (water) compartment in the rat can be reasonably estimated from the data available. Based on differences in glomerular filtration rate/weight relationships between rat and man, the k of a rat was reduced from $0.80 \times 24 \text{ hr}^{-1}$ to $0.25 \times 24 \text{ hr}^{-1}$. This is a moderate estimate which should also allow for known higher rates of biotransformation in the rat when compared to man.

The volume of distribution (V_D) of the compounds was assumed to be in total body water plus fat. $V_D = V_{TBW} + (V_F \times W/F)$ where V_{TBW} = volume of total body water (36 liters in 70 kg man); V_F = volume of fat (10 liters in 70 kg man); $W/O = O/F$ = blood/water partition coefficient (taken as octanol/water partition coefficient).

A major consideration is the time necessary for the blood to reach equilibrium with the fat. Because this process is slow, the possibility exists for significant elevation of X_b, if V_D as calculated above is used.

To account for this, it was recognized that the NOAEL inhalation exposures were based on 7 to 8 hours of exposure. Consequently, a safety factor was incorporated in the V_D calculation such that the lipid space was corrected to include only that apparent fat volume which would be filled during 8 hours to exposure. Thus, $V_D = V_{TBW} + (V_F \times O/W \times F_{sh})$ where F_{sh} = fraction of final equilibrium level of substance fat after 8 hours; $F_{sh} = 1 - e^{-kt}$;

1n $(1-F) = -kt$; where k = plasma flow rate per minute in fat (0.11); $V_F O/W$ t = 480 minutes. Dichloropropane: O/W = 105; F_{sh} = 0.05; and V_D = 36 + (10 x 105 x 0.05) = 89; Dichloropropene: O/W = 43; F_{sh} = 0.11; and V_D = 36 + (10 x 43 x 0.11) = 83.

As stated above:

$$ADI = \frac{\text{Ingestion NOAEL}}{\text{Uncertainty factor}}$$

The uncertainty factor for both PDC and DCP was taken as 100 based on the fact that the inhalation data utilized appears highly reliable and conversions to ingestion NOAEL have built in underestimation factors. Finally,

$$CR = \frac{ADI}{2 + (BCF \times 0.0187)}$$

where CR = water quality criterion; 2 = liters of water consumed per day; BCF = bioconcentration faction in edible portion fish (obtained from USEPA Duluth Laboratory); and 0.0187 = estimated consumption (kg) by an individual daily.

Dichloropropane: The inhalation NOAEL for PDC is 75 ppm (350 mg/m^3) which is the ACGIH TLV; λ = 5.5; X_a = 0.35 mg/l; X_b = 5.5 x 0.35 = 1.9 mg/l; V_D = 89 liters; and k = 0.25 x 24 hr^{-1}

$$ADI = \frac{0.25 \times 1.9 \times 89}{100} = 420 \ \mu g/day$$

$$BCF = 5.8$$

$$CR = \frac{420}{2 + (5.8 \times 0.0187)} = 200 \ \mu g/l$$

Dichloropropene: The inhalation NOAEL for DCP is 1 ppm (4.5 mg/m^3) which is that recommended by Torkelson and Oyen (29-3); λ = 1.4; X_a = 4.5; X_b = 1.4 x 4.5 = 6.3 $\mu g/l$; V_D = 83; k = 0.25 x 24 hr^{-1}.

$$ADI = \frac{0.25 \times 6.3 \times 83}{100} = 1.3 \ \mu g/day$$

$$BCF = 2.9$$

$$CR = \frac{1.3 \ \mu g}{2 + (2.9 \times 0.0187)} = 0.63 \ \mu g/l$$

In summary, based upon the use of an inhalation no-observed-adverse-effect-level in rats, (DCP), and an uncertainty factor of 100, the criterion level corresponding to the estimated acceptable daily intake of 1.3 $\mu g/day$ for DCP and 420 $\mu g/day$ for PDC is 0.6 $\mu g/l$ and 200 $\mu g/l$, respectively. Drinking water accounts for 95% of the assumed exposure for PDC and 98% for DCP. The criterion level can alternatively be expressed as 3.9 mg/l for PDC and 24 $\mu g/l$ for DCP if exposure is assumed to be from the consumption of fish and shellfish products alone.

These criterion formulations assume that 100% of man's exposure is assigned to the ambient water pathway as information on other likely exposure situations is unavailable.

References

(29-1) Am. Conf. of Govt. Ind. Hygienists, *Threshold Limit Values for Chemical Substances in Workroom Air*, Cincinnati, Ohio (1979).

(29-2) Heppel, L.A., et al, "Toxicology of 1,2-dichloropropane (propylene dichloride), 1, studies on effects of daily inhalation," *J. Ind. Hyg. Toxicol.*, 28, 1 (1946).

(29-3) Torkelson, R.R. and Oyen, F., "The toxicity of 1,3-dichloropropene as determined by repeated exposure of laboratory animals," *Jour. Am. Ind. Hyg. Assoc.*, 38, 217 (1977).

DIELDRIN

See "Aldrin/Dieldrin" (4).

DIETHYL PHTHALATE

See "Phthalate Esters" (53).

2,4-DIMETHYLPHENOL (#30)

2,4-DMP is also known as m-xylenol, 2,4-xylenol or m-4-xylenol, and has the empirical formula $C_6H_{10}O$. This discussion is intended to deal specifically with 2,4-dimethylphenol; however, three methylphenol isomers and six dimethylphenol isomers generally occur together in nature, in several industrial processes, commercial products, and phenolic wastes. It is unlikely that any large segment of the population would be exposed to 2,4-dimethylphenol alone. Because quantitative and qualitative data are not available for human exposure to 2,4-dimethylphenol, it is very difficult to establish a direct relationship between this compound and health effects in humans (30).

Occurrence: 2,4-Dimethylphenol (2,4-DMP) is a naturally occurring, substituted phenol derived from the cresol fraction of petroleum or coal tars by fractional distillation and extraction with aqueous alkaline solutions.

The compound also occurs naturally in plants and has been detected in tea, tobacco, and cigarette smoke.

A large number of products utilize 2,4-DMP as a feedstock or constituent. Hence, disposal of chemical and industrial process wastes and distribution from normal product applications represent feasible modes of entry of 2,4-DMP into the environment. Examples of the latter mode include pesticide applications, asphalt and roadway runoff, and the washing of dyed materials (30-1).

No quantitative information is available on the presence of 2,4-DMP in industrial and municipal effluents, natural waters, soils and sediments, drinking water supplies, or finished drinking water.

Physical Properties: 2,4-DMP has a molecular weight of 122.17 and in its normal state exists as a colorless, crystalline solid. It has a melting point of 27 to 28°C, a boiling point of 210°C (760 mm Hg), a vapor pressure of 1 mm Hg at 52.8°C, and a specific gravity of 0.9650 at 20°C.

2,4-DMP is slightly soluble in water and as a weak acid (pKa, 10.6); it is also soluble in alkaline solutions. 2,4-DMP readily dissolves in organic solvents such as alcohol and ether.

Chemical Properties: 2,4-DMP can be oxidized to form pseudoquinone. However, the conditions required for this reaction generally are not found in the environment. 2,4-DMP reacts with aqueous alkaline solutions to form the corresponding salt. Such salts are readily soluble in water, provided that an alkaline pH is maintained. The free position on the aromatic ring, ortho to the hydroxyl group, may be alkylated or halogenated. However, such reactions under normal environmental conditions have not been reported.

Virtually no information is available on the persistence of 2,4-DMP in the environment. Nevertheless, the biooxidation of 2,4-DMP by *Pseudomonas testosteroni* grown on p-cresol has been reported by Dagley and Patel (30-2). In addition, laboratory studies by Chapman (30-3) demonstrated the ability of a strain of *Pseudomonas* sp. isolated from estuarine water to utilize 2,4-DMP as the sole carbon source in liquid enrichment cultures. Although the microbial metabolic pathways for the aerobic degradation of 2,4-DMP to β-ketoadipic acid have been reported (30-4), these laboratory studies provide little information for its persistence in the environment. The complete biodegradation of 2,4-DMP has been reported to occur in approximately 2 months although the conditions were not stated.

Uses: 2,4-DMP finds use commercially as an important chemical feedstock or constituent for the manufacture of a wide range of commercial products for industry and agriculture. 2,4-Dimethylphenol is used in the manufacture of phenolic antioxidants, disinfectants, solvents, pharmaceuticals, insecticides, fungicides, plasticizers, rubber chemicals, polyphenylene oxide, wetting agents, and dyestuffs, and is an additive or constitutent of lubricants, gasolines, and cresylic acid.

Toxic Effects: Toxicity data on freshwater aquatic organisms for 2,4-DMP exist in the literature; however, there are no corresponding data on saltwater aquatic organisms. Studies have demonstrated acute toxic effects of 2,4-DMP on freshwater plants, invertebrates and vertebrate species. Chronic toxic effects have also been demonstrated in 2 freshwater vertebrate species. Studies on various species of freshwater microorganisms exposed to 2,4-DMP demonstrate either growth inhibition and/or lethality in the 2,4-DMP concentration range of 0.2×10^6 μg/l to 2.5×10^6 μg/l (30-5)(30-6).

2,4-DMP demonstrates both oral and topical toxicity to several mammalian species at doses ranging from 809 mg/kg (oral LD_{50}, mouse) (30-7) to 5,600 mg/kg (topical tumor formation, mouse)(30-8).

No data on mutagenic or teratogenic effects for 2,4-DMP on mammalian species were found in the literature. No reports of epidemiologic studies on workers exposed to 2,4-DMP or on a general population exposed to small amounts of 2,4-DMP which relate cancer incidence to exposure level were found.

Current Levels of Exposure: Data are not available for estimating the exposure of humans to 2,4-dimethylphenol.

Information regarding the concentration, persistence, fate and effects of 2,4-DMP in the environment is limited. However, its presence in petroleum fractions and coal tars, together with its use as a chemical feedstock or constituent for the manufacture of numerous products, clearly indicates the potential for both point and nonpoint source water contamination.

Special Groups at Risk: Workers involved in the fractionation and distillation of petroleum or coal and coal tar products comprise one group at risk. Workers who are intermittently exposed to certain commercial degreasing agents containing cresol may also be at risk. Cigarettes and marijuana smoking groups and those exposed to cigarette smoke inhale μg quantities of 2,4-dimethylphenol.

The National Institute for Occupational Safety and Health has estimated that 11,000 people in the United States are occupationally exposed to cresol containing 2,4-dimethylphenol.

Existing Guidelines and Standards: Standards have not been promulgated for 2,4-dimethylphenol for any sector of the environment or workplace.

Summary of Proposed EPA Criteria: *Freshwater Aquatic Life* — For 2,4-dimethylphenol, the criterion to protect freshwater aquatic life, as derived using the Guidelines, is 38 μg/l as a 24-hour average and the concentration should never exceed 86 μg/l at any time.

Saltwater Aquatic Life — For saltwater aquatic life, no criterion for 2,4-dimethylphenol can be derived using the Guidelines and there are insufficient data to estimate a criterion using other procedures.

Human Health — Due to a lack of sufficient definitive data on mammalian toxicology and human health effects, a criterion to protect human health from toxic effects due to exposure to 2,4-dimethylphenol ingested through water and through contaminated aquatic organisms cannot be set at this time. In order to protect public health, exposure to this compound should be minimized as soon as possible.

Basis for Proposed Human Health Criteria: In quantitative assessment of carcinogenicity, there are a number of special conditions which render the extrapolation of animal carcinogenesis data to man inappropriate. In the present case, the condition which applies is that the route of administration is inappropriate in terms of conceivable human exposure.

Only one study was found which indicated that 2,4-dimethylphenol could be carcinogenic in mammals; Sutter mice, a strain highly susceptible to skin carcinomas, were used.

In these experiments, 5 mg or 2.5 mg of 2,4-dimethylphenol in benzene, applied twice a week to the backs of shaved mice, produced papillomas and carcinomas of the skin at the site of application. Even though the compound is known to be rapidly absorbed, systemic effects or internal tumors were not reported. Additionally, the possible contribution of other chemicals to the response observed cannot be discounted. A solvent control (benzene) was not run, and the mice were housed in wood cages treated with creosote, which may have initiated the carcinogenic response.

In addition, the Carcinogen Assessment Group, U.S. EPA, Washington, D.C. concluded that the above data regarding possible carcinogenic effects (via initiation) of 2,4-dimethylphenol are inconclusive. The report did indicate that 2,4-dimethylphenol was a promoting agent. Although promoters have a potential carcinogenic risk to humans, there is no dose-response data with which to formulate a quantitative risk extrapolation.

It is inappropriate to extrapolate from results obtained from the use of high concentrations in skin painting studies to an estimate of the possible carcinogenic effects of the ingestion of small amounts of 2,4-dimethylphenol in water. The only data found for the ingestion of 2,4-dimethylphenol were an LD_{50} for mice of 809 mg/kg, and an LD_{50} for rats of 3,200 mg/kg.

The National Academy of Sciences concluded the following concerning drinking water and health. 2,4-Dimethylphenol appears to be a topical cocarcinogen, but its role as a primary cancer-producing agent is uncertain. Its potential role in cancer production warrants consideration of further testing. An in vitro mutagenicity assay should be carried out to further evaluate its mutagenic potential.

In view of the relative paucity of data on the mutagenicity, carcinogenicity, teratogenicity and long-term oral toxicity of 2,4-dimethylphenol, estimates of the effects of chronic oral exposure at low levels cannot be made with any confidence. It is recommended that studies to produce such information be conducted before limits in drinking water are established.

We recommend that a criterion should not be set for 2,4-dimethylphenol in water until definitive data are obtained. In order to protect public health, exposure of humans to this compound should be minimized.

References

(30-1) U.S. EPA, *Identification of organic compounds in effluents from industrial sources*, Prepared for U.S. Environ. Prot. Agency, Report by Versar, Inc., Springfield, Va. (1975).

(30-2) Dagley, S. and Patel, M.D., "Oxidation of p-cresol and related compounds by a *Pseudomonas*," *Biochem. Jour.*, 66, 227 (1957).

(30-3) Chapman, P.J., "An outline of reaction sequences used for the bacterial degradation of phenolic compounds," in *Degradation of synthetic organic molecules in the biosphere*, Washington, D.C., Natl. Acad. Sci.,(1971).

(30-4) Ornston, L.N. and Stanier, R.Y., "The conversion of catechol and protocatechuate to β-keto-adipate by *Pseudomonas putida*," *Jour. Biol. Chem.*, 241, 3776 (1966).

(30-5) Zsolnai, T., "Action of new fungicides. I. Phenol derivatives," *Biochem. Pharmacol.*, 5, 1 (1960).

(30-6) von Oettingen, W.F., *Phenol and its derivatives: the relation between their chemical constitution and their effect on the organism*, Natl. Inst. Health Bull. No. 190, Washington, D.C., U.S. Government Printing Office (1949).

(30-7) Uzhdovini, E.R., et al, "Acute toxicity of lower phenols," *Gig. Tr. Prof. Zabol.*, 18, 58 (1974).

(30-8) Boutwell, R.K. and Bosch, D.K., "The tumor-producing action of phenol and related compounds for mouse skin," *Cancer Res.*, 19, 413 (1959).

DIMETHYL PHTHALATE

See "Phthalate Esters" (53).

4,6-DINITRO-o-CRESOL

See "Nitrophenols" (49).

2,4-DINITROPHENOL

See "Nitrophenols" (49).

DINITROTOLUENES (#31)

The name given by the Chemical Abstracts Service for this compound is 1-methyl-2,4-dinitrobenzene. Other synonyms include 2,4-dinitrotoluol, toluene-2,4-dinitro and DNT.

Occurrence: DNT is produced by nitration of toluene to nitrotoluene to dinitrotoluene in a nitric and sulfuric acid solution. In 1975, the production of 2,4- and 2,6-DNT in the United States was 264,030 metric tons. There are six isomers of dinitrotoluene, with the 2,4-isomer being the most important. Often this isomer alone is referred to as DNT or dinitrotoluol.

2,4-DNT is encountered chiefly as a major component in the wastewater from munitions industries. The general population may experience exposure as a result of this discharge of 2,4-DNT into rivers and streams from munition plants (31-1).

DNT has been shown to enter the body through inhalation of vapors or dust particles, ingestion of contaminated food, and absorption through the skin.

Physical Properties: 2,4-Dinitrotoluene (2,4-DNT) is a pale yellow crystalline solid. 2,4-DNT has a molecular weight of 182.14, a melting point of 71°C, a boiling point of 300°C with decomposition, and a Sp. Gr. of 1.3208 at 71°C. Its solubility in water is 270 mg/l water at 22°C; 94 g/l ether at 22°C and 21.9 g/l carbon disulfide at 17°C. It is also readily soluble in ethanol at 15°C (30.5 g/l).

2,6-DNT has a melting point of 66°C, a Sp. Gr. of 1.2833 at 111°C, and is soluble in alcohol.

Chemical Properties: Except for their tendency to decompose at elevated temperatures, dinitrotoluenes are relatively stable. At 250°C, commercial grades of dinitrotoluene decompose at nonsustaining rates. However, at approximately 280°C rapid self-sustaining decomposition occurs. Dinitrotoluenes may burn safely if unconfined, but if confined may result in an explosion. Decomposition may occur at lower temperatures in the presence of impurities.

Uses: Dinitrotoluene (DNT) is an ingredient of explosives for commercial and military use because of its waterproofing action and explosive potential. Use is also made of DNT as a chemical stabilizer in the manufacture of smokeless powder. DNT is also widely used as a raw material for dyestuffs and for urethane polymers through a conversion to the corresponding diamine and then to diisocyanate.

Toxic Effects: As a result of exposure to DNT, workers have experienced muscular weakness, headaches, and dizziness; this exposure also has been suspected of causing pallor, cyanosis, and anemia.

Aromatic nitro compounds are one of several classes of chemicals thought to contribute to the increased cancer risk in dye and explosive manufacturing industries (31-2). The structural relationship of 2,4-DNT to the known carcinogen 2,4-toluenediamine (2,4-TDA) is also a factor in its selection for testing as a possible carcinogen (31-1).

Current Levels of Exposure: No data on the extent of human exposure to 2,4-DNT are available in the literature. However, a study of the concentration of explosives in air by isotope dilution analysis (31-3) reported a concentration of 184 ppb V/V (= 1.384 mg/m^3) of 2,4-DNT in air at 25°C, which is very close to the TLV-TWA value noted in a section which follows.

Special Groups at Risk: The main group expected to be at high risk for exposure to 2,4-DNT is industrial workers involved in the manufacturing or handling of 2,4-DNT in places such as ammunition, dye, and polyurethane plants.

Existing Guidelines and Standards: At present, no standard for exposure to 2,4-DNT in drinking or ambient water has been set in the United States. However, a Russian study (31-4) recommends that a maximum permissible concentration in the surface waters should be set at a level of 0.5 mg/l for each DNT isomer.

The American Conference of Governmental Industrial Hygienists recommends a threshold limit value-time weighted average (TLV-TWA) concentration of 1.5 mg of 2,4-DNT/m^3 of air (1.5 mg/m^3) including dermal exposure for a normal eight-hour workday of 40-hour workweek. This value represents the highest level to which nearly all workers may be repeatedly exposed, day after day, without adverse effect. This TLV-TWA was set by analogy with chemically similar nitro aromatic compounds. A threshold limit value-short term exposure level (TLV-STEL) of 5 mg of 2,4-DNT/m^3 of air was also set by the ACGIH. The TLV-STEL is defined as the maximal allowable concentration to which workers can be exposed for a period of up to 15 minutes continuously without suffering from (1) irritation, (2) chronic or irreversible tissue change, or (3) narcosis of sufficient degree to increase accident proneness, impair self-rescue, or materially reduce work efficiency. No more than four exposures to the TLV-STEL per day are permitted, with at least 60 minutes between exposure periods, and the daily TLV-TWA must also not be exceeded.

Summary of Proposed EPA Criteria: *Freshwater Aquatic Life* — For 2,3-dinitrotoluene the criterion to protect freshwater aquatic life as derived using the Guidelines is 12 µg/l as a 24-hour average and the concentration should not exceed 27 µg/l at any time.

For 2,4-dinitrotoluene the criterion to protect freshwater aquatic life as derived using procedures other than the Guidelines is 620 µg/l as a 24-hour average and the concentration should not exceed 1,400 µg/l at any time.

Saltwater Aquatic Life — For 2,3-dinitrotoluene the criterion to protect saltwater aquatic life as derived using procedures other than the Guidelines is 4.4 μg/l as a 24-hour average and the concentration should not exceed 10 μg/l at any time.

For saltwater aquatic life, no criterion for 1,4-dinitrotoluene can be derived using the Guidelines, and there are insufficient data to estimate a criterion using other procedures.

Human Health — For the maximum protection of human health from the potential carcinogenic effects of exposure to 2,4-dinitrotoluene through ingestion of water and contaminated aquatic organisms, the ambient water concentration is zero. Concentrations of 2,4-dinitrotoluene estimated to result in additional lifetime cancer risks ranging from no additional risk to an additional risk of 1 in 100,000 are presented in the Criterion Document. The EPA is considering settling criteria at an interim target risk level in the range of 10^{-5}, 10^{-6}, or 10^{-7} with corresponding criteria of 740 ng/l, 74.0 ng/l, and 7.4 ng/l, respectively.

Basis for the Proposed Human Health Criteria: The data from the bioassay of 2,4-DNT for possible carcinogenicity obtained by the National Cancer Institute (31-1) and Lee, et al (31-5) were used for the determination of a water quality criterion for the protection of human health. The criterion was developed from the animal carcinogenicity data utilizing a linear nonthreshold model.

The rat carcinogenicity studies with dietary administration of 2,4-DNT showed increased incidences of fibroadenomas of the subcutaneous tissue and inanition in male rats and fibroadenomas of the mammary gland and inanition in female rats.

Under the Consent Decree in *NRDC vs Train*, criteria are to state "recommended maximum permissible concentrations (including where appropriate, zero) consistent with the protection of aquatic organisms, human health, and recreational activities." 2,4-DNT is suspected of being a human carcinogen. Because there is no recognized safe concentration for a human carcinogen, the recommended concentration of 2,4-DNT in water for maximum protection of human health is zero.

Because attaining a zero concentration level may be infeasible in some cases and in order to assist the Agency and States in the possible future development of water quality regulations, the concentrations of 2,4-DNT corresponding to several incremental lifetime cancer risk levels have been estimated. A cancer risk level provides an estimate of the additional incidence of cancer that may be expected in an exposed population. A risk of 10^{-6} indicates one additional case of cancer for every million people exposed, etc.

In the *Federal Register* notice of availability of draft ambient water quality criteria, EPA stated that it is considering setting criteria at an interim target risk level of 10^{-5}, 10^{-6} or 10^{-7} as shown in Table 55.

Table 55: Possible Alternative Criteria for Dinitrotoluene

Exposure Assumptions (per day)	Risk Levels and Corresponding Criteria			
	0	10^{-7}	10^{-6}	10^{-5}
2 liters of drinking water and consumption of 18.7 g of fish and shellfish*, ng/l	0	7.4	74.0	740
Consumption of fish and shellfish only, μg/l	0	0.156	1.56	15.6

*Approximately 5% of the DNT exposure results from the consumption of aquatic organisms which exhibit an average bioconcentration potential of 5.5-fold. The remaining 95% of DNT exposure results from drinking water.

Source: Reference (31)

The risk levels are calculated by applying a modified "one-hit" extrapolation model described in the Methodology Document and is directly proportional to the water concentration. Since the extrapolation model is linear at low doses, the additional lifetime risk

Concentration levels were derived assuming a lifetime exposure to various amounts of DNT (1) occurring from the consumption of both drinking water and aquatic life grown in waters containing the corresponding DNT concentrations and, (2) occurring solely from consumption of aquatic life grown in the waters containing the corresponding DNT concentrations. Although total exposure information for chloroform is discussed and an estimate of the contributions from other sources of exposure can be made, this data will not be factored into ambient water quality criteria. The criteria presented, therefore, assume an incremental risk from ambient water exposure only.

Summary of Pertinent Data — The water quality criterion for 2,4-dinitrotoluene is derived from the oncogenic effects observed in the mammary gland and liver of female Charles River CD rats fed 200 ppm in the diet. The time-weighted average dose of 45 mg/kg/day was given in the feed for 24 months, with the surviving animals sacrificed one month later. The mammary tumor incidence was 11/23 and 33/35 in the control and treated groups, respectively. The incidence of hepatocellular carcinomas and neoplastic nodules was 0/23 and 24/34 in the control and treated groups, respectively. Assuming a fish bioconcentration factor of 5.5, the criterion is calculated from the following parameters: n_t mammary, 33; N_t mammary, 35; n_C mammary, 11; N_C mammary, 28; n_t liver, 24; N_t liver, 34; n_C liver, 0; N_C liver, 23; le, 24 months; Le, 25 months; d, 45mg/kg/day; R, 5.5; L, 25 months; W, 0.464 kg; and F, 0.0167 kg/day.

Based on these parameters the one-hit slope, ^{B}H, is 2.95×10^{-1} for mammary tumors and 1.53×10^{-1} for hepatocellular carcinomas and hepatocellular neoplastic nodules. The resulting water concentration of 2,4-dinitrotoluene calculated to keep the individual lifetime cancer risk below 10^{-5} is 740 ng/l.

References

(31-1) National Cancer Institute, *Bioassay of 2,4-Dinitrotoluene for Possible Carcinogenicity*, Carcinogenesis Tech. Rept. Series No. 54, DHEW (NIH) Publ. No. 78-1360, Wash., D.C. (1978).

(31-2) Wynder, E.L., et al, "An epidemiological investigation of cancer of the bladder," *Cancer*, 16, 1388 (1963).

(31-3) St. John, G.A., et al, "Determination of the concentration of explosives in air by isotope dilution analysis," *Forensic Sci.*, 6, 53 (1975).

(31-4) Korolev, A.A., et al, "Experimental data for hygienic standardization of dinitrotoluene and trinitrobenzene in reservoir waters," *Gig. Sanit. Iss.*, 10, 17 (1977).

(31-5) Lee, C.C., et al, *Mammalian toxicity of munition compounds. Phase III: Effects of lifetime exposure. Part I: 2,4-Dinitrotoluene*, U.S. Army Medical Research and Development Command Contract No. DAMD-17-74-C-4073, Report No. 7 (September 1978).

DI-n-OCTYL PHTHALATE

See "Phthalate Esters" (53).

DIPHENYLHYDRAZINE (#32)

Diphenylhydrazine exists as an unsymmetrical isomer, 1,1-diphenylhydrazine, and a symmetrical isomer, 1,2-diphenylhydrazine (hydrazobenzene). The diphenylhydrazines have the following formulas:

$$C_6H_5{\diagdown} \atop C_6H_5{\diagup}\ NNH_2 \text{ (unsymmetrical)}$$

and

$$C_6H_5NHNHC_6H_5 \text{ (symmetrical)}$$

Occurrence: Industrial exposure to 1,2-diphenylhydrazine is primarily limited to workers in the dye manufacturing industry and in the pharmaceutical industry. No data were found on the environmental presence or persistence of diphenylhydrazines, except for one report of detection in drinking water at a concentration of 1 μg/l (32-1).

Physical Properties: The physical data for 1,2-diphenylhydrazine are as follows: molecular weight, 184.24; melting point, 131°C; boiling point, 220°C; and solubility—slightly soluble in water and very soluble in benzene, ether, alcohol.

Chemical Properties: The reaction of 1,2-diphenylhydrazine with acid results in the benzidine rearrangement. In addition to benzidine, other products formed include diphenyline, o-benzidine, and o-semidine. In the stomach, 1,2-diphenylhydrazine can be converted into benzidine, a human carcinogen.

Uses: 1,2-Diphenylhydrazine (DPH) is a precursor in the manufacture of benzidine, an intermediate in the production of dyes. 1,2-Diphenylhydrazine is used in the synthesis of phenylbutazone, a potent antiinflammatory (antiarthritic) drug.

The commercial production of 1,2-diphenylhydrazine per se in 1977 was in excess of 1,000 pounds. However, this figure is probably an underestimate of the amount of diphenylhydrazine that was actually available. Diphenylhydrazine is produced in several synthetic processes as an intermediate and a contaminant but there is no way of estimating these quantities which are substantial.

Toxic Effects: Experimental data indicate that 1,2-diphenylhydrazine is toxic to freshwater aquatic organisms and reported LC_{50} values range from 0.27 to 4.1 mg/l (32-2). Rats and mice developed a variety of malignancies after dermal exposures to 1,2-diphenylhydrazine (32-3)(32-4). Oral doses of 1,2-diphenylhydrazine did not produce malignancies (32-5). The documented carcinogenicity of 1,2-diphenylhydrazine is of primary concern to industrial workers, who are exposed to higher concentrations than other segments of the population.

Although there are few data describing the fate of diphenylhydrazines in water, the carcinogenic effects of 1,2-diphenylhydrazine warrant its regulation, to protect humans and aquatic organisms from possible water-related hazards associated with this chemical.

Derivatives of hydrazine are reported to be hepatotoxic, hemolytic, convulsants, and irritants. They are absorbed from all routes (32-6).

The basis for concern over 1,2-diphenylhydrazine includes: (1) its presence in drinking water (highest concentration reported was 1 μg/l (1 ppb) (32-1); (2) the likely production of benzidine from DPH in the stomach due to gastric acidity (32-7); (3) the documented carcinogenicity of hydrazine and selected substituted hydrazines (32-8); (4) the increased incidence of bladder cancer among workers involved in the manufacture of dyes (32-9)(32-10); and (5) the carcinogenicity of azobenzene, a metabolite of DPH, as well as the established carcinogenicity of benzidine to which DPH is converted.

Current Levels of Exposure: No information is available on the concentration of 1,2-diphenylhydrazine in the atmosphere. 1,2-Diphenylhydrazine has been found to be present in drinking water at levels of 1 μg/l = 1 ppb (32-1). 1,2-Diphenylhydrazine has not been found to be a natural constituent of food.

Special Groups at Risk: Manufacturers of dyes and pharmaceuticals are subject to occupational exposure. Groups working in the laboratory and forensic medicine may also be subject to 1,2-diphenylhydrazine exposure.

Existing Guidelines and Standards: No existing guidelines or standards were found for 1,2-diphenylhydrazine.

Summary of Proposed EPA Criteria: *Freshwater Aquatic Life* — For 1,2-diphenylhydrazine the criterion to protect freshwater aquatic life as derived using the Guidelines is 17 μg/l as a 24-hour average and the concentration should not exceed 38 μg/l at any time.

Saltwater Aquatic Life — For saltwater aquatic life, no criterion for 1,2-diphenylhydrazine can be derived using the Guidelines, and there are insufficient data to estimate a criterion using other procedures.

Human Health — For the maximum protection of human health from the potential carcinogenic effects of exposure to 1,2-diphenylhydrazine through ingestion of water and contaminated aquatic organisms, the ambient water concentration is zero. Concentrations of 1,2-diphenylhydrazine estimated to result in additional lifetime cancer risks ranging from no additional risk to an additional risk of 1 in 100,000 are presented in the Criterion Formulation section of this document. The EPA is considering setting criteria at an interim target risk level in the range of 10^{-5}, 10^{-6}, or 10^{-7} with corresponding criteria of 0.4 μg/l, 0.04 μg/l and 0.004 μg/l, respectively.

Basis for the Proposed Human Health Criteria: An evaluation of the subacute, acute and chronic toxicity, with the exception of carcinogenicity is impossible because of only scanty data. No current guidelines or standards presently exist for DPH.

Diphenylhydrazine has been shown to produce carcinogenic responses in rats and mice (32-11)(32-4). Since the NCI study (32-11) represents the only report in which all the data can be analyzed, it will be used as a basis for formulating a criterion.

More specifically, the data on the induction of cancer in male and female rats and female mice were chosen for analysis because they all had significantly increased tumor formation following DPH treatment (i.e., dietary). The respective criterion levels obtained from applying the standard water quality dose extrapolation/criteria calculation methodology are given in Table 56.

Table 56: 1,2-Diphenylhydrazine Induction of Tumors in Mice and Rats

Species	Sex	Estimated Criterion Level at 10^{-5} Risk (μg/l)
Mouse	female	1.43
Rat	female	1.32 (liver)
Rat	female	1.32 (mammary gland)
Rat	male	5.14 (Zymbal gland)
Rat	male	0.38 (liver)

It can be seen that male rats appear to have the lowest tolerance for DPH.

Under the Consent Decree in *NRDC vs Train*, criteria are to state "recommended maximum permissible concentrations (including where appropriate, zero) consistent with the protection of aquatic organisms, human health, and recreational activities." DPH is suspected of being a human carcinogen. Because there is no recognized safe concentration for human carcinogens the recommended concentration of DPH in water for maximum protection of human health is zero.

Because attaining a zero concentration level may be infeasible in some cases and in order to assist the EPA and States in the possible future development of water quality regulations, the concentrations of DPH corresponding to several incremental lifetime cancer risk levels have been estimated. A cancer risk level provides an estimate of the additional incidence of cancer that may be expected in an exposed population. A risk of 10^{-5}, e.g., indicates a probability of one additional case of cancer for every 100,000 people exposed; a risk of 10^{-6} indicates one additional case of cancer for every million people exposed, etc.

In the *Federal Register* notice of availability of draft ambient water quality criteria, EPA stated that it is considering setting criteria at an interim target risk level of 10^{-5}, 10^{-6} or 10^{-7} as shown in Table 57.

Table 57: Possible Alternative Criteria for Diphenylhydrazine

Exposure Assumptions (per day)	Risk Levels and Corresponding Criteria			
	0	10^{-7}	10^{-6}	10^{-5}
2 liters of drinking water and consumption of 18.7 g of fish and shellfish*, ng/l	0	4	40	400
Consumption of fish and shellfish only, ng/l	0	19	190	1,900

*21% of the DPH exposure results from the consumption of aquatic organisms which exhibit an average bioconcentration potential of 29-fold. The remaining 79% of DPH exposure results from drinking water.

Source: Reference (32)

The risk levels are calculated by applying a modified "one-hit" extrapolation model described in the *FR* 15926, 1979. Since the extrapolation model is linear to low doses, the additional lifetime risk is directly proportional to the water concentration. Therefore, water concentrations corresponding to other risk levels can be derived by multiplying or dividing one of the risk levels and corresponding water concentrations shown in the table by factors such as 10, 100, 1,000, etc.

Concentration levels were derived assuming a lifetime exposure to various amounts of DPH, (1) occurring from the consumption of both drinking water and aquatic life grown in water containing the corresponding DPH concentrations and, (2) occurring solely from consumption of aquatic life grown in the waters containing the corresponding DPH concentrations.

Although a total exposure evaluation for DPH is desirable there are no data to support a total exposure analysis. The criteria presented, therefore, assume an incremental risk from assumed ambient water exposure only.

For DPH the case for criterion development is based upon the existence of carcinogenicity responses in animals (rats and mice).

Because of the lack of investigations for other chronic and acute responses, there is no information on other effects in either human or animal systems. Thus, the criterion proposed should be considered as precautionary until further studies can be used in the overall toxicity evaluations.

Summary of Pertinent Data — The water quality criterion for 1,2-diphenylhydrazine is based on the induction of hepatocellular carcinomas and neoplastic nodules in male Fischer 344 rats, exposed to 0.03% (300 ppm) 1,2-diphenylhydrazine in the diet ad libitum for 78 weeks (32-11). The incidence of hepatocellular carcinomas and neoplastic nodules was 37/49 and 1/48 in the treated and control groups, respectively. The criterion was calculated from the following parameters: $n_t = 37$; $N_t = 49$; $n_c = 1$; $N_c = 48$; Le = 104 weeks; le = 78 weeks; L = 104 weeks; d = 15 mg/kg/day; F = 0.0187 kg/day; R = 29; and W = 0.375 kg. The dose d (expressed as mg/kg body wt/day) is based on the assumption that the amount of diet consumed by rats each day was 5% of their body weight; 0.05 x 0.375 kg = 0.0187 kg diet/day; 0.01875 kg diet/day x 300 mg/kg = 5.625 mg 1,2-DPH/day; 5.625 mg 1,2-DPH/day/0.375 kg = 15 mg/kg/day.

Based on these parameters, the "one-hit" slope (B_H is 0.715 $(mg/kg/day)^{-1}$. The resulting water concentration of 1,2-diphenylhydrazine, calculated to keep the individual lifetime cancer risk below 10^{-5}, is 0.40 $\mu g/l$.

References

(32-1) U.S. EPA, *Preliminary assessment of suspected carcinogens in drinking water*, Washington, D.C., Off. Tox. Subs. (1975).

(32-2) U.S. EPA, *In-depth studies on health and environmental impacts of selected water pollutants*, Report on Contract No. 68-01-4646, Wash., D.C. (1978).

(32-3) Spitz, S., et al, "The carcinogenic action of benzidine," *Cancer*, 3, 789 (1950).

(32-4) Pliss, G., "Carcinogenic properties of hydrazobenzene," *Vop. Onkol.*, 20, 53 (1974).

(32-5) Marhold, Jr., et al, "The possible complexity of diphenylene in the origin of tumors in the manufacture of benzidine," *Neoplasma*, 15, 3 (1968).

(32-6) Sutton, W.L., "Heterocyclic and miscellaneous nitrogen compounds. Industrial hygiene and toxicology" in Patty, F.A., Ed., *Toxicology*, New York, Interscience (1967).

(32-7) International Agency for Research in Cancer, *Aromatic Amines*, Monographs on Carcinogenic Risk of Chemicals to Man, 1, 69 (1972).

(32-8) International Agency for Research on Cancer, *Hydrazine and its Derivatives*, Monographs on the Evaluation of Carcinogenic Risk of Chemicals to Man, 4, 81 (1974).

(32-9) Wynder, E.L., et al, "An epidemiological investigation of cancer in the bladder," *Cancer*, 16, 338 (1963).

(32-10) Anthony, A.M., et al, "Tumors of the urinary bladder: an analysis of the occupations of 1030 patients in Leeds, England," *Jour. Nat. Cancer.Inst.*, 45, 879 (1970).

(32-11) National Cancer Institute, *Bioassay of Hydrazobenzene for Possible Carcinogenicity*, DHEW Publ. No. (NIH)78-1342 (1978).

E

ENDOSULFAN (#33)

Endosulfan is a chlorinated cyclodiene insecticide having the molecular formula $C_9Cl_6H_6O_3S$ and the following structural formula:

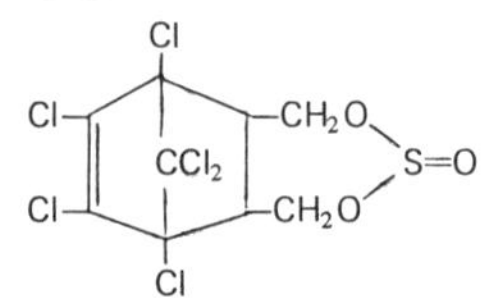

$$Cl-\!\!\!\!\!\!\underset{\displaystyle Cl}{\overset{\displaystyle Cl}{\underset{\big|}{\overset{\big|}{\bigcirc}}}}\!\!\!\!\!\!-CH_2O,\; CCl_2,\; CH_2O \Big/ S\!=\!O$$

Occurrence: Endosulfan is a broad spectrum insecticide. It was discovered and developed in 1954 by Farbwerke Hoechst AG in Germany. The chemical name for endosulfan is 6,7,8,9,10,10-hexachloro-1,5,5a,6,9,9a-hexahydro-6,9-methano-2,4,3-benzodioxathiepin-3-oxide. It is prepared through the Diels-Alder addition of hexachlorocyclopentadiene with cis-butene-1,4-diol to form the bicyclic dialcohol, followed by esterification and cyclization with $SOCl_2$.

Physical Properties: Endosulfan is a light to dark brown crystalline solid with a terpene-like odor, a molecular weight of 406.95, and a vapor pressure of 9×10^{-3} mm Hg at 80°C. It exhibits a solubility in water of 60 to 150 μg/l and is readily soluble in organic solvents.

Technical grade endosulfan has a purity of 95% and is composed of a mixture of two stereoisomers referred to as alpha and beta or I and II. It has a melting point range of 70° to 100°C and a density of 1.745 at 20°C. The endosulfan isomers are present in the ratio 70% isomer I to 30% isomer II. Impurities present in technical grade endosulfan consist mainly of the degradation products and may not exceed 2% endosulfandiol and 1% endosulfandiol and 1% endosulfan ether.

Chemical Properties: Endosulfan is stable to sunlight, but is susceptible to oxidation and the formation of endosulfan sulfate in the presence of growing vegetation. Technical grade endosulfan is sensitive to moisture, bases, and acids and decomposes slowly by hydrolysis to SO_2 and endosulfan alcohol. In the environment, endosulfan is metabolically converted by microorganisms, plants, and animals to endosulfan sulfate, endosulfandiol, endosulfan ether, endosulfan hydroxyether, and endosulfan lactone. Of these conversion products, endosulfan sulfate is of toxicologic importance.

Uses: Endosulfan is commercially available in the form of wettable powders, emulsifiable concentrates, granules, and dusts of various concentrations. It is a powerful contact and stomach insecticide used to control a wide spectrum of insects.

Annual production of endosulfan in the United States was estimated in 1974 at three million pounds. It is presently on the Environmental Protection Agency's restricted list which limits its usage. However, significant commercial use of endosulfan for insect control on vegetables, fruits, and tobacco continues.

Toxic Effects: Endosulfan has been demonstrated to be highly toxic to fish and marine invertebrates and is readily adsorbed by sediments. It therefore represents a potential hazard in the aquatic environment.

Current Level of Exposure: Endosulfan has been detected in water samples from the United States and Canada. Maximum values reported from various studies include:

0.02 μg/l in streams of the western United States (1 positive sample out of 546).

0.032 μg/l in drainage ditches from treated agricultural fields near Lake Erie.

0.011 μg/l in Canadian water systems.

0.083 μg/l in Ontario municipal water samples.

0.014 μg/l in surface and bottom water samples from Lake Erie.

0.060 μg/l in the St. Lawrence River.

The detection limit for endosulfan in water, using electron capture gas chromatography, is ~0.005 μg/l. Residues in food (α-endosulfan, β-endosulfan, and endosulfan sulfate) result from the use of endosulfan on over 60 food and nonfood crops. During the 1965 to 1970 period, daily U.S. intake of endosulfan residues was estimated using market basket samples from the total diet program of the FDA. These samples showed a daily intake of endosulfan (α-, β-, and sulfate) of from <0.001 to 0.001 mg/day.

The acceptable daily intake of endosulfan (i.e., the daily intake which during an entire lifetime appears to be without appreciable risk), as established by FAO/WHO, is 0.0075 mg/kg. This value corresponds to an intake of 0.525 mg/day for a 70-kg person. Endosulfan has also been shown to bioconcentrate in the tissue of aquatic species.

Endosulfan residues (α-endosulfan, β-endosulfan, and endosulfan sulfate) have been found in most types of U.S. tobacco products in recent years. The following data summarize the average residue levels (milligram residue per kilogram processed tobacco) detected in several independent studies.

	Year	Average Residue (mg/kg)
Cigarettes	1971	0.2
	1972	0.38
	1973	0.83
Cigars	1971	0.4
	1972	0.41
	1973	0.37
Little cigars	1971	0.4
	1973	0.22
Smoking or pipe tobacco	1971	<0.2
	1973	0.37
Chewing tobacco	1971	0.2
	1973	0.36
Snuff	1971	<0.2
	1973	<0.12

Air samples from 16 states in 1970 showed an average level of 13.0 ng/m^3 α-endosulfan and 0.2 ng/m^3 β-endosulfan. None of the air samples collected in 1971 or 1972, however, contained detectable levels of either isomer.

Special Groups at Risk: Data on the presence of endosulfan residues (α-endosulfan, β-endosulfan, and endosulfan sulfate) in food, tobacco, water, and air have been briefly summarized in the preceding subsection. These data indicate the following three areas present risks to humans:

(1)   Residues in foods as a result of the use of endosulfan on food crops and feedstuff; bioconcentration in aquatic species; residues in air adjacent to sites of manufacture or application; and residues in water.

(2) Residues in processed tobacco products (cigarettes, cigars, snuff, etc.)
     resulting from the field use of endosulfan.

(3) Dermal and respiratory exposure occurring during manufacture,
     formulation/packaging, field application, and harvesting.

Existing Guidelines and Standards: The National Technical Advisory Committee on Water
Quality Criteria (33-1) did not establish a permissible limit of endosulfan in raw suface
waters for public water supply purposes. The Committee stated, however, that the 48 hr
TLM (median tolerance level) of endosulfan in shrimp is 0.2 μg/l and therefore classified
endosulfan as acutely toxic to shrimp at concentrations of 5 μg/l or less. On the assumption that 1/100 of this level represents a reasonable application factor, the Committee recommended that environmental levels of endosulfan should not be permitted to rise above
0.05 μg/l. This level is so low that endosulfan should not be applied directly in or near
the marine habitat without danger of causing damage.

In the 1972 report of the Committee on Water Quality Criteria (33-2) a maximum concentration of 0.003 μg/l of endosulfan is recommended for whole (unfiltered) fresh water sampled at any time and at any place. This concentration was determined by multiplying the
acute toxicity value of endosulfan for the most sensitive native aquatic species (rainbow
trout, *Salmo gairdneri*) (33-3) by an application factor of 0.01. The marine criterion of
0.001 μg/l was similarly determined using LC_{50} values of the most sensitive marine species
(striped bass, *Morone saxatilis,* (33-4).

Revision of the above-recommended standards may be indicated by more recent data. For
example, the 96 hr LC_{50} value of 0.04 μg/l on pink shrimp (*Penaeus duorarum*) would, if
incorporated, reduce the saltwater criterion from 0.001 μg/l to 0.0004 μg/l, using a theoretical application factor of 0.01 (33-5). This theoretical ratio is used in the absence of
an empirically derived factor.

Macek, et al (33-6) have empirically derived application factors from their work on two
fresh water species, fathead minnows *(Pimephales promelas)* and water fleas *(Daphnia magna)*.
The seven-day incipient LC_{50} of 0.86 μg/l and the maximum acceptable toxicant concentration (MATC) limits of 0.20 to 0.40 μg/l for fathead minnows give a derived application
factor (ratio of chronic toxicity to acute or subacute) range of 0.23 to 0.47. MATC limits
are the highest concentration for which there is no effect and the lowest concentration
showing an adverse effect. The 48 hr LC_{50} of 166 μg/l and the MATC limits of 2.7 to
7.0 μg/l for *Daphnia magna,* however, give a derived factor range of 0.016 to 0.042.

The recent National Academy of Sciences report on drinking water (33-7) did not address
water standards for endosulfan.

Summary of Proposed EPA Criteria: *Freshwater Aquatic Life* — For endosulfan the criterion
to protect freshwater aquatic life as derived using the Guidelines is 0.042 μg/l as a 24 hr
average and the concentration should not exceed 0.49 μg/l at any time.

Saltwater Aquatic Life — For saltwater aquatic life, no criterion for endosulfan can be derived using the Guidelines, and there are insufficient data to estimate a criterion using other
procedures.

Human Health — For the protection of human health from the toxic properties of endosulfan ingested through water and through contaminated aquatic organisms, the ambient water
criterion is determined to be 0.1 mg/l.

Basis for the Proposed Human Health Criteria: Establishing a scientific basis for evaluating
the hazard of endosulfan to man is difficult. At very high levels of acute exposure, humans
show central nervous system (CNS) symptoms and may die. Several studies report endosulfan has been used for suicides.

Workers who failed to use good safety practices (i.e., to cover skin and use respiratory protection) have died from endosulfan exposure. In one incident, three persons exposed showed CNS symptoms; two of them died. It therefore appears that the most toxic potential effect to man is that of CNS toxicity since the available data indicate a lack of carcinogenic, mutagenic, or teratogenic potential. The absence of reports on toxic effects associated with the proper use of endosulfan (particularly such effects as skin sensitization or other human symptoms) has been noted.

There appears to be considerable species variation in toxic effects. Of the species tested with endosulfan, cattle are the most sensitive to the neurotoxic effects and would therefore be a worst case model for human toxicity. There are much more controlled toxicity data on rodents, but cattle appear to be closer in sensitivity and effects to man. Data on CNS toxicity to cattle are presented in Table 58.

Table 58: Lethality and CNS Toxicity of Endosulfan in Cattle

Dose, Route	Number Animals Exposed	Time to CNS Toxicity (hours)	Percent Exposed Showing CNS Effects	Time to Death (days)	Percent Exposed Dying
12.5 mg/kg, oral	2	10	100	6	50
0.12% formulation, dermal	250	5	20	1	4
4% dust, dermal	5	2	100	1	80
35% powder, dermal	30	5	*	**	50

*apparently 100%
**hours to days

Source: Reference (33)

The relevance of these high exposure levels to a water quality criterion presents additional sources of calculation error. The CNS toxicity in these studies is an acute symptom of high exposure. All reported human poisonings, however, have resulted from accident, human error, or suicidal intention. The reported poisonings of man and the most sensitive other mammal, cattle, have occurred after acute, high level exposure to concentrated endosulfan. These levels will not occur in drinking water. The key question then is, "Are there any data in the toxicology reports or studies to indicate that CNS effects can occur after chronic, very low level exposure to endosulfan?"

Tiberin, et al reported occasional EEG alteration in one of three men one year after a convulsive seizure following exposure to endosulfan. Terziev, et al report that autopsy on an endosulfan suicide case showed changes in the neurons among lesions in other organs. In female rats, exposed for 78 weeks and then autopsied or necropsied, cause of death was not indicated in the report. Rats, although more resistant to toxicity than man or cattle, demonstrate no histopathological changes in the brain after receiving high doses of endosulfan orally for 78 weeks, or most of a lifetime.

Cerebral hemorrhage was reported in seven female rats that died early in the study (week 21) but the absence of lesions at even higher and more long-term dosage suggested to the authors that these deaths were not compound related. Several lesions were present in the male rats and mice that died early in these endosulfan feeding studies. The most prevalent lesions included nephropathy, parathyroid hyperplasia and testicular atrophy, all without clear dose response pattern.

An important question is, "Do the apolar metabolites of endosulfan remain in the body to produce chronic effects if endosulfan is ingested in low-level quantities over a long term?" No controlled metabolic studies in man have been reported, although Demeter and Heyndrickx report (33-9) that endosulfan sulfate is a metabolite in humans. This metabolite is approximately as toxic to mice as the parent isomers but no specific CNS effects were reported (based on toxicity trials on the pure compound).

The toxicity of endosulfan is somewhat greater in animals with deficiencies of dietary protein. The differences in even a dose as high as an LD_{50} are not great enough, however, to ascribe any potential human hazard to this mechanism or to suggest that protein-deprived humans would be more sensitive to chronic exposure to endosulfan in drinking water. It can be concluded that (a) the controlled studies uniformly report CNS toxicity following acute high level exposure and (b) there has been no indication reported of specific lesions in mammals related to mortality following chronic exposure.

A water quality criterion could be based on the lowest no-effect level (NOEL) reported for endosulfan in test species. Available data on no-effect levels are summarized in Table 59.

Table 59: No-Effect Dose Levels for Endosulfan on Different Species and Biochemical Parameters

Species	Organ/Tissue	Effect Observed	No-Effect Dose	Route Administered*
Rat	—	lethality	$\cong 55$ mg/kg = LD_0	acute oral (intragastric)
Rat	—	lethality	40 mg/kg = LD_0	acute oral
Rat	liver	cholinesterase inhibition	68 mg/kg minimum	acute oral
Rat	liver	microsome enzyme function	50 ppm diet	diet (2 weeks)
Rat	embryo	teratogenicity	10 mg/kg	oral (gestation day 7-14)
Rat **	—	lethality	445 ppm diet	diet (78 weeks)
Hamster	—	lethality	70 mg/kg	acute oral
Hamster	liver	enzyme inhibition: GPT, LDH	134 mg/kg minimum	acute oral
Mice	—	weight depression	3.2 ppm diet	diet (6 weeks)
Mice***	—	lethality	2.0 ppm diet	diet (78 weeks)
Rabbit	eye	inflammation and irritation	1:1,000 aqueous	instillation
Rabbit	eye	inflammation and irritation	20% aqueous solution	instillation
Rabbit	skin	irritation	100 mg/kg	dermal
Chicken	egg	hatchability	0.07 mg/egg	yolk injection
Dog	—	gross and microscopic lesions	0.75 mg/kg/day	oral (52 weeks)
Salmonella typhimunium (Strains TA 98, 100, 1534 and 1978)	—	base-pair substitution (mutagenicity)	1.0 mg/plate	—

*Single dose unless otherwise noted.
**Female Osborne-Mendel.
***Female B6C3F1.

Source: Reference (33)

The lowest NOEL reported in the published literature is 2.0 mg endosulfan per kilogram feed when fed to mice for 78 weeks (33-10). This dose corresponds to 0.4 mg endosulfan per kilogram body weight per day for a typical 25 g mouse consuming 5 g feed per day;

$$\frac{2.0 \text{ mg endosulfan}}{1,000 \text{ g feed}} \times \frac{5 \text{ g feed}}{\text{mouse-day}} \times \frac{\text{mouse}}{0.025 \text{ kg}} = 0.4 \text{ mg/kg/day}$$

Applying a 0.01 animal-to-human uncertainly factor to this dosage gives an upper limit for nonoccupational daily exposure (ADI) of 0.28 mg/kg body weight for a 70 kg person:

$$\frac{0.4 \text{ mg}}{\text{kg-day}} \times 0.01 \times \frac{70 \text{ kg}}{\text{person}} = 0.28 \text{ mg/day}$$

For the purpose of establishing a water quality criterion, human exposure to endosulfan is considered to be based on ingestion of 2 liters of water and 18.7 g of fish per day. The amount of water ingested is approximately 100 times greater than the amount of fish consumed. The fish bioconcentration factor for endosulfan of 28 has been established. The equation for calculating the criterion for endosulfan content of water is:

$$2X \ + \ (0.0187)(F)(X) \ = \ ADI$$

where: 2 is the amount of drinking water consumed, liters/day; X is the endosulfan concentration in water, mg/l; 0.0187 is the amount of fish consumed, kg/day; F is the bioconcentration factor, mg endosulfan/kg fish per mg endosulfan/liter water and ADI is the limit on daily exposure for a 70 kg person.

For the case where F is 28,

$$2X \ + \ (0.0187)(28)(X) \ = \ 0.28$$
$$2.5236 \ X \ = \ 0.28$$
$$X \ = \ 0.1 \ mg/l$$

References

(33-1) Federal Water Pollution Control Admin., *"Water Quality Criteria,"* Nat. Tech. Advisory Committee, Wash., D.C. (1968).

(33-2) National Academy of Sciences/Nat. Academy of Engineering, *Water Quality Criteria,* Wash, D.C. (1972).

(33-3) Schoettger, R.A., "Toxicology of thiodan in several fish and aquatic invertebrates," U.S. Dept of the Interior, Fish and Wildlife Service, *Invest. Fish Control* 35, 1 (1970).

(33-4) Korn, S. and Earnest, R., "Acute toxicity of twenty insecticides to striped bass, *Morone saxatilis,"* *Calif. Fish Game,* 60, 128 (1974).

(33-5) Schimmel, S.C. et al, *Acute Toxicity to and Bioconcentration of Endosulfan by Estuarine Animals,* Proc. ASTM Symp. Aquatic Toxicol, ASTM Report STP 634 (1977).

(33-6) Macek, K.J. et al, *Toxicity of Four Pesticides to Water Fleas and Fathead Minnows,* Report EPA-600/3-76-099, Wash, D.C., U.S. Envir. Prot. Agency (1976).

(33-7) National Academy of Sciences, *Drinking Water and Health, Wash., D.C. (1977).*

(33-8) Terziev, G. et al, "Forensic medical and forensic chemical study of acute lethal poisonings with thiodan," *Folea Med. (Plovdiv)* 16, 325 (1974).

(33-9) Demeter, J. and Heyndrickx, A., "Two lethal endosulfan poisonings in man", *Jour. Anal. Toxicol.* 2, 68 (1978).

(33-10) Weisburger, J.H. et al, *Bioassay of Endosulfan for Possible Carcinogenicity,* DHEW Publ (NIH) 78-1312, Wash., D.C., National Cancer Institute (1978).

ENDRIN (#34)

Endrin is the common name of one member of the cyclodiene group of pesticides. It is a cyclic hydrocarbon having a chlorine-substituted methano bridge structure as follows:

Occurrence: Endrin enters the environment primarily as a result of direct applications to soil and crops. Waste material discharge from endrin manufacturing and formulating plants and disposal of empty containers also contribute significantly to observed residue levels.

Endrin was introduced into the United States in 1951. The endrin sold in the United States is a technical grade product, containing not less than 95% active ingredient, available in a variety of diluted formulations.

Human exposure to endrin occurs through the diet, from inhalation, and through dermal contact. The average dietary intake in the United States in 1973 was 0.033 μg/day (0.0005 μg/kg/day) for a 69.1 kg man. This is far below the maximum daily intake of 138.2 μg/day (2 μg/kg/day) established by the World Health Organization. Respiratory and/or dermal exposure to endrin occurs during manufacture and distribution but is more likely to result from agricultural uses.

Background concentrations in the atmosphere, hydrosphere, and lithosphere, far removed from agricultural areas where endrin is used and industrialized areas where endrin is manufactured, are generally below the levels of detection.

Physical Properties: Endrin is a white crystalline solid, mp 226 to 230°C with decomposition, vp 2×10^{-7} torr at 25°C. It is practically insoluble in water, sparingly soluble in alcohols and petroleum hydrocarbons, moderately soluble in acetone, benzene. The technical product is a light tan powder of not less than 92% w/w endrin.

Chemical Properties: Endrin is isomeric with dieldrin. [See also the criteria document on aldrin/dieldrin (4).] It is stable to alkali and acids but strong acids or heating above 200°C causes a rearrangement to a less insecticidal derivative. It is compatible with other pesticides.

Uses: Known uses of endrin in the United States are as an avicide, rodenticide, and insecticide, the latter being the most prevalent. The largest single use of endrin domestically is for the control of lepidopteron larvae attacking cotton crops in the southeastern and Mississippi delta states. Its persistence in soil led to its discontinuation for control of tobacco worms. In the past several years, endrin utilization has been increasingly restricted and production has continued to decline. In 1978, endrin production was approximately 400,000 lb (34-1).

Toxic Effects: In the aquatic environment endrin is acutely toxic to carp at 0.046 μg/l (34-2) and to the pink shrimp at 0.037 μg/l (34-3). It is chronically toxic to the fathead minnow at 0.187 μg/l (34-4) and at 0.038 μg/l to the grass shrimp (34-5). Endrin has been reported to bioconcentrate by factors as high as 15,000 in freshwater fish (34-6) and 6,400 in marine fish (34-7). Endrin is toxic to mammals, but a no-effect level of 1 mg/kg for the rat and the dog has been established by Brooks (34-8).

Endrin is highly toxic to all animals regardless of the route of exposure (34-9). The primary toxic effect of acute exposure is on the central nervous system. When lethal concentrations are administered to experimental animals, convulsions may occur as soon as 30 min after exposure, and may culminate in death through respiratory failure in about 48 hr. The dose lethal to 50% of the experimental animals ranges from 3 mg/kg for the monkey to 50 mg/kg for the goat.

Many cases of mammalian fatalities have been reported outside the laboratory. For example, field application of endrin at rates of 0.55 to 2.75 kg/ha resulted in the death of 33 to 100% of various species of wild mice inhabiting the target area (34-10). The chronic toxicity of endrin to mammals is greater than that of other organochlorine pesticides. Sublethal effects in wild animals manifest primarily as behavioral and reproductive disorders, i.e., improper maternal care, temporary loss of normal activity, increased vulnerability to predators, reduced reproductive potential, increased postnatal mortality and fetal death. Chronic exposure to endrin may also be fatal. Five to eight mg/kg in the diet was fatal to dogs in 18 to 44 days. Twelve mg/kg in the diet for life decreased the survival time for mice. Deer mice succumbed to a diet which contained only 2 mg/kg endrin.

No malignancies attributable to endrin exposure have been reported in the literature; however, endrin has been found to cause chromosomal aberrations in rats following intratesticular injection. Teratogenesis, growth retardation and increases in fetal mortality have been observed in mice and hamsters following endrin administration.

Quantitative data on endrin toxicity to humans are not available. However, outbreaks of human poisoning have resulted from accidental contamination of foods and have been traced to doses as low as 0.2 mg/kg body weight. Endrin toxicity seems to result primarily from the effects of endrin and its metabolites on the central nervous system. Symptoms usually observed in victims of endrin poisoning were convulsions, vomiting, abdominal pain, nausea, dizziness, and headache. Respiratory failure was the most common cause of death. Significantly increased activity of the hepatic microsomal drug-metabolizing enzymes has occurred in individuals employed in the manufacture of endrin. No irreversible adverse effects of occupational exposure to endrin have been reported in the literature so far. The National Cancer Institute has recently published a bioassay of endrin for possible carcinogenicity (34-11).

Current Levels of Exposure: While no recent data are available on levels of exposure of humans to endrin it appears that the risk of exposure is decreasing because of the decreased usage of the pesticide. In a survey of over 500 drinking water samples, the number of samples containing concentrations of endrin in excess of 0.1 μg/l, which has been established as a maximum reasonable stream allowance, decreased from 23 in the period 1964 to 1965 to 0 in the period 1966 to 1967. The most recent study found only 4 ng/l in contaminated drinking water.

In a series of analyses of total diets, the average daily intake of endrin remained at trace levels (<0.001 mg) during the period 1965 to 1970, but the frequency of occurrence decreased considerably. Exposure of the general populace to endrin in the air decreased from a maximum level of 25.6 μg/m^3 in 1971 at Greeley, Colorado, to a maximum of 0.5 μg/m^3 in 1975 in Jackson, Mississippi.

Special Groups at Risk: Agricultural workers, home gardeners, and those involved in endrin manufacture and distribution are the most likely to be exposed to endrin. They may be exposed through inhalation or dermal exposure. The most significant occupational exposure comes during spraying of fields, and dermal exposure is almost always greater than respiratory exposure. Probably the greatest hazard associated with the use of endrin occurs when measuring and pouring the emulsifiable concentrate material. Because endrin has been shown to cause teratogenic effects, pregnant women, particularly those whose diets may contain large amounts of fish, must also be considered a special group at risk. Evidence that endrin may cause chromosomal damage in germinal tissue suggests that men and women of child-bearing intent may also be a special risk group.

Endrin concentrations are highest in the atmospheres over agricultural areas and probably reach their peak levels during the pesticide use season. Of all urban communities, those surrounded by farm lands run the highest risk of atmospheric contamination. Endrin absorbed to particulates could not be detected in the air over representative communities but may perhaps be present at very low concentrations in the vapor phase. Urban communities far removed from agricultural areas are unlikely to experience significant contamination. The homes of occupationally exposed workers have higher levels of atmospheric contamination than do those of the general populace.

Existing Guidelines and Standards: In 1965, maximum permissible levels were assigned to each of the organochlorine compounds based on the "maximum acceptable concentrations" suggested on July 9, 1965, by the subcommittee on toxicology to the Public Health Service Advisory Committee on Drinking Water Standards. This concentration for endrin was 0.001 ppm. In 1967, the "maximum reasonable stream allowance" for endrin of 0.1 ppb was suggested by Ettinger and Mount (34-12) and was accepted as a guideline.

A maximum acceptable level of 0.002 mg/kg body weight/day was established by a Joint FAO/WHO Meeting on Pesticide Residues in Food held in Rome, November, 1972. A threshold limit value of 100 μg/m^3 has been set for atmospheric levels of endrin by the

American Conference of Governmental Industrial Hygienists. A threshold limit value of 100 $\mu g/m^3$ for an 8 hr time-weighted average occupational exposure has also been established by the Occupational Safety and Health Administration. Toxic pollutant effluent standards (34-13) have been promulgated by the U.S. EPA. These allow an effluent concentration of 1.5 $\mu g/l$ per average working day calculated over a period of one month, not to exceed 7.5 $\mu g/l$ in any sample representing one working day's effluent. In addition, discharge is not to exceed 0.0006 kg per 1,000 kg of production.

Summary of Proposed EPA Criteria: *Freshwater Aquatic Life* — For endrin the criterion to protect freshwater aquatic life as derived using the Guidelines is 0.0020 $\mu g/l$ as a 24 hr average and the concentration should not exceed 0.10 $\mu g/l$ at any time.

Saltwater Aquatic Life — For endrin the criterion to protect saltwater aquatic life as derived using the Guidelines is 0.0047 $\mu g/l$ as a 24 hr average and the concentration should not exceed 0.031 $\mu g/l$ at any time.

Human Health — For the protection of human health from the toxic properties of endrin ingested through water and contaminated organisms, the ambient water criterion is determined to be 1 $\mu g/l$.

Basis for the Proposed Human Health Criteria: The limited teratogenic and mutagenic studies on endrin suggest that effects are induced with high endrin doses. However, an unusual administration route was used and unrealistically high endrin levels were employed in these studies. Such levels do not occur in water supplies under normal circumstances; therefore, the results of these studies were not used as the basis for the criterion. More toxicological data must be gathered about these potential effects of endrin before a final conclusion can be reached. The available data do not indicate that endrin is carcinogenic.

On the basis of long-term dietary studies in mammals and occupational exposures in man, a realistic water criterion may be proposed. Maximum no-effect dietary levels of endrin reported for experimental animals are:

Species	Dose Level (mg/kg)	Duration
Mouse	1	lifetime
Rat	1	2 years
Rat	1	established no-effect level
Hamster	1.5	no-effect level (1 day)
Dog	0.1	128 days
Dog	1	established no-effect level

Extrapolation of the 0.1 mg/kg no-effect dietary level for the dog to man is reasonable. Since experimental studies of chronic human ingestion are not available (but acute exposure data are), and valid long-term animal feeding studies have been done in more than one species, an uncertainty factor of 100 may be used in the absence of any indication of carcinogenicity in arriving at a water criterion. In deriving a water quality criterion, human exposure to endrin was assumed to come from daily ingestion of 2-liters of water and 18.7 g of fish with a bioconcentration factor of 1,900 for endrin. Using a no-effect dose level of 0.1 mg/kg, the total allowable intake for a 70 kg man is:

$$0.1 \text{ mg endrin/kg} \times 70 \text{ kg} = \frac{7 \text{ mg/day}}{100 \text{ (uncertainty factor)}} = 70 \text{ } \mu g/day$$

The criterion for endrin is thus:

$$x = \frac{70 \text{ } \mu g/day}{2 \text{ liters } + (0.0187 \text{ kg} \times 1{,}900)} = 1.87 \text{ } \mu g/day$$

This approximates closely the 1 $\mu g/l$ maximum allowable concentration for endrin proposed by the Public Health Service for drinking water. It is therefore, recommended that the endrin criterion be established at 1 μg endrin/liter of ambient water (1.0 ppb).

This calculation assumes that 100% of man's exposure is assigned to the ambient water pathway. Although it is desirable to establish a criterion based upon total exposure potential, the data for other exposure conditions have not been factored into this analysis.

In summary, based upon the use of toxicologic data for dogs, and an uncertainty factor of 100, the initial level for endrin corresponding to daily intake of 70 μg/day, is 1.9 μg/l. Since the existing 1 μg/l allowable concentration in the drinking water standards is reasonably close to 1.9 μg/l, it is recommended that 1.0 μg/l be used as the criterion with notation that there are special groups at risk. Drinking water contributes 5% of the assumed exposure while eating contaminated fish products accounts for 95%. The criterion level for endrin can alternatively be expressed as 1.1 μg/l if exposure is assumed to be from the consumption of fish and shellfish alone.

It should be noted that, if endrin was present in waters from which edible fish were obtained and if these fish concentrate endrin by a factor of 1,900, this criterion may not be sufficient to protect a special high risk group (i.e., pregnant women who consume a single dose of endrin-contaminated fish). Given the bioconcentration factor, fish in water at the maximum recommended concentration of 1 μg/l, may contain 1.9 μg/g endrin. A 250 g portion of fish would contain approximately 0.5 mg endrin (or 0.01 mg/kg for a 50 kg female). This dose provides a margin of safety of only 150 over the NOEL of 1.5 mg/kg for teratogenicity in the hamster. The adequacy of this margin of safety is highly questionable, especially given the likelihood of consumption of more than 250 g of fish at a given time.

The recommended water quality criterion of 1 μg/l was based on a chronic exposure study; teratologic outcomes are more likely to occur with acute exposures at critical times in gestation.

References

(34-1) U.S. EPA. *Endrin–Position Document* Washington D.C., Office of Pesticide Programs (1978).

(34-2) Iyatomi, K.T., et al "Toxicity of endrin to fish" *Prog. Fish. Cult.* 20, 155 (1958).

(34-3) Schimmel, S.C., et al "Endrin: Effects on several estuarine organisms." *Proc. 28th Annu. Conf. S.E. Assoc. Game and Fish Comm.,* 1974, 187 (1975).

(34-4) Jarvinen, A W., and R.M. Tyo. "Toxicity of fathead minnows of endrin in food and water." *Arch. Environ. Contam. Toxicol.* 7, 1 (In press-1979).

(34-5) Tyler-Schroeder, D.B. "Use of grass shrimp, *Palaemonetes pugio,* in a life-cycle toxicity test." In *Proceedings of a Symposium on Aquatic Toxicology and Hazard Evaluation.* L.L. Marking and R.A Kimerle, eds. Am. Soc. Testing and Materials (ASTM), October 31-November 1, (in press 1977).

(34-6) Hermanutz, R. "Endrin and malathion toxicity to flagfish, *Jordanella floridae.*" *Arch Environ Contam. Toxicol.* 7, 159 (1978).

(34-7) Hansen, D J., et al "Endrin: Effects on the entire life-cycle of saltwater fish, *Cyprinodon variegatus.*" *Jour. Toxicol. Environ. Health* 3, 721 (1977).

(34-8) Brooks, G.T. *Chlorinated insecticides. Vol. II: Biological and environmental aspects.* Cleveland, Ohio, CRC Press (1974).

(34-9) Treon, J.F. et al, "Toxicity of Endrin for laboratory animals", *Agric. Food. Chem.* 3, 842 (1955).

(34-10) Dana, R.H. and Shaw, D.H, *Meadow Mouse Control in Holly,* Calif. Dept. Agric. Bull. 47, 224 (1958).

(34-11) National Cancer Institute, *Bioassay of Endrin for Possible Carcinogenicity,* DHEW Publ. No. (NIH) 79-812, Wash, D.C. (1979).

(34-12) Ettinger, M.B. and Mount, D.L., "A wild fish should be safe to eat", *Envir. Sci. Tech.* 1, 203 (1967).

(34-13) 40 *CFR* Part 129.102.

ETHYLBENZENE (#35)

Ethylbenzene, $C_6H_5CH_2CH_3$, has a molecular weight of 106.16.

Occurrence: EB is present in drinking waters and in the atmosphere. It has been shown to persist in man for days after exposure. It is present in the respiratory tract, umbilical cord and maternal blood and subcutaneous fat of exposed humans. There is little reason to suspect that the current sources of EB in our environment will be abated. The sources of EB include: (1) commercial, e.g., petroleum and petroleum by-products; (2) motor vehicle exhaust, and (3) cigarette smoke.

Significant quantities of EB are present in mixed xylenes. These are used as diluents in the paint industry, in agricultural sprays for insecticides and in gasoline blends (which may contain as much as 20% EB). In light of the large quantities of EB produced and the diversity of products in which it is found, there exist many environmental sources for ethylbenzene, e.g., vaporization during solvent use, pyrolysis of gasoline and emitted vapors at filling stations.

Physical Properties: Ethylbenzene is a flammable, colorless liquid with a boiling point of 136.25°C and a freezing point of –95.01°C. Its density at 25°C (relative to water at the same temperature) is 0.866 and it has a specific gravity of 0.8669. Vapor pressures range from 7 to 15.3 mm Hg at 20°C to 20 mm Hg at 38.6°C. Ethylbenzene is slightly soluble (less than 0.1% or 866 mg/l) in water, but it is freely soluble in organic solvents.

Chemical Properties: The major commercial use for ethylbenzene is based on the dehydrogenation of ethylbenzene to styrene. This may be carried out by catalytic dehydrogenation or by oxidative dehydrogenation. Ethylbenzene may also be oxidized to a variety of products. Indeed, one alternative route to styrene involves oxidation to a mixture of acetone and phenylmethylcarbinol; the mixture is reduced catalytically to give all phenylmethylcarbinol which is dehydrated to styrene in a subsequent step.

Uses: The two primary commercial uses of EB are in the plastic and rubber industries where it is utilized as an initial reactant in the production of styrene. The majority of these commercial sites of production are geographically clustered in Texas and Louisiana. The amount of EB produced in the United States in 1976 was approximately 6 to 7 billion pounds of which about 98% was used in the manufacture of styrenes.

Toxic Effects: The paucity of information available on the biological effects of ethylbenzene (EB) in man and other mammalian species is rather surprising considering the degree of exposure to EB in our environment. In man and in animals, EB is an irritant of mucous membranes. It is this response which forms the basis for the current Threshold Limit Values (TLVs). The EPA proposed to evaluate the carcinogenic potential of EB in 1976, but test results are not yet available. Similarly, no data exist for mutagenicity and teratogenicity of ethylbenzene. The potential adverse human health effects following exposure to EB were stated (35-1):

> Kidney disease, liver disease, chronic respiratory disease, skin disease—and the facts in brief are as follows: EB is not nephrotoxic. Concern is expressed because the kidney is the primary route of excretion of EB and its metabolites. EB is not hepatotoxic. Since EB is metabolized by the liver, concern is expressed for this tissue. Exacerbation of pulmonary pathology might occur following exposure to EB. Individuals with impaired pulmonary function might be at risk. EB is a defatting agent and may cause dermatitis following prolonged exposure. Individuals with preexisting skin problems may be more sensitive to EB.

Current Levels of Exposure: *Air* – Several investigators have reported that ethylbenzene is present in the ambient atmosphere at a level of approximately 0.01 ppm.

Water – Shackelford and Keith (35-2) reviewed the literature on EB contamination and concluded that it was found in most of the potable waters tested. No data were reported on levels of EB in potable waters.

Food – Except for the report by Kinlan, et al (35-3), EB has not been reported in food.

Industrial – EB can be found in a number of volatile compounds with widespread industrial use (including gasoline and solvents).

Special Groups at Risk: Those individuals who are involved in the use of petroleum by-products, e.g., polymerization workers involved in styrene production, may be at risk. In a study of 494 styrene workers, Lilis, et al (35-4) reported various neurotoxic manifestations. These included prenarcotic symptoms, incoordination, dizziness, headache and nausea (13% of worker group) and a decrease in a radial and peroneal nerve conduction velocity (19% of workers). In 50% of the workers, distal hypoesthesia involving the lower limbs was observed. It is difficult to assess occupational reports evaluating such a situation since these workers are exposed to a number of different precursors, by-products and end products.

In this particular study, toxic effects were reported but there was a general lack of symptoms among workers who were exposed for many years, suggesting that the risk of severe neurologic deficiencies may be minimal. Recently, however, Harkonen, et al (35-5) reported on the relationship between styrene exposure and symptoms of central nervous system dysfunction in 98 occupationally exposed workers. Urinary mandelic acid concentration was used as an index of exposure intensity. Although no exposure-response relationship was observed between symptoms of ill health and urinary mandelic acid concentration, the exposed group expressed significantly more symptoms than the unexposed group. Symptoms included abnormal electroencephalograms, and impaired psychological functions such as visuomotor accuracy and psychomotor performance.

A NIOSH report by Rivera and Rostand (35-6) on worker exposure to various lacquer constituents including EB in a baseball bat manufacturing facility concluded that no health hazard existed with the exception of mucous membrane irritation and the potential for contact dermatitis under the conditions at the plant. This occupational situation again illustrates the fact that these workers were exposed to more than one chemical besides EB.

Cigarettes contain 7 to 20 x 10^{-6} g of EB per cigarette. It has been reported that moderate cigarette smokers expired up to 14 x 10^{-6} g/hr of EB (during an 8 hr measurement).

Groups of individuals who are exposed to EB to the greatest extent and could represent potential pools for the expression of EB toxicity include: (1) individuals in commercial situations where petroleum products or by-products are manufactured (e.g., rubber or plastics industry); (2) individuals residing in areas with high atmospheric smog generated by motor vehicle emissions.

Existing Guidelines and Standards: The U.S. Occupational Standard for "permissible exposure has been set at 100 ppm (435 mg/m³) by ACGIH with a STEL value of 125 ppm (545 mg/m³). At this level of exposure eye irritation is minimal. The Soviet standards (TLV) for EB are approximately eight-fold less than current U.S. TLV standards.

Summary of Proposed EPA Criteria: *Freshwater Aquatic Life* — For freshwater aquatic life, no criterion for ethylbenzene can be derived using the Guidelines, and there are insufficient data to estimate a criterion using other procedures.

Saltwater Aquatic Life — For saltwater aquatic life, no criterion for ethylbenzene can be derived using the Guidelines, and there are insufficient data to estimate a criterion using other procedures.

Human Health — For the protection of human health from the toxic properties of ethylbenzene ingested through water, the ambient water quality criterion is 1.1 mg/l.

Basis for Proposed Human Health Criteria: The TLV of 435 mg/m³ (100 ppm) EB represents what is believed to be a maximal concentration to which a worker may be exposed for 8 hr per day, 5 days per week over his working lifetime without hazard to health or well-being (35-7). To the TLV, Stokinger and Woodward (35-8) apply terms expressing respiratory volume during an 8 hr period (assumed to be 10 m³) and a respiratory absorption coefficient appropriate to the substance under consideration. In addition, the 5 day per week occupational exposure is often converted to a 7 day per week equivalent in keeping with the more continuous pattern of exposure to drinking water. According to the model, the amount of ethylbenzene that may be taken into the bloodstream and presumed to be noninjurious and which, hence, may be taken in water each day is:

$$435 \text{ mg/m}^3 \quad \times \quad 10 \text{ m}^3 \quad \times \quad 0.5 \quad \times \quad {}^5\!/_7 \text{ week} \quad = \quad 1{,}555 \text{ mg/day}$$

TLV	respiratory intake term	respiratory adsorption coefficient	proportion of week exposed	maximum noninjurious intake

A safety factor of 1,000 is used since no long-term or acute human data are available, and there is very little information from experimental animals (35-9). Thus, 1,555 mg/day divided by 1,000 = 1.555 or 1.6 mg/day. To calculate an acceptable amount of EB in ambient water, the methodology assumes a maximal daily intake of 2 liters of water per day, the consumption of 18.7 g of fish/shellfish per day, a bioconcentration factor of 42 for fish and 50% absorption.

$$(X) \quad \times \quad [2 + 42\,(0.0187)] \quad \times \quad 0.5 \quad = \quad 1.6 \text{ mg/day}$$

upper intake limit	oral intake term	gastrointestinal absorption coefficient	maximum noninjurious intake

Solving for X, the value derived is 1.1 mg/l. According to Stokinger and Woodward (35-8), "This derived value represents an approximate limiting concentration for a healthy adult population; it is only a first approximation in the development of a tentative water quality criterion. . . several adjustments in this value may be necessary. . .Other factors, such as taste, odor and color may outweigh health considerations because acceptable limits for these may be below the estimated health limit." It should also be noted that the basis for the above-recommended limit, the TLV for EB, is the avoidance of irritation, rather than chronic effects (35-7). Should chronic effects data become available, both TLVs and recommendations based on them will warrant reconsideration.

In summary, based on a TLV, and an uncertainty factor of 1,000, the criterion level for ethylbenzene corresponding to the calculated acceptable daily intake of 1.6 mg/day, is 1.1 mg/l. Drinking water contributes 72% of the assumed exposure while eating contaminated fish products accounts for 28%. The criterion level can alternatively be expressed as 2.0 mg/l if exposure is assumed to be from the consumption of fish and shellfish products alone.

References

(35-1) 40 *FR* 1910 1034.

(35-2) Shackelford, W.M. and Keith, L.H. *Frequency of Organic Compounds Identified in Water,* Report EPA 600/4-76-002, Wash , D.C., U.S. Environmental Protection Agency (1976).

(35-3) Kinlan, T.E. et al, "Volatile compounds in roasted filberts," *Journ. Agric. Food Chem.* 20, 1021 (1972)

(35-4) Lilis, R et al, "Neurotoxicity of styrene in production and polymerization workers," *Environ. Res.* 15, 133 (1978).

(35-5) Harkonen, H. et al, "Exposure-response relationship between styrene exposure and central nervous functions," *Scand. Jour. Work Envir. Health* 4, 53 (1978).

(35-6) Rivera, R O. and Rostand, R.A., *Health Hazard Evaluation/Toxicity Determination Report,* Report No 74-121-203, Wash., D.C., Nat. Inst. for Occup. Safety and Health (1975).

(35-7) American Conference of Governmental Industrial Hygienists. 1977. "Threshold limit values for chemical substances and physical agents in the workroom environment with intended changes for 1979" Cincinnati, Ohio (1979).

(35-8) Stokinger, H.E., and R.L. Woodward. "Toxicologic methods for establishing drinking water standards" *Jour. Am. Water Works Assoc.* 50, 515 (1958).

(35-9) National Academy of Sciences. "*Drinking water and health.*" Wash. D.C. (1977).

ETHYL CHLORIDE

See "Chlorinated Ethanes" (15).

ETHYLENE DICHLORIDE

See "Chlorinated Ethanes" (15).

F

FLUORANTHENE (#36)

Fluoranthene, $C_{16}H_{10}$ has the structural formula:

It has a common name, idryl and is properly designated 1,2-benzacenaphthene. It has a molecular weight of 202.

Occurrence: Fluoranthene, a polynuclear aromatic hydrocarbon, is produced from the pyrolytic processing of organic raw materials such as coal and petroleum at high temperatures. It is also known to occur naturally as a product of plant biosynthesis. Fluoranthene is ubiquitous in the environment and has been detected in U.S. air, in foreign and domestic drinking waters and in foodstuffs. It is also contained in cigarette smoke.

Physical Properties: Fluoranthene has a melting point of 111°C, a boiling point of approximately 375°C and a vapor pressure of 0.01 mm Hg at 25°C. It is soluble in water to the extent of 265 μg/l.

Chemical Properties: Fluoranthene is oxidized only with difficulty. In common with other polynuclear aromatics, it may be halogenated. There is virtually no information in the literature on the chemical properties of this compound.

Uses: Fluoranthene is not an article of commerce and hence has no uses as such.

Toxic Effects: There is concern about the toxicity of fluoranthene because it is widespread in the human environment and belongs to a class of compounds (polynuclear aromatic hydrocarbons) that contain numerous potent carcinogens. Experimentally, fluoroanthene does not exhibit properties of a mutagen or primary carcinogen but it is a potent cocarcinogen (36-1, 36-2, 36-3). In the laboratory, fluoranthene has also demonstrated toxicity to various freshwater and marine organisms (36-4). This finding, coupled with the cocarcinogenic properties of the compound, points out the need to protect humans and aquatic organisms from the potential hazards associated with fluoranthene in water.

Current Levels of Exposure: Quantitative estimates of human exposure to fluoranthene require numerous assumptions concerning routes of exposure, extent of absorption, conformity of lifestyle, and lack of geographic-, sex-, and age-specific variables. Nevertheless, working with estimates developed for PAH as a class, certain extrapolations are possible to arrive at an admittedly crude estimate of fluoroanthene exposure.

An estimate of fluoranthene intake from drinking water may be derived from data obtained in a survey of 16 U.S. cities (36-5). By arbitrarily assigning the lower limit of detectability for fluoranthene to those samples where none was detected, and using the measured values of fluoranthene in the four positive samples found, the estimated average fluoroanthene level in drinking water would be 8.6 ng/l. Thus, the daily intake of fluoranthene in drinking water may be calculated:

$$8.6 \text{ ng/l} \times 2 \text{ l/day} = 17.2 \text{ ng/day}$$

Borneff (36-6) estimates that the daily dietary intake of PAHs is about 8 to 11 μg/day. As a check on this estimate, fluoranthene intake may be calculated based on reported concentrations of fluoranthene in various foods and the per capita estimates of food consumption by the International Commission on Radiological Protection. Taking a range of 1 to 10 ppb as a typical concentration for fluoranthene in various foods, and 1,600 g/day as the total daily food consumption by man from all types of foods (i.e., fruits, vegetables, cereals, dairy products, etc.), the intake of fluoranthene from the diet would be in the range of 1.6 to 16 μg/day.

It has recently been reported that fluoranthene concentrations in ambient air average about 4 μg/1,000 m^3 (36-7). If it is assumed that 100% of the fluoranthene which is inhaled is adsorbed, and that the average amount of air inhaled by a human each day is about 10 to 20 m^3, then fluoranthene intake via the air would be in the range of 40 to 80 ng/day. However, in certain indoor environments, particularly in the presence of sidestream tobacco smoke, PAH exposure from inhaled air may be considerably higher (36-8).

In summary, a crude estimate of total daily exposure to fluoranthene would be as follows:

Source	Estimated Exposure (μg/day)
Water	0.017
Food	1.6–16
Air	0.040–0.080

The figures presented above make it quite clear that foods are by far the greatest source of fluoranthene to humans. The present levels of fluoranthene in drinking water would be expected to contribute very little to the total human intake.

It is important to note two factors which are not taken into account in the above estimate. First, it is known that tobacco smoking can contribute greatly to fluoranthene exposure in man. It is estimated that smoking one cigarette will increase exposure to fluoranthene via the lungs by about 0.26 μg (36-9). The sum of methylfluoranthenes in the smoke of a nonfiltered cigarette is about 0.18 ng (36-9). Second, it is assumed that the possibility of dermal absorption for fluoranthene contributes only a negligible amount to the total exposure. It is expected that only in certain occupational situations would dermal exposure be a quantitatively important route of exposure.

Special Groups at Risk: Individuals living in areas which are heavily industrialized, and in which large amounts of fossil fuels are burned, would be expected to have greatest exposure from ambient sources of fluoranthene. In addition, certain occupations (e.g., coke oven workers, steelworkers, roofers, automobile mechanics) would also be expected to have elevated levels of exposure relative to the general population.

Exposure to fluoranthene will be considerably increased among tobacco smokers or those who are exposed to smokers in closed environments (i.e., indoors).

Existing Guidelines and Standards: There have been no standards developed for fluoranthene in air, water, and food, or in the workplace. The only existing standard which takes fluoranthene into consideration is a drinking water standard for PAHs. The 1970 World Health Organization European Standards for Drinking Water recommends a concentration of PAHs not exceeding 0.2 μg/l. This recommended standard is based upon the analysis of six PAHs in drinking water as follows:

Fluoranthene	Benzo[b]fluoranthene
Benzo[a]pyrene	Benzo[k]fluoranthene
Benzo[g,h,i]perylene	Indeno[1,2,3-cd]pyrene

The designation of the above six PAHs for analytical monitoring of drinking water was not made on the basis of potential health effects or bioassay data on these compounds (36-10). Thus, it should not be assumed that these six compounds have special significance in determining the likelihood of adverse health effects resulting from absorption of any particular PAH. They are, instead, considered to be a useful indicator for the presence of PAH pollutants. Borneff and Kunte (36-10) found that PAHs were present in ground water at concentrations up to 50 ng/l, and in drinking water at concentrations up to 100 ng/l. Based on these data they suggested that water containing more than 200 ng/l should be rejected. However, as data from a number of U.S. cities indicate, levels of PAHs in raw and finished waters are typically much less than the 0.2 µg/l criterion.

Summary of Proposed EPA Criteria: *Freshwater Aquatic Life* — For fluoranthene, the criterion to protect freshwater aquatic life as derived using procedures other than the Guidelines is 250 µg/l as a 24 hour average and the concentration should not exceed 560 µg/l at any time.

Saltwater Aquatic Life — For fluoranthene, the criterion to protect saltwater aquatic life as derived using the Guidelines is 0.30 µg/l as a 24 hour average and the concentration should not exceed 0.69 µg/l at any time.

Human Health — For the protection of human health from the toxic properties of fluoranthene exposure through water, the ambient water quality criterion is determined to be 200 µg/l.

Basis for the Proposed Human Health Criteria: Calculation of the criterion takes into consideration the contribution of dietary and airborne sources of fluoranthene. Once these factors are accounted for, this procedure leads to the conclusion that 200 µg/l of fluoranthene in drinking water would represent an acceptable level of exposure.

It must be emphasized, however, that the criterion is based on chronic toxicity data with mortality being the endpoint, and applies only to situations where exposure occurred to fluoranthene alone. In environmental situations, it is well established that fluoranthene is found in the presence of numerous PAHs, a situation having important implications for potential toxic interactions.

Several studies have clearly shown that fluoranthene possesses no carcinogenic activity, and is neither a tumor initiator nor a tumor promoter. However, two carefully conducted studies have shown that fluoranthene when applied to mouse skin together with much smaller quantities of benzo[a]pyrene could act as a cocarcinogen to increase tumorigenic response. These data do not permit a quantitative estimation of health risks incurred by this type of biological phenomenon. Nevertheless, because fluoranthene is present in environmental mixtures together with other PAHs (including several carcinogens), it may pose an additional risk to the population exposed. In view of the cocarcinogenic and anticarcinogenic properties of several environmental PAHs, the degree of added risk, if one exists, cannot be easily determined on the basis of our present scientific knowledge.

Inadequacies in the current scientific data base, prevent the formulation of a drinking water criterion for fluoranthene based on potential cocarcinogenicity. However, it would seem prudent to temporarily limit the level of fluoranthene in drinking water to no more than the acceptable concentration of the sum of all nonfluoranthene PAHs. In addition, since environmental exposures to fluoranthene will almost certainly involve concomitant exposure to carcinogenic PAHs, their potential interaction should be considered in future research and health criteria development.

References

(36-1) VanDuuren, B.L., and Goldschmidt, B.M. "Cocarcinogenic and tumor-promoting agents in tobacco cocarcinogenesis." *Jour. Natl. Cancer Inst. 56,* 1237–1242. (1976)

(36-2) Tokiwa, H., et al. "Detection of mutagenic activity in particulate air pollutants." *Mutat. Res. 48,* 237. (1977).

(36-3) LaVoie, E., et al. "A comparison of the mutagenicity, tumor initiating activity and complete carcinogenicity of polynuclear aromatic hydrocarbons." Unpublished report. (1978). Cited in Reference (36).

(36-4) U.S. EPA. *In-depth studies on health and environmental impacts of selected water pollutants.* Report on Contract no. 68-01-4646, Wash., D.C. (1978).

(36-5) Basu, D.K., and Saxena, J. "Polynuclear aromatic hydrocarbons in selected U.S. drinking waters and their raw water sources." *Environ. Sci. Technol. 12,* 795. (1978).

(36-6) Borneff, J. "Fate of carcinogens in the aquatic environment" (Paper in Press-1979) (Cited in Reference 36).

(36-7) Santodonato, J. et al. "Health assessment document for polycyclic organic matter." Wash., D.C., Office of Research and Development, U.S.E.P.A. (In draft-1978).

(36-8) Grimmer, G. et al. "Passive smoking: intake of polycyclic aromatic hydrocarbons by breathing cigarette smoke containing air." *Int. Arch. Occup. Envir. Health 40,* 93. (1977).

(36-9) Hoffmann, D. et al. "Fluoranthenes: quantitative determination in cigarette smoke, formation by pyrolysis and tumor-initiating activity," *Jour. Nat. Cancer Inst. 49,* 1165. (1972).

(36-10) Borneff, J. and Kunte, H. "Carcinogenic substances in water and soil, XXVI: a routine method for the determination of PAH in water." *Arch. Hyg. Bakt. 153,* 220. (1969).

FLUORENE

See "Polynuclear Aromatic Hydrocarbons" (55).

FLUOROCARBONS

See "Halomethanes" (38).

H

HALOETHERS (#37)

Haloethers are compounds which contain an ether moiety and halogen atoms attached to the aryl or alkyl groups. Chloroethers appear to be the most important haloethers used commercially and can be divided into two categories, alpha- and nonalpha-chloroethers (37-1). This category overlaps with "Chloroalkyl Ethers (#16) and the reader is referred to that section as well.

Occurrence: The β-chloroethers are widespread environmental contaminants. It has been suggested that they are produced or may be formed as by-products in sizable quantities, released to and appear to persist in the environment, can pass through drinking water treatment plants, and may be carcinogenic.

Physical Properties: The haloethers exist within a wide range of physical properties. For example, boiling points may range from $43.2°C$ (2,2,2-trifluoroethyl vinyl ether) to $310°C$ (4-bromophenyl phenyl ether). Melting points can range from $103.5°C$ (chloromethyl methyl ether) to $-3°C$ (chloromethyl phenyl ether). The haloethers are very soluble in benzene, carbon tetrachloride, and acetone, and miscible in all oils. Chlorine substitution on ethers tends to increase their density, boiling point, and odor while decreasing their flammability and altering their solubility properties. The fluorine substituted compounds are much more volatile than their chlorinated analogues (37-1).

Chemical Properties: The α-haloethers are more reactive than β-haloethers due to the two electronegative atoms (oxygen and halogen) which are bonded to the same carbon (37-2). This difference in reactivity is evident by the different rates of hydrolysis.

Uses: Bis(2-chloroethyl) ether (BCE) is used as a dewaxing agent for lubricating oils and is a useful solvent for naphthenic components. BCE has also been used to separate butadiene from butylene. The second major use of bis(2-chloroethyl) ether is in the textile industry as a cleaning agent, a wetting agent and penetrant in combination with diethylene glycol, sulfonated oils, etc. The compound generally is a good solvent for tars, fats, waxes, oils, resins and pectins, and will dissolve cellulose esters when used with 10 to 30% ethanol. Chloromethyl methyl ether (CMME) is the only α-haloether of commercial significance and is used primarily in the synthesis of strong base ion exchange resins used in water conditioning and for chemical separation processes.

Toxic Effects: Bis(chloromethyl) ether (BCME) has been demonstrated to be a potent carcinogen.

Current Levels of Exposure: Only limited information is available on the extent of human exposure to haloethers in water and no information is available on ambient levels of haloethers in air or food. Quantitative estimates of human exposure cannot be made.

Special Groups at Risk: Individuals working with haloethers or living in areas where these haloethers are produced are probably at greater risk than the general population.

Existing Guidelines and Standards: The Occupational Safety and Health Administration (37-3) has set a time-weighted average value of 500 $\mu g/m^3$ for the following aromatic chloroethers in the air of the working environment: monochlorophenyl phenyl ether, dichloro-phenyl phenyl ether, trichlorophenyl phenyl ether, tetrachlorophenyl phenyl ether, and pentachlorophenyl phenyl ether. This value has also been adopted by the American Conference of Governmental and Industrial Hygienists for "Chlorinated Diphenyl Oxide" as of 1979. A STEL value of 2.0 $\mu g/m^3$ is also specified by ACGIH. Again, the reader is referred to the section on "Chloroalkyl Ethers" (#16) for guidelines and standards on bis-(chloromethyl) ether (BCME), bis(2-chloroethyl) ether (BCEE), and bis(2-chlorosiopropyl) ether (BCIE). The standard is designed to prevent the formation of chloracne in exposed workers.

Summary of Proposed EPA Criteria: *Freshwater Aquatic Life* — For 4-bromophenyl phenyl ether the criterion to protect freshwater aquatic life as derived using the guidelines is 6.2 $\mu g/l$ as a 24 hour average and the concentration should not exceed 14 $\mu g/l$ at any time.

Saltwater Aquatic Life — For saltwater aquatic life, no criterion for 4-bromophenyl phenyl ether can be derived using the guidelines, and there are insufficient data to estimate a criterion using other procedures.

Human Health — Because of a lack of adequate toxicological data on nonhuman mammals and humans, protective criteria cannot be derived at this time for any haloether discussed, according to EPA (37). This is confusing and apparently in direct contrast with another criteria document (16) which does present limits for chloroalkyl ethers (specifically, bis-(chloromethyl) ether, bis(2-chloroethyl) ether and bis(2-chloroisopropyl) ether.

Basis for the Proposed Human Health Criteria: (1) Bis(2-chloroisopropyl) ether. A reliable criterion cannot be calculated for this ether according to EPA (37) because a long-term "no adverse effect" level cannot be established for mammals. A criterion might be derived from a bioassay described in the criteria document using nontumor pathology. However, in the low dose groups, both male and female mice evidenced an increased incidence of centrilobular necrosis of the liver which was not seen in the high dose groups. The reader should contrast this general statement with the much more specific and quantitative discussion of bis-(2-chloroisopropyl) ether (BCIE) in the earlier section on chloroalkyl ethers referencing another criteria document (16).

(2) Chlorinated aromatic ethers. The TLV for chlorophenyl phenyl ether is 500 $\mu g/m^3$. By a process analogous to that used by Stokinger and Woodward, this standard could be used to calculate a water criterion. However, since the TLV for these compounds is based on preventing chloracne, rather than chronic toxicity, such a calculation would not be appropriate. Because of the lack of data on both toxicologic effects and environmental contamination, the hazard posed by these compounds cannot be estimated according to EPA (37).

References

(37-1)   U.S. EPA *Investigation of Selected Potential Environmental Contaminants: Haloethers.* Wash., D.C., Off. Tox. Subst. (1975).
(37-2)   Summers, L. "The Alpha-Haloalkyl Ethers". *Chem. Rev. 55*, 301 (1955).
(37-3)   38 *FR* 23540.

HALOMETHANES (#38)

The halomethanes are a subclass of halogenated aliphatic hydrocarbon compounds, some of whose members constitute important or potentially hazardous environmental contaminants. The seven halomethane compounds selected for discussion in this document are listed in Table 60. Many other halogenated methane derivative chemicals exist, including various combinations of halogen (bromine, chlorine, fluorine, iodine) substitutions on one, two, three, or all four of the hydrogen positions of methane. Of these, two other particularly important halomethanes, trichloromethane (chloroform) and tetrachloromethane (carbon tetrachloride) are subjects of separate criteria documents. Several recent reviews are available which present extensive discussions of health effects related to halomethane exposure (38-1, 38-2, 38-3).

Table 60: Halomethanes*

Names and CAS Registry Number	Formula
Bromomethane, *methyl bromide*, monobromo- methane, Embafume, Iscobrome, Rotox; 74–83–9	CH_3Br
Chloromethane, *methyl chloride*, monochloromethane; 74–87–3	CH_3Cl
Dichloromethane, *methylene chloride*, methane di- chloride, methylene dichloride, methylene bi- chloride; 75–09–2	CH_2Cl_2
Tribromomethane, *bromoform*, methyl tribromide; 75–25–2	$CHBr_3$
Bromodichloromethane, *dichloromethyl bromide*; 75–25–4	$BrCHCl_2$
Dichlorodifluoromethane, *fluorocarbon 12*, F–12, Arcton 6, Freon 12, Frigen 12, Genetron 12, Halon, Isotron 12, difluorodichloromethane; 75–71–8	CCl_2F_2
Trichlorofluoromethane, *fluorocarbon 11*, F–11, Arcton 9, Freon 11, Frigen 11, Algofrene type 1, trichloromonofluoromethane, fluorotrichloro- methane; 75–69–4	CCl_3F

*Chemical names, common names (italicized), some trade names (capitalized) and synonyms are provided.

Occurrence: Humans are exposed to halomethanes by any of three primary routes: (a) intake in water or other fluids; (b) ingestion in food; and (c) inhalation. In certain circumstances (e.g., occupational), exposure by skin absorption may be significant. Halomethanes have been identified in air, water and food, but information concerning relative exposure for specific compounds via the different media is incomplete. Inhalation and/or ingestion of fluids are probably the most important routes of human exposure (38-1). Presence of the halomethanes in the environment is generally the result of natural, anthropogenic, or secondary sources. The monohalomethanes (bromo-, chloro-, iodomethane) are believed natural in origin with the oceans as a primary source. Natural sources have also been proposed for dichloromethane, tribromomethane, and certain other halomethanes (38-1). Anthropogenic sources of environmental contamination, such as manufacturing and use emissions are important for several halomethanes. (See the section on "Uses" which follows.)

Secondary sources of halomethanes include such processes as the use of chlorine to treat municipal drinking water and some industrial wastes, and the combustion and thermal degradation of products or waste materials, wherein secondary formation reactions or incidental contamination occur (38-1).

The relatively high water solubilities of chloromethane and bromomethane and their relatively high vapor pressures indicate that they have a low potential to bioconcentrate in aquatic species. The predicted bioconcentration factors are 2 and 6, respectively.

Methylene chloride is a major halogenated pollutant with a large potential for delivery of chlorine to the stratosphere. The photooxidation of the compound in the troposphere probably proceeds with a half-life of several months, similar to the case of methyl chloride. The principal oxidation product of methylene chloride is phosgene which results from the two hydrogens being abstracted from the molecule. It is conceivable that this phosgene may be photolyzed to yield chlorine atoms in the ozone-rich region of the stratosphere. It thus appears that there is some potential for ozone destruction by methylene chloride since the generated chlorine atoms will attack ozone (38-4).

Similarly, fully halogenated substances such as trichlorofluoromethane and dichlorodifluoromethane migrate to the stratosphere where they are photodissociated, adversely affecting the ozone balance (38-4). Trichlorofluoromethane does not significantly bioconcentrate in aquatic organisms. There are few data in the literature relating to the environmental fate or degradation of bromodichloromethane and tribromomethane.

Physical Properties: The physical characteristics of the halomethanes are listed in Table 61.

Table 61: Physical Characteristics of Halomethanes

Compound	Physical State Under Ambient Conditions*	MP (°C)	BP (°C)	Specific Gravity	Vapor Pressure (mm Hg)	Solubility in Water (μg/l)	Solubility in Organic Solvents
Chloro-methane	Gas	-97.73	-24.2	0.973**		5.38×10^6	Alcohol, ether, acetone, benzene, chloroform, acetic acid
Bromo-methane	Gas	-93.6	3.56	1.737**		1×10^6	Alcohol, ether, acetic acid
Dichloro-methane	Liquid	-95.1	40	1.327***	362.4***	13.2×10^6†	Alcohol, ether
Trichloro-fluoromethane	Liquid	-111	23.82	1.467†	667.4***	1.1×10^6***	Alcohol, ether
Dichloro-difluoromethane	Gas	-158	-29.79	1.75††	4,306***	2.8×10^5†	Alcohol, ether
Tribromo-methane	Liquid	8.3	149.5	2.890***		Slightly sol.	Alcohol, ether, benzene, chlorform, ligroin
Bromo-dichloromethane	Liquid	-57.1	90	1.980***		Insoluble	Alcohol, ether, acetone, benzene, chloroform

*All compounds are colorless.
**10°C.
***20°C.
†25°C.
††115°C.

Source: Reference (38).

Chemical Properties: Monohalomethanes can be hydrolyzed slowly in neutral waters forming methanol and hydrogen halide. The rate of hydrolysis increases with size of the halogen moiety. In seawater iodomethane can react with chloride ion to yield chloromethane and this reaction occurs as fast as the exchange of iodomethane into the atmosphere (exchange rate, 4×10^{-7}/sec). The monohalomethanes are not oxidized readily under ordinary conditions. Bromomethane at 14.5% concentrations in air and intense heat will produce a flame. Chloromethane in contact with a flame will burn, producing CO_2 and HCl. Monohalomethanes undergo photolysis in the upper atmosphere where ultraviolet radiation is of sufficient energy to initiate a reaction.

Prolonged heating of dichloromethane with water at 180°C results in the formation of formic acid, methyl chloride, methanol, hydrochloric acid and some carbon monoxide. In contact with water at elevated temperatures, methylene chloride corrodes iron, some stainless steels, copper, and nickel.

Trichlorofluoromethane is nonflammable. Decomposition of tribromomethane is accelerated by air and light.

Uses: These include: chloromethane (chemical intermediate in production of silicone, gasoline antiknock, rubber, herbicides, plastics, and other materials); bromomethane (soil, seed, feed, and space fumigant agents); dichloromethane (paint remover, solvent, aerosol sprays, plastics processing); tribromomethane (chemical intermediate); bromodichloromethane (used as a reagent in research); dichlorodifluoromethane and trichlorofluoromethane (refrigerant and aerosol propellant uses) (38-1, 38-2).

Toxic Effects: Chloromethane has been demonstrated to be toxic to aquatic organisms at levels of 270,000 to 550,000 μg/l (96 hr LC_{50} values) in controlled laboratory tests (38-5). Corresponding acute toxicity values for bromomethane range from 11,000 to 12,000 μg/l. Dichloromethane LC_{50} values range from 224,000 to 331,000 μg/l (38-6). Tribromomethand LC_{50} values range from 17,900 to 46,500 μg/l. The latter compound demonstrates aquatic organism chronic toxicity effects at 14,000 to 24,000 μg/l.

The toxic nature of methyl chloride on humans is thought to act on the central nervous system. In a mild to moderate intoxication, the symptoms consist of blurring of vision, headache, vertigo, loss of coordination, slurring of speech, staggering, mental confusion, nausea, and vomiting. A severe exposure involves rapid loss of consciousness leading to death (38-7).

Chloromethane is highly mutagenic to the bacteria, *Salmonella typhimurium* TA 1535 (38-8) and to the bacteria, *Salmonella typhimurium* TA 100 (38-9).

Inhalation of bromomethane is the usual route of systemic poisoning, but gastrointestinal absorption is a possibility (38-10). Following exposure, irritation of eyes and mucous membranes may be noticeable. Within a few hours, malaise, headache, and nausea develop. After 2 to 16 hours, the more serious symptoms develop, including visual disturbance, speech disturbance, irrational behavior, drunkenness and drowsiness. Under serious exposure, neurologic and psychiatric abnormalities may persist for months or years. As with chloromethane, bromomethane has been reported to be mutagenic in *Salmonella* bacterial test systems (38-9).

In nonhuman mammals, methylene chloride inhalation at levels of 1,000 and 5,000 ppm (3,477 and 17,383 mg/m^3) for not more than 14 hours resulted in severe weight losses, liver injury, hepatic failures, and death (38-11). In humans, methylene chloride is a central nervous system depressant resulting in narcosis at high concentrations (38-12). Inhalation levels of 500 to 1,000 ppm (1,738 to 3,477 mg/m^3) resulted in elevated carboxyhemoglobin saturation levels as well as signs and symptoms of central nervous system depression (38-13).

Dichloromethane demonstrated mutagenic properties in *Salmonella typhimurium* TA 100 and in immunosuppressed mice (38-9). The compound also demonstrated a carcinogenic response in mice (38-14), but the significance of results from this test are open to question. The carcinogenicity of dichloromethane was reported to be under study by the National Cancer Institute as of 1977.

Trichlorofluoromethane has completely inhibited the growth of several species of microorganisms at vapor concentrations of 5.62 x 10^4 to 5.62 x 10^6 mg/m^3 (38-15). In atmospheric ambient conditions of a 1:1 mixture of oxygen and dichlorodifluoromethane, a significant increase in the mutation rate of the yeast, *Neurospora crassa*, was noted (38-16). Slater (38-17) administered trichlorofluoromethane to the stomach of rats and noted no effect on serum-β-glucuronidase activity or liver NADPH levels. Taylor (38-18) noted that exposure to 7% oxygen and 15% trichlorofluoromethane caused cardiac arrhythmias in all rabbits exposed. Only a slight hyperglycemia with hyperlacticacidemia was noted in rats, rabbits, and dogs exposed to ambient atmospheric conditions of 5% trichlorofluoromethane (38-19). In dogs, trichlorofluoromethane caused a depression of myocardial function (38-20) and in the upper respiratory tract lead to an initial apnea, bradycardia, and a fall in aortic blood pressure (38-21). Azar, et al. (38-22), noted that human inhalation of 1,000 ppm (4,949 mg/m^3) dichlorodifluoromethane did not reveal any adverse effect, while exposure to 10,000 ppm (49,489 mg/m^3) resulted only in a 7% reduction in a standardized psycho-motor test score.

Tribromomethane is considered to be highly toxic to both nonhuman mammalian species and humans. The compound has been shown to be mutagenic in the *Salmonella typhimurium* TA 100 and TA 1535 test systems (38-9) and carcinogenic in mice (38-14), with the same qualifications for result significance as for dichloromethane noted. Cantor, et al. (38-23), have reported positive correlations between cancer mortality rates and levels of brominated trihalomethanes in drinking water in epidemiological studies.

Bromodichloromethane is acutely toxic to mice (38-24). It was mutagenic in the *Salmonella typhimurium* TA 100 bacterial test system (38-9) and carcinogenic in mice (38-14) with the same qualification for result significance as for dichloromethane noted. Cantor, et al. (38-23), have reported positive correlations between cancer mortality rates and levels of brominated trihalomethanes in drinking water in epidemiological studies.

Current Levels of Exposure: Data on current levels of the halomethanes in water, food, and ambient air are not sufficient to permit adequate estimates of total human exposures from these media. Available data discussed earlier in the section "Occurrence" indicate that the greatest human exposure to the trihalomethanes occurs through the consumption of liquids (including drinking water and beverages containing it), and that exposure to chlorofluorocarbons, chloromethane, dichloromethane, and bromomethane occurs primarily by inhalation.

Special Groups at Risk: Perhaps the greatest concern for special risk considerations among the halomethanes is that for dichloromethane. In this case, the added threat is for those such as smokers or workers in whom significant COHb levels exist, or those with preexisting heart disease, for whom COHb formation by dichloromethane metabolism would present an added stress or precipitate an episode from disturbed oxygen transport. NIOSH, recognizing this combined stress hazard, has recommended lowering the existing TLV for dichloromethane and tying it with existing CO exposure levels.

A second possible special risk concerns exposure to fluorocarbon vapors. In this case there is evidence that a characteristic toxicity involves sensitization to cardioarrhythmogenic effects of endogenous or administered epinephrine and related catecholamines. An individual with cardiac disease taking certain medication or in an acutely stressed state may be especially susceptible to fluorocarbon cardiotoxicity.

Existing Guidelines and Standards: *Chloromethane* —

1. Warning label required by Federal Insecticide, Fungicide and Rodenticide Act (FIFRA). Interpretation with respect to warning, caution, and antidote statements required to appear on labels of economic poisons.

2. Food tolerance requirements of Federal Food, Drug and Cosmetic Act—chloromethane is permitted as propellant in pesticide formulations up to 30% of finished formulation when used in food storage/processing areas not contacting fatty foods.

3. Human exposure—A maximum permissible concentration (MPC) of 5 mg/m^3 in industrial plant atmospheres was established in Russia based on rat studies of chronic poisoning; and OSHA has established the maximum acceptable time-weighted average air concentration for daily 8 hour occupational exposure at 210 mg/m^3 with ceiling and peak (5 minutes during or in any 3 hours) concentration values of 413 and 620 mg/m^3, respectively.

4. Other—Chlorinated hydrocarbons are under consideration for addition to the list of compounds for Toxic Effluent Standards.

5. Multimedia Environmental Goals, (MEG), Estimated Permissible Concentrations (EPC): 0.5 mg/m^3 air, health; 2.9 to 7.5 mg/l water,

health; and 5.8 mg/kg land, health.

Bromomethane —

1. A warning and antidote labeling required by FIFRA. Interpretation with respect to warning, caution, and antidote statements required to appear on labels of economic poisons.

2. Food tolerance limits required under Federal Food, Drug and Cosmetic Act Tolerances for residues of inorganic bromides resulting from fumigation with methyl bromide. Regulations set inorganic bromide residue concentration limits for many food commodities at levels ranging from 20 to 400 mg/kg.

3. Human exposure—Occupational exposure during 8 hour work day limited to 78 mg/m^3 by the Texas State Department of Health; also regulated are use periods for respirators. OSHA has established the 8 hour air concentration ceiling for occupational exposure at 80 mg/m^3, with an added warning of skin exposure hazard. The American National Standards Institute has set a standard of 58 mg/m^3 time-weighted average air concentration for an 8 hour day, with interlocking period ceilings of 97 mg/m^3, and 194 mg/m^3 (5 minutes). The industrial TLV (threshold limit value) of 78 mg/m^3 to prevent neurotoxic and pulmonary effects was established by the American Conference of Governmental Industrial Hygienists.

Dichloromethane —

1. As an oil and fat solvent, dichloromethane is allowed in spice oleoresins at up to 30 mg/kg and in decaffeinated coffee at up to 10 mg/kg.

2. Human exposure—OSHA has established occupational exposure standards as follows: 8 hour time weighted average (TWA), 1,737 mg/m^3; acceptable ceiling concentration, 3,474 mg/m^3; and acceptable maximum peak above ceiling, 6,948 mg/m^3 (5 minutes in any 3 hours). However, in recognition of metabolic formation of COHb and additive toxicity with CO, NIOSH (38-28) has recommended a 10 hour workday TWA exposure limit of 75 ppm (261 mg/m^3) in the presence of no more CO than 9.9 mg/m^3 TWA and a 1,737 mg/m^3 peak (15 minute sampling); in the case of higher CO levels, lower levels of dichloromethane are required. Permissible exposure levels in several other countries range from 49 up to 1,737 mg/m^3 (maximum allowable concentration) or 2,456 mg/m^3 (peak). The maximum permissible concentration for dichloromethane in water in the USSR is 7.5 mg/l; this is intended to be proportionately reduced in the presence of other limited compounds.

3. MEG values for Estimated Permissible Concentrations (EPC): 0.619 mg/m^3 air, health; 3.59 to 9.18 mg/l water, health; and 7.2 mg/kg land, health.

Trihalomethanes — The U.S. EPA has considered the available health and exposure data for trihalomethanes as a group, determined that they represent a potential yet reducible hazard to public health, and proposed regulations establishing a maximum contaminant level (MCL) of 0.100 mg/l for total trihalomethanes (TTHM) in finished drinking water of cities greater than 75,000 (served population) employing added disinfectants.

Tribromomethane — The OSHA Occupational Exposure Standard for workroom air (8 hour TWA) is 5 mg/m^3, with a dermal absorption warning notation. Tribromomethane is one of four trihalomethanes comprising the total trihalomethanes group for which the U.S. EPA has proposed to regulate a maximum contaminant level in drinking water (0.100 mg/l).

Bromodichloromethane –

Human exposure: (1) There is no currently established occupational exposure standard for bromodichloromethane in the U.S.

(2) Bromodichloromethane, along with chlorodibromomethane, trichloromethane (chloroform) and tribromomethane form the group of halomethanes termed total trihalomethanes (TTHM), which are to be regulated in finished drinking water in the U.S. The maximum permissible concentration set for TTHM in the proposed regulations is 0.100 mg/l.

Trichlorofluoromethane and Dichlorodifluoromethane –

Food use: FDA regulations permit use of dichlorodifluoromethane (F-12) as a direct contact freezing agent for food, and specify labeling and instructions for use.

Human exposure: (1) The current OSHA 8 hour TWA occupational standards for F-11 and F-12 are 5,600 and 4,950 mg/m^3, respectively.

(2) Underwriters Laboratories classify F-11 and F-12 in groups 5 and 6, respectively.

Other Considerations –

(1) F-11, F-12, and several other fluorocarbons have been exempted from regulation under the Texas Clean Air Act.

(2) The U.S. EPA can control fluorocarbon uses in pesticide applications and has requested formulators to seek suitable alternative propellants for products dispensed as aerosols, in view of the ozone depletion concern.

(3) Pressurized containers must meet ICC regulations for compressed gases to be shipped.

Summary of Proposed EPA Criteria: *Freshwater Aquatic Life* – For methyl chloride the criterion to protect freshwater aquatic life as derived using procedures other than the Guidelines is 7,000 µg/l as a 24 hour average and the concentration should never exceed 16,000 µg/l at any time.

For methyl bromide the criterion to protect freshwater aquatic life as derived using procedures other than the Guidelines is 140 µg/l as a 24 hour average and the concentration should never exceed 320 µg/l at any time.

For methylene chloride the criterion to protect freshwater aquatic life as derived using procedures other than the Guidelines is 4,000 µg/l as a 24 hour average and the concentration should never exceed 9,000 µg/l at any time.

For bromoform the criterion to protect freshwater aquatic life as derived using procedures other than the Guidelines is 840 µg/l as a 24 hour average and the concentration should never exceed 1,900 µg/l at any time.

Saltwater Aquatic Life – For methyl chloride the criterion to protect saltwater aquatic life as derived using procedures other than the Guidelines is 3,700 µg/l as a 24 hour average and the concentration should never exceed 8,400 µg/l at any time.

For methyl bromide the criterion to protect saltwater aquatic life as derived using procedures other than the Guidelines is 170 µg/l as a 24 hour average and the concentration should never exceed 380 µg/l at any time.

For methylene chloride the criterion to protect saltwater aquatic life as derived using procedures other than the Guidelines is 1,900 µg/l as a 24 hour average and the concentration should never exceed 4,400 µg/l at any time.

For bromoform the criterion to protect saltwater aquatic life as derived using the Guidelines is 180 μg/l as a 24 hour average and the concentration should never exceed 420 μg/l at any time.

Human Health — For the protection of human health from the toxic properties of halomethanes ingested through water and through contaminated aquatic organisms, the ambient water criteria for the halomethanes are:

Compound	Criterion level (μg/l)
Chloromethane (methyl chloride)	2
Bromomethane (methyl bromide)	2
Dichloromethane (methylene chloride)	2
Bromodichloromethane	2
Tribromomethane (bromoform)	2
Dichlorodifluoromethane	3,000
Trichlorofluoromethane	32,000

Basis for the Proposed Human Health Criteria: Data on current levels of the halomethanes in water, food, and ambient air are not sufficient to permit adequate estimates of total human exposures from these media.

Available data discussed in an earlier section of this report "Occurrence" indicate that the greatest human exposure to the trihalomethanes occurs through the consumption of liquids (including drinking water and beverages containing it), and that exposure to chlorofluoro-carbons, chloromethane, dichloromethane and bromomethane occurs primarily by inhalation.

Observed correlations among concentrations of trihalomethanes in finished water are attributed to the presence of common organic precursor materials in raw water. Among the halomethanes considered in this report, bromodichloromethane seems to predominate in drinking waters. Concentrations of bromodichloromethane in raw and finished water samples are generally in the area of 6 μg/l or less, and thus represent a reasonable upper limit for anticipated levels of any halomethane in water (excluding chloroform and carbon tetrachloride).

Recent reports showing that chloromethane, bromomethane, tribromomethane, dichloromethane and bromodichloromethane exhibit carcinogenic and/or mutagenic effects in certain bioassay systems suggest the need for conservation in the development of water quality criteria for the protection of human health. Since the presently available carcinogenicity data base for these compounds is judged qualitatively informative but quantitatively inadequate for risk extrapolation, an alternative approach is necessary for criteria development.

At present levels in relatively unpolluted raw and finished waters (10 μg/l), the halomethanes pose little threat for the production of noncarcinogenic toxic effects in humans. However, the possibility of carcinogenic effects must be evaluated in light of current and past exposures to halomethanes via water supplies. Limited epidemiologic studies have failed to show a clear association between cancer mortality and bromine-containing trihalomethanes at levels in water of about 5 to 10 μg/l.

Since the possible association between human cancers and halomethanes cannot presently be disproven, it would be wise to limit their presence in water to no more than the median levels which are currently encountered (pending better human risk data). Thus, a maximum level of 6 μg/l in raw and finished waters could be considered as acceptable for bromomethane, chloromethane, dichloromethane, tribromomethane, and bromodichloromethane. From the limited animal bioassay data which are available in the strain A mouse lung tumor system, a daily human intake of halomethanes at 12 μg/day (6 μg/l x 2 l/day) represents a dose which is about 100,000 fold less than the minimum daily dose of tribromomethane which caused a significant increase in tumor formation in mice. Since there exists considerable uncertainty over the human carcinogenic risks of halomethanes, a safety factor of 100,000 seems prudent for the development of an interim standard for all halomethanes pending the results of further research.

The 6 μg/l maximum acceptable concentration for bromomethane, chloromethane, tribromomethane, dichloromethane and bromodichloromethane does not take into consideration the contribution to total exposure from air and food. Exposure via these media cannot be accurately predicted, although it is likely that it is sufficiently large for chloromethane, dichloromethane and bromomethane to warrant the recommendation of a water quality criterion below 6 μg/l. Present levels of these three compounds are generally much less than 6 μg/l and it is not likely that current anthropogenic sources would significantly increase their level in water.

For criteria setting purposes it is recommended that a criterion of 2 μg/l be adopted for this group of halomethanes, based upon analogy to the structure and biological activity of chloroform. Despite the presently inadequate data base for most of these compounds, it can nevertheless be predicted that similar biological effects, including neoplastic transformation, may be encountered. Since the recommended criterion for chloroform was derived from reliable experimental data, it represents the most applicable value for all of the halomethanes which are suspected carcinogens.

Evidence for mutagenicity of dichlorodifluoromethane is equivocal and there is no evidence as yet for carcinogenicity as a result of direct exposure. Chronic toxicity data for dichlorofluoromethane are quite limited. In the only long-term (two years) feeding study reported (38-3) which cites (38-25), the maximum dose level producing no observed adverse effect (in dogs) was 80 mg/kg/day. Applying an uncertainty factor of 1,000 (38-26) to this data yields a presumptive "acceptable daily intake" of 0.08 mg/kg/day. For a man weighing 70 kg, consuming 2 liters of water per day and absorbing at 100% efficiency, and assuming that the water is the sole source of exposure, this acceptable intake level translates into a criterion level as follows: (0.08) (70)/2 = 2.8 mg/l.

There is no evidence for mutagenicity of trichlorofluoromethane, and no evidence as yet for carcinogenicity as a result of direct exposure. The only data on toxicity testing using prolonged exposure at relatively low test concentrations are from a report (38-27) which showed no observed adverse effects in rats and guinea pigs exposed continuously by inhalation for 90 days at 5,610 mg/m^3. If the reference man weighing 70 kg breathed this atmosphere and absorbed the compound at 50% efficiency, his estimated exposure dose would be 5,610 x 23 x 0.5 = 64,515 mg/day or 922 mg/kg/day. Applying an uncertainty factor of 1,000 (38-26) to this data yields a presumptive "acceptable daily intake" of 0.922 mg/kg/day for trichlorofluoromethane. Assuming man's weight to be 70 kg and his absorption of ingested compound to be 100% efficient, and that his sole source of exposure is water consumed at 2 l/day, the acceptable intake is translated into a criterion level as follows: (0.922) (70)/2 = 32.3 mg/l.

Criterion levels intended to protect the public against unacceptable risk of toxicity mutagenicity, or carcinogenicity from exposure to selected halomethanes in water for consumption, derived as described in the foregoing text, are summarized above under "Summary of Proposed EPA Criteria."

Adoption of the presently recommended criterion for chloroform (2μg/l) as the recommended level for other possibly carcinogenic halomethanes should provide an adequate margin of safety in the absence of sufficient data for quantitative risk assessment. This criterion is intended to reduce carcinogenic risks to the public, and takes into account the fact that exposure to halomethanes also occurs through foods and via inhalation. Although the potential carcinogenicity of bromodichloromethane, tribromomethane, dichloromethane, bromomethane and chloromethane cannot be adequately assessed at present, the adoption of an interim water quality standard in excess of 2 μg/l may be interpreted as approval to discharge larger quantities of these substances than of chloroform. Such a practice is clearly unwarranted until such time that concerns over possible carcinogenic activity have been resolved.

References

(38-1)   National Academy of Sciences. *Nonfluorinated Halomethanes in the Environment*, Washington, D.C. (1978).

(38-2)   Davis, C.N. et al., *Investigation of Selected Potential Environmental Contaminants: Monohalomethanes,* Report EPA 560/2-77-007, Washington, D.C. (1977).

(38-3)   Howard, P.H. et al., *Environmental Hazard Assessment of One and Two Carbon Fluorocarbons,* Report EPA 560/2-75-003, Washington, D.C. (1974).

(38-4)   U.S. EPA *Report on the Problem of Halogenated Air Pollutants and Stratospheric Ozone.* Report No. EPA 600/9-75-008. Washington, D.C. (1975).

(38-5)   Dawson, G.W. et al., "The Acute Toxicity of 47 Industrial Chemicals to Fresh and Saltwater Fishes." *Jour. Hazard. Mater. 1,* 303 (1977).

(38-6)   U.S. EPA *In-depth Studies on Health and Environmental Impacts of Selected Water Pollutants.* Report on Contract No. 68-01-4646. Washington, D.C. (1978).

(38-7)   MacDonald, J.D.C. "Methyl Chloride Intoxication." *Jour. Occup. Med. 6,* 81 (1964).

(38-8)   Andrews, A.W. et al., "A Comparison of the Mutagenic Properties of Vinyl Chloride and Methyl Chloride." *Mutat. Res. 40,* 273 (1976).

(38-9)   Simmon, V.F. et al., "Mutagenic Activity of Chemicals Identified in Drinking Water." Presented at 2nd Int. Conf. Environ, Mutagens. Edinburgh, Scotland (July, 1977).

(38-10) Collins, R.P. "Methyl Bromide Poisoning." *Calif. Med. 103,* 112 (1965).

(38-11) Haun, C.C. et al., *Continuous Animal Exposure to Methylene Chloride.* Aerospace Med. Res. Lab. Wright Patterson Air Force Base, Ohio (1971).

(38-12) Berger, M. and Fodor, G.G., "Zentralnervose Storunger inter Einfluso Dichloromethanhaltiger Luftgemische-2b1." *Bakt.,* Abt. 1, Ref. 215, 1963, 503 (1969).

(38-13) Stewart, R.D. et al., "Experimental Human Exposure to Methylene Chloride." *Arch. Environ. Health 25,* 342 (1972).

(38-14) Theiss, J.C. et al., "Test for Carcinogenicity of Organic Contaminants of United States Drinking Waters by Pulmonary Tumor Response in Strain A Mice." *Cancer Res. 37,* 2717 (1977).

(38-15) Van Auken, et al., "Comparison of the Effects of Three Fluorocarbons on Certain Bacteria." *Can. Jour. Microbiol. 21,* 221 (1975).

(38-16) Stephens, S. et al., "Phenotypic and Genetic Effects of *Neurospora Crassa* Produced by Selected Gases and Gases Mixed with Oxygen." *Dev. Ind. Microbiol. 12,* 346 (1971).

(38-17) Slater, T.F. "A Note on the Relative Toxic Activities of Tetrachloromethane and Trichlorfluoromethane on the Rat." *Biochem. Pharmacol. 14,* 178 (1965).

(38-18) Taylor, G.J. "Cardiac Arrhythmias in Hypoxic Rabbits During Aerosol Propellant Inhalation." *Arch. Environ. Health 30,* (1975).

(38-19) Paulet, G. et al., "Fluorocarbons and General Metabolism in the Rat, Rabbit, and Dog." *Toxicol. Appl. Pharmacol. 34,* 197 (1975).

(38-20) Aviado, D.M. and Belej, M.A., "Toxicity of Aerosol Propellants in the Respiratory and Circulatory Systems. Ventricular Function in the Dog." *Toxicology 3,* 79 (1975).

(38-21) Aviado, D.M., "Cardiopulmonary Effects of Fluorocarbon Compounds." Aerospace Med. Res. Lab. Wright Patterson Air Force Base, Ohio (1971).

(38-22) Azar, A. et al., "Experimental Human Exposure to Fluorocarbon 12 (Dichlorodifluoromethane." *Am. Ind. Hyg. Assoc. Jour. 33,* 207 (1972).

(38-23) Cantor, K.P. et al., 1977. Associations of Halomethanes in Drinking Water with Cancer Mortality. *Jour. Natl. Cancer Inst.* (In press) (1977).

(38-24) Bowman, F.G. et al., "The Toxicity of Some Halomethanes in Mice." *Toxicol. Appl. Pharmacol. 44,* 213 (1978).

(38-25) Sherman, H., "Long Term Feeding Studies in Rats and Dogs with Dichlorodifluoromethane (Freon 12 Food Freezant)." Unpublished Report, Haskell Laboratory, Wilmington, Delaware, E.I. DuPont de Nemours and Company (1974).

(38-26) National Academy of Sciences, *Drinking Water and Health,* Washington, D.C. (1977).

(38-27) Jenkins, L.J. et al., "Repeated and Continuous Exposure of Laboratory Animals to Trichlorofluoromethane," *Toxicol. Appl. Pharmacol.16,* 133 (1970).

(38-28) National Institute for Occupational Safety and Health, *Criteria for a Recommended Standard: Occupational Exposure to Methylene Chloride,* DHEW Publ. No. (NIOSH) 76-138, Washington, D.C. (1976).

HEPTACHLOR (#39)

Heptachlor is a chlorinated cyclodiene insecticide having the structural formula:

It has the molecular formula $C_{10}H_5Cl_7$ and the chemical name of 1,4,5,6,7,8,8-heptachloro-3a,4,7,7a-tetrahydro-4,7-methanoindene. It has a molecular weight of 373.35.

Occurrence: Heptachlor is produced by means of a Diels-Alder addition reaction which joins cyclopentadiene to hexachlorocyclopentadiene. Heptachlor was tentatively identified at levels greater than 0.002 µg/l in 15 of 96 river water samples tested by Weaver, et al. (39-1).

Heptachlor and/or heptachlor epoxide have been reported present in plankton-algae and aquatic insects, crayfish, crabs, shellfish and fish. Heptachlor and heptachlor epoxide will bioconcentrate in numerous species and will accumulate in the food chain. Heptachlor/heptachlor epoxide bioconcentration factors as high as 17,600 in the oyster, *Crassostrea virginica*, have been reported.

Heptachlor epoxide is readily stored in the adipose tissue of rats and dogs but may also be found in liver, brain, and other tissues. It has been found in human milk samples and has also been detected in fetal blood and placenta.

The persistence of heptachlor and heptachlor epoxide in the environment is well known. Heptachlor also has been shown to be converted to the more toxic metabolite, heptachlor epoxide, in various soils and plants.

Physical Properties: Pure heptachlor is a white crystalline solid with a camphorlike odor and a vapor pressure of 3×10^{-4} mm Hg at 25°C. It has a solubility in water of 0.056 mg/l at 25° to 29°C and is readily soluble in relatively nonpolar solvents.

Technical grade heptachlor has the typical composition of approximately 73% heptachlor, 21% trans (gamma) chlordane, 5% heptachlor and 1% chlordene isomers. Technical heptachlor is a tan, soft, waxy solid with a melting point range of 46° to 74°C. It has a vapor pressure of 4×10^{-4} mm Hg at 25°C and a density of 1.65 to 1.67 g/ml at 25°C.

Chemical Properties: In general, heptachlor is quite stable to chemical reactions such as dehydrochlorination, autooxidation, and thermal decomposition. However, in the environment, heptachlor undergoes numerous microbial, biochemical, and photochemical reactions.

Microbial conversion yields heptachlor epoxide which exhibits equal or greater toxicity than the parent compound. Photochemical conversion yields photoheptachlor which is more toxic than heptachlor. Biological conversion yields metabolites of lesser toxicity than the starting material.

Uses: Heptachlor is a broad spectrum insecticide. It was introduced in 1948 as a contact insecticide as E 3314 and Velsicol 104. During the period 1971 to 1975 the most important use of heptachlor was to control soil insects for corn cultivation and other crop production. Since 1975 both the applications and production volume of heptachlor have undergone dramatic changes as a result of the sole producer's voluntary restriction of domestic use and subsequent issuance by the Environmental Protection Agency of a registration suspension notice for all food crops and home use of heptachlor, effective August 2, 1976. However, significant commercial use of heptachlor for termite control or nonfood plants continues and numerous formulation plants and packaging facilities have remained in operation.

Toxic Effects: Heptachlor has been demonstrated to be highly toxic to aquatic life, to persist for prolonged periods in the environment, to bioconcentrate in organisms at various trophic levels, and to exhibit carcinogenic activity in mice.

Current Levels of Exposure: Various investigators have detected heptachlor and/or heptachlor epoxide in the major river basins of the United States with a mean concentration of 0.0063 μg/l for those instances of detection.   Food can add to man's exposure to heptachlor and metabolites through biomagnification in the food chain.

The FDA showed that in their market basket study covering August 1974 to July 1975 for 20 different cities, 3 of 12 food classes contained residues of heptachlor epoxide ranging from 0.0006 to 0.003 ppm.

A national study by the U.S. Department of Interior in 1967 and 1968 reported that heptachlor and/or heptachlor epoxide were found in 32% of 590 fish samples examined with whole fish residues of from 0.01 to 8.33 mg/kg.   Schimmel, et al., (39-2) reported an average bioconcentration factor of 12,000 for the sheepshead minnow which will subsequently be used in risk calculations as being representative of fish bioconcentration potential.

Nisbet (39-3) calculated the typical human exposure to heptachlor to be 0.01 μg/individual/day based on an ambient air mean concentration of 0.5 ng/m^3 and breathing 20 m^3 of air per day.   Nisbet further states that even in Jackson, Miss., which has a mean air level as high as 6.3 ng/m^3, the average individual would inhale only 0.13 μg/day of heptachlor.

The significance of these figures is dependent upon the efficiency of lung absorption which does not appear to be reported for humans (39-3).   Based on this, it appears that inhalation is not a major route for human exposure to heptachlor.

Special Groups at Risk: Infants have been exposed to heptachlor and heptachlor epoxide through mothers' milk, cows' milk, and commercially prepared baby foods.   It appears that infants raised on mothers' milk run a greater risk of ingesting heptachlor epoxide than if they were fed cows' milk and/or commercially prepared baby food.

Nisbet (39-3) found that persons living and working in or near heptachlor treated areas had a particularly high inhalation exposure potential.

Existing Guidelines and Standards: Table 62 summarizes the status of published standards for heptachlor exposure in various countries.

Table 62:   Published Standards for Heptachlor Exposure

Agency	Published Standard	Reference
OSHA	500 μg/m^3 * on skin from air	(39-4)
ACGIH (TLV)	500 μg/m^3 inhaled	(39-5)
Fed. Rep. Germany	500 μg/m^3 inhaled	(39-6)
Soviet Union	10 μg/m^3 ceiling value inhaled	(39-6)
WHO**	0.5 μg/kg/day acceptable daily intake in diet	(39-7)
U.S. Pub. Health Serv. Adv. Comm.	Recommended drinking water std. (1968) 18 μg/l of heptachlor and 18 μg/l heptachlor epoxide	(39-7)

   *Time weighted average.

  **Maximum residue limits in certain foods can be found in Food Agric.Organ./ World Health Organ. reports for 1977 and 1978.

Source: Reference (39)

Summary of Proposed EPA Criteria: *Freshwater Aquatic Life* — For heptachlor the criterion to protect freshwater aquatic life as derived using the Guidelines is 0.0015 μg/l as a 24 hour average and the concentration should not exceed 0.45 μg/l at any time.

Saltwater Aquatic Life — For heptachlor the criterion to protect saltwater aquatic life as derived using the Guidelines is 0.0036 μg/l as a 24 hour average and the concentration should not exceed 0.05 μg/l at any time.

Human Health — For the maximum protection of human health from the potential carcinogenic effects of exposure to heptachlor through ingestion of water and contaminated aquatic organisms, the ambient water concentration is zero. Concentrations of heptachlor estimated to result in additional lifetime cancer risks ranging from no additional risk to an additional risk of 1 in 100,000 are presented in the Criterion Formulation section of this document.

The EPA is considering setting criteria at an interim target risk level in the range of 10^{-5}, 10^{-6}, or 10^{-7} with corresponding criteria of 0.23 ng/l, 0.023 ng/l, and 0.0023 ng/l, respectively.

Basis for the Proposed Human Health Criterion: The proposed criterion for heptachlor-heptachlor epoxide in drinking water was derived from the extrapolation of the data presented by Davis (39-8) using a linear, nonthreshold model. The extrapolation methodology can be found in the Methodology Document (39). From this extrapolation the calculated dose of heptachlor/heptachlor epoxide in drinking water was found to be 0.23 ng/l.

Under the Consent Decree in *NRDC vs Train,* criteria are to state "recommended maximum permissible concentrations (including where appropriate, zero) consistent with the protection of aquatic organisms, human health, and recreational activities." Heptachlor is suspected of being a human carcinogen. Because there is no recognized safe concentration for a human carcinogen, the recommended concentration of heptachlor in water for maximum protection of human health is zero.

Because attaining a zero concentration level may be infeasible in cases and in order to assist the Agency and States in the possible future development of water quality regulations, the concentrations of heptachlor corresponding to several incremental lifetime cancer risk levels have been estimated. A cancer risk level provides an estimate of the additional incidence of cancer that may be expected in an exposed population. A risk of 10^{-5} for example, indicates a probability of one additional case of cancer for every 100,000 people exposed, a risk of 10^{-6} indicates one additional case of cancer for every million people exposed, and so forth.

In the *Federal Register* notice of availability of draft ambient water quality criteria, EPA stated that it is considering setting criteria at an interim target risk level of 10^{-5}, 10^{-6} or 10^{-7} as shown in Table 63. The risk levels and corresponding criteria in Table 63 are calculated by applying a modified "one-hit" extrapolation model described in the Methodology Document. Since the extrapolation model is linear at low doses, the additional lifetime risk is directly proportional to the water concentration. Therefore, water concentrations corresponding to other risk levels can be derived by multiplying or dividing one of the risk levels and corresponding water concentrations shown in the table by factors such as 10, 100, 1,000, and so forth.

Table 63: Possible Alternative Criteria for Heptachlor

Exposure Assumptions (per day)	Risk Levels and Corresponding Criteria (ng/l)			
	0	10^{-7}	10^{-6}	10^{-5}
2 liters of drinking water and consumption of 18.7 g fish and shellfish*	0	0.0023	0.023	0.23

(continued)

Table 63: (continued)

Exposure Assumptions (per day)	Risk Levels and Corresponding Criteria (ng/l)			
	0	10^{-7}	10^{-6}	10^{-5}
Consumption of fish and shellfish only	0	0.0023	0.023	0.23

*98% of the heptachlor exposure results from the consumption of aquatic organisms which exhibit an average bioconcentration potential of 5,200-fold. The remaining 2% of heptachlor exposure results from drinking water.

Source: Reference (39)

Concentration levels were derived assuming a lifetime exposure to various amounts of heptachlor, (1) occurring from the consumption of both drinking water and aquatic life grown in waters containing the corresponding heptachlor concentrations and, (2) occurring solely from consumption of aquatic life grown in the waters containing the corresponding heptachlor concentrations.

Although total exposure information for heptachlor is discussed and an estimate of the contributions from other sources of exposure can be made, these data will not be factored into ambient water quality criteria formulation until additional analysis can be made. The criteria presented, therefore, assume an incremental risk from ambient water exposure only.

Summary of Pertinent Data — The FDA lifetime carcinogenicity study (39-8) of heptachlor epoxide at 10 ppm in the diet of C3Heb/Fe/J strain mice resulted in liver carcinomas in females in 77 of 81 treated animals and 2 of 54 controls. Using a fish bioaccumulation factor of 5,200, the water concentration estimated to result in a lifetime risk of 10^{-5} is calculated from the extrapolation model using the following parameters:

$$nt = 77$$
$$NT = 81$$
$$nc = 2$$
$$NC = 54$$
$$Le = 104 \text{ weeks}$$
$$le = 104 \text{ weeks}$$
$$d = 10 \times 10^{-6} \times 0.13 \times 10^{-6} \text{ mg food per day/kg body weight} = 1.3 \text{ mg/kg/day}$$
$$w = 0.030 \text{ kg}$$
$$L = 104 \text{ weeks}$$
$$R = 5,200$$

The result is that the water concentration corresponding to a lifetime risk of 10^{-5} is 0.23 (0.233) ng/l.

References

(39-1)   Weaver, L. et al., *Chlorinated Hydrocarbon Pesticides in Major U.S. River Basins.* Publ. Health Rep. 80, 481 (1965).

(39-2)   Schimmel, S.C. et al., "Heptachlor: Uptake, Depuration, Retention and Metabolism by Spot, *Leistomus xanthurus,*" *Jour. Toxicol. Envir. Health, 2, 169 (1976).*

(39-3)   Nisbet, L.C.T., "Human Exposure to Chlordane, Heptachlor and their Metabolites," Unpublished Review Prepared for EPA Cancer Assessment Group, Washington, D.C. (1977).

(39-4)   National Institute for Occupational Safety and Health, *Agricultural Chemicals and Pesticides: A Subfile of the Registry of Toxic Effects of Chemical Substances*, Washington, D.C. (1977).

(39-5)   Amer. Conf. of Govt. Ind. Hygienists, *Threshold Limit Values for Chemical Substances and Physical Agents in the Workroom Environment*, Cincinnati, Ohio (1979).

(39-6)   Winell, M.A., "An International Comparison of Hygienic Standards for Chemicals in the Work Environment," *Ambio 4*, 34 (1975).

(39-7)   National Academy of Sciences, *Drinking Water and Health,* Washington, D.C. (1977).

(39-8)   Davis, K.J., "Pathology Report on Mice Fed Aldrin, Dieldrin, Heptachlor, or Heptachlor Epoxide for Two Years." Internal Memorandum to Dr. A.J. Lehman, U.S. Food Drug Admin. (1965) [Cited in Reference (39)].

HEXACHLOROBENZENE

See "Chlorinated Benzenes" (#14).

HEXACHLOROBUTADIENE (#40)

Hexachlorobutadiene, C_4Cl_6, has the following chemical structure:

$$\begin{array}{cccc}
Cl & & & Cl \\
| & & & | \\
C & = C - C = & C \\
| & | & | & | \\
Cl & Cl & Cl & Cl
\end{array}$$

It is also known as perchlorobutadiene and has a molecular weight of 260.74.

Occurrence: Hexachlorobutadiene (HCBD) is not produced in the United States but is a significant by-product of the manufacture of chlorinated hydrocarbons such as tetrachloroethylene, trichloroethylene, and carbon tetrachloride. Secondary production estimates range from 7.3 to 14.5 million pounds per year (40-1). In 1974, approximately 0.5 million pounds were imported into the U.S. (40-1).

Environmental contamination by HCBD results primarily during the disposal of wastes containing HCBD from chlorinated hydrocarbon industries (40-2). Disposal methods include landfill, high temperature incineration, deep-well injection, and lagoon storage (40-1).

HCBD has been detected in a limited number of surface waters that serve as U.S. drinking water supplies (40-3). Highest levels have been measured in air, water, soil and sediment in the vicinity of chlorinated hydrocarbon industries (40-4).

HCBD appears to be rapidly adsorbed to soil and sediment from contaminated water and is known to concentrate in sediment from water by a factor of 100 (40-5). The presence of HCBD in aquatic life ranges from relatively high levels in freshwater organisms from industrially polluted inland waters (40-4) to considerably less in organisms from marine environments (40-6).

Physical Properties: HCBD, a colorless liquid with a faint turpentinelike odor, has a water solubility of only 5 μg/ml at 20°C, a melting point of –21°C and a vapor pressure of 0.15 mm Hg.

Chemical Properties: Little is known of the chemical properties of hexachlorobutadiene but it is presumably quite inert because of its perchlorinated structure.

Uses: HCBD is used as a solvent for many organic substances; its low vapor pressure gives it a distinct advantage over some other chlorohydrocarbons for this purpose. The largest domestic users of HCBD are chlorine producers, which use it to recover chlorine from "sniff" gas which is cleaned by passage through HCBD.

Other applications of HCBD include its use as an intermediate in the manufacture of rubber compounds and lubricants and as a fluid for gyroscopes (40-1). It is also used as an additive for transformer oils.

Toxic Effects: Studies of the toxicity of HCBD to aquatic organisms indicate that levels below one part per million are biologically significant as indicated by reported LC_{50} values (40-4, 40-5, 40-6).

Experimental evidence in nonhuman mammals shows that HCBD is fetotoxic, neurotoxic, nephrotoxic and is carcinogenic at severely toxic levels (40-7, 40-8, 40-9, 40-10, 40-11).

Current Levels of Exposure: The analytical data available on the distribution of HCBD in the environment suggest that exposure is a localized problem, potentially affecting those living in areas with nearby chemical plants producing parent compounds for which HCBD is a by-product. However, due to the limited number of air and water samples taken, it is difficult to estimate the level of exposure even to those populations living in areas where the heaviest exposure might be encountered.

Special Groups at Risk: A special group at risk would be those workers in an industrial environment where concentrations of HCBD in the air might be present.

Existing Guidelines and Standards: There are no guidelines or standards of record other than a standard of 10 $\mu g/m^3$ for inhalation referenced by Poteryaeva of the Soviet Union (40-7).

Summary of Proposed EPA Criteria: *Freshwater Aquatic Life* — For freshwater aquatic life, no criterion for hexachlorobutadiene can be derived using the Guidelines, and there are insufficient data to estimate a criterion using other procedures.

Saltwater Aquatic Life — For saltwater aquatic life, no criterion for hexachlorobutadiene can be derived using the Guidelines, and there are insufficient data to estimate a criterion using other procedures.

Human Health — For the maximum protection of human health from the potential carcinogenic effects of exposure to hexachlorobutadiene through ingestion of water and contaminated aquatic organisms, the ambient water concentration is zero.

Concentration of hexachlorobutadiene estimated to result in additional lifetime cancer risks ranging from no additional risk to an additional risk of 1 in 100,000 are presented in the "Criterion Formulation" section of this document.

The EPA is considering setting criteria at an interim target risk level in the range of 10^{-5}, 10^{-6}, or 10^{-7} with corresponding criteria of 0.77 $\mu g/l$, 0.077 $\mu g/l$, and 0.0077 $\mu g/l$, respectively.

Basis for the Proposed Human Health Criteria: HCBD exhibits acute, subacute and chronic toxicity in animal test systems. The kidney appears to be the organ most sensitive to HCBD. Chronic effects are observed at doses as low as 2 to 3 mg/kg/day in rats.

Renal tubular neoplasms were observed during a 2 year study in which 20 mg/kg/day were administered to rats in their diet. Single oral doses as low as 8.4 mg/kg have been observed to have a deleterious effect on the kidney. The carcinogenic effects of renal tubular adenomas and adenocarcinomas were strongly demonstrated at the 20 mg/kg/day dosage.

In addition, a dose-dependent increase in reversion rate was observed upon adding HCBD without activation to cultures of *S. typhimurium*. Although the observed rate was not quite double the background rate a mutagenic potential for HCBD is indicated.

The evidence of carcinogencity is sufficient to conclude that HCBD is a suspect human carcinogen. As carcinogens are generally assumed to have a nonthreshold dose/response characteristic, the carcinogenic effect is the most significant exposure effect from which to estimate an ambient water quality criterion value.

Under the Consent Decree in *NRDC vs Train,* criteria are to state "recommended maximum permissible concentrations (including where appropriate, zero) consistent with the protection of aquatic organisms, human health, and recreational activities."

Hexachlorobutadiene is suspected of being a human carcinogen. Because there is no recognized safe concentration for a human carcinogen, the recommended concentration of hexachlorobutadiene in water for maximum protection of human health is zero.

Since attaining a zero concentration level may be infeasible in some cases and in order to assist the EPA and States in the possible future development of water quality regulations, the concentrations of hexachlorobutadiene corresponding to several incremental lifetime cancer risk levels have been estimated.

A cancer risk level provides an estimate of the additional incidence of cancer that may be expected in an exposed population. A risk of 10^{-5} for example, indicates a probability of one additional case of cancer for every 100,000 people exposed, a risk of 10^{-6} indicates one additional case of cancer for every million people exposed, and so forth.

In the *Federal Register* notice of availability of draft ambient water quality criteria, EPA stated that it is considering setting criteria at an interim target risk level of 10^{-5}, 10^{-6} or 10^{-7} as shown in Table 64.

In the table the risk levels and corresponding criteria are calculated by applying a modified "one-hit" extrapolation model described in the Methodology Document to animal bioassay data present in "Summary of Pertinent Data."

Since the extrapolation model is linear at low doses, the additional lifetime risk is directly proportional to the water concentration. Therefore, water concentrations corresponding to other risk levels can be derived by multiplying or dividing one of the risk levels and corresponding water concentrations shown in the table by factors such as 10, 100, 1,000 and so forth.

Table 64: Possible Alternative Criteria for Hexachlorobutadiene

Exposure Assumptions (per day)	Risk Levels and Corresponding Criteria (μg/l)			
	0	10^{-7}	10^{-6}	10^{-5}
2 liters of drinking water and consumption of 18.7 g fish and shellfish*	0	0.0077	0.077	0.77
Consumption of fish and shellfish only	0	0.0087	0.087	0.87

*Approximately 89% of the hexachlorobutadiene exposure results from the consumption of aquatic organisms which exhibit an average bioconcentration potential of 870-fold. The remaining 11% of hexachlorobutadiene exposure results from drinking water.

Source: Reference (40)

Concentration levels were derived assuming a lifetime exposure to various amounts of hexachlorobutadiene, (1) occurring from the consumption of both drinking water and aquatic life grown in waters containing the corresponding hexachlorobutadiene concentrations and, (2) occurring solely from consumption of aquatic life grown in the waters containing the corresponding hexachlorobutadiene concentrations. Because data indicating other sources of hexachlorobutadiene exposure and their contributions to total body burden are inadequate for quantitative use, the figures reflect the incremental risks associated with the indicated routes only.

Summary of Pertinent Data — In a 2 year feeding study in rats, Kociba (40-9) observed renal tubular adenomas and carcinomas in males with significantly higher incidence in animals fed 20 mg/kg/day (7/39) than control animals (1/90). Using a fish bioaccumulation factor of 870, the parameters of the extrapolation model are:

$$n_t = 7$$
$$N_t = 39$$
$$n_c = 1$$
$$N_c = 9$$
$$Le = 730 \text{ days}$$
$$le = 669 \text{ days}$$
$$d = 20 \text{ mg/kg/day}$$
$$w = 0.610 \text{ kg}$$
$$L = 730 \text{ days}$$
$$R = 870$$

The result is that the water concentration should be less than 0.77 μg/l in order to keep the individual lifetime risk below 10^{-5}.

References

(40-1)   U.S. EPA, *Survey of Industrial Processing Data. Task I - Hexachlorobenzene and Hexachlorobutadiene Pollution from Chlorocarbon Processing.* Report by Midwest Res. Inst., Kansas City, Mo. Report No. EPA 560/3-75-003. Off. Toxic Subst., Washington, D.C. (1975).

(40-2)   U.S. EPA, *Sampling and Analysis of Selected Toxic Substances. Task IB - Hexachlorobutadiene.* EPA Rep. No. 560/6-76-015. Off. Toxic Subst., Washington, D.C. (1976).

(40-3)   U.S. EPA, *Preliminary Assessment of Suspected Carcinogens in Drinking Water.* In Report to Congress. EPA Report No. 560/4-75-003. Washington, D.C. (1975).

(40-4)   Laseter, J.L., et al., *An Ecological Study of Hexachlorobutadiene (HCBD).* Report No. EPA 560/6-76-010. Off. Toxic Subst., Washington, D.C. (1976).

(40-5)   Leeuwangh, P., et al., "Toxicity of Hexachlorobutadiene in Aquatic Organisms." *Sublethal Effects of Toxic Chemicals on Aquatic Animals.* Proc. Swedish-Netherlands Symp., September 2-5, New York. Elsevier Scientific Publishing Co., Inc. (1975).

(40-6)   Pearson, C.R. and McConnell, G., "Chlorinated C_1 and C_2 Hydrocarbons in the Marine Environment." Proc. R. Soc. London Ser. B 189, 305 (1975).

(40-7)   Poteryaeva, G.E., "Toxicity of Hexachlorobutadiene During Entry into the Organism through the Gastrointestinal Tract." *Gig. Tr. 9*, 98 (1973).

(40-8)   Murzakaev, F.G., "Effect of Small Doses of Hexachlorobutadiene on the Activity of the Central Nervous System and the Morphological Changes in the Organism of Animals Poisoned by it." *Gig. Tr. Prof. Zabol. 11*, 23 (1967).

(40-9)   Kociba, R.J., et al., "Results of a Two-year Chronic Toxicity Study with Hexachlorobutadiene (HCBD) in Rats." *Am. Ind. Hyg. Assoc. 38*, 589 (1977).

(40-10) Schwetz, B., et al., "Results of a Reproduction Study in Rats Fed Diets Containing Hexachlorobutadiene." *Toxicol. Appl. Pharmacol. 42*, 387 (1977).

(40-11) Gage, J., "The Subacute Inhalation Toxicity of 109 Industrial Chemicals." *Br. Jour. Ind. Med. 27*, 1 (1970).

HEXACHLOROCYCLOHEXANE (BHC) (HCH) (#41)

BHC is the common name approved by the International Standards Organization for the mixed configurational isomers of 1,2,3,4,5,6-hexachlorocyclohexane, although the terms BHC and benzene hexachloride are misnomers for this aliphatic compound and should not be confused with aromatic compounds of similar structure, such as the aromatic compound hexachlorobenzene. Lindane is the common name approved by the International Standards

Organization for the insecticidally-active γ-isomer of 1,2,3,4,5,6-hexachlorocyclohexane.

Occurrence: Hexachlorocyclohexane is a broad spectrum insecticide of the group of cyclic chlorinated hydrocarbons called organochlorine insecticides. It consists of a mixture of five configurational isomers and was introduced in 1942 as a contact insecticide as BHC, benzene hexachloride, and 666.

Since its introduction, both the uses and production volume of technical grade BHC have undergone dramatic changes as a result of the discovery that virtually all of the insecticidal activity of BHC resides with its γ-isomer.

By voluntary action, the principal domestic producer of technical grade BHC requested cancellations of its BHC registrations on September 1, 1976. As of July 21, 1978, all registrants of pesticide products containing BHC voluntarily cancelled their registrations or switched their former BHC products to lindane formulations.

On the other hand, significant commercial use of the purified γ-isomer of BHC (lindane) continues. As of January 17, 1977, there were 557 Federal registrations for pesticide products containing lindane and 87 formerly State-registered products containing lindane for which Federal registration has been requested.

Physical Properties: Hexachlorocyclohexane, commonly referred to as BHC or benzene hexachloride, is a brownish-to-white crystalline solid with a phosgenelike odor, a molecular formula of $C_6H_6Cl_6$, a molecular weight of 290.0, a melting point of 65°C, and a solubility in water of 10 to 32 mg/l.

Chemical Properties: The isomers of BHC are not susceptible to photolysis or strong acids but are, with the exception of the β-isomer, dehydrochlorinated by alkalies to form primarily 1,2,4-trichlorobenzene.

Lindane has been shown to be slowly degraded (10% degradation after six weeks) by soil microorganisms and is capable of isomerization to α- and/or Δ-BHC by microorganisms and plants.

Uses: The major commercial usage of HCH is based upon its insecticidal properties. As indicated previously, the γ-isomer has the highest acute toxicity, but the other isomers are not without activity. It is generally advantageous to purify the γ-isomer from the less active isomers. The γ-isomer acts on the nervous system of insects, principally at the level of the nerve ganglia.

As a result, lindane has been used against insects in a wide range of applications including treatment of animals, buildings, man for ectoparasites, clothes, water for mosquitoes, living plants, seeds and soils. Some applications have been abandoned due to excessive residues, e.g., stored foodstuffs.

Toxic Effects: HCH is a persistent stomach poison and contact insecticide with some fumigant action, the activity of which is determined by the content of the γ-isomer. It is nonphytotoxic, except to cucurbits, at insecticidal concentrations, but, at higher concentrations, may cause root deformation and polyploidy. It taints certain crops seriously, especially blackcurrent and potato.

The mammalian toxicities of the isomers differ: alpha, low acute, chronic and cumulative toxicities; beta, low acute, but high chronic and cumulative toxicities; gamma, see below; and delta, low acute and chronic toxicities but irritant to mucous membrances.

Gamma-HCH is the main insecticidal component of HCH and has a strong stomach poison action, high contact toxicity and some fumigant activity on a wide range of insects. It is nonphytotoxic at insecticidal concentrations and of lower tainting propensities than HCH. The acute oral LD_{50} for male rats is 88 mg/kg, for female rats 91 mg/kg; the acute dermal LD_{50} for male rats is 1,000 mg/kg, for female rats 900 mg/kg.

Current Levels of Exposure: Considering the steady decline in the use of organochlorine insecticides, it is likely that HCH concentrations will continue to fall. This should also lower the amount of human exposure of HCH by oral ingestion. Dermal and inhalation, however, are recognized sources of contamination for those involved in the manufacture, use, and formulation of HCH and its isomers.

There is considerable pressure in the European countries to ban all organochlorine insecticides except lindane (γ-HCH). It is strongly believed by many that γ-HCH does not represent a pollution problem. It is recognized by these scientistis that α- and β-HCH do represent a significant hygienic problem. α- and β-HCH are accumulated up the food chain, e.g., Japanese rice → rice straw → cattle → cattle products → man.

The t-HCH contains a significant amount of the α- and β-isomers, so production of t-HCH should be restricted and only production of γ-HCH allowed. The presence of the α-, and β-isomers has in part given rise to the hypothesis that the γ-isomer can be transformed to the unwanted isomers.

Experimental isomerization has occurred, but only under anaerobic aquatic conditions and probably by microorganisms. There is a lack of bioisomerization in mammals. It should not be overlooked that α-HCH, despite its relatively short half-life, will be detected for a long time following the use of t-HCH, in which it is present in high proportion (60 to 70%).

Practical proof of this theory is shown by the fact that in countries where the use of technical (t-) HCH was terminated (and no γ-HCH had been used), residues of α- and β-HCH were found for many years. It is known that in such cases, the relative share of β-HCH of the total HCH residues is increasing. If γ-HCH is used exclusively in an area, then the share of γ-HCH of the total HCH residues will vary in accordance with the extent of application, and the other isomers will show a downward trend.

Special Groups at Risk: No t-HCH or γ-HCH is currently manufactured in the U.S. Use of t-HCH has been banned but γ-HCH is still approved for usage. All γ-HCH used in the U.S. is currently imported; there is no exposure during manufacture in this country. Formulators, distributors and users of the product certainly represent a special risk group. The major use of γ-HCH in recent years has been to pretreat seeds (42% in 1974), representing a source of exposure for employees of the seed companies. Agricultural workers could be exposed during handling and planting of the seed and during application to crops.

Existing Guidelines and Standards: The FAO/WHO Allowable Daily Intake (ADI) is set at 1 μg/kg/day and was revised down to that figure from 12.5 mg/kg/day originally set by FAO/WHO in 1972. The average daily intake of HCH for U.S. citizens was estimated in 1969 to be 0.002 μg/kg/day from the air and 0.07 μg/kg/day for foodstuffs, clearly below the established level of 1 μg/kg/day.

The EPA set the tolerance for animal fats at 7 ppm, and 0.3 ppm for milk. 1 ppm is the tolerance level for most fruits and vegetables. Finished drinking water should contain no more than 0.004 ppm. The maximum air concentration that is allowed by the EPA is 0.5 mg/m^3 of air. Cases of HCH poisoning in Japan have shown concentrations of 23 and 59 mg/m^3 at factories involved in the manufacture of HCH. In both cases a number of workers became ill with convulsions. It is clear that research is needed concerning the effects of long term, low level air concentrations of the HCH isomers.

The ACGIH, as of 1979, has set a TWA value of 0.5 mg/m^3 and a STEL value of 1.5 mg/m^3 for lindane.

Summary of Proposed EPA Criteria: *Freshwater Aquatic Life* — For lindane the criterion to protect freshwater aquatic life as derived using the Guidelines is 0.21 µg/l as a 24 hour average and the concentration should not exceed 2.9 µg/l at any time.

For freshwater aquatic life, no criterion for a mixture of isomers of BHC can be derived using the Guidelines, and there are insufficient data to estimate a criterion using other procedures.

Saltwater Aquatic Life — For saltwater aquatic life, no criterion for lindane can be derived using the Guidelines, and there are insufficient data to estimate a criterion using other procedures.

For saltwater aquatic life, no criterion for a mixture of isomers of BHC can be derived using the Guidelines, and there are insufficient data to estimate a criterion using other procedures.

Human Health — For the maximum protection of human health from the potential carcinogenic effects of exposure to α-HCH, β-HCH, and γ-HCH through ingestion of water and contaminated aquatic organisms, the ambient water concentration is zero. Concentrations of α-HCH, β-HCH, and γ-HCH estimated to result in additional lifetime cancer risks ranging from no additional risk to an additional risk of 1 in 100,000 are presented in the Criterion document.

The EPA is considering setting criteria at an interim target risk level in the range of 10^{-5}, 10^{-6}, or 10^{-7}, with corresponding criteria as follows:

Isomer	. .Criteria (ng/l) at the Following Risk Levels . .		
	10^{-5}	10^{-6}	10^{-7}
α-HCH	16	1.6	0.16
β-HCH	28	2.8	0.28
γ-HCH	54	5.4	0.54
t-HCH	21	2.1	0.21

There are insufficient data to establish criteria for the δ- and ϵ-isomers of HCH. A criterion for technical BHC has been proposed as 21.0 ng/l.

Basis for the Proposed Human Health Criteria: The animal carcinogenicity data (41-1, 41-2, 41-3, 41-4) have been used to develop water quality criteria for α-, β-, γ-, and t-HCH, respectively. These criteria have been developed by the Carcinogen Assessment Group of EPA. The assessment is given in the Criterion Document.

Under the Consent Decree in *NRDC vs Train*, criteria are to state "recommended maximum permissible concentrations (including where appropriate, zero) consistent with the protection of aquatic organisms, human health, and recreational activities."

α-HCH, β-HCH, γ-HCH and t-HCH are suspected of being human carcinogens. Because there is no recognized safe concentration for a human carcinogen, the recommended concentration of α-HCH, β-HCH and t-HCH in water for maximum protection of human health is zero.

Since attaining a zero concentration level may be infeasible in some cases and in order to assist the EPA and States in the possible future development of water quality regulations, the concentrations of α-HCH, β-HCH, γ-HCH and t-HCH corresponding to several incremental lifetime cancer risk levels have been estimated.

A cancer risk level provides an estimate of the additional incidence of cancer that may be expected in an exposed population. A risk of 10^{-5} for example, indicates a probability of one additional case of cancer for every 100,000 people exposed, a risk of 10^{-6} indicates one additional case of cancer for every million people exposed, and so forth.

In the *Federal Register* notice of availability of draft ambient water quality criteria, EPA stated that it is considering setting criteria at an interim target risk level of 10^{-5}, 10^{-6}, or 10^{-7} as shown in Table 65. The risk levels and corresponding criteria shown in the table are calculated by applying a modified "one-hit" extrapolation model described in the *FR* 15926, 1979. Appropriate bioassay data used in the calculation of the model are presented in the "Summary of Pertinent Data." Since the extrapolation model is linear at low doses, the additional lifetime risk is directly proportional to the water concentration. Therefore, water concentrations corresponding to other risk levels can be derived by multiplying or dividing one of the risk levels and corresponding water concentrations shown in the table by factors such as 10, 100, 1,000, and so forth.

Approximately 88% of the α-HCH, β-HCH, γ-HCH and t-HCH exposure results from the consumption of aquatic organisms which exhibit an average bioconcentration potential of 780 fold. The remaining 12% of α-HCH, β-HCH, γ-HCH and t-HCH exposure results from drinking water.

Table 65: Possible Alternative Criteria for Hexachlorocyclohexane Isomers

Exposure Assumptions (per day)	Risk Levels and Corresponding Criteria (ng/l)			
	0	10^{-7}	10^{-6}	10^{-5}
α-HCH				
2 liters of drinking water and consumption				
of 18.7 g fish and shellfish	0	0.16	1.6	16
Consumption of fish and shellfish only	0	0.18	1.8	18
β-HCH				
2 liters of drinking water and consumption				
of 18.7 g fish and shellfish	0	0.28	2.8	28
Consumption of fish and shellfish only	0	0.32	3.2	32
γ-HCH				
2 liters of drinking water and consumption				
of 18.7 g fish and shellfish	0	0.54	5.4	54
Consumption of fish and shellfish only	0	0.61	6.1	61
t-HCH				
2 liters of drinking water and consumption				
of 18.7 g fish and shellfish	0	0.21	2.1	21
Consumption of fish and shellfish only	0	0.24	2.4	24

Concentration levels were derived assuming a lifetime exposure to various amounts of HCH, (1) occurring from the consumption of both drinking water and aquatic life grown in waters containing the corresponding HCH concentrations and, (2) occurring solely from consumption of aquatic life grown in the waters containing the corresponding HCH concentrations. Although total exposure information for HCH is discussed and an estimate of the contributions from other sources of exposure can be made, these data will not be factored into ambient water quality criteria formulation until additional analyses can be made. The criteria presented, therefore, assume an incremental risk from ambient water exposure only.

Water quality criteria for the δ- and ϵ-isomers of HCH have not been established because of insufficient data. These isomers have not been detected in the environment, however, and would not appear to be a health risk.

Summary of Pertinent Data — The water quality criterion of α-hexachlorocyclohexane is derived from the oncogenic effects observed in the liver of male DDY mice fed 500 ppm α-HCH in the diet (41-1). The time-weighted average dose of 65 mg/kg/day was given in the feed for 24 weeks. The liver tumor incidence was 0/18 and 20/20 in the control and treated groups, respectively. Assuming a fish bioconcentration factor of 780, the criterion is calculated from the following parameters:

n_t = 20 (used 19.5 for calculation)
N_t = 20
n_c = 0
N_c = 18
le = 24 weeks
Le = 90 weeks
d = 500 ppm x 0.12 = 65 mg/kg/day
R = 780
L = 90 weeks
w = 0.0357 kg
F = 0.0187 kg/day

Based on these parameters, the one-hit slope, B_H, is 2.6637. The resulting water concentration of α-hexachlorocyclohexane calculated to keep the individual lifetime cancer risk below 10^{-5} is 16 ng/l.

The water quality criterion for β-hexachlorocyclohexane is derived from the oncogenic effects observed in the liver of male ICR-JCL mice fed 600 ppm β-HCH in the diet (41-2). The time-weighted average dose of 78 mg/kg/day was given in the feed for 26 weeks. The liver tumor incidence was 0/10 and 10/10 in the control and treated groups, respectively. Assuming a fish bioconcentration factor 780, the criterion is calculated from the following parameters:

n_t = 10 (used 9.5 for calculation)
N_t = 10
n_c = 0
N_c = 10
le = 26 weeks
Le = 90 weeks
d = 600 ppm x 0.13 = 78 mg/kg/day
R = 780
L = 90 weeks
w = 0.0475 kg
F = 0.0187 kg/day

Based on these parameters, the one-hit slope, B_H, is 1.5129. The resulting water concentration of β-hexachlorocyclohexane calculated to keep the individual lifetime cancer risk below 10^{-5} is 28 ng/l.

The water quality criterion for γ-hexachlorocyclohexane is derived from the oncogenic effects observed in the liver of male CF1 mice fed 400 ppm γ-HCH in the diet (41-3). The time-weighted average dose of 52 mg/kg/day was given in the feed for 110 weeks. The liver tumor incidence was 11/45 and 27/28 in the control and treated groups, respectively. Assuming a fish bioconcentration factor of 780, the criterion is calculated from the following parameters:

n_t = 27
N_t = 28
n_c = 11
N_c = 45
le = 110 weeks
Le = 110 weeks
d = 400 ppm x 0.13 = 52 mg/kg/day
R = 780
L = 110 weeks
w = 0.030 kg
F = 0.0187 kg/day

Based on these parameters, the one-hit slope, B_H, is 7.7844 x 10^{-1}. The resulting concentration of γ-hexachlorocyclohexane calculated to keep the individual lifetime cancer risk below 10^{-5} is 54 ng/l.

The water quality criterion for t-hexachlorocyclohexane is derived from the oncogenic effects observed in the liver of male dd mice fed 660 ppm t-HCH in the diet (41-4). The time-weighted average dose of 85.8 mg/kg/day was given in the feed for 24 weeks. The liver tumor incidence was 0/14 and 20/20 in the control and treated groups, respectively. Assuming a fish bioconcentration factor of 780, the criterion is calculated from the following parameters:

$$n_t = 20 \text{ (used 19.5 for calculation)}$$
$$N_t = 20$$
$$n_c = 0$$
$$N_c = 14$$
$$le = 24 \text{ weeks}$$
$$Le = 90 \text{ weeks}$$
$$d = 660 \text{ ppm} \times 0.13 = 85.8 \text{ mg/kg/day}$$
$$R = 780$$
$$L = 90 \text{ weeks}$$
$$w = 0.0364 \text{ kg}$$
$$F = 0.0187 \text{ kg/day}$$

Based on these parameters, the one-hit slope, B_H, is 2.0050. The resulting water concentration of t-hexachlorocyclohexane calculated to keep the individual lifetime cancer risk below 10^{-5} is 21 ng/l.

References

(41-1)   Ito, N., et al., "Development of Hepatocellular Carcinomas in Rats Treated with Benzene Hexachloride," *Jour. Nat. Cancer Inst. 54*, 801 (1975).

(41-2)   Goto, M., et al., "Ecological Chemistry. Toxizitat von α-HCH in Mausen," *Chromosphere 1*, 153 (1972).

(41-3)   Thorpe, E. and Walker, A.I., "The Toxicology of Dieldrin (HEOD), II, In Mice with Dieldrin, DDT, Phenobarbitone, beta-BCH and gamma-BCH," *Food Cosmet. Toxicol. 11*, 433 (1973).

(41-4)   Nagasak, H., et al., "Carcinogenicity of Benzene Hexachloride (BHC)," *Top. Chem. Carcinog.*, Proc. 2nd Int. Symp. (1972).

HEXACHLOROCYCLOPENTADIENE (#42)

Hexachlorocyclopentadiene, C_5Cl_6, is also known in the trade as Hex and as C-56. It is 1,2,3,4,5,5'-hexachlorocyclopentadiene.

Occurrence: Environmental monitoring data for Hex are lacking except for measured levels in the vicinity of industrial sites. Hex has been identified and/or quantified in wastewater, receiving streams, rivers, fish, soil, sediment, and air surrounding pesticide plants (42-1).

An incident involving the improper disposal of Hex-containing industrial wastes in a Louisville, KY sewer system, resulted in no apparent widespread environmental release of the chemical (42-2).

Physical Properties: Hexachlorocyclopentadiene is a pale to greenish yellow liquid with the molecular formula C_5Cl_6. Other physical properties include a molecular weight of 272.66; a solubility in water of 0.805 mg/l; a vapor pressure of 1 mm Hg at 78° to 79°C, and a specific gravity of 1.7119 (20°/4°C).

Chemical Properties: Six active chlorines and two double bonds make Hex a highly reactive compound which readily undergoes substitution and addition reactions. Its versatility is based upon its reactivity as a diene with a variety of decomposition.

Data from isooctane solutions revealed no degradation after 24 hours, but a multipeak spectrum indicating the presence of degradation products was obtained after 7 to 21 days' exposure. This spectrum suggested to the investigators that the compound may be susceptible to atmospheric oxidation and/or photodecomposition.

Hex, unlike some of the pesticides derived from it, degrades rapidly by photolysis, giving water-soluble degradation products. Tests on its stability towards hydrolysis at ambient temperature indicated a half-life of about 11 days at pH 3 to 6, which was reduced to 6 days at pH 9.

Uses: Hex was used as a chemical intermediate in the manufacture of numerous widely used chlorinated pesticides. Recent governmental bans on the use of chlorinated pesticides have restricted the use of Hex as a pesticide intermediate to the endosulfan (Thiodan) and decachlorobi-2,4-cyclopentadiene-1-yl (Pentac) industries.

The major use of Hex is as an intermediate in the synthesis of commercially important flame retardants. Hex, though commercially important as a chemical intermediate (production levels approximate 50 million pounds per year), has no end uses of its own (42-3).

Toxic Effects: Hex has proven to be a potent irritant. Industrial workers have experienced irritation of the eye, irritation of the upper airway passages and headaches upon exposure to Hex vapors and burns upon contact of skin with the liquid (42-2, 42-4). Long-term exposure to hazardous concentrations results in systemic poisoning of laboratory animals (42-5).

In the laboratory, Hex has exhibited toxicity to fish and mammals (42-1, 42-5). Hex has been reported to be nonmutagenic in unpublished laboratory tests and there are no data available to evaluate the carcinogenicity of the compound.

Current Levels of Exposure: As indicated previously, it is unknown whether ingestion or inhalation of Hex (through ingestion of Hex-contaminated food, water, or air) constitute significant sources of exposure among the general population. Although it is not likely this is the case, data on the environmental occurrence of Hex are so sketchy that this possibility cannot be ruled out.

Special Groups at Risk: Occupational exposures appear to constitute the only documented source of human exposure to Hex. Oral contact does not appear to be a likely mode of occupational exposure.

Dermal and inhalation exposures are recognized hazards for the following groups: (1) workers engaged directly in Hex manufacture; (2) those engaged in the formulation and use of other related pesticides where Hex may be present as an impurity; (3) flame retardant workers; and (4) those having "quasi-occupational" exposure such as sewage treatment workers, industrial hygienists, etc.

Existing Guidelines and Standards: The Occupational Safety and Health Administration (OSHA) has not set a standard for occupational exposure to Hex. On the other hand, the American Conference of Governmental Industrial Hygienists (ACGIH) has adopted both a threshold limit value (TLV) and a Short Term Exposure Limit (STEL) for hexachlorocyclopentadiene.

The current (1979) occupational TLV for Hex is set at 0.01 ppm (0.11 mg/m^3), which, according to ACGIH "represents a time-weighted average concentration for a normal 8 hour workday or 40 hour workweek to which nearly all workers may be repeatedly exposed, day after day, without adverse effect."

The Short Term Exposure Limit (STEL) for Hex is set at 0.03 ppm (0.33 mg/m^3). This level represents the maximal concentration to which workers can be exposed for a period up to 15 minutes without suffering from irritation, chronic or irreversible tissue damage, or narcosis of sufficient degree to increase accident proneness, impair self-rescue, or materially reduce work efficiency.

The STEL should be considered a maximum allowable concentration or absolute ceiling not to be exceeded at any time in the 15 minutes. Up to four excursions up to the STEL are permitted per day provided that there are at least 60 minutes between excursions up to the STEL.

In selecting the TLV and STEL values for Hex, the ACGIH emphasizes that these particular levels were selected on the basis of preventing irritant effects rather than chronic toxicity. The U.S.S.R. has recommended a tenfold lower limit (0.001 ppm) for occupational workers.

No nonoccupational exposure limits have been established or recommended except for one Soviet study which proposed a maximum concentration of 0.001 mg/l in water to prevent "organoleptic effects" (i.e., adverse effects on the taste and odor of water). There is a serious lack of data to support nonoccupational exposure limits or environmental criteria for Hex. Specifically lacking are: (1) epidemiologic studies of individuals having known and quantifiable Hex exposures; (2) long-term animal studies (e.g., 2 year chronic feeding studies) suitable for evaluating chronic effects, especially carcinogenicity; (3) data on current levels of human exposure from various media; and (4) suitable methods for interpreting the significance of in vitro assays and their applicability to actual environmental conditions.

Without these essential data it is not possible to use the model proposed by U.S. EPA's Carcinogen Assessment Group (CAG) to derive recommended exposure criteria for humans. In fact, the CAG states that "there is insufficient evidence to categorize this compound as a carcinogen or noncarcinogen." Consequently, other toxic endpoints must form the basis for recommended exposure criteria until a more adequate information base on Hex is developed.

Summary of Proposed EPA Criteria: *Freshwater Aquatic Life* — For hexachlorocyclopentadiene, the criterion to protect freshwater aquatic life, as derived using the Guidelines is 0.39 µg/l as a 24 hour average and the concentration should not exceed 7.0 µg/l at any time.

Saltwater Aquatic Life — For saltwater aquatic life, no criterion can be derived using the Guidelines, and there are insufficient data to estimate a criterion using other procedures.

Human Health — For the prevention of adverse effects due to the organoleptic properties of hexachlorocyclopentadiene in water, the criterion is 1.0 µg/l.

Basis for the Proposed Human Health Criteria: As indicated earlier, there are no epidemiologic studies nor suitable chronic toxicity studies in mammals from which threshold levels for chronic effects could be derived. Very little is known regarding potential Hex exposures through ingestion of contaminated food or water.

In the environment Hex has been detected only in specific bodies of water near points of industrial discharges. There is no data on Hex levels in drinking or untreated water.

Based on the available and cited literature, there is insufficient evidence to categorize this compound as a carcinogen or noncarcinogen. There has not been a satisfactory study of the effects of chronic oral exposure to Hex.

One test consisted of only one species (rats) with a duration of exposure of only six months. No neoplasms were reported, however the duration of the study would not have been sufficient for a proper evaluation of carcinogenicity.

Hex has been tested for mutagenicity and reported nonmutagenic in both short-term in vitro mutagenic assays and in a mouse dominant lethal study. No epidemiologic studies or case reports examining the relationship between exposure to Hex and cancer incidences could be found in the literature. Therefore, there is virtually no information regarding the carcinogenic potential of chronic exposure to Hex. In selecting Hex for future chronic toxicity testing, National Cancer Institute recognized these data voids.

Although one study reported the effects of chronic low-dose inhalation of Hex, its applicability in deriving water quality guidelines is unclear. Furthermore, with the exception of very limited data on Hex in water near points of discharge, there appears to be no information on Hex levels in water bodies. What is needed is a method for converting the results of respiratory exposure experiments into equivalent dosages from water.

There is a model by which the threshold limit values (TLVs) for industrial substances in air may be used in establishing drinking water standards. The model assumes that, for any given inhaled dose, an equivalent ingested dose from ingested water can be derived using reasonable estimates of daily air and water intakes and corresponding respiratory and gastrointestinal absorption rates. In the absence of suitable chronic ingestion studies of Hex, this model will be used to estimate suitable limits for Hex in water based on the established threshold limit value expressed as milligrams per cubic meter of air.

The threshold limit of 0.11 mg/m^3 (0.01 ppm) Hex represents what is believed to be a maximal concentration to which a worker may be exposed for 8 hours per day, 5 days per week over his working lifetime without hazard to health or well-being. To the TLV, are applied terms expressing respiratory volume during an 8 hour period (assumed to be 10 m^3) and a respiratory absorption coefficient appropriate to the substance under consideration. As in the case of Hex where absorption rates are unknown, 100% absorption is assumed. In addition, the 5 day per week occupational exposure is often converted to a 7 day per week equivalent in keeping with the more continuous pattern of exposure to drinking water.

According to the model, the amount of Hex that may be taken into the bloodstream and presumed to be noninjurious and which, hence, may be taken in water each day is:

0.11 mg/m^3	x	10 m^3	x	1.0	x	5/7 week	=	0.7857 mg/d
(TLV)		Respiratory Intake Term		Respiratory Absorption Coefficient		Proportion of week Exposed		Maximum Noninjurious Intake

To calculate the equivalent amount of Hex in ambient water, the model assumes a maximal daily intake of 2 liters of water per day, the consumption of 18.7 grams of fish/shellfish per day, a bioconcentration factor of 3.2 for fish, and 100% absorption.

(X)	x	[2 + 3.2(0.0187)]	x	1.0	=	0.7857
Upper Intake Limit		Oral Intake Term		Gastrointestinal Absorption Coefficient		Maximum Noninjurious Intake

Solving for X, the value derived is 0.38 mg/l or 380 μg/l. According to Stokinger and Woodward (42-6) who developed the model, "This derived value represents an approximate limiting concentration for a healthy adult population; it is only a first approximation in the development of a tentative drinking water criterion . . . several adjustments in this value may be necessary . . . Other factors, such as taste, odor and color may outweigh health considerations because acceptable limits for these may be below the estimated health limit."

It should also be noted that the basis for the above recommended limit, the TLV for Hex, is set on the basis of avoidance of irritation, rather than chronic effects. Should chronic effects data become available, both TLVs and recommendations based on them will warrant reconsideration.

A single study of chronic oral toxicity in white rats reported no adverse effects (specifically changes in peripheral blood cells, ascorbic acid content of the adrenals, conditioned reflexes of the animals, or histological structure of the organs) following daily oral administration of doses up to 4 μg/l of Hex in aqueous solution. Animals receiving the highest dosage, 40 μg/l, showed neutropenia and lymphocytosis which the investigators thought possibly attributable to mobilization of the protective forces of the organism in response to this dose.

Such findings imply adverse effects at levels as low as 10% of the tentative drinking water standard based on the Stokinger and Woodward model. Hex in concentrations of 1.4 to 1.6 μg/l is capable of altering the smell and taste of water. Based on these organoleptic effects, these investigators proposed a maximum permissible concentration of 1 μg/l. Stokinger and Woodward themselves noted that oftentimes "other factors, including taste, odor and color may outweigh health considerations because acceptable limits for these may be well below the estimated health limit."

Because chronic effects in a mammalian species (rats) have been documented at water concentrations of Hex as low as 40 μg/l, it is obvious that an acceptable water quality criterion should be well below this level. Thus, a reasonable safety factor of 10 to 100 applied to 40 μg/l would place an appropriate criterion recommendation in the range of 4.0 to 0.4 μg/l in water.

No adverse effects on humans or mammals have been reported to be caused by Hex concentrations lower than approximately 1.0 μg/l. Therefore, based on avoidance of alteration in smell and aftertaste in water, a criterion of 1.0 μg/l of Hex in water is tentatively suggested. This level should be adequate for protection of public health. It is to be stressed that this criterion is based on inadequate chronic effects data and should be reevaluated upon completion of chronic oral toxicity studies.

References

(42-1)   Spehar, R.L., et al., "Toxicity and Bioaccumulation of Hexachlorocyclopentadiene, Hexachloro-norbornadiene and Heptachloronorbornene in Larval and Early Juvenile Fathead Minnows, *Pimephales promelas*." *Bull. Environ. Contam. Toxicol.* (In Press - 1979).

(42-2)   Carter, M.R., "The Louisville Incident." Internal Report (Unpublished), Athens, Ga. Serveillance and Analysis Division, Region IV, U.S. EPA, (1977).

(42-3)   Bell, M.A., et al., "Review of the Environmental Effects of Pollutants XI. Hexachlorocyclopentadiene." Unpublished report by Battella Columbus Lab. for U.S. EPA Health Res. Lab, Cincinnati, Ohio (1978).

(42-4)   Ingle, L., "The Toxicity of Chlordane Vapor." *Science 118*, 213 (1953).

(42-5)   Treon, J.F., et al., "The Toxicity of Hexachlorocyclopentadiene." *Arch. Ind. Health 11*, 459 (1955).

(42-6)   Stokinger, H.E. and Woodward, R.L., "Toxicologic Methods for Establishing Drinking Water Standards," *Jour. Am. Water Works Assoc. 50*, 515 (1958).

HEXACHLOROETHANE

See "Chlorinated Ethanes" (#15).

HEXACHLORONAPHTHALENES

See "Chlorinated Naphthalenes (#17).

I

INDENO (1,2,3-cd) ANTHRACENE

See "Polynuclear Aromatic Hydrocarbons" (55)

ISOPHORONE (#43)

Isophorone (γ-isophorone) has the chemical name 3,5,5-trimethyl-2-cyclohexen-1-one, and is also known as trimethyl cyclohexanone or isoacetophorone. Although isophorone is normally produced as the γ-isomer, it may exist also as a β-isomer having the chemical name 3,5,5-trimethyl-3-cyclohexen-1-one. The technical or industrial grade of isophorone normally contains 3.0% or less of the β-isomer, causing a slight deviation in the melting and boiling points reported for pure isophorone (γ-isomer).

Occurrence: Although isophorone has been reported in drinking water, the Delaware River, and effluents of several industrial facilities, little or no information is available regarding bioconcentration, persistence, or fate of isophorone under environmental conditions. However, its broad application as a solvent or cosolvent or chemical feedstock for industrial and agricultural products clearly suggests that the potential for both point source and non-point source water contamination exists (39 *FR* 37195).

In the environment, isophorone has been detected in a few samples of drinking water, but not in ambient air, soil, or food.

Physical Properties: The pure compound (γ-isophorone) is a water-white liquid which exhibits low volatility, possesses a camphor or peppermint-like odor, and turns yellow upon standing. It has the empirical formula $C_9H_{14}O$ and a molecular weight of 138.21. The physical properties include: melting point, $-8.1°C$; boiling point, $215.2°C$; vapor pressure, 0.31 Hg at $20°C$ and 1 mm Hg at $38°C$; and a density of 0.9229 at $20°C$. The compound is soluble in water up to 1.2 gm/100 ml at $20°C$ and is readily soluble in fats, oils, and other hydrophobic substances.

Chemical Properties: Isophorone is considered chemically stable. At $150°C$, however, it will form salts with sulfuric acid and a tricyclic γ-, β-unsaturated ketone in the presence of 60% aqueous sodium hydroxide. Such reactions may be of little significance since the conditions required for their completion are generally not found in the environment.

In aqueous solutions, isophorone forms three different tricyclic diketodimers when exposed to direct sunlight (43-1). The molecular weights of these compounds are double that of isophorone and the melting points range from 182 to 186.5°C. Following ultraviolet irradiation for one and ten days, conversions to the dimer were 10 and 50%, respectively. In a similar study, irradiation for 40 and 80 days resulted in dimer conversions of 76 and 83%, respectively (43-2). The significance of these laboratory studies with respect to the stability of isophorone in the environment is not known.

The microbiological degradation of isophorone, measured as percent biooxidation, was investigated by Price, et al (43-3) in domestic waste water and synthetic saltwater using a modification of the standard BOD test. The observed biooxidation levels of isophorone were 13, 47, and 42% in the domestic waste water at 10, 15, and 20 days, respectively. The biooxidation in synthetic saltwater reached only 9% after 20 days incubation.

Uses: Isophorone is an industrial chemical synthesized from acetone and used commercially as a solvent or cosolvent for finishes, lacquers, polyvinyl and nitro cellulose resins, pesticides, herbicides, fats, oils, and gums. It is also used as a chemical feedstock for the synthesis of 3,5 xylenol, 2,3,5-trimethyl-cyclohexanol, and 3,5-dimethylaniline.

Isophorone production was estimated at a level of 28 million pounds for 1973.

Toxic Effects: Isophorone has been reported to be toxic to aquatic life, particularly saltwater invertebrate species. Isophorone also has been shown to be toxic to experimental mammals in acute, subacute, and chronic toxicity tests.

Current Levels of Exposure: Only limited monitoring data are available regarding levels of isophorone in water, and virtually no information is available on ambient levels in air or food. Since there is a lack of extensive monitoring data on isophorone levels in drinking water, it is difficult to predict the magnitude or extent of human population exposure.

Although isophorone has been detected at levels of less than 3 ppt in several water samples, a maximum daily intake can be calculated from the highest reported level (9.5 μg/l) (43-4), by assuming that 100% exposure comes from the ingestion of water and fish and shellfish from contaminated waters. Assuming: (a) an average daily consumption of 2 liters of water plus 18.7 g fish/shellfish; (b) a bioconcentration factor of 16; and (c) 100% gastrointestinal absorption of the ingested isophorone; then the daily intake of isophorone from water would be 21.8 μg/day ⟨9.5 μg/l x [2 liters + (16 x 0.0187)] x 1.0⟩.

Special Groups at Risk: Certain occupations (particularly individuals who are exposed to isophorone as a solvent) have elevated levels of exposure relative to the general population.

NIOSH (43-5) estimates that more than 1.5 million workers are exposed to isophorone. In the industrial handling of isophorone inhalation of the vapors is the most likely mode of contact, although skin and eye contact with the liquid may also occur. Because of the odor and taste of isophorone, ingestion is not expected unless by accident.

Existing Guidelines and Standards: The current eight-hour time-weighted average threshold limit value (TLV) for isophorone established by the American Conference of Governmental Industrial Hygienists, as of 1979 is 5 ppm ($\sim$28 mg/m^3). The TLV was lowered from 25 ppm ($\sim$140 mg/m^3) to 5 ppm in response to a June 1973 communication from the Western Electric Company to the TLV committee regarding fatigue and malaise among workers exposed to levels of 5 to 8 ppm for one month (43-6). When isophorone levels in air were lowered to 1 to 4 ppm ($\sim$6 to 23 mg/m^3) by increasing exhaust ventilation, no further complaints were received.

The current U.S. Federal standard for occupational exposure to isophorone is 25 ppm (140 mg/m^3) as an eight-hour time-weighted average concentration limit in the air of the working environment. This standard is based on the TLV adopted by the ACGIH in 1968, and is intended to prevent irritative and narcotic effects. The National Institute for Occupational Safety and Health (NIOSH) currently recommends a permissible exposure limit of 4 ppm (23 mg/m^3) as a TWA concentration for up to a 10-hour workshift, 40-hour work week (43-5). The NIOSH recommended standard is essentially based on the 1974 ACGIH TLV documentation.

Isophorone was exempted from the requirement of a tolerance under the Federal Food, Drug and Cosmetic Act when used as an inert solvent or cosolvent in pesticide formulations before a crop emerges from the soil, and for post-emergence use both on rice before the crop begins to head and on sugar and table beets.

Basis for Proposed EPA Criteria: *Freshwater Aquatic Life* — The data base for freshwater aquatic life is insufficient to allow use of the Guidelines. The following recommendation is inferred from toxicity data for saltwater organisms.

For isophorone the criterion to protect freshwater aquatic life as derived using the Guidelines is 2,100 μg/l as a 24-hour average and the concentration should not exceed 4,700 μg/l at any time.

Saltwater Aquatic Life — For isophorone the criterion to protect saltwater aquatic life as derived using the Guidelines is 97 μg/l as a 24-hour average and the concentration should not exceed 220 μg/l at any time.

Human Health — For the protection of human health from the toxic properties of isophorone ingested through water, the criterion is 460 μg/l.

Basis for the Proposed Human Health Criteria: Based on the available data on the toxicological effects of isophorone absorption in both man and experimental animals, a calculated water quality criterion for isophorone can only be based upon a noncarcinogenic effect. Water quality criteria may therefore be derived from the TLV, acute oral LD_{50} values, or from subacute oral toxicity data using noncarcinogenic biological responses. Criteria derivations based on all three approaches are presented below.

Criterion Based on TLV — Stokinger and Woodward (43-7) presented a method for calculating water quality criteria from TLV's. Essentially, this method consists of deriving an acceptable daily intake (ADI) from the TLV by making assumptions on breathing rate, and respiratory and gastrointestinal absorption. Stokinger and Woodward assumed that the daily total pollutant uptake from air at the TLV concentration can be safely tolerated, and that this safe quantity of pollutant per day can be similarly tolerated in drinking water. The ADI is then partitioned into permissible amounts from drinking water and from other sources.

The International Commission on Radiological Protection has estimated that the "reference man" breathes 7.6 m^3 of air during eight hours of "light activity". Since respiratory absorption rates are unknown, 50% absorption of inhaled isophorone will be assumed. In addition, the five day per week TLV may be converted to a seven day per week equivalent to reflect the more continuous pattern of exposure via drinking water. An ADI for man can be thus calculated from the TLV by multiplying by these factors:

$$28 \text{ mg/m}^3 \times 7.6 \text{ m}^3 \times 0.5 \times 5 \text{ days/7 days} = 76 \text{ mg/day}$$

Since estimates of isophorone exposure from nonwater sources are not available, it will be assumed that total isophorone exposure is attributable to the ingestion of drinking water and fish and shellfish. For the purpose of estimating a criterion it will be further assumed that the maximal daily intake of water is 2 liters, that the consumption of fish/shellfish amounts to 18.7 g/day, and that the gastrointestinal absorption of isophorone is 100%. Also a bioconcentration factor of 16 has been calculated for fish by EPA. A water quality criterion may then be calculated as:

$$\frac{76 \text{ mg/man}}{[2 + (16 \times 0.0187)] \times 1.0} = 33 \text{ mg/l}$$

It should be noted that the TLV is based on the prevention of the irritant effects of isophorone on inhalation exposures, rather than on chronic effects. Consequently, the calculation of a criterion by this approach probably has little validity in this case.

Criterion Based on Acute Oral Toxicity Data — McNamara (43-8) has suggested that data from acute exposures can be used to estimate chronic no-effect levels for toxic responses to chemical absorption. Based on an extensive review of the literature comparing the results of acute and chronic toxicity bioassays, McNamara noted that "for 95 percent of chemical compounds . . .(on which data were available) . . . $LD_{50}/1000$ will produce no effects in a lifetime." Using this approximation for isophorone, and an average oral LD_{50} value of 2 g/kg (Effects section), the no observable effect level for isophorone in rats can be estimated at 2 mg/kg/day. This value may be converted into an ADI by applying an appropriate uncertainty factor to account for species extrapolation and limitations of the data. Since the chronic no-effect dose is merely an estimate based on observed relationships between acute and chronic toxicity, an uncertainty factor of 1,000 is recommended (43-9). Thus, the estimated ADI for man is 2 μg/kg or 140 μg/man, assuming a 70 kg body weight. By assuming that man consumes 2 liters of water per day, that man is additionally exposed daily to 18.7 g of fish and shellfish which bioaccumulate isophorone from water by a factor of 16, and that gastrointestinal absorption is 100%, the corresponding no adverse effect level in water can be calculated as:

$$\frac{140 \ \mu g/day}{[2 \ + \ (16 \ \times \ 0.0187)] \ \times \ 1.0} \ = \ 61 \ \mu g/l$$

Based on these calculations, the criterion for isophorone should not exceed 0.06 mg/l.

Criterion Based on Subacute Oral Data — As summarized in the Effects section, no significant effects were produced in beagle dogs by feeding isophorone in gelatin capsules at levels up to 150 mg/kg/day for 90 days (EPA, 1979a). Due to the fact that this study did not involve a truly chronic exposure, the NAS guidelines for establishing an acceptable daily intake for man (43-9) are not directly applicable. McNamara (43-8) has suggested, however, that subacute exposures can be used to estimate chronic no-effect exposure levels.

McNamara (43-8) found that for 95% of chemical compounds for which data were available, a three month no-effect dose/10 will yield a level which should produce no adverse effects in a lifetime. By using this relationship, the chronic no-effect dose for dogs is calculated to be:

$$\frac{150 \ mg/kg}{10} \ = \ 15 \ mg/kg$$

The application of an uncertainty factor of 1,000 is suggested to convert this value to an ADI (43-9). Therefore, an estimated ADI for man is 15 μg/kg or 1,050 μg/man, assuming a 70 kg body weight. Consumption of 2 liters of water daily and of 18.7 g of contaminated aquatic organisms which have a bioconcentration factor of 16 would result in, assuming gastrointestinal absorption of isophorone, a maximum permissible concentration of 0.46 mg/l for the ingested water:

$$\frac{1050 \ \mu g/day}{[2 \ + \ (16 \ \times \ 0.0187)] \ \times \ 1.0} \ = \ 457 \ \mu g/l$$

In conclusion, permissible levels for isophorone in water have been derived on the basis of a TLV (33 mg/l), acute oral toxicity data (0.06 mg/l) and a 90 day feeding study in dogs (0.46 mg/l). Although this exercise has yielded figures which may have some utility in the protection of human health, the available scientific data base is inadequate to support a reliable criterion. The most prudent approach at this time would be to recommend only an interim criterion pending the results of future research, including the planned NCI bioassay.

An interim criterion of 0.46 mg/l could be recommended in cases where water is the sole source of exposure to isophorone, because the basis for this value is a well defined no-effect level derived from a higher vertebrate species (dog) subjected to subchronic oral exposure. Since current levels of isophorone in drinking water are usually less than 3 μg/l, although amounts as high as 9.5 μg/l have been reported, an ample margin of safety apparently exists.

References

(43-1)   Jennings, P.W., "Photochemistry of isophorone. I," Dissertation Abstr. 26: 698, (1965)

(43-2)   Craven, E.C., "Isophorone," *Jour. Appl. Chem.* (London), 12, 120 (1962).

(43-3)   Price, K.S., et al, "Brine shrimp bioassay and BOD of petrochemicals," *Jour. Water Pollut. Control Fed.* 46, 63 (1974).

(43-4)   U.S. Environmental Protection Agency, *Preliminary assessment of suspected carcinogens in drinking water: report to Congress,* Wash. D.C. (1975).

(43-5)   Nat. Inst. for Occupational Safety & Health, *Criteria for a recommended standard: occupational exposure to ketones,* DHEW (NIOSH) Publ. No. 78-173, Wash., D.C. (1978).

(43-6)   Am. Conf. of Govt. Ind. Hygienists, *Documentation of the threshold limit values for substances in workroom air,* 3rd Ed. (1971), 4th Printing, Cincinnati, Ohio (1977).

(43-7)   Stokinger, H.E. and Woodward, R.L., "Toxicologic methods for establishing drinking water standards," *Jour. Am. Water Works Assoc.* 50, 515 (1958).

(43-8)   McNamara, B.P., "Concepts in health evaluation of commercial & industrial chemicals" in Mehlman, M.A., et al, Eds., *Advances in modern toxicology,* New York, John Wiley & Sons (1976).

(43-9)   National Academy of Sciences, *Drinking water and health,* Wash., D.C. (1977).

L

LEAD (#44)

Lead, symbol Pb, is an element in Group IV of the periodic table. It has an atomic number of 82 and an atomic weight of 207.21.

Occurrence: Lead concentrations in seawater have been reported at 0.03 μg/l and in fresh waters from 2 to 140 μg/l, with a mean of 23 μg/l. Lead reaches the aquatic environment through precipitation, fallout of lead dust, leaching from soil, street runoff, and both industrial and municipal wastewater discharges.

Lead is ubiquitous in nature, being a natural constituent of the earth's crust. The usual concentration in rocks and in soils from natural sources ranges from 10 to 30 mg/kg. Most natural groundwaters have concentrations ranging from 1 to 10 μg/l. This is well below the U.S. drinking water standard of 50 μg/l. It is much easier to specify natural levels of lead in rocks and soil than in vegetation since long-range transport of lead from man-made sources via the air inevitably contaminates both surface soil and plants growing thereon. The normal concentration of lead in rural vegetation, however, ranges from 0.1 to 1.0 mg/kg dry weight, or 2 to 20 mg/kg ash weight.

Thus, nutrient movement from soil to the organic matter in plants via water does not result in any noticeable degree of biomagnification. Again, because of the impact of long-range transport of lead via air from man-generated sources, it is only possible to specify lowest concentrations found over areas of the globe most remote from human activity. These are of the order of 0.0001 to 0.001 μg/m^3, mostly measured over Greenland and over remote oceans.

Areas of abnormally high concentrations of lead occur in natural ores, usually in conjunction with high concentrations of cadmium and zinc. There is essentially no transfer from natural ore beds into overlying streams. There is none if the soil is even slightly alkaline.

Physical Properties: Lead is a soft gray, acid-soluble metal. The solubility of lead compounds in water depends heavily on pH and ranges from about 10,000,000 μg/l of lead at pH 5.5 to 1 μg/l at pH 9.0.

Chemical Properties: Inorganic lead compounds are most stable in the plus two valence state, while organolead compounds are more stable in the plus four state.

Bacterial action has been shown capable of converting inorganic lead to organic forms. Algae reportedly can concentrate lead in their tissues to levels as much as 31,000 times ambient water concentrations. Since lead is an element, it will not be destroyed and may be expected to persist indefinitely in the environment in some form.

Uses: Lead consumption in the U.S. has been fairly stable from year to year at about 1.3 x 10^6 metric tons. Approximately half of that consumption has been for the manufacture of storage batteries and one-fifth has been for the manufacture of gasoline antiknock additives, notably tetraethyl- and tetramethyllead. Pigments and ceramics account for about 6% of annual production. All other major uses are for metallic lead products or for lead-containing alloys. The consumption of tetraethyl- and tetramethyllead is declining. Other uses that have significant potential for input into man are for paint pigment and solder. Paints applied to surfaces will eventually crack, flake or peel. Children are known to ingest this type of deteriorating paint. Solder also is a potential source of lead exposure either when used to seal water pipe joints or for joining seams in metal food and beverage containers.

Toxic Effects: In the aquatic environment, lead has been reported (44-1) to be acutely toxic to invertebrates at concentrations as low as 450 μg/l and chronically toxic at less than 100 μg/l. The comparable figures for vertebrates are 900 μg/l for acute toxicity (44-2) and 7.6 μg/l for chronic toxicity (44-3). Toxicity is also affected by water hardness (44-4, 44-5). Hard water is protective of organisms exposed to lead.

Lead has been shown to be teratogenic in animals (44-6). Lead exposure has been reported to decrease reproductive ability in men (44-7) and women (44-8). It has also been shown to cause disturbances of blood chemistry (44-9), neurological disorders (44-10, 44-11), kidney damage (44-12) and adverse cardiovascular effects (44-13).

Current Levels of Exposure: Approximately 1% of tap water samples have been found to exceed the current standard of 50 μg/l. This is generally a problem in soft water areas, particularly where lead pipes convey the water supply to the tap from the surface connection. The contribution of the diet is approximately 200 μg/day for adults. For children (ages 3 months to 9 years) the diet contributes 40 to 200 μg of lead per day. On the basis of current information, it is impossible to judge how much dietary lead is attributable to the water used in food preparation. The concentration of lead in ambient air ranges from approximatley 0.1 μg/m^3 in rural areas to as much as 10 μg/m^3 in areas of heavy automotive traffic.

Special Groups at Risk: In addition to these usual levels of exposure from environmental media, there exist miscellaneous sources which are hazardous. The level of exposure resulting from contact is highly variable. Children with pica for paint chips or for soil may experience elevation in blood lead ranging from marginal to sufficiently great to cause clinical illness. Certain adults may also be exposed to hazardous concentrations or lead in the workplace, notably in lead smelters and storage battery manufacturing plants. Again, the range of exposure is highly variable. Women in the workplace are more likely to experience adverse effects from lead exposure than men due to the fact that their hematopoietic system is more lead-sensitive than men's.

Existing Guidelines and Standards: Since lead is ubiquitous in the environment, several government agencies have become involved in regulating its use. The most recent action was taken by the Consumer Product Safety Commission (CPSC). In 1977, the CPSC lowered the maximum allowable concentration of lead in house paint to 0.06%. Similarly, the U.S. EPA has set an ambient air lead standard. The U.S. Food and Drug Administration also has prepared new guidelines for the regulation of sources of lead in foods and cosmetics. Given the multimedia nature of lead exposure to man, it is essential that any action taken in regard to one source, such as water, be coordinated with similar actions being taken for other media such as air and diet.

The Federal standard for lead and its inorganic compounds was 0.2 mg/m^3 as a time-weighted average. The NIOSH Criteria Document (44-14) recommends a time-weighted average value of 0.15 mg Pb/m^3. On November 14, 1978, OSHA (44-15) set a final standard in which industries will be given 1 to 3 years to reach a 0.1 mg (100 μg)/m^3 level and from 1 to 10 years to reach a final standard of 0.05 mg (50 μg)/m^3.

Summary of Proposed EPA Criteria: *Freshwater Aquatic Life* — For lead, the criterion to protect freshwater aquatic life as derived using the Guidelines is

$$e^{[1.51 \ln(\text{hardness}) - 3.37]}$$

as a 24-hour average and the concentration should not exceed

$$e^{[1.51 \ln(\text{hardness}) - 1.39]}$$

at any time.

Saltwater Aquatic Life — For saltwater aquatic life, no criterion for lead can be derived using the Guidelines, and there are insufficient data to estimate a criterion using other procedures.

Human Health — For the protection of human health from the toxic properties of lead ingested through water and through contaminated aquatic organisms, the ambient water criterion for lead is 50 μg/l.

Basis for the Proposed Human Health Criteria: The approach that will be taken here in assessing the impact of lead in water on human health is basically the same as has been taken by the U.S. EPA for lead in air (44-16). The critical target organ or system must first be identified. Then, the highest internal dose of lead that can be tolerated without injury to the target organ must be specified. Finally, the impact of lead in water on the maximum tolerated internal dose must be estimated, as well as the likely consequences of specific reductions in the maximum allowable concentration of lead in water.

In identifying the critical organ or system, great reliance is placed on the concentration of lead in the blood (PbB) as an index of internal dose. Such an indirect measurement is necessary because of the multimedia character of lead intake. It is virtually impossible to measure total lead input in people in any meaningful way. To do so would require long-term balance studies because past experience has shown that intake and output fluctuate greatly from day to day. Furthermore, it would be necessary to conduct such studies on large numbers of free-living subjects, given the influences of chemical and physical variables in the numerous environmental forms of lead.

Variables have a substantial influence on the rate and degree of lead uptake from the external environment. Some groups have proposed alternatives to PbB as a measure of internal dose, e.g., FEP and tooth lead. FEP is not suitable because it is a biological response to lead. As such, it is subject to influences other than lead, notably iron deficiency. Tooth lead is a potentially useful index of lead exposure, but with the present state of art being what it is, tooth lead is difficult to interpret. It only provides an integrated profile of past lead exposure. One is not able to say when the exposure occurred. It has the additional limitation of not being available on demand. Teeth are shed spontaneously only in childhood. Beyond all that is the fact that there is only a very small data base for dose-effect and dose-response using any measure of dose other than PbB. The use of PbB as a measure of internal dose is widely accepted, simply because nothing better is available.

Having specified that PbB is the best measure of internal dose currently available, the next question concerns the least PbB at which adverse health effects occur. Two recent documents have been published (44-16, 44-17) in which judgements were rendered in this regard (Table 66). It will be noted that the estimates are strikingly similar. The estimated no-effects levels are based on limited populations and probably are lower to some indefinable degree in the total population at risk.

The expert panels that made these estimates were largely composed of different individuals, although there was some overlap. Slightly more information was available to the U.S. EPA panel than to the World Health Organization panel since it reviewed literature only through mid-1977 whereas the World Health Organization expert groups reviewed literature through much of 1976. In addition, the U.S. EPA performed statistical calculations based on the known distribution of blood lead levels in the U.S.

Both sets of data in Table 66 are in error in one regard. They use the term anemia inappropriately under the "Effect" column. What they really mean is "decrement in hemoglobin." Anemia is a clinical term used to denote a degree of hemoglobin decrement which is below the normal range for that class of individuals, e.g., men or children.

The question that arises in considering Table 66 is which is the critical effect? Precisely the same issue confronted the U.S. EPA in its deliberations concerning establishment of a national ambient air quality standard for lead (44-16). It focused on the lead effects in children since they are more sensitive than adults.

Table 66: Summary of Lowest PbBs Associated with Observed Biological Effects in Various Population Groups

Lowest Observed Effect Level (μg Pb/100 ml blood)	Effect	Population Group
10	ALAD inhibition	children and adults
15-20	erythrocyte protoporphyrin elevation	women and children
25-30	erythrocyte protoporphyrin elevation	adult males
40	increased urinary ALA excretion	children and adults
40	anemia	children
40	coproporphyrin elevation	adults and children
50	anemia	adults
50-60	cognitive (CNS) deficits	children
50-60	peripheral neuropathies	adults and children
80-100	encephalopathic symptoms	children
100-120	encephalopathic symptoms	adults

No-Detected Effect Levels in Terms of PbB

No-Detected Effect Level (μg Pb/100 ml blood)	Effect	Population Group
10	erythrocyte ALAD inhibition	adults and children
20-25	FEP	children
20-30	FEP	female adults
25-35	FEP	male adults
30-40	erythrocyte ATPase inhibition	general
40	ALA excretion in urine	adults and children
40	CP excretion in urine	adults
40	anemia	children
40-50	peripheral neuropathy	adults
50	anemia	adults
50-60	minimal brain dysfunction	children
60-70	minimal brain dysfunction	adults
60-70	encephalopathy	children
80	encephalopathy	adults

Source: Reference (44)

Quite properly, it ruled that the maximum safe blood lead level for any given child should be somewhat lower than the threshold for a decline in hemoglobin level (40 μg Pb/dl). In considering how much lower this limit should be, the U.S. EPA cited the opinion of the Center for Disease Control, as endorsed by the American Academy of Pediatrics, that the maximum safe blood lead level for any given child should be 30 μg/dl. Based upon epidemiological and statistical considerations, the U.S. EPA estimated that if the geometric mean PbB were kept at 15 μg/dl, 99.5% of children would have PbBs $\geq$ 30 μg/dl. This position seems prudent and reasonable. It provides a substantial margin of safety which accommodates minor excursions in lead exposure due to adventitious sources.

Controls on lead in obligatory media (e.g., air and water) do not, of course, protect children from the hazards of pica for lead-base paint chips or soil and dust contaminated with lead from such sources as fallout from the smoke zone of lead smelters. These, however, are separate problems which must be dealt with appropriately by responsible agencies.

In its deliberations concerning an ambient air lead standard, the U.S. EPA estimated that the contribution of sources other than air to PbB is 10 to 12 μg/dl. This is presumably composed overwhelmingly of dietary sources which, in turn, is composed of both food and water.

The next question concerns the contribution of water to lead exposure. It is unfortunate that only three useful studies of the interrelationship between PbB and lead in drinking water are available. There is an obvious need for more such work. Overall, the Moore, et al study, (44-18) the one by Hubermont, et al, (44-19) and the calculations made from U.S. EPA data collected in the Boston area (44-20) are credible because they are consistent with other information concerning the curvilinear relationship between PbB and Pb. The implication of the equation describing the relationship between PbB and water lead is that with increasing lead in water the incremental rise in PbB becomes progressively smaller as with air lead vs PbB and dietary lead vs PbB.

The water lead vs PbB relationship differs in one significant respect, however, from the air lead vs PbB relationship in that the baseline PbB (0 water PbB) is independent of the contribution of water lead to PbB. Thus, regardless of whether one starts with a baseline PbB of 11 μg/dl, as was indicated in the Moore, et al study, (44-18) or whether one starts at some other PbB level, e.g., 20 μg/dl, the add-on PbB from any given level in water will be the same. Such is not the case in the Azar analysis of air Pb vs PbB. Here, the higher the baseline, the less the contribution of any specific air Pb. This is because log PbB (not PbB) is proportional to baseline PbB + log air concentration.

Future research may provide better insight into whether this discrepancy is real and, if so, why. The question is of some practical importance. For instance, if you have a baseline PbB (no lead in water) of 30 μg/dl such as in a child acquiring lead from paint, it would be of some importance to know whether an additional increment of lead in water would have the same impact on PbB as it would in a child having a baseline PbB of 10 μg/dl. An Azar-type model would suggest a lesser impact starting from the higher baseline PbB.

So far as a specific recommendation regarding a revised water standard for lead is concerned, one is tempted to avoid the whole issue by simply recommending more research. However, that might defer the recommendation indefinitely. A position must be taken using available data. Beginning with the assumption that a PbB of 12 μg/dl is essentially attributable to food and water and that the average lead content of water consumed is 10 μg/l, approximately 5 μg Pb/dl blood is attributable to the water that is used in food and beverage preparation and in direct consumption. If the water Pb were consistently consumed at the present Pb standard of 50 μg/l instead of at 10 μg/l, an additional contribution of approximately 3.4 μg/dl to PbB would result. This would yield a total PbB of 12 + 3.4 or 15.4 μg/dl, the approximate maximum geometric mean PbB compatible with keeping 99.5% of the population under PbB = 30 μg/dl. Thus, based on most recent data, the present water standard of 50 μg Pb/l may be viewed as representing the upper limit of acceptability.

All the assumptions that have been made in arriving at an estimate of the impact of lead in water on PbB have been on the conservative side. For instance, unpublished data from the Commission of the European Communities suggest that the impact of lead in water on PbB is appreciably less than has been estimated from published data used in this document.

Furthermore, data from a study of the effect of lead in water on the PbB of a population of children in a relatively small town are reassuring (44-18). They indicate that among children whose water supply contained 50 to 180 μg Pb/l, PbBs averaged 17.2 μg/dl.

Finally, there remains the issue of the carcinogenic effects of lead. Using data from one species of laboratory animal (the rat) it was possible to construct a seemingly valid dose-response curve and to calculate a level of lead intake which would predict an incidence of cancer of 1:100,000 people. This calculated level of lead intake, 29 μg/kg of diet, poses some problems which must be confronted by the EPA Carcinogen Assessment Group. Since this estimate includes lead from all sources, its implications are beyond the scope of this document. It should be noted, however, that the International Agency for Research on Cancer, (IARC), Lyon, France considers the experimental animal evidence to be of dubious significance with regard to man. The IARC summary statement is as follows:

> There is no evidence to suggest that exposure to lead salts causes cancer of any site in man. However, only one epidemiological study of the relationships between exposure to lead and the occurrence of cancer has been reported. It must be noted that the level of human exposure equivalent to the levels of lead acetate producing

renal tumors in rats is 810 mg per day (550 mg Pb). This level appears to exceed by far the maximum tolerated dose for man.

References

(44-1) Biesinger, K.E., and G.M. Christensen. "Effect of various metals on survival, growth, reproduction, and metabolism of *Daphnia magna*." *Jour. Fish. Res. Board Can. 29,* 1691. (1972).

(44-2) Brown, V.M. "Calculation of the acute toxicity of mixtures of poisons to rainbow trout." *Water Res. 2,* 723. (1968).

(44-3) Davies, P.H., et al. "Acute and chronic toxicity of lead to rainbow trout, *Salmo gairdneri,* in hard and soft water." *Water Res. 10,* 199. (1976).

(44-4) Tarzwell, C.M., and C. Henderson. "Toxicity of less common metals to fishes." *Ind. Wastes 5,* 12. (1960).

(44-5) Pickering, Q.H., and C. Henderson. "The acute toxicity of some heavy metals to different species of freshwater fishes." *Air Water Pollut. Int. Jour. 10,* 453. (1966).

(44-6) McLain, R.M., and B.A. Baker. "Teratogenicity, fetal toxicity and placental transfer of lead nitrate in rats." *Toxicol. Appl. Pharmacol. 31,* 72. (1975).

(44-7) Lancranjan, I. et al. "Reproductive ability of workmen occupationally exposed to lead." *Arch. Environ. Health 30,* 396. (1975).

(44-8) Lane, R.E. "The care of the lead worker." *Br. Jour. Ind. Med. 6,* 1243. (1949).

(44-9) Roels, H.A., et al. "Lead and cadmium absorption among children near a nonferrous metal plant. A follow-up study of a test case." *Environ. Res. 15,* 290. (1978).

(44-10) Perlstein, M.A., and R. Atlala. "Neurologic sequelae of plumbism in children." *Clin. Pediat. 6,* 266. (1966).

(44-11) Byers, R.K. and E.E. Lord. "Late effects of lead poisoning on mental development." *Am. Jour. Child. 66,* 471. (1943).

(44-12) Clarkson, T.W., and J.E. Kench. "Urinary excretion of amino acids by men absorbing heavy metals." *Biochem. Jour. 62,* 361. (1956).

(44-13) Dingwall-Fordyce, J., and R.E. Lane. "A follow-up study of lead workers." *Br. Jour. Ind. Mech. 30,* 313. (1963).

(44-14) National Inst. for Occup. Safety and Health, *Criteria for a recommended standard: occupational exposure to inorganic lead,* NIOSH Doc. No. 73–11010, Wash. D.C. (1973).

(44-15) Occupational Safety and Health Admin., "Occupational exposure to lead: final standard," *Federal Register 43,* 53952-53014 (Nov. 14, 1978).

(44-16) U.S. Environmental Protection Agency, *A quality criteria for lead,* Report No. EPA 600/8-77-017, Wash., D.C. (1977).

(44-17) World Health Organization, *Environmental health criteria: lead,* Geneva. (1977).

(44-18) Moore, M.R. et al, "Contribution of lead in water to blood lead," *Lancet 11,* 661 (1977).

(44-19) Hubermont, G. et al, "Placental transfer of lead, mercury and cadmium in women living in a rural area." *Int. Arch. Occup. Envir. Health 41,* 117. (1978).

(44-20) Greathouse, D.G. and Craun, G.F., "Epidemiologic study of the relationship between lead in drinking water and blood levels" in D.D. Hemphill, Ed., *Trace Substances in Environmental Health,* Univ. of Missouri Press. (1976).

(44-21) Azar, A. et al, "An epidemiologic approach to community air lead exposure using personal air samples," *Environ. Qual. Safe. Suppl. II. (1975).*

M

MERCURY (#45)

Mercury, symbol Hg, is an element in Group II-B of the periodic table. It has an atomic number of 80, and an atomic weight of 200.59.

Occurrence: Several forms of mercury, ranging from elemental to dissolved inorganic and organic species, are expected to occur in the environment. The finding that certain micro-organisms have the ability to convert inorganic and organic forms of mercury to the highly toxic methyl or dimethyl mercury has made any form of mercury potentially hazardous to the environment (45-1). In water, under naturally occurring conditions of pH and temperature, inorganic mercury can be converted readily to methyl mercury (45-2).

The Department of the Interior carried out a nationwide reconnaissance of mercury in U.S. water in the summer and fall of 1970. Of the samples from the industrial wastewater category, 30% contained mercury at greater than 10 μg/l; nearly 0.5% of the samples in this group contained more than 1,000 μg/l. Only 4% of the surface water samples contained more than 1,000 μg/l. The higher mercury concentrations were generally found in small streams. About half the 43 samples from the Mississippi River contained less than 0.1 μg/l. The mercury content of lakes and reservoirs was between 0.1 and 1.8 μg/l. With few exceptions, the mercury content of groundwater samples was below detection (0.1 μg/l).

In a survey by the EPA Division of Water Hygiene, 273 community, recreation, and federal installation water supplies were examined. Of these, 261 or 95.5% showed either no detectable mercury or less than 1.0 μg/l in the raw and finished water. Eleven of the supplies had mercury concentrations of 1.0 to 4.8 μg/l and one supply exceeded 5.0 μg/l. When this one supply was extensively reexamined, the mercury concentration was found to be less than 0.8 μg/l.

Seawater contains 0.03 to 2.0 μg/l, depending on the sampled area, the depth, and the analyst. In a study of Pacific waters, mercury concentrations were found to increase from surface values of near 0.10 μg/l to 0.15 to 0.27 μg/l at greater depths. In an area seriously affected by pollution (Minamata Bay, Japan), values ranged from 1.6 to 3.6 μg/l. The National Research Council (45-3) has shown typical oceanic mercury values to be 0.01-0.03 μg/l. Oceanic mercury is generally present as an anionic complex ($HgCo^-$), which does not have as pronounced a tendency to bind to particulate substances and then settle out as do mercury compounds found in freshwater.

Mercury can be bioconcentrated many fold in fish and other aquatic organisms because of rapid uptake and the relative inability of fish to excrete methyl mercury from their tissues. Freshwater values of 63,000 have been found as well as saltwater bioconcentration values of 10,000.

Physical Properties: Mercury is a silver-white metal. A liquid at room temperature, its melting point is $-38.87°C$ and its boiling point ranges from $356°$ to $358°C$. The metal is insoluble and is not attacked by water. At $20°C$, the specific gravity is 13.546, and the vapor pressure is 0.0012 mm Hg.

The more commonly found mercuric salts (with their solubilities in water) are $HgCl_2$ (1 g/13.5 ml water), $Hg(NO_3)_2$ (soluble in a small amount of water), and $Hg(CH_3COO)_2$

(1 g/2.5 ml water). Mercurous salts are much less soluble in water. $HgNO_3$ will solubilize only in 13 parts water containing 1% HNO_3. Hg_2Cl_2 is practically insoluble in water. Because of this, mercurous salts are much less toxic than the mercuric forms.

Chemical Properties: Mercury is able to form a series of organometallic compounds with alkyl, phenyl, and methoxyethyl radicals. Short-chained alkyl mercurials are toxicologically important because the carbon-mercury bond can be broken in vivo, with the subsequent disappearance of the organic radical.

Uses: A major use of mercury has been as a cathode in the electrolytic preparation of chlorine and caustic soda; this accounted for 33% of total demand in the U.S. in 1968. Electrical apparatus (lamps, arc rectifiers, and mercury battery cells) accounted for 27%, and industrial and control instruments (switches, thermometers, and barometers), and general laboratory applications accounted for 14% of demand. Use of mercury in antifouling and mildew-proofing paints (12%) and mercury formulations used to control fungal diseases of seeds, bulbs, plants, and vegetation (5%) were other major utilizations; however, mercury is no longer registered by the EPA for use in antifouling paints or for the control of fungal diseases of bulbs. The remainder (9%) was for dental amalgams, catalysts, pulp and paper manufacture, pharmaceuticals, and metallurgy and mining.

Toxic Effects: Nonhuman mammals have been shown to suffer central nervous system damage as well as teratogenesis and spontaneous tumorigenesis (45-4, 45-5). There is no data available on the teratogenicity or mutagenicity of inorganic mercury in human populations. Furthermore, there is no evidence of mercury exposure producing carcinogenicity.

In humans, mercurials have been associated with neurological disorders, sensory impairment, tremors, buccal ulceration, gastrointestinal complaints and multisystem involvement due to general encephalopathy (45-6, 45-7, 45-8, 45-9, 45-10). Mercurials will damage the bronchial epithelium and interrupt respiratory function in freshwater invertebrates. Rainbow trout will suffer loss of equilibrium, and trout fry are more susceptible to mercury poisoning than fingerlings. Mercurial compounds may interfere with receptor membranes in fish.

Current Levels of Exposure: Evidence indicates that the predominant form of mercury in freshwater (and probably marine water also) is Hg^{++}, present as chelates and complexes with a variety of inorganic and organic ligands. However, the data are not sufficiently detailed or accurate to exclude the possibility of the presence of other forms of mercury, especially in contaminated areas. Methyl mercury compounds may be present due to biomethylation of inorganic mercury in sediment, elemental mercury (Hg°) due to discharge from industry, and aryl and alkoxy mercurials due to their use in the paint industry. Although it is highly probable that the proportions of organomercurials and elemental mercury vapor are small compared to inorganic divalent mercury (Hg^{++}) compounds, it will be assumed that the species most toxic to man accounts for 100% of the total mercury in water because methyl mercury compounds are the forms of mercury which are most toxic to man and present the greatest risk of irreversible functional damage.

Special Groups at Risk: The evidence indicates that intake of mercury from drinking water is toxicologically negligible. Human exposure to the most hazardous form of this metal, methyl mercury, is almost exclusively via consumption of fish. Thus, the population most likely to be at risk is heavy consumers of fish containing the highest mercury concentrations. The stage of the human life cycle subject to the greatest hazard from mercury intake is probably prenatal.

Other forms of mercury probably do not present a significant risk, except in the case of mercury vapor. The latter may present a health risk if occupational exposures are not maintained below acceptable limits. Unfortunately, the stage of the life cycle most susceptible to the toxic effects of mercury vapor has not yet been identified.

An unusual and rare reaction to inorganic mercury forms, called acrodynia or Pink's disease has been described. This disease has occurred in children receiving oral doses of medications containing inorganic mercury, or inhaling mercury vapor. Only a small number of children develop acrodynia when exposed to mercury. It is unlikely that a small amount of inorganic mercury ingested in drinking water would cause this disease.

Existing Guidelines and Standards: A World Health Organization expert group has recommended an international standard for drinking water of 1 μg Hg/l (45-12); the U.S. Environmental Protection Agency recommended a standard of 2 μg Hg/l in 1973.

The ACGIH, as of 1979, has adopted a TWA value of 0.05 mg/m^3 for all forms of mercury except alkyl mercury. The tentative STEL value for that same category is 0.15 mg/m^3.

For alkyl mercury compounds, ACGIH has adopted a TWA value of 0.001 ppm (0.01 mg/m^3) and has set forth a tentative STEL value for alkyl mercury compounds of 0.003 ppm (0.03 mg/m^3).

NIOSH (45-11) has recommended a standard of 0.05 mg/m^3 as a TWA for inorganic mercury.

Summary of Proposed EPA Criteria: *Freshwater Aquatic Life* — The data base for freshwater aquatic life and inorganic mercury is insufficient to allow use of the Guidelines. The following recommendation is inferred from toxicity data for saltwater organisms.

For inorganic mercury, the criterion to protect freshwater aquatic life as derived using procedures other than the Guidelines is 0.064 μg/l as a 24-hour average and the concentration should not exceed 3.2 μg/l at any time.

For methyl mercury the criterion to protect freshwater aquatic life as derived using the Guidelines is 0.016 μg/l as a 24-hour average and the concentration should not exceed 8.8 μg/l at any time.

Saltwater Aquatic Life — For inorganic mercury, the criterion to protect saltwater aquatic life as derived using the Guidelines is 0.19 μg/l as a 24-hour average and the concentration should not exceed 1.0 μg/l at any time.

The data base for saltwater aquatic life and methyl mercury is insufficient to allow use of the Guidelines. The following recommendation is inferred from toxicity data for freshwater organisms.

For methyl mercury, the criterion to protect saltwater aquatic life as derived using procedures other than the Guidelines is 0.025 μg/l as a 24-hour average and the concentration should not exceed 2.6 μg/l at any time.

Human Health — For the protection of human health from the toxic properties of mercury ingested through water and through contaminated aquatic organisms the ambient water criterion is determined to be 0.2 μg/l.

Basis for the Proposed Human Health Criteria: From a health effects perspective and recognition of exposure potential the organomercury compounds are the most important, especially methyl mercury. However, inorganic compounds of mercury should also be recognized because of their toxicity potential, but perhaps more importantly because with alkylation from environmentally present biological systems, the inorganic mercury can be converted to methyl and dimethyl mercury.

The approach that has been adopted by this criterion document involves the following steps:

    (1) Identify those organs or tissues most sensitive to damage by the different chemical and physical forms of mercury, damage being defined as an effect that adversely changes normal function or diminishes an individual's reserve capacity to deal with harmful agents or diseases;

(2) Determine the lowest body burden known to be associated with functional damage in man and, if possible, determine the highest body burden tolerated by man;

(3) Estimate the potential human intake from ingesting water and eating contaminated fish products; and

(4) Estimate the effect on body burden of mercury by establishing a criterion for mercury in ambient water based on human health effects.

Table 67 taken from the review by the World Health Organization expert group indicates long-term daily intakes of methyl mercury which relates to the earliest effect on the central nervous system. This system is more sensitive to damage from methyl mercury than other functional systems in the human body. The conclusions represented in Table 67 were recently endorsed by the National Academy of Sciences.

Evidence reviewed in the criterion document is essentially the same as the evidence reviewed by the WHO group with regard to adult exposures to methyl mercury.

Table 67: The Concentration of Total Mercury in Indicator Media and the Equivalent Long-Term Daily Intake of Mercury as Methyl Mercury Associated with the Earliest Effects in the Most Sensitive Group in the Adult Population*

| Concentrations in Indicator Media | | Equivalent Long-Term |
Blood (μg/100 ml)	Hair (μg/g)	Daily Intake (μg/kg body weight)
20-50	50-125	3-7

*The risk of the earliest effects can be expected to be between 3 to 8%. The table should not be considered independently of the text.

Source: Reference (45-13)

Effects on the adult nervous system have been estimated to occur at blood concentrations in the range of 200 to 500 ng Hg/ml, corresponding to a long-term daily intake of methyl mercury in the diet of 3 to 7 μg/kg body weight. The risk of effects at this intake level is probably less than 8% (1 in 12 chances).

Since the WHO document (45-13) was written, new evidence has been documented. As reported in the criterion document, females who had experienced maximum hair concentrations during pregnancy in the range of 99 to 384 μg Hg/g had a high probability of having children liable to retarded development. Unfortunately, the population size was too small to establish a lower limit to effects of prenatal exposure. A hair concentration of 99 μg/g is equivalent to a blood concentration of about 400 ng Hg/ml.

The most recent information on effect of mercury on human health has come from the study of the Iraq outbreak of 1971-1972. The follow-up of the cases of prenatal exposure is still in progress. As noted by the National Academy of Sciences (45-3), "continued careful evaluation of this very important cohort of prenatally exposed individuals will provide the most sensitive assessment of human methyl mercury toxicity."

Thus, at this stage of knowledge of the dose-effect relationship of mercury in man, it appears that the earliest detected effects in man are at blood concentrations between 200 and 500 ng Hg/ml for both pre- and postnatal exposures. Blood concentrations of methyl mercury correspond to body burdens in the range of 30 to 50 mg Hg/70 kg body weight, and to long-term daily intakes in the range of 200 to 500 μg Hg/70 kg.

Mercury intake from drinking water, according to data reviewed in the document is less than 1 μg Hg/day, and is considerably less than the diet portion (Table 68). Assuming that the concentration of methyl mercury in all samples of drinking water is at the current U.S. EPA standard of 2 μg Hg/l, the maximum daily intake would only be 4 μg Hg, assuming 2 liters of drinking water are consumed per person each day. This maximum intake would amount to only about 1 to 2% of the minimum toxic intake given in Table 68. Thus, from the toxicological standpoint, exposure to mercury via drinking water only would be negligible.

Table 68: Estimate of Average and Maximum Daily Intake of Mercury by the 70 kg Standard Adult in the U.S. Population*

| Media | . . Mercury Intake (μg/day/70 kg) . . | | Predominate Form |
	Average	Maximum**	
Air	0.3	0.8	Hg°
Water	0.1	0.4	Hg^{++}
Food	3.0	5.0	CH_3Hg^{+}

*For details on the calculation of these numbers see the Exposure Section of the Criteria Document (45).
**Approximate figures indicating 95% of population have intakes less than these figures. Occupational exposures are not included.

The ingestion of water has been assumed to be the main pathway of direct intake of mercury from water. The transport of mercury through skin is another possible route of intake. Indirect transfer of mercury from water to man is much more important than transfer from direct routes. This conclusion is based on the assumption that fish bioaccumulate a significant amount of methyl mercury from water. In theory, it should be possible to calculate the maximum concentration of methyl mercury in water which would assure that concentrations in edible tissues of fish do not exceed the Food and Drug Administration Guidelines of 1.0 μg Hg/g fresh tissue.

Thus, if the bioaccumulation factor is known for each species of edible fish, it is arithmetically simple to estimate the maximum concentration of methyl mercury in water. For example, the U.S. EPA in 1978 calculated bioconcentration factors (concentration in fish/concentration in water) for methyl mercury compounds based on literature reports. These factors are for edible fish species: 4,525 to 8,376 for rainbow trout *Salmo gairdneri,* 20,000 for brook trout *Salvelinus fontinalis,* and 900 to 1,640 for clams *Anodanta grandis, Lampsitis radiata, Lasmigona complanta.* Thus, if the maximum bioaccumulation factor of 20,000 is adopted, the maximum concentration of methyl mercury in freshwater that would prevent fish from exceeding the current FDA guideline would be 0.05 μg/l.

Unfortunately, both practical and theoretical difficulties thwart any accurate calculation. First, quantitative information is inadequate with regard to the role of direct uptake from water vs accumulation from food chains as contributors to the total amount of methyl mercury in fish. Differences may be expected between fish at lower and upper ends of the food chain. Second, the accumulation factors for methyl mercury uptake by fish are only known for few species. Third, the concentration of methyl mercury in water is probably a variable fraction of total mercury in water. The proportion of methyl to total mercury will probably vary in different bodies of water, being influenced by such factors as water pH, degree of oxygenation, the amount of biota and the sedimentary concentrations of mercury. Fourth, in most cases, the concentration of methyl mercury in water will be so low as to defy accurate measurement even by the most modern technology.

When more information is available on the behavior of mercury in aquatic environments, it might be possible to calculate a reliable criterion based on acceptable concentrations of mercury in fish. In the meantime, a more pragmatic approach will have to be used. The discharge of mercury into bodies of water must be carefully controlled.

Those bodies of freshwater supporting edible fish with mercury concentrations above the acceptable levels will have to be identified, and anthropogenic discharge of mercury curtailed. It is also possible that nonanthropogenic sources are predominant (for example, in ocean waters) so that control is not possible. This empirical approach, although the only one available, is unsatisfactory as it allows mainly after-the-fact corrections. Development of procedures for estimating maximum safe concentrations of mercury in ambient water that will prevent unacceptable bioaccumulation of methyl mercury by fish is clearly desirable.

Methyl Mercury – Two approaches could be used to derive a criterion for methyl mercury. One approach is to use the existing U.S. drinking water standard of 2 μg/l and the typical water quality exposure assumptions (2 liters water/day, 0.0187 kg fish products/day) along with an estimated fish and shellfish bioconcentration factor of 6,200 to calculate a potential uptake. This can then be compared to the Lowest Observable Effect Level (LOEL) to determine the range of safety. A second approach is to use the LOEL as a basis for establishing an acceptable daily intake (ADI) and calculate a criterion level using the typical water quality assumptions.

$$\text{Given:} \quad \text{Fish and shellfish consumption} = 0.0187 \text{ kg fish/person/day}$$

$$\text{Bioconcentration factor for methyl mercury} = 6,200 = \frac{\text{mg Hg/kg fish}}{\text{mg Hg/liter water}}$$

$$\text{Water consumption} = 2 \text{ liters/person/day}$$

(1) Assume:

$$
\begin{aligned}
\text{Criterion} &= 2 \text{ μg/l} \\
\text{Human Exposure} &= 2 \text{ liters/day} + (6,200 \times 0.0187) \\
&= 2 \,(2+115.9) \\
&= 235.8 \text{ μg/day}
\end{aligned}
$$

Recognizing that the LOEL range is 200 to 500 μg Hg/day, it could be hypothesized that there is little or no margin of safety at the 2 μg/l criterion level especially where realizing that dietary sources other than fish products may be contributing to the body burden.

(2) Derive ADI using typical water quality exposure and LOEL

LOEL range = 200 to 500 μg/day

Use 200 μg Hg/day to assure marginal safety

$$
\begin{aligned}
\text{ADI} &= 200 \text{ μg/day} \\
&= C \,[2 \text{ liters/day} + (6,200 \times 0.0187)] \\
200 &= C \,(2 + 115.9) \\
200/117.9 &= C \\
1.7 \text{ μg/l} &= C
\end{aligned}
$$

According to the National Academy of Science (45-3) an uncertainty factor of ten can be applied to the ADI as the 200 to 500 data results from studies on prolonged ingestion by man, with no indication of carcinogenicity.

$$
\begin{aligned}
200/10 &= C \,(2+115.9) \\
0.17 \text{ μg/l} &= C \\
0.2 \text{ μg/l} &\sim C
\end{aligned}
$$

Whereas, approach No. 1 has an estimated narrow margin of safety, if any, and given that LOELs do exist, it is reasonable to focus on the ADI-based criterion with an uncertainty factor as the preferred basis for establishing a criterion.

References

(45-1) Jensen, S., and A. Jernelov. "Biological methylation of mercury." *Nature. 223,* 753. (1969).

(45-2) Bisogni, J.J., and A.W. Lawrence. *Methylation of mercury in aerobic and anaerobic environments.* Tech. Rep. 63. Cornell Univer. Resour. Mar. Sci. Center, Ithaca, New York. (1973).

(45-3) National Research Council. *An assessment of mercury in the environment.* Wash., D.C. National Academy of Sciences. (1977).

(45-4) Robbins, E.B., and K.K. Chen. "A new mercurial diuretic." *Jour. Am. Pharma. Assoc. 40,* 249. (1951)

(45-5) Spann, J.W., et al. "Ethyl mercury p-toluene sulfonanilide: lethal and reproductive effects on pheasants." *Science 175,* 328. (1972).

(45-6) Matsumoto, H., et al. "Fetal minamata disease. A neuropathological study of two cases of intrauterine intoxication by a methyl mercury compound." *Jour. Neuropathol. Exp. Neurol. 24,* 563. (1965).

(45-7) Chang, L.W., et al. "Minamata disease." *Acta Neuropathol. 26,* 275. (1973).

(45-8) Davis, L.E., et al. "Central nervous system intoxication from mercurous chloride laxatives." *Arch. Neurol. 30,* 428. (1974).

(45-9) Rustam, H., et al. *Arch. Environ. Health, 30,* 190. (1975).
(45-10) Weiss, B., and R.A. Doherty. "Methylmercury poisoning." *Teratology 12,* 311. (1976).
(45-11) Nat. Inst. for Occup. Safety and Health, *Criteria for a recommended standard: occupational exposure to inorganic mercury,* NIOSH Doc. No. 73-11024 (1973).
(45-12) World Health Organization, *International standards for drinking water,* 3rd Ed., Geneva (1971).
(45-13) World Health Organization, *Environmental health criteria: mercury,* Geneva (1976).

METHYL BROMIDE

See "Halomethanes" (38).

METHYL CHLORIDE

See "Halomethanes" (38).

METHYLENE CHLORIDE

See "Halomethanes" (38).

MONOCHLOROBENZENE

See "Chlorinated Benzenes" (14).

N

NAPHTHALENE (#46)

Naphthalene is a bicyclic aromatic hydrocarbon with the chemical formula $C_{10}H_8$ and a molecular weight of 128.16.

Occurrence: Naphthalene is the most abundant single constituent of coal tar (46-1). In 1974, 1.8×10^5 metric tons of naphthalene were produced from coal tar, and 1.1×10^5 metric tons were produced from petroleum. Naphthalene has a varied environmental distribution and has been detected in ambient water (up to 2.0 μg/l), sewage plant effluents (up to 22 μg/l), and drinking water supplies (up to 1.4 μg/l). Recent studies have determined that naphthalene will accumulate in sediments by more than 100 times the concentration in the overlying water.

Naphthalene has been shown to bioconcentrate in both invertebrate and vertebrate species of aquatic organisms. It has also been suggested that much of the naphthalene taken up by aquatic organisms returns to the ecosystem in fecal matter without being metabolized.

Physical Properties: Pure naphthalene forms a white crystalline solid at room temperature whereas the crude or technical grades may range in color from brown to tan. Naphthalene vapor and dust can form explosive mixtures with air. Pure naphthalene melts at 80.2°C; the less pure forms of the compound will melt at temperatures ranging from 74° to 80°C. The boiling point of naphthalene is 217.96°C at atmospheric pressure. At 15.5°C, the density is 1.145 and at 100°C, the density is 0.9625. At 19.8°C, the vapor pressure of solid naphthalene is 0.0492 mm Hg.

The solubility of naphthalene in water has been reported to range between 30,000 and 40,000 μg/l at 25°C. The solubility of naphthalene in seawater will vary according to the degree of chlorosity; in seawater of average composition, the solubility of naphthalene is approximately 33,000 μg/l. Naphthalene has also been reported to be soluble in organic solvents.

Chemical Properties: Naphthalene can oxidize in the presence of light and air, and it was determined that 50% of the theoretical CO_2 was liberated after 14 days. The process involves initial conversion to naphthaquinone with subsequent rupture of one of the aromatic rings and the release of CO_2. However, this oxidation process occurs only at elevated temperatures.

When combined with alcohol and ozone, cyclic alkoxyhydroxyperoxides are formed. In an acidic medium, these peroxides will be converted to methyl phthalaldehydate; in a basic medium, they are converted to phthalaldehydic acid. When combined with metal nitrate within a temperature range of 55° to 180°C, naphthalene can be nitrated at the alpha position. In the presence of oxygen, K_2SO_4, and a vanadium oxide catalyst, naphthalene can be converted to phthalic anhydride.

Microorganisms can degrade naphthalene to 1,2-dihydro-1,2-dihydroxynaphthalene and ultimately to carbon dioxide and water. Studies have indicated a degradation rate under laboratory conditions of up to 3.3 μg/l.

Uses: This compound is used as an intermediate in the production of dye compounds and the formulation of solvents, lubricants, and motor fuels. One of the principal uses of naphthalene as a feedstock in the United States is for the synthesis of phthalic anhydride. It has also been used directly as a moth repellent and insecticide as well as an anthelminthic, vermicide, and an intestinal antiseptic.

Toxic Effects: Naphthalene has been shown to be toxic to microorganisms and has been reported to reduce photosynthetic rates in algae. It has also been reported to be acutely toxic to various invertebrate and vertebrate species of aquatic organisms. In laboratory mammals and humans, naphthalene has been linked to blood disorders and is suspected of traversing the placental membrane in humans following naphthalene ingestion by the mother.

Current Levels of Exposure: Natural waters have been found to contain up to 2 μg/l of naphthalene while drinking water supplies have been found to contain up to 1.4 μg/l of naphthalene. Ambient air levels have been measured at 0.00035 μg/m^3 in an urban area and 0.00006 μg/m^3 in a small town. Industrial exposures can range as high as 1.1 x 10^6 μg/m^3 for naphthalene-using industries with exposures up to 1,120 μg/m^3 for coke oven workers and 310 μg/m^3 for aluminum reduction plant workers. No measurements of naphthalene have been reported for market-basket foods.

Special Groups at Risk: Approximately 100 million people worldwide have G6PD deficiency which would make them more susceptible to hemolytic anemia on exposure to naphthalene. At present, more than 80 variants of this enzyme deficiency have been identified (46-2). The incidence of this deficiency is 0.1% in American and European Caucasians, but can range as high as 20% in American blacks and greater than 50% in certain Jewish groups.

Newborn infants have a similar sensitivity to the hemolytic effects of naphthalene, even without G6PD deficiency. Zinkham and Childs (46-3) surveyed 26 normal white and black newborn infants and found that their blood reduced glutathione levels dropped moderately to severely in all of the samples tested when incubated with acetylphenylhydrazine, suggestive of a glutathione reductase deficiency. Brown and Burnett (46-4) also noted that newborn infants have a decreased capacity to conjugate chemical metabolites with glucuronide secondary to an absolute decrease in the activity of UDP-glucuronyl dehydrogenase and transferase. Such a lack in glucuronidation can allow the build-up of toxic amounts of 1,2-dihydroxynaphthalene and 1,2-naphthaquinone.

A small percentage of the population might have an allergic hypersensitivity to naphthalene. Fanburg (46-5) described a 43-year-old physician with a generalized exfoliative dermatitis who was found to be allergic to naphthalene. Both the clinical and histologic picture resembled a malignancy, mycosis fungoides. A patch test with naphthalene was positive, resulting in urticaria. When all exposure to naphthalene was discontinued, the skin condition cleared rapidly and did not recur over a 3-year period of followup.

Existing Guidelines and Standards: The only existing United States standard for naphthalene is the Occupational Safety and Health Administration standard of 10 ppm (50 mg/m^3) of vapor exposure for a time-weighted industrial exposure (46-6). This standard was adopted from the American Conference of Governmental Industrial Hygienists' Threshold Limit Value which, in turn, was based on an irritant threshold for naphthalene of 15 ppm. At present, the ACGIH also suggests a maximum 15-minute exposure value of 15 ppm (75 mg/m^3). The maximum permissible concentration of naphthalene in fishery water bodies of the USSR is 4 μg/l.

Summary of Proposed EPA Criteria: *Freshwater Aquatic Life* — For freshwater aquatic life, no criterion for naphthalene can be derived using the Guidelines, and there are insufficient data to estimate a criterion using other procedures.

Saltwater Aquatic Life — For saltwater aquatic life, no criterion for naphthalene can be derived using the Guidelines, and there are insufficient data to estimate a criterion using other procedures.

Human Health — For the protection of human health from the toxic properties of naphthalene ingested through water and through contaminated aquatic organisms, the ambient water criterion is determined to be 143 μg/l.

Basis for the Proposed Human Health Criteria: All chronic toxicity studies using naphthalene have failed to demonstrate any carcinogenic activity except for those performed by Knake (46-7). This author found an excess occurrence of lymphosarcoma when naphthalene was given by the subcutaneous route to rats, and lymphocytic leukemia when naphthalene was chronically painted on the skin of mice using benzene as a solvent. However, the naphthalene used in this study was derived from coal tar and contained 10% or more unidentified impurities. Furthermore, a known experimental carcinogen, carbolfuchsin, was applied prior to each injection of naphthalene in the former study. In light of these defects, carcinogenicity data derived from this study cannot be used as a basis for a naphthalene water criterion.

No other chronic toxicity studies are available that can be used as an adequate basis for a naphthalene criterion. Furthermore, there are no adequate epidemiologic studies that can be used as a basis.

The ACGIH has recommended a time-weighted threshold limit value for an industrially exposed population of 50 mg/m^3 (50 μg/l) of naphthalene vapor in air. This value was set to prevent workers with exposure to naphthalene vapors from getting eye irritation. It is unclear, however, whether exposures to water containing naphthalene in excess of this level (50 μg/l) might also result in mucous membrane irritation. Until further information is available on the direct irritant properties of naphthalene in water, the ACGIH threshold limit value cannot be used as a basis for a naphthalene water criterion.

Mahvi et al (46-8) noted a dose-related response by C57 B1/6J mice given intraperitoneal injections of naphthalene in sesame oil. No bronchiolar epithelial changes were noted in two control groups. The authors noted minimal bronchiolar epithelial changes in the treated group receiving 6.4 mg/kg body weight of naphthalene. Severe, reversible damage to bronchiolar epithelial cells was noted among two higher dosage groups. The results of this study can be used as the basis for the criterion. The minimal effect level of 6.4 mg/kg of body weight is equivalent to a 448-mg dose for a 70-kg man and can reasonably be used as a basis for calculating an acceptable daily dosage if it is reduced by a factor of 1,000, which equals 448 μg, to protect sensitive individuals (46-9).

No pharmacokinetic data are available on the absorption of naphthalene by the oral route. Because of its high octanol:water partition coefficient (46-10), it is reasonable to expect that naphthalene in water should be nearly completely absorbed and an absorption efficiency of 100% can be assumed.

For the purposes of establishing a water quality criterion, human exposure to naphthalene is considered to be based on ingestion of 2 liters of water and 18.7 g of fish. Fish bioaccumulate naphthalene from water by a factor of 60. With these considerations in mind, the following equation has been established:

$$2 \text{ liters} \times X + (0.0187 \times 60) \times X = 448 \, \mu g$$

where:

$$448 \, \mu g = \text{limit on daily exposure for a 70 kg person (ADI)}$$

2 liters = amount of drinking water consumed

0.0187 kg = amount of fish consumed

60 = bioaccumulation factor

Solving for X:

$$X = 143 \, \mu g/l$$

Thus, the water level would have to be limited to 143 μg/l to limit the daily intake of naphthalene to 448 μg.

References

(46-1)   Schmeltz, I. et al, "The role of naphthalenes as carcinogens," A paper presented at the 16th Annu. Meet. Soc. Toxicol., Toronto, Canada (March 27–30, 1977).

(46-2)   Wintrobe, M.M. et al, *Clinical Hematology*, 7th Ed., Phila., Lea & Febiger (1974).

(46-3)   Zinkham, W.J. and Childs, B., "A defect of glutathione metabolism in erythrocytes from patients with a naphthalene-induced hemolytic anemia," *Pediatrics* 22, 461 (1958).

(46-4)   Brown, A.K. and Burnett, H., "Studies on the neonatal development of the glucuronide conjugating system," *Am. Jour. Dis. Child.* 94, 510 (1957).

(46-5)   Fanburg, S.J., "Exfoliative dermatitis due to naphthalene," *Arch. Dermt. Syph.* 42, 53 (1940).

(46-6)   39 *FR* 23540.

(46-7)   Knake, E., "Uber schwache geschwulsterzengende wirkung von naphthalin und benzol," *Virchows Archiv. Pathol. Anat. Physiol.* 329, 141 (1956).

(46-8)   Mahvi, D. et al, "Morphology of a naphthalene-induced bronchiolar lesion," *Am. Jour. Pathol.* 86, 559 (1977).

(46-9)   National Academy of Sciences, *Drinking Water & Health*, Wash., D.C. (1977).

(46-10)   Krishnamurthy, T. and Wasik, S.P., "Fluorometric determination of partition coefficients of naphthalene homologs in octanol-water mixtures," *Jour. Envir. Sci. Health* A-13, 595 (1978).

NICKEL (#47)

Nickel, symbol Ni, is an element in Group VIII of the periodic table. It has an atomic number of 28 and an atomic weight of 58.69.

Occurrence: Nickel enters the environment via both natural and anthropogenic activity, and a detailed description of sources and prevalence of nickel in the environment is given in a comprehensive National Academy of Sciences (NAS) review (47-1). Nickel levels in United States drinking waters are typically less than 10 μg/l.

Physical Properties: Nickel is a bright, silver metal of the iron-cobalt-nickel triad. It is a hard and malleable metal with a high tensile strength and is used in electroplating and virtually all areas of metallurgy.

Chemical Properties: Nickel is a divalent metal, with characteristic divalent metal chemistry, although it does not readily form chloro-complexes and, under environmental conditions, would not be expected to form significant amounts of sulfate complexes.

Uses: In 1972, United States consumption of nickel, exclusive of scrap, was estimated to total about 160,000 tons. The estimate consisted mainly of commercially pure nickel (about 110,000 tons). The main uses for this commercially pure nickel were stainless steel, various other alloys, and electroplating. Presumably, the commercial utility of nickel is such that growth in the use of nickel is assured.

Toxic Effects: In the aquatic environment, nickel is acutely toxic to fishes at concentrations as low as 2,480 μg/l. Chronic toxicity to fishes has been reported at 433 μg/l. Water quality also affects nickel toxicity. For instance, Lind et al (47-2) found the lowest effect level for fathead minnows to lie between 109 and 433 μg/l in embryo-larval tests in water with a hardness of 44 mg/l as calcium carbonate, while Pickering (47-3) reported a range 380 to 730 μg/l in a life cycle test with the same species at a water hardness of 210 mg/l as calcium carbonate.

The human health criterion is calculated on the basis of adverse effects seen in rats provided with drinking water containing 5 ppm nickel. These effects included reduction of litter size, increased numbers of runts, and increased neonatal mortality (47-4).

Current Levels of Exposure: The route by which most people in the general population receive the largest portion of daily nickel intake is through food. Based on the available data from composite diet analysis, between 300 to 600 μg nickel per day are ingested. Fecal nickel analysis, a more accurate measure of dietary nickel intake, suggests about 300 μg per day. The highest level of nickel observed in water was 75 μg/l. Average drinking water levels are about 5 μg/l. A typical consumption of 2 liters daily would yield an additional 10 μg of nickel, of which up to 1 μg would be absorbed.

Special Groups at Risk: Occupational groups, such as nickel workers and other workers handling nickel, comprise the individuals at the highest risk. Women, particularly housewives, are at special risk to nickel-induced skin disorders. Approximately 47 million individuals, comprising the smoking population of the United States, are potentially at risk for possible co-factor effects of nickel in adverse effects on the respiratory tract.

Existing Guidelines and Standards: The threshold limit values (TLV) for a work day exposure has been set at 0.1 mg/m^3 on a TWA basis for soluble nickel compounds (as Ni) with a tentative STEL value of 0.3 mg/m^3 for such compounds.

Nickel metal has a TWA value of 1.0 mg/m^3 adopted by ACGIH as of 1979. Nickel sulfide roasting fume and dust also has a 1.0 mg/m^3 TWA value assigned, but that category is also listed under Human Carcinogens.

NIOSH (47-5) quotes a current OSHA environmental standard of 1.0 mg/m^3 as a TWA value but recommend 15 μg/m^3 on a TWA basis. NIOSH, in a special hazard review in 1977, defines the allowable TWA value for nickel carbonyl as 7.0 μg/m^3 (1.0 ppb).

Summary of Proposed EPA Criteria: *Freshwater Aquatic Life* — For nickel, the criterion to protect freshwater aquatic life as derived using the Guidelines is $e^{[1.01 \cdot \ln(hardness) - 1.02]}$ as a 24-hour average and the concentration should not exceed $e^{[0.47 \cdot \ln(hardness) + 4.19]}$ at any time.

Saltwater Aquatic Life — For nickel, the criterion to protect saltwater aquatic life as derived using procedures other than the Guidelines is 220 μg/l as a 24-hour average and the concentration should not exceed 510 μg/l at any time.

Human Health — For the protection of human health based on the toxic properties of nickel ingested through water and through contaminated aquatic organisms, the ambient water criterion is determined to be 133 μg/l/day.

Basis for the Proposed Human Health Criteria: In arriving at a criterion for nickel, several factors must be taken into account. There is little evidence for accumulation of nickel in various tissues. Absorption through the gastrointestinal tract is minimal. Acute exposure of man to nickel is chiefly of concern in workplaces where nickel carbonyl or nickel dust are present at high levels. In these situations, inhalation is the main route of entry and the lung is the critical organ although, in some instances of high exposure, the central nervous system may also be involved.

The major problem posed by nickel for the United States population at large is nickel hypersensitivity, mainly via contact with many nickel-containing commodities. Nickel could play a role in altering defense mechanisms against xenobiotic agents in the respiratory tract, leading to enhanced risk for respiratory tract infections.

While nickel has a possible role as a co-carcinogen in producing respiratory cancer, as suggested by animal studies, this remains to be demonstrated. There is no evidence for carcinogenicity due to the presence of nickel in water. The role of nickel as an essential element is a confounding factor in any risk estimate.

In order to develop a risk assessment based on toxicological effects other than carcinogenicity, dose-response data would be most helpful. However, while the frequency or extent of various effects of nickel are related to the level or frequency of nickel exposure in man, the relevant data do not permit any quantitative estimation of dose-response relationships. The lowest levels of nickel associated with adverse health effects, therefore, must be used in establishing a criterion level for nickel in drinking water. To arrive at a risk estimate for nickel, a modification of the approach used for nonstochastic effects (47-6) has been adopted. The studies cited in this document have not demonstrated a no-observable effect level (NOEL). Therefore, the study demonstrating the lowest observable effect level (LOEL) for nickel in drinking water has been used to arrive at a nonstochastic risk estimate.

In the study of Schroeder and Mitchener (47-4), adverse effects in rats were demonstrated at a level of 5 ppm in drinking water. Three generations of rats were continuously exposed to 5 ppm of nickel in drinking water. In each of the generations, increased numbers of runts and enhanced neonatal mortality were seen. A significant reduction in litter size and a reduced proportion of males in the third generation also were observed.

To adapt the LOEL into an Acceptable Daily Intake (ADI) for man, the LOEL is divided by an uncertainty factor of 100, as detailed in a recent National Academy of Sciences report (47-7) and adopted by the United States Environmental Protection Agency (47-6). The choice of this factor is based on the absence of long-term or acute human data, scanty results on experimental animals, and an absence of evidence for carcinogenicity.

If the 5.0 mg/l were used in the standard water quality criteria, the criterion can be determined to be 133 μg/l.

$$\frac{5 \text{ (mg/l)} \times 25 \text{ ml/day/rat}}{0.3 \text{ (kg/av. rat)}} = \frac{125}{0.3}$$

$$= 416.67 \ \mu g$$

$$= 420 \ \mu g \text{ dose/day/av. rat}$$

$$\frac{420}{100} = 4.2 \ \mu g \text{ (ADI)}$$

$$4.2 \times 70 = 294 \ \mu g \text{ (ADI for 70 kg/man)}$$

$$2(X) + \text{(Av. fish intake)(BCF)(X)} = \text{Daily Intake}$$

$$2(X) + (0.0187)(11)(X) = 294 \ \mu g$$

$$2.205X = 294 \ \mu g$$

$$X = 133 \ \mu g/l \text{ (criterion)}$$

$$2 = \text{amount of water ingested (l/day)}$$

$$X = \text{Ni concentration (mg/l)}$$

$$0.0187 = \text{amount of fish and shellfish products consumed (kg/day)}$$

$$F = 11 \text{ (BCF)} \frac{\text{mg Ni/kg fish}}{\text{mg Ni/l of water}}$$

Drinking water contributes 91% of the assumed exposure while eating contaminated fish products accounts for 9%. The criterion level for nickel can alternatively be expressed as 1.4 μg/l, if exposure is assumed to be from the consumption of fish and shellfish products alone.

$$X \times 0.0187 \times 11 = 294 \ (\mu g/l)$$

$$X \times 0.2057 = 294$$

$$X = 1.429 \text{ mg}$$

$$X = 1.4 \text{ (mg/l)}$$

References

(47-1)   National Academy of Sciences, *Report on Medical and Biological Effects of Environmental Pollutants: Nickel,* Wash., D.C. (1975).

(47-2)   Lind, D. et al, *Regional Copper-Nickel Study, Aquatic Toxicology Study*, Minneapolis/St. Paul, Minnesota Environmental Quality Board (Undated).

(47-3)   Pickering, Q.H., Chronic toxicity of nickel to the fathead minnow, *Jour. Water Poll. Control Fed.* 46, 760 (1974).

(47-4)   Schroeder, H.A. and Mitchener, M., Toxic effects of trace elements on the reproduction of mice and rats, *Arch. Envir. Health* 23, 102–6 (1971).

(47-5)   Nat. Inst. for Occup. Safety and Health, *Criteria for a Recommended Standard: Occupational Exposure to Inorganic Nickel*, NIOSH Doc. No. 77-164 (1977).

(47-6)   44 *FR* 15980 (Mar. 15, 1979).

(47-7)   National Academy of Sciences, *Drinking Water and Health*, Wash., D.C. (1977).

NITROBENZENE (#48)

Nitrobenzene, $C_6H_5NO_2$, is the simplest nitroaromatic compound. It is also known as nitrobenzol and sometimes as oil of mirbane or oil of bitter almonds.

Occurrence: Nitrobenzene is stored in closed containers and is not usually released to the open air. Atmospheric contamination is usually prevented in plants manufacturing or using nitrobenzene by the use of activated charcoal absorbers or a carbon dioxide blanket. There is no industrial monitoring of nitrobenzene in the atmosphere. The greatest loss of nitrobenzene during production (estimated as eight million pounds annually) occurs at the acid extraction step in the purification of the crude reaction mixture, when nitrobenzene is lost to the effluent wash (48-1). Thus, greatest exposure to nitrobenzene occurs inside plants and most cases of chronic nitrobenzene exposure in man are nitrobenzene workers. Today, plant levels of nitrobenzene are usually kept below the threshold limit value (TLV) of 5 mg/m^3 (48-2) but much higher levels have been reported in the past (48-3). Nitrobenzene may also form spontaneously in the atmosphere from the photochemical reaction of benzene with oxides of nitrogen.

Physical Properties: Nitrobenzene is a pale yellow oily liquid with an almond-like odor. The color of the liquid varies from pale yellow to yellowish brown depending on the purity of the compound. In the solid state, it forms bright yellow crystals. Nitrobenzene $C_6H_5NO_2$, has a molecular weight of 123.11 g.

The physical properties of nitrobenzene are as follows: a boiling point of 210° to 211°C at 760 mm Hg, a melting point of 6°C, a density of 1.205 at 15°C, a refractive index of 1.5529, and a flash point of 89°C. It is steam volatile and, at 25°C nitrobenzene has a vapor pressure of 0.340 mm Hg.

Nitrobenzene is miscible with most organic solvents, such as ethanol, diethyl ether, acetone, and benzene. It is slightly soluble in water, 0.1 per 100 parts of water (1,000 mg/l) at 20°C. In aqueous solutions, nitrobenzene has a sweet taste.

Chemical Properties: Nitrobenzene undergoes substitution reactions but requires more vigorous conditions than does benzene. Substitution takes place at either the meta position or the ortho and para positions depending on the physical conditions. Nitrobenzene undergoes photoreduction when irradiated with ultraviolet light in organic solvents that contain abstractable hydrogen atoms.

Nitrobenzene is a fairly strong oxidizing agent. Since the compound can act as an oxidizing agent in the presence of aqueous solutions of alkali hydroxides, it has the capability of oxidizing compounds containing free phenolic hydroxyl groups without effectively changing these groups. Nitrobenzene is reactive and will undergo nitration, halogenation, and sulfonation by the same methods used for benzene. However, these reactions are unlikely to occur in environmental conditions.

Uses: Estimates of annual nitrobenzene production range from 200 to over 700 million pounds (48-1, 48-4). The principal use of nitrobenzene is for reduction to aniline, which is widely used as an ingredient for dyes, rubber, and medicinals. The commercial applications of nitrobenzene are: reduction to aniline (97%), solvent for Friedel-Crafts reaction, metal polishes, shoe black, perfume, dye intermediates, crystallizing solvent for some substances, and as a combustible propellant (48-1).

Toxic Effects: The great toxicity of nitrobenzene impairs its usefulness as an organic solvent. It is readily absorbed by contact with the skin, inhalation of the vapor, or by ingestion. The absorption of nitrobenzene into the body produces cyanosis.

Nitrobenzene has been found to have a metabolic turnover slow enough to result in distinct accumulation under conditions of daily exposure (48-5). Complications could arise from the possible accumulation of either nitrobenzene or p-nitrophenol. The half-life of the excretion of the p-nitrophenol is approximately 60 hours (48-6).

The toxicological data on the effects of nitrobenzene are limited primarily to mammalian, especially human, studies and case histories. There are few data on the toxic effects of nitrobenzene to aquatic organisms. A freshwater fish acute value for nitrobenzene was found to be 42,600 μg/l with a chronic value of more than 16,000 μg/l. A saltwater acute value was 58,539 μg/l. In the case of mammals, nitrobenzene is highly toxic when ingested, inhaled, or absorbed through the skin. Exposure by any of these routes can result in headaches, drowsiness, nausea, vomiting, and methemoglobinemia with cyanosis.

Current Levels of Exposure: A worker exposed to the current occupational standard of 5 mg/m^3 (1 ppm) nitrobenzene for an eight-hour workday would absorb approximately 24 mg by inhalation and 9 mg cutaneously. The maximum eight-hour uptake would be 33 mg, which is less than the reasonable safe level of 35 mg/day (48-1). Doses of up to 70 mg/day have been reported for factory workers and up to 80 mg/day have been reported in a dyestuff factory in England.

Nitrobenzene can be a contaminant in industrial wastewater, and companies utilizing or making nitrobenzene are required to monitor its level in their effluent waste. The minimum detectable level of nitrobenzene in drinking water by gas chromatography is 0.7 ng.

Nitrobenzene may be vented to the atmosphere. The vents are usually equipped with absorbers or scrubbers, but some nitrobenzene vapors can escape. Atmospheric nitrobenzene levels outside a plant are not monitored by industry. Since inner plant levels are below the TLV of 5 mg/m^3 (1 ppm) and nitrobenzene vapors accumulate at the floor level due to their high density, the external air nitrobenzene concentrations are expected to be very low (48-1).

Special Groups at Risk: Workers in plants producing or using nitrobenzene have the greatest risk of toxic exposure. At the current TLV level of 5 mg/m^3 (1 ppm), a worker could absorb as much as 33 mg/day. This is enough to produce symptoms of chronic toxicity in some susceptible individuals (48-1). The amount of nitrobenzene absorbed by a worker via inhalation and cutaneous absorption can be estimated from the level of total (free and conjugated) p-nitrophenol in urine as described by Piotrowski (48-5).

Due to the current widespread use of disposable diapers and underpads in hospitals, nitrobenzene poisoning in infants from laundry marking dyes is no longer a problem.

Pregnant women may be especially at risk with respect to nitrobenzene as with many other chemical compounds, due to transplacental passage of the agent. Individuals with glucose-6-phosphate dehydrogenase deficiency may also be special risk groups. Additionally, because alcohol ingestion or chronic alcoholism can lower the lethal or toxic dose of nitrobenzene, individuals consuming alcoholic beverages may be at risk.

Existing Guidelines and Standards: The maximum allowable concentration of nitrobenzene in air in industrial plants is 5 mg/m^3. This value was set by the joint ILO/WHO Committee on Occupational Health in 1975 (48-2). The OSHA (Occupational Safety and Health Administration) standard for nitrobenzene in air is 5 mg/m^3 (1 ppm) set in 1977. This is also the threshold limit value (TLV) in Germany and Sweden, while the TLV in the USSR is 3 mg/m^3 (48-1).

There are no standards for nitrobenzene levels in water. Nitrobenzene was not listed among the substances for which a maximum concentration has been set.

Summary of Proposed EPA Criteria: *Freshwater Aquatic Life* — For nitrobenzene, the criterion to protect freshwater aquatic life as derived using the Guidelines is 480 µg/l as a 24-hour average and the concentration should not exceed 1,100 µg/l at any time.

Saltwater Aquatic Life — For nitrobenzene, the criterion to protect saltwater aquatic life as derived using procedures other than the Guidelines is 53 µg/l as a 24-hour average and the concentration should not exceed 120 µg/l at any time.

Human Health — For the prevention of adverse effects due to the organoleptic properties of nitrobenzene in water, the criterion is 30 µg/l.

Basis for the Proposed Human Health Criteria: There is no established criterion for nitrobenzene in water. Because there are little or no data available on the toxicity of nitrobenzene ingested in drinking water, or on the teratogenic, mutagenic, or carcinogenic effects of nitrobenzene in general, experimental testing is necessary before an oral-ingestion-based criterion can be derived. It is recommended that testing in these areas of toxicity be implemented so that the effects of nitrobenzene on mammals may be better understood.

Using the methodology of Stokinger and Woodward (48-7), a water quality criteria (WQC) is derived using the organoleptic level and the TLV. Organoleptic level: minimum detectable odor level in water is 0.03 µg/l = 30 µg/l.

Assuming a daily intake of 2 liters of water, the total intake of nitrobenzene based on this criteria would be 60 µg/day. Recommended WQC = 30 µg/l.

A calculation of the percentage of exposure attributable to fish and shellfish products is not applicable to a criterion based upon organoleptic effects. Since an organoleptic effect is not based on a toxicological assessment, it would be inappropriate to apportion a percentage of exposure to the consumption of toxicologically contaminated fish.

TLV = 5 mg/m^3, air intake = 10 m^3/day. Assuming 80% absorption:

(5 mg/m^3) x (10 m^3/day) x (0.8) = 40 mg/day average over 7 days:

40 mg/day x 5/7 = 29 mg/day

Assuming 100% gastrointestinal absorption of nitrobenzene, consuming 2 liters of water daily and 18.7 g of contaminated fish having a bioconcentration factor of 4.3 would result in a maximum permissible concentration of 13.9 mg/l for the ingested water:

$$\frac{29 \text{ mg/day}}{2 \text{ liters} + (4.3 \times 0.0187) \times 1.0} = 13.9 \text{ mg/l}$$

WQC using TLV = 13.9 mg/l.

Since the WQC using TLV is well above the detectable odor level of nitrobenzene, water containing this concentration of nitrobenzene would not be esthetically acceptable for drinking. Even though the limitations of using organoleptic data as a basis for establishing a WQC are recognized, it is recommended that a WQC of 30 µg/l be established at the present time. This level may be altered as more data are developed upon which to calculate a WQC.

The analysis and recommendations generated in this document are based on the literature available to date. If future reports indicate that nitrobenzene may be carcinogenic, mutagenic or teratogenic, a reassessment of the WQC will be necessary.

References

(48-1)   Dorigan, J. and Hushon, J., *Air pollution assessment of nitrobenzene*, Wash., D.C., U.S. Environ. Prot. Agency (1976).

(48-2)   Goldstein, I., "Studies on MAC values of nitro- and amino-derivatives of aromatic hydrocarbons. Adverse Affects," *Environ. Chem. Psychotropic Drugs* 1, 153 (1975).

(48-3)   Pacseri, I. and Magos, L., "Determination of the measure of exposure to aromatic nitro and amino compounds," *Jour. Hyg. Epidemiol. Microbiol. Immunol.* 2, 92 (1958).

(48-4)   Lu, P.Y. and Metcalf, R., "Environmental fate and biodegradability of benzene derivatives as studied in a model aquatic ecosystem," *Environ. Health Perspect.* 19, 269 (1975).

(48-5)   Piotrowski, J., "Further investigations on the evaluation of exposure to nitrobenzene," *Br. Jour. Ind. Med.* 24, 41 (1967).

(48-6)   Salmowa, J. et al, "Evaluation of exposure to nitrobenzene," *Br. Jour. Ind. Med.* 20, 41 (1963).

(48-7)   Stokinger, H.E. and Woodward, R.L., "Toxicological methods for establishing drinking water standards," *Jour. Am. Water Works Assoc.* 517 (1958).

NITROPHENOLS (#49)

Mononitrophenol has three isomeric forms, distinguished by the position of the nitro group on the phenolic ring. Three isomeric forms are possible, namely, 2-nitrophenol, 3-nitrophenol, and 4-nitrophenol. The compounds are also commonly referred to as o-nitrophenol, m-nitrophenol, and p-nitrophenol, respectively. Six isomeric forms of dinitrophenol are possible, distinguished by the position of the nitro groups on the phenolic ring.

Five isomeric forms of trinitrophenol are possible, distinguished by the position of the nitro groups relative to the hydroxy group on the six carbon benzene ring. The isomers are: 2,3,4-, 2,3,5-, 2,3,6-, 2,4,5-, 2,4,6- and 3,4,5-trinitrophenol.

Dinitro-ortho-cresol is a yellow crystalline solid derived from o-cresol. There are six possible isomers but the 4,6-dinitro-o-cresol isomer is the only one of any commercial importance.

Occurrence: Commercial synthesis of 2-nitrophenol and 4-nitrophenol is accomplished through the hydrolysis of the appropriate chloronitrobenzene isomers with aqueous sodium hydroxide at elevated temperatures (49-1). Production of 3-nitrophenol is achieved through the diazotization and hydrolysis of m-nitroaniline.

Commercial synthesis of 2,4-dinitrophenol is accomplished by the hydrolysis of 2,4-dinitro-1-chlorobenzene with sodium hydroxide at 95° to 100°C.

Picric acid (2,4,6-trinitrophenol) is not made by the direct nitration of phenol because too many oxidation products are formed. It is made instead by the mixed acid nitration of mixed phenol sulfonates.

Dinitro-o-cresol is made by nitration of o-cresol in glacial acetic acid at low temperatures or by nitration of o-cresol sulfonate.

The major source for environmental release of mononitrophenols and dinitrophenols is likely from production plants and chemical firms where the compounds are used as intermediates. The mononitrophenols and dinitrophenols may also be inadvertently produced via microbial or photodegradation of pesticides which contain mononitrophenol moieties or those containing the dinitrophenol moiety, such as parathion.

Information regarding the mobility and persistence of nitrophenols in natural soil and water environments is limited. Based upon experimentally determined solubilities and sorption characteristics, the persistence of some of the nitrophenols might be estimated. For example, although 2-nitrophenol is soluble in water, it has also been shown to be strongly attracted through hydrogen bonding to montmorillonite clays, perhaps reducing its movement through the groundwater regime. However, these estimates do not consider the data available on microbial, photolytic, and oxidative degradation available in the literature.

No measured steady-state data are available regarding the bioconcentration of nitrophenols. Only limited data are available on the levels of nitrophenols in municipal effluents or treated drinking waters.

Physical Properties: Physical properties of the mononitrophenols are summarized in Table 69.

Table 69: Properties of Mononitrophenols

	2-Nitrophenol	3-Nitrophenol	4-Nitrophenol
Formula	$C_6H_5NO_3$	$C_6H_5NO_3$	$C_6H_5NO_3$
Molecular weight	139.11	139.11	139.11
Melting point, °C	44–45	97	113–114
Boiling point, °C	214–216	194	279
Specific gravity	1.485	1.485	1.479
Water solubility, g/100 g	0.32 at 38°C	1.35 at 25°C	0.804 at 15°C
	1.08 at 100°C	13.3 at 90°C	1.6 at 25°C
Vapor pressure	1 mm Hg at 49.3°C	—	—
K_a	7.5×10^{-8}	5.3×10^{-9}	7×10^{-8}

Source: Reference (49)

The physical and chemical properties of the dinitrophenol isomers are summarized in Table 70.

Table 70: Properties of Dinitrophenol Isomers

Isomer	MP (°C)	K_a (at 25°C)	Water Solubility (g/l)	Specific Gravity
2,3-Dinitrophenol	144	1.3×10^{-5}	2.2	1.681
2,4-Dinitrophenol	114–115*	1.0×10^{-4}	0.79	1.683
2,5-Dinitrophenol	104	7×10^{-6}	0.68	—
2,6-Dinitrophenol	63.5	2.7×10^{-4}	0.42	—
3,4-Dinitrophenol	134	4.3×10^{-5}	2.3	1.672
3,5-Dinitrophenol	122–123	2.1×10^{-4}	1.6	1.702

*Sublimes.

Source: Reference (49)

The physical properties of trinitrophenols are found in Table 71.

Table 71: Properties of Trinitrophenols

2,3,4-Trinitrophenol	
Molecular weight	229.11
2,3,5-Trinitrophenol	
Molecular weight	229.11
Melting point	119°–120°C

(continued)

2,3,6-Trinitrophenol
  Molecular weight 229.11
  Melting point .... 119°C
  Water solubility
    Room temperature .... Slightly soluble
    Hot water .... Very soluble
2,4,5-Trinitrophenol
  Molecular weight 229.11
  Melting point .... 96°C
  Water solubility
    Room temperature .... Slightly soluble
    Hot water .... Soluble
2,4,6-Trinitrophenol (Picric acid)
  Molecular weight 229.11
  Melting point .... 122°–123°C
  Boiling point .... Sublimates: explodes at 300°C
  Vapor pressure .... 1 mm Hg at 195°C
  Density .... 1.763 g/cm^3
  Water solubility
    Room temperature .... 1.28 g/l
    100°C .... 6.7 g/l

Source: Reference (49)

Some important chemical and physical properties of DNOC are shown in Table 72.

Table 72: Properties of 4,6-Dinitro-o-Cresol

Molecular weight	198.13
Appearance	Yellow solid
Melting point	85.8°C
Vapor pressure	0.000052 mm Hg at 20°C
Water solubility	100 mg/l at 20°C
pKa	4.46

Source: Reference (49)

Chemical Properties: Few data are available regarding the breakdown of nitrophenols by natural communities of microorganisms. A number of researchers have isolated microorganisms capable of using nitrophenols as a sole source of carbon in pure culture. However, the significance of such studies as related to the stability of nitrophenols in the environment is not known.

Several investigators have shown that individual species of aerobic and anaerobic bacteria, including *Azotobacter chroococcum* and *Clostridium butyricum*, and the fungus *Fusarium*, are capable of reducing 2,4-dinitrophenol in culture. However, the precise pathway for metabolic degradation is not known. It has been found that *Arthrobacter simplex*, *Pseudomonas*, and *Arthrobacter* were able to metabolize 2,4-dinitrophenol and 2,4,6-trinitrophenol, forming nitrites.

The actual degradation pathway of dinitro-o-cresol has been investigated in pure cultures of microorganisms. It was reported that in *Pseudomonas* sp. degradation proceeded by way of formation of an aminocresol. In *Arthrobacter simplex*, a hydroxylated catechol is formed prior to ring cleavage.

Uses: Approximately 10 to 15 million pounds of 2-nitrophenol are produced annually for uses including synthesis of o-aminophenol, o-nitroanisole, and other dyestuffs (49-1). Although production figures for 3-nitrophenol are not available, it has been estimated that production is less than 1 million pounds annually. 3-Nitrophenol is used in the manufacture of dye intermediates such as anisidine and m-aminophenol. 4-Nitrophenol is probably the most important of the mononitrophenols in terms of quantities used and potential environmental contamination. Demand for 4-nitrophenol was 35,000,000 pounds in 1976 and production was projected to increase to 41,000,000 pounds by 1980. Most of the 4-nitrophenol produced (87%) is used in the manufacture of ethyl and methyl parathions. Other uses (13%) include the manufacture of dyestuffs and n-acetyl-p-aminophenol (APAP) and leather treatments.

Of the six possible dinitrophenol isomers, 2,4-dinitrophenol is by far the most important. Approximate consumption per year is estimated at 1,000,000 pounds (49-1). 2,4-dinitrophenol is used primarily as a chemical intermediate for the production of sulfur dyes, azo dyes, photochemicals, pest control agents, wood preservatives, and explosives.

Production figures and usage data for the remaining five dinitrophenol isomers are not available. It is reasonable to assume that production and usage of these compounds are extremely limited in the United States.

Usage of the trinitrophenol isomers is apparently limited to 2,4,6-trinitrophenol, otherwise known as picric acid. In fact, a comprehensive search of the literature failed to detect a single citation dealing with any of the trinitrophenol isomers except picric acid.

Picric acid has found usage as: a dye intermediate, explosive, analytical reagent, germicide, fungicide, staining agent and tissue fixative, tanning agent, photochemical, pharmaceutical, and a process material for the oxidation and etching of iron, steel and copper surfaces. The extent to which picric acid finds usage in any of these applications at the present time is unknown.

DNOC is used primarily as a blossom-thinning agent on fruit trees and as a fungicide, insecticide, and miticide on fruit trees during the dormant season. DNOC usage in the U.S. has declined in recent years because the compound is highly toxic to plants in the growing stage and nonselectively kills both desirable and undesirable vegetation. Additionally, the compound is highly toxic to humans and is considered one of the more dangerous agricultural pesticides.

Toxic Effects: None of the nitrophenols addressed here is found to be carcinogenic, mutagenic, or teratogenic; however, because of their widespread use as agricultural chemicals, their toxicity to microorganisms, fish, and mammals, the nitrophenols pose a potential threat to aquatic and terrestrial life, including man.

An excellent review of the toxicological effects of DNOC on human and laboratory animals has recently been published by the National Institute for Occupational Safety and Health (49-2).

Current Levels of Exposure: Human exposure to the nitrophenols or dinitro-o-cresols has not been monitored. Unspecified amounts of 4-nitrophenol have been detected in samples of urban ambient particulate matter.

The photochemical reaction between benzene vapor and nitrogen monoxide results in the production of 2-nitrophenol, 4-nitrophenol, 2,4-dinitrophenol, and 2,6-dinitrophenol under laboratory conditions and 4-nitrophenol has been detected in rainwater in Japan. Available data indicate that the general public may be exposed to nitrophenols in the atmosphere when severe photochemical fog conditions develop. Quantitative estimates of such exposures are not possible at the present time.

4-Nitrophenol has been detected in the urine of 1.7% of the general population at levels as high as 0.1 mg/l (with a mean urinary level of 10 μg/l).

If it is assumed that urinary residues of 4-nitrophenol reflect direct exposure to the compound, a pharmacokinetic estimate of exposure based on steady-state conditions can be made. The exposure level leading to the 1.7 μg/l residue can be calculated as follows:

$$\text{Exposure} = \frac{(10\ \mu\text{g/l})\ (1.4\ \text{l of urine/day})}{(70\ \text{kg/man})} = 0.20\ \mu\text{g/kg/day}$$

A similar calculation using the maximum urine residue level observed (113 μg/l) gives an exposure of 2.26 μg/kg/day.

These urine levels are not believed to result from direct exposure to 4-nitrophenol, however. A number of widely used pesticides, including parathion, are readily metabolized to 4-nitrophenol in the human body and are believed to be the source of 4-nitrophenol residues in human urine.

Current levels of human exposure to the nitrophenols or dinitrocresols (with the possible exception of 4-nitrophenol) are either very low, nonexistent, or have gone undetected. In the absence of data, any of the above could be operative.

Special Groups at Risk: The only individuals expected to be at risk for high exposure to the nitrophenols are industrial workers involved in the manufacture of compounds for which the nitrophenols are intermediates. Since picric acid (2,4,6-trinitrophenol) may find some usage as an explosive, germicide, tanning agent, fungicide, tissue fixative, and industrial process material, a higher risk of exposure exists among personnel engaged in such operations.

Although 4,6-dinitro-o-cresol (DNOC) is no longer manufactured in the United States, a limited quantity is imported and used as a blossom-thinning agent on fruit trees and as a fungicide, insecticide, and miticide on fruit trees during the dormant season. Hence, individuals formulating or spraying the compound incur the highest risk of exposure to the compound.

NIOSH (49-2) estimates that 3,000 workers in the United States are potentially exposed to DNOC. In view of the small amount of DNOC used in the United States, exposure of the general public is expected to be minimal.

Existing Guidelines and Standards: No United States standards for exposure to the nitrophenols or dinitrocresols in drinking or ambient water have been set.

The following limits for toxic substances in drinking water has been set in the U.S.S.R. (49-3):

	Milligram/Liter
2-Nitrophenol	0.06
3-Nitrophenol	0.06
4-Nitrophenol	0.02
2,4-Dinitrophenol	0.03

Based on organoleptic considerations, a limit of 0.5 mg/l for 2,4,6-trinitrophenol has been set by the U.S.S.R. (49-3).

The maximum air concentration established by the American Conference of Governmental Industrial Hygienists is 0.1 mg/m^3 for 2,4,6-trinitrophenol and 0.2 mg/m^3 for 4,6-dinitro-o-cresol for an 8-hour exposure (TLV).

The Code of Federal Regulations (40 CFR Part 180) establishes a tolerance of 0.02 mg/kg for residues of 4,6-dinitro-o-cresol and its sodium salt in or on apples resulting from applications to apple trees at the blossom stage as a fruit-thinning agent.

Summary of Proposed EPA Criteria: *Freshwater Aquatic Life* — For 2-nitrophenol, the criterion to protect freshwater aquatic life as derived using procedures other than the Guidelines is 2,700 μg/l as a 24-hour average and the concentration should not exceed 6,200 μg/l at any time.

For 4-nitrophenol, the criterion to protect freshwater aquatic life as derived using procedures other than the Guidelines is 240 μg/l as a 24-hour average and the concentration should not exceed 550 μg/l at any time.

For 2,4-dinitrophenol, the criterion to protect freshwater aquatic life as derived using procedures other than the Guidelines is 79 μg/l as a 24-hour average and the concentration should not exceed 180 μg/l at any time.

For 2,4-dinitro-6-methylphenol, the criterion to protect freshwater aquatic life as derived using procedures other than the Guidelines is 57 μg/l as a 24-hour average and the concentration should not exceed 130 μg/l at any time.

For 2,4,6-trinitrophenol, the criterion to protect freshwater aquatic life as derived using procedures other than the Guidelines is 1,500 μg/l as a 24-hour average and the concentration should not exceed 3,400 μg/l at any time.

Saltwater Aquatic Life — For saltwater aquatic life, no criterion for 2-nitrophenol can be derived using the Guidelines, and there are insufficient data to estimate a criterion using other procedures.

For 4-nitrophenol, the criterion to protect saltwater aquatic life as derived using the Guidelines is 53 μg/l as a 24-hour average and the concentration should not exceed 120 μg/l at any time.

For 2,4-dinitrophenol, the criterion to protect saltwater aquatic life as derived using procedures other than the Guidelines is 37 μg/l as a 24-hour average and the concentration should not exceed 84 μg/l at any time.

For saltwater aquatic life, no criterion for 2,4-dinitro-6-methylphenol can be derived using the Guidelines, and there are insufficient data to estimate a criterion using other procedures.

For 2,4,6-trinitrophenol, the criterion to protect saltwater aquatic life as derived using procedures other than the Guidelines is 150 μg/l as a 24-hour average and the concentration should not exceed 340 μg/l at any time.

Human Health — To protect human health from the adverse effects of various nitrophenols ingested in contaminated water and fish, suggested criteria are as follows: mononitrophenols, no criterion; dinitrophenols, 68.6 μg/l; trinitrophenols, 10 μg/l; and dinitrocresols, 12.8 μg/l.

Basis for the Proposed Human Health Criteria: Uncertainty factors used for criteria formulation have been loosely adapted from *Drinking Water and Health* (49-4).

In the absence of data on chronic mammalian effects, no water criteria for human health can be established for the mononitrophenol isomers at this time.

Information on the dinitrophenol isomers is limited to 2,4-dinitrophenol. Spencer et al (49-5), in a 6-month feeding study with rats, demonstrated the no-observable-effect level (NOEL) for 2,4-dinitrophenol to be between 5.4 and 20 mg/kg. Taking the lower of the two figures and assuming a 70-kg man consumes 2 liters of water daily and 18.7 g of contaminated fish having a BCF of 2.4, the NOEL for humans based on the results obtained in rats may be calculated as follows:

$$5.4 \text{ mg/kg} \times 70 \text{ kg} = 378 \text{ mg}$$

$$\frac{378 \text{ mg}}{2 \text{ liters} + (2.4 \times 0.0187) \times 1.0} = 185.3 \text{ mg/l}$$

Based on these calculations, no biological effect would be predicted in a man drinking water containing 185.3 mg/l 2,4-DNP.

Experience with the use of 2,4-DNP as an antiobesity drug in the 1930s indicates that adverse effects, including cataract formation, may occur in humans exposed to as little as 2 mg/kg/day. The drug was frequently used in an uncontrolled manner and the available data do not allow the calculation of a no-adverse-effect level in humans. It is clear, however, that ingestion of 2 mg/kg/day 2,4-DNP for a protracted period may result in adverse effects, including cataracts, in a small proportion of the population. Assuming a 70-kg man consumes 2 liters of water daily and 18.7 g of contaminated fish having a BCF of 2.4 and assuming 100% gastrointestinal absorption of 2,4-DNP, a 2 mg/kg dose of 2,4-DNP would result if drinking water contained 68.6 mg/l of 2,4-DNP.

$$\frac{140 \text{ mg/day}}{2 \text{ liters} + (2.4 \times 0.0187) \times 1.0} = 68.6 \text{ mg/l}$$

These data taken together with the demonstrated bacterial mutagenicity of 2,4-DNP (49-6) and the suspected ability of the compound to induce chromosomal breaks in mammals (49-7) suggest that an uncertainty factor of 1,000 should be used in criteria formulation. The suggested water criterion for 2,4-DNP is, therefore:

$$\frac{68.6 \text{ mg/l}}{1,000} = 68.6 \text{ }\mu\text{g/l}$$

The available data are insufficient to enable calculation of water criterion levels for the remaining dinitrophenol isomers. For the present, it seems reasonable to assume that the 2,4-dinitrophenol criterion would be appropriate for the other isomers.

Chronic mammalian toxicology data for the trinitrophenols are absent from the literature. An outbreak of microscopic hematuria among shipboard U.S. Navy personnel exposed to 2,4,6-trinitrophenol in drinking water has been reported, however. Although it is not possible to precisely estimate either the 2,4,6-trinitrophenol water level or duration of exposure required for the development of hematuria, 2,4,6-trinitrophenol levels of 10 and 20 mg/l were detected in drinking water aboard two ships at the time of the outbreak.

Based on the presumed development of hematuria in humans at drinking water levels of 10 mg/l and the evidence indicating mutagenic activity in bacteria, an uncertainty factor of 1,000 is suggested for formulation of the 2,4,6-trinitrophenol water criteria:

$$\frac{10 \text{ mg/l}}{1,000} = \text{ }\mu\text{g/l}$$

Since available data are insufficient to enable calculation of water criterion levels for the remaining trinitrophenol isomers, it seems reasonable to assume, for the present, that the 2,4,6-trinitrophenol criterion is appropriate for the other isomers.

Although 4,6-dinitro-o-cresol (DNOC) is considered a cumulative poison in humans, probably as a result of slow metabolism and inefficient excretion, true chronic or subacute effects have never been reported in either humans or experimental animals. Since DNOC is not a cumulative poison in experimental animals, extrapolation to humans from long-term animal studies is of questionable value.

The no-observable-effect level (NOEL) for DNOC respiratory exposure in humans has been reported as 0.2 mg/m^3 air (49-2). NIOSH has, in fact, recommended that the current federal workplace environmental limit of 0.2 mg/m^3 be retained, based on the available data.

It is possible to calculate the anticipated daily exposure of a 70-kg human male exposed to 0.2 mg/m^3 for an 8-hour period. If one assumes the average minute volume is 28.6 liters of air/minute (average minute volume for a man doing light work—NIOSH), the anticipated daily exposure is 39 μg/kg/day. Since the NOELs calculated from long-term experimental animal studies are considerably higher than this value, it will be used as a basis for the suggested water criterion.

If one assumes that absorption of DNOC across the respiratory tract is identical to gastro-intestinal absorption and that a 70-kg human male consumes 2 liters of water daily and 18.7 g of contaminated fish having a BCF of 7.5, the following calculations indicate the maximum allowable levels of DNOC in drinking water based on the NIOSH air standard values:

$$39 \; \mu g/kg/day \times 70 \; kg \; = \; 2.73 \; mg/day$$

$$\frac{2.73 \; mg/day}{(2 \; liters \; + \; (7.5 \times 0.0187) \times 1.0} = 1.28 \; mg/l$$

In view of the lack of data indicating chronic effects and the existence of a very recent federal guideline for human exposure, an uncertainty factor of 100 is chosen for the protection of the general public. The suggested criterion for 4,6-dinitro-o-cresol (and in the absence of adequate data, the other dinitrocresol isomers) is:

$$\frac{1.28 \; mg/l}{100} = \; 12.8 \; \mu g/l$$

References

(49-1)   Howard, H. et al, *Investigation of selected potential environmental contamination: Nitroaromatics*, Washington, D.C., Off. Tox. Subs. U.S. Environ. Prot. Agency (1976).

(49-2)   National Institute for Occupational Safety and Health, *Criteria for a recommended standard: Occupational exposure to dinitro-ortho-cresol*, NIOSH Publ. No. 78-131, Washington, D.C. (1978).

(49-3)   Stofen, D., "The maximum permissible concentrations in the U.S.S.R. for harmful substances in drinking water," *Toxicology* 1, 187 (1973).

(49-4)   National Academy of Sciences, *Drinking water and health*, Washington D.C. (1977).

(49-5)   Spencer, H.C. et al, "Toxicological studies on laboratory animals of certain alkyl dinitrophenols used in agriculture," *Jour. Ind. Hyg. Toxicol.* 30, 10 (1948).

(49-6)   Demerec, M. et al, "A survey of chemicals for mutagenic action on *E. coli*," *The Am. Natur.* 85, 119 (1951).

(49-7)   Mitra, A.B. and Manna, G.K., "Effect of some phenolic compounds on chromosomes of bone marrow cells of mice.," *Indian Jour. Med. Res.* 59, 1442 (1971).

NITROSAMINES (#50)

The nitrosamines belong to a large group of chemicals generally called N-nitroso compounds. Also, included in this group are the structurally related nitrosamides. Because they frequently coexist with N-nitrosamines in the environment, nitrosamides are addressed also in the criteria document (50).

Nitrosamines are characterized by the functional group $\diagdown N-N{=}O$ and nitrosamides are characterized by the functional group $-C(O)-NH-N{=}O$. Depending on the nature of the radical group, nitrosamines exist in several forms, including symmetrical dialkyl-nitrosamines, asymmetrical dialkyl-nitrosamines, nitrosamines with functional groups, cyclic nitrosamines and acylalkylnitrosamines with functional groups, cyclic nitrosamines and acylalkyl-nitrosamines or nitrosamides.

Occurrence: N-nitrosamines are widespread in the environment, and anthropogenic sources contribute negligibly to these levels.

The most significant source of N-nitrosamines and N-nitrosamides in the environment is probably nitrosation of amine and amide precursors (50-1). These reactions may occur in air, soil, water, food, and animal systems, when the precursors occur simultaneously (50-2, 50-3, 50-4). Concentrations in the nanogram to microgram per unit volume or mass range have been recorded in air, water, soil, plants, and foodstuffs (50-2). Laboratory tests show that N-nitroso-diphenylamine bioconcentrates in the bluegill sunfish by a factor of 217. A survey of U.S. waters and industrial effluents, conducted by U.S. EPA (50-5), recorded levels of various nitrosamines ranging from less than 0.1 μg/l in industrial pipe sources to less than 10 μg/l in ambient streams. The extent of exposure of the general population of N-nitrosamines and N-nitrosamides is unknown. The most significant exposures, resulting from anthropogenic sources, are probably restricted to limited industrial areas (50-2, 50-3, 50-4).

Physical Properties: The nitrosamines vary widely in their physical properties and may exist as solids, liquids, or gases. They are soluble in water and organic solvents. Nitrosamines of low molecular weight are volatile at room temperature, and high molecular weight nitrosamines are steam volatile (50-6).

Chemical Properties: N-dealkylation of N-nitrosodimethylamine and N-nitrosodiethylamine by tissue specific microsomal mixed-function oxidases is believed to generate alkylating intermediates that are responsible for the mutagenic, toxic and carcinogenic effects of the parent compounds in vivo and in vitro according to Fishbein (50-17).

R_2NNO compounds are decomposed by mineral acids; thus hydrochloric acid reacts to give a secondary amine salt, $R_2NH \cdot HCl$ plus nitrous acid HONO. They may also be reduced to substituted hydrazines by such agents as zinc dust in acid. Although stable to light in neutral solution, N-nitrosamines can rearrange to the corresponding amidoximes in acid solution (50-18).

Uses: Synthetic production of N-nitrosamines is limited to small quantities, and the only nitrosamine produced in quantities greater than 450 kg per year is N-nitrosodiphenylamine. It is used as a vulcanizing retarder in rubber processing and in the manufacture of pesticides. Other N-nitroso compounds are produced primarily as research chemicals and not for commercial purposes (50-6).

Toxic Effects: Nearly 70% of all N-nitrosamines studied have been found to be carcinogenic in a wide range of laboratory animals including various aquatic organisms (50-6). The carcinogenic and toxic properties are well established; and both N-nitrosamines and N-nitrosamides are considered to be among the most potent of all mutagenic, teratogenic, and carcinogenic agents known (50-7, 50-8). They have been demonstrated to induce tumors in essentially all vital organs via all routes of administration (50-9). Since tumor production can occur after long-term exposure to small doses, there is concern about human exposure to these agents in water (50-10, 50-11, 50-12, 50-13).

It is interesting to note that in November 1979 workers at Oak Ridge National Laboratory reported that ethylnitrosourea (ENV) causes 15 times more genetic damage in mice than any other known chemical. It is the only chemical more potent (in fact five times more) than radiation in causing mammalian mutations.

Current Levels of Exposure: For the general population, information is very limited. It has been estimated that air, diet and smoking all play a roughly equivalent role in direct human exposure, contributing a few micrograms per day, with direct intake from ingested water, probably much less than 1 μg per day (50-6).

There is even greater uncertainty with regard to the significance of exposure to precursors. The chief source of the nitrate body burden, except in the newborn, is ingested vegetables, unless rural well water high in nitrate is consumed. Food and water normally contribute a few hundred milligrams per day. Inhalation may also contribute several hundred micrograms per day (50-5). On a daily basis, the major source of nitrite is saliva. However, salivary nitrite is presented to the body as a continuous, low-level input, in comparison with the relatively high concentrations over short periods resulting from ingestion of cured meats. This may be significant since the rate of nitrosation is a function of the square of the nitrite concentration (50-5).

The concentrations of nitrite (and its precursors, ammonia and nitrate) and nitrosatable compounds can be much greater in soils heavily fertilized with organic waste matter or in waters receiving runoff from agricultural areas or discharges of industrial or municipal wastewaters containing substantial amounts of amines. Levels of nitrate or municipal drinking water in the United States seldom exceed 10 mg/l nitrate N, although some private supplies contain much more.

Significant concentrations of nitrosamines have been reported for a limited number of samples of ocean water, river water and waste treatment plant effluent adjacent to or receiving wastewater from industries using nitrosamines or secondary amines in production operations. Nitrosodimethylamine has been reported at the 3 to 4 ng/l level in these samples. Nitrosamines, however, are rapidly decomposed by photolysis and do not persist for a significant time in water exposed to sunlight.

Although it is difficult to analyze this wide spectrum of exposure potential, it must be concluded that ingested water is a relatively minor source of exposure when compared with other potential sources of either preformed N-nitroso compounds or their precursors.

Special Groups at Risk: Because of the ubiquitous nature of nitrosatable compounds and nitrosating agents in the environment (food, air, drugs, tobacco, water, soil), special risk groups would have to include those individuals who are exposed to multiple exposure situations. To quantify this, however, is almost impossible at this point because of the need to create exposure scenarios for which the bounding factors are unknown or relatively wide ranging.

Existing Guidelines and Standards: The American Conference of Governmental Industrial Hygienists simply says that, because of extremely high toxicity and presumed carcinogenic potential of nitrosodimethylamine, contact should not be permitted by any route.

Summary of Proposed EPA Criteria: *Freshwater Aquatic Life* — For freshwater aquatic life, no criterion for N-nitrosodiphenylamine can be derived using the Guidelines, and there are insufficient data to estimate a criterion using other procedures.

Saltwater Aquatic Life — For saltwater aquatic life, no criterion for N-nitrosodiphenylamine can be derived using the Guidelines, and there are insufficient data to estimate a criterion using other procedures.

Human Health — For the maximum protection of human health from the potential carcinogenic effects of exposure to N-nitrosodimethylamine through ingestion of water and contaminated aquatic organisms, the ambient water concentration is zero. Concentrations of N-nitrosodimethylamine, N-nitrosodiethylamine, N-nitrosodibutylamine and N-nitrosopyrrolidine effecting additional lifetime cancer risks ranging from no additional risk to an additional risk of 1 in 100,000 are presented in Table 73.

Table 73: Concentrations in Water Estimated to Induce No More than One Excess Cancer per 100,000 Individuals Exposed over a Lifetime

Compound	Estimated Concentration (μg/l)	Data Base
N-nitrosodimethylamine	0.026	rats (female) (50-9)
N-nitrosodiethylamine	0.0092	rats (male?) (50-14)
N-nitrosodi-n-butylamine	0.013	mice (male) (50-15)
N-nitrosopyrrolidine	0.11	rats (mixed sexes) (50-16)

Source: Reference (50)

Basis for the Proposed Human Health Criteria: Both N-nitrosamines and N-nitrosamides exhibit acute toxicity, teratogenicity, mutagenicity and/or carcinogenicity. For most, it is the last capability which demands consideration in the context of human exposure since the toxicological evidence is such that they must be treated as potential human carcinogens. Thus, nitrosamines are included in the American Conference of Governmental Industrial Hygienists' list of "Industrial Substances Suspect of Carcinogenic Potential for Man." No Threshold Limit Value is given. The guidelines which follow are based upon the assumption that N-nitrosamines are human carcinogens.

Adequate dose-response data to permit an assessment of the carcinogenic risk to man are available from studies involving lifetime exposure of rats or mice to four nitrosamines (N-nitrosodimethylamine, N-nitrosodiethylamine, N-nitrosodi-n-butylamine, and N-nitrosopyrrolidine) in their drinking water or food. These data have been used to derive estimates of the concentrations in water which, if used as the source for man of drinking water and edible fish and shellfish, would increase the risk of a tumor by not more than 1 in 100,000 individuals exposed for the duration of their lifespan. The method of extrapolation was based on a linear, nonthreshold mathematical model. The water criteria numbers given in Table 73 are based upon the tumor incidence, at the organ which is the chemical's principal site of action, in the most sensitive sex, at the lowest dose level which yields a response significantly greater than in the control animals. The actual parameters used are given in Summary of Pertinent Data which follows.

The only nitrosamine for which any data on bioaccumulation in fish or shellfish are available is N-nitrosodiphenylamine. One test in bluegill yielded a maximum bioconcentration factor (BCF) of 217 for the whole fish. Using this, a weighted BCF for all species was calculated to be 500. These values are believed not to be representative for the nitrosamines for which carcinogenicity data are available and another approach has therefore been attempted. A relationship has been described between the BCF and the n-octanol/water partition coefficient, log BCF = 0.76 log P–0.23. The equation can be used to estimate the BCF for aquatic organisms that contain about 8% lipids from the partition coefficient P. The partition coefficients for N-nitrosodimethylamine, N-nitrosodiethylamine, N-nitrosodi-n-butylamine and N-nitrosopyrrolidine are 0.27, 3, 83, and 0.65, respectively.

Values of BCF calculated using this equation are 0.2, 1.4, 17, and 0.42, respectively, for N-nitrosodimethylamine, N-nitrosodiethylamine, N-nitrosodi-n-butylamine, and N-nitrosopyrrolidine, respectively. An adjustment factor of 2.3/8.0 = 0.2875 can be used to adjust the estimated BCF from the 8.0% lipids on which the equation is based to the 2.3% lipids that is the weighted average for consumed fish and shellfish. The adjusted BCF values are 0.06, 0.39, 4.9, and 0.12, respectively.

Other empirical procedures can be used to estimate BCFs from partition coefficients. The values obtained are of the same order of magnitude.

For purposes of calculating criteria, the estimated BCFs for the methyl, ethyl, butyl, and pyrrolidine compounds are judged to be rough estimates of the bioconcentration potential. As the influence of these values ranges from 0.05 to 4% of the exposure uptake from fish consumption, for simplicity the assumed BCF for criteria level purposes is zero.

The relative carcinogenic potential of N-nitrosodiethylamine (3.20) is exceeded by only that for N-nitrosomethyl-2-chloroethylamine (3.21) and approached by only the values for N-nitroso-methylbenzylamine (3.10) and N-nitrosomethyl-(2-phenylethyl)amine (3.01). Hence, N-nitrosodiethylamine can reasonably be considered to be one of the most carcinogenic nitrosamines. It is, therefore, appropriate to base the water criterion number for any individual nitrosamine on the number obtained for N-nitrosodiethylamine, viz 9.2 ng/l.

This criterion number has been derived by considering only the excess cancer risk imposed by exposure to contaminated drinking water, fish, and shellfish. However, the average daily intake of preformed nitrosamines from other sources (air, diet, and smoking) is estimated to be in the order of a few micrograms per day. There is an additional and, at the present time, ill-defined contribution to the body burden from the in vivo nitrosation of precursors. This contribution has been variously estimated to range from a few micrograms to several hundred micrograms daily. Thus, present evidence suggests that control of exposure to N-nitrosamines should take into account both preformed nitrosamines and their precursors in the environment.

Under the Consent Decree in NRDC v. Train, criteria are to state recommended maximum permissible concentrations (including where appropriate, zero) consistent with the protection of aquatic organisms, human health, and recreational activities. Nitrosamines are suspected of being human carcinogens. Because there is no recognized safe concentration for a human carcinogen, the recommended concentration of nitrosamines in water for maximum protection of human health is zero.

Because attaining a zero concentration level may be infeasible in some cases and in order to assist the Agency and States in the possible future development of water quality regulations, the concentrations of nitrosamines corresponding to several incremental lifetime cancer risk levels have been estimated. A cancer risk level provides an estimate of the additional incidence of cancer that may be expected in an exposed population. A risk of 10^{-5}, for example, indicates a probability of one additional case of cancer for every 100,000 people exposed, a risk of 10^{-6} indicates one additional case of cancer for every million people exposed, and so forth.

In the *Federal Register* notice of availability of draft ambient water quality criteria, EPA stated that it is considering setting criteria at an interim target risk level of 10^{-5}, 10^{-6} or 10^{-7} as shown in Table 74. In Table 74, the risk levels and corresponding criteria are calculated by applying a modified one-hit extrapolation model described in the methodology document to the animal bioassay data presented in summary of pertinent data. Since the extrapolation model is linear at low doses, the additional lifetime risk is directly proportional to the water concentration. Therefore, water concentrations corresponding to other risk levels can be derived by multiplying or dividing one of the risk levels and corresponding water concentrations shown in the table by factors such as 10, 100, 1,000, and so forth.

Table 74: Possible Alternative Criteria for Nitrosamines

Exposure Assumptions (per day)	. . .Risk Levels and Corresponding Criteria . . .			
	0	10^{-7}	10^{-6}	10^{-5}
	. . . .(μg/l)			
2 liters of drinking water and consumption of 18.7 g fish and shellfish*				
N-nitrosodimethylamine	0	0.00026	0.0026	0.026
N-nitrosodiethylamine	0	0.000092	0.00092	0.0092
N-nitrosodi-n-butylamine	0	0.00013	0.0013	0.013
N-nitrosopyrrolidine	0	0.0011	0.011	0.11
Consumption of fish and shellfish only				
N-nitrosodimethylamine	0	—	—	—
N-nitrosodiethylamine	0	—	—	—
N-nitrosodi-n-butylamine	0	—	—	—
N-nitrosopyrrolidine	0	—	—	—

*Approximately 0% of nitrosamine exposure results from the consumption of aquatic organisms which exhibit an average bioconcentration potential of zero. The remaining 100% of nitrosamine exposure results from drinking water.

Source: Reference (50)

Concentration levels were derived assuming a lifetime exposure to various amounts of nitrosamines, (1) occurring from the consumption of both drinking water and aquatic life grown in waters containing the corresponding nitrosamines concentrations and, (2) occurring solely from consumption of aquatic life grown in the waters containing the corresponding nitrosamines concentrations. Because data indicating other sources of nitrosamines exposure and their contributions to total body burden are inadequate for quantitative use, the figures reflect in incremental risks associated with the indicated routes only.

Summary of Pertinent Data — Druckery (50-9) summarized a series of experiments in which a large series of nitrosamine compounds were given to B-D rats for a lifetime. He found that the incidence of liver tumors increased with daily dose, d, and that the median time when tumors were observed, t_{50}, was less at higher doses and the relationship between d and t_{50} was $d(t_{50})2.3 = k$, where k is a constant equal to 0.81×10^4 mmol/kg/day when t_{50} is expressed in units of days. The extrapolation model used the dose units of mg/kg/day and the time units of fractions of a lifetime. Converting k to these units by using 728 days as the lifetime and a molecular weight of 74 mg/mmol gives the following:

$$k = \frac{0.81 \times 10^4 \text{ mmol/kg/day} \times 74 \text{ mg/mmol}}{(728)\,2.2} = 0.3746$$

Therefore, the parameters of the dose-response model are:

$$n_t/N_t = 0.05$$
$$n_c/N_c = 0$$
$$w = 0.35 \text{ kg}$$
$$L = 728 \text{ days}$$
$$dt^n = 0.3746$$
$$R = 0$$

The result is that the water concentration should be less than 0.026 μg/l in order to keep the individual lifetime risk below 10^{-5}.

Druckery et al (50-14) administered diethylnitrosamine to B-D rats via drinking water in nine dose groups ranging from 0.075 to 14.2 mg/kg/day. They found that the incidence of liver tumors increased with daily dose, d, and that the median time when tumors were observed, t_{50}, was less at higher doses and the relationship between d and t_{50} was $d(t_{50})^{2.3} = k$, where k is a constant. At a dose of 0.6 mg/kg/day, the incidence of tumors reached 50% (30 animals with liver tumors out of 60 animals initially) at 355 days. Using a bioaccumulation factor of zero, the parameters of the extrapolation model are:

$$n_t = 30$$
$$N_t = 60$$
$$nc/N_c = 0$$
$$Le = 355 \text{ days}$$
$$le = 355 \text{ days}$$
$$d = 0.6 \text{ mg/kg/day}$$
$$w = 0.28 \text{ kg}$$
$$L = 730 \text{ days}$$
$$m = 2.3 \text{ instead of 3 in the standard model}$$
$$dt^m = 0.6\ (3\ dd/730^{2.3}) = 0.114$$
$$R = 0$$

The result is that the water concentration should be less than 0.0092 μg/l in order to keep the individual lifetime risk below 10^{-5}.

Bertram and Craig (50-15) administered dibutylnitrosamine via drinking water to C57BL/6- mice at dose levels of about 8 and 30 mg/kg/day until the animals became moribund or died. They found that all of the 179 animals reaching autopsy had tumors of the bladder or esophagus except 3, which had tumor induction at either site. These were the males given 7.6 mg/kg/day, where the mean tumor induction time was 261 days. Assuming a bioaccumulation factor of zero, the parameters of the extrapolation model are:

$$n_t/N_t = 0.5$$
$$N_c/n_c = 0$$
$$Le = 261 \text{ days}$$
$$le = 261 \text{ days}$$
$$d = 7.6 \text{ mg/kg/day}$$
$$L = 728 \text{ days}$$
$$w = 0.028 \text{ kg}$$
$$R = 0$$

The result is that the water concentration should be less than 0.013 μg/l in order to keep the individual lifetime risk below 10^{-5}.

Preussman et al (50-16) found a dose-related incidence of hepatocellular carcinomas in Sprague-Dawley rats in a lifetime feeding study at levels of 0.3, 1.0, 3.0, and 10 mg/kg/day. The total tumor incidence was equal to controls at the 0.3 mg/kg/day level, but was 46, 84 and 32% at the successively higher doses. Animals at the highest dose had a smaller tumor incidence because of early deaths from pneumonia. At 3 mg/kg/day, the incidence of liver tumors was 31/38 whereas the 61 controls had no tumors. With a negligible fish accumulation, the parameters of the dose-response model are:

$$nt = 31$$
$$N_t = 38$$
$$n_c = 0$$
$$N_c = 61$$
$$Le = 104 \text{ weeks}$$
$$le = 104 \text{ weeks}$$
$$d = 3 \text{ mg/kg/day}$$
$$w = 0.35 \text{ kg}$$
$$L = 104 \text{ weeks}$$
$$R = 0$$

The result is that the water concentration should be less than 0.11 μg/l in order to keep the individual lifetime risk below 10^{-5}.

References

(50-1) Bogovski, P. et al, "N-nitroso compounds, analysis and formation," IARC Sci. Pub. No. 3, Lyon, France, Int. Agency Res. Cancer (1972).

(50-2) Fine, D.H. et al, "Human exposure to N-nitroso compounds in the environment," In H.H. Hiatt et al, eds., *Origins of human cancer*, Cold Spring Harbor, New York, Cold Spring Harbor Lab. (1977).

(50-3) Fine, D.H. et al, "Formation in vivo of volatile N-nitrosamines in man after ingestion of cooked bacon and spinach," *Nature* 265, 753 (1977).

(50-4) Fine, D.H. et al, "Determination of dimethylnitrosamine in air, water and soil by thermal energy analysis: measurements in Baltimore, Md.," *Environ. Sci. Technol.* 11, 581 (1977).

(50-5) U.S. EPA, *Scientific and assessment report on nitrosamines*, Report No. EPA 600/6-77-001, Washington, D.C., Off. Res. Dev. (1977).

(50-6) U.S. EPA, *Environmental assessment of atmospheric nitrosamines*, Report by Mitre Corp., McLean, Va. on Contract No. 68-02-1495, Washington, D.C. (1976).

(50-7) Montesano, R. and Bartsch, H., "Mutagenic and carcinogenic N-nitroso compounds; possible environmental hazards," *Mutat. Res.* 32, 179 (1976).

(50-8) Czygan, P.H. et al, "Cytochrome P-450 content and the ability of liver microsomes from patients undergoing abdominal surgery to alter the mutagenicity of a primary and a secondary carcinogen," *Jour. Natl. Cancer Inst.* 51, 1761 (1973).

(50-9) Druckery, H. et al, "Organotropic carcinogenic action of 65 different N-nitroso compounds in BD rats," *Z. Krebsforsch.* 69, 103 (1967).

(50-10) Druckery, H., "Specific carcinogenic and teratogenic effects of 'indirect' alkylating methyl and ethyl compounds and their dependency on stages of oncogenic development," *Xenobiotica* 3, 271 (1973).

(50-11) Druckery, H., "Mechanisms of transplacental carcinogenesis," In Tomatis, L. and U. Mohr, eds., *Transplacental carcinogenesis*, IARC Sci. Pub. No. 6, Lyon, France, Int. Agency Res. Cancer (1973).

(50-12) Magee, P.N. et al, "N-nitroso compounds and related carcinogens," In C.S. Searle, ed., *Chemical carcinogens*, ACS Monograph No. 1973, Washington, D.C., Am. Chem. Soc. (1976).

(50-13) Lijinsky, W. and Taylor, H.W., "Nitrosamines and their precursors in food," In H.H. Hiatt et al, eds., *Origins of human cancer*, Cold Spring Harbor, N.Y., Cold Spring Harbor Lab. (1977).

(50-14) Druckery, H. et al, "Quantitative analysis of the carcinogenic action of diethylnitrosamine," *Arzneimittel-Forsch* 13, 841 (1963).

(50-15) Bertram, J.S. and Craig, A.W., "Induction of bladder tumors in mice with dibutylnitrosamine," *Br. Jour. Cancer* 24, 352 (1970).

(50-16) Preussmann, R. et al, "Carcinogenicity of N-nitrosopyrrolidine: dose-response study in rats," *Z. Krebsforsch.* 90, 161 (1977).

(50-17) Fishbein, L. (National Center for Toxicological Research), *Potential Industrial Carcinogens and Mutagens*, Report EPA-560/5-77-005, Washington, D.C., Office of Toxic Substances (May 5, 1977).

(50-18) Anselme, J.P., Ed., "N-Nitrosamines," ACS Symposium Series No. 101, Washington, D.C., American Chemical Society (1979).

O

OCTACHLORONAPHTHALENES

See "Chlorinated Naphthalenes" (17).

P

PCBs

See "Polychlorinated Biphenyls" (54).

PENTACHLOROBENZENE

See "Chlorinated Benzenes" (14).

PENTACHLOROETHANE

See "Chlorinated Ethanes" (15).

PENTACHLORONAPHTHALENES

See "Chlorinated Naphthalenes" (17).

PENTACHLOROPHENOL (#51)

Pentachlorophenol (PCP) is a substituted phenol prepared by the chlorination of phenol in the presence of a catalyst. It has the empirical formula C_6Cl_5OH and a molecular weight of 266.35. It has been shown that commercial preparations of PCP contain certain "caustic insolubles" or "nonphenolic, neutral impurities," such as tetra-, penta-, hexa-, hepta-, and octachlorodibenzofurans and the octachlorodibenzo-p-dioxins. The chemically pure PCP used in comparative studies had no detectable concentrations of any chlorinated dioxins.

Occurrence: Although PCP and its sodium salt, Na-PCP, are both highly toxic and widely disseminated in the environment, there is a paucity of data of their environmental concentration, fate, and effects. Their principal use as a wood preservative results in both point source water contamination at manufacturing and wood preservation sites and, conceivably, nonpoint source water contamination through runoff wherever there are PCP-treated lumber products exposing PCP or Na-PCP to soil. Raw and finished drinking waters have been found to have PCP levels of 0.17 and 0.06 $\mu g/l$, respectively. It has also been noted that PCP persisted in warm, moist soils for a period of 12 months. Studies of PCP bioconcentration by aquatic life indicate factors ranging from 13 to 1,000 for freshwater and marine vertebrates.

Physical Properties: PCP has specific gravity of 1.978, and a vapor pressure of 0.12 mm Hg at 100°C. The melting point of pentachlorophenol ranges between 190° and 191°C for the anhydrous form. PCP is slightly soluble in water (14 mg/l at 20°C) while its alkaline salts such as sodium pentachlorophenate (Na-PCP) are highly soluble in water.

Chemical Properties: PCP decomposes at its boiling point of 309° to 310°C. PCP behaves as a weak acid and is readily disassociated to form the corresponding salt in an alkaline solution.

PCP is known to undergo photochemical degradation in solution in the presence of sunlight with the subsequent formation of several chlorinated benzoquinones, 2,4,5,6-tetrachloro-resorcinol, and chloranilic acid. Na-PCP is decomposed directly by sunlight with the formation of numerous products including oxidized monomers, dimers, a trimer, and chloranilic acid. Studies have reported the degradation by sunlight or ultraviolet light of dilute solutions of pentachlorophenol to lower chlorophenols, tetrachlorodihydroxyl benzenes, and nonaromatic fragments such as dichloromaleic acid. The irradiation of Na-PCP in relatively high concentrations in aqueous solutions has been reported to form octachlorodibenzo-p-dioxin (51–1).

Although one investigator observed no alteration of Na-PCP by activated sludge microbes after 4 days of incubation, another reported the growth of an isolated species of *Pseudomonas* from PCP-perfused culture samples using PCP as the sole carbon source. Other microorganisms also have been isolated and reported to metabolize PCP. The microbial degradation of Na-PCP to carbon dioxide and chloride ions has been demonstrated using mixed microbial communities and an axenic bacterial culture.

Uses: Pentachlorophenol (PCP) is a commercially produced bactericide, fungicide, and slimicide used primarily for the preservation of wood, wood products, and other materials. As a chlorinated hydrocarbon, its biological properties have also resulted in its use as an herbicide, insecticide, and molluscicide.

Toxic Effects: PCP and its sodium salt, sodium pentachlorophenate (Na-PCP), have been demonstrated to be highly toxic to man, mammals, and aquatic life. As a result of their toxic nature, accumulation in tissues, and widespread industrial and agricultural applications, both PCP and Na-PCP pose a potential threat to terrestrial and aquatic life.

Current Levels of Exposure: Based on an assumed food consumption of 1.5 kg and a water intake of 2.0 kg, a food PCP residue of 10 μg/kg, and a water PCP residue of 60 ng/kg, the resulting maximum total daily exposure for a 70 kg person would likely be 15 μg from food and 120 ng from water. The exposure rate would be 0.21 μg/kg/day from food and 1.7 ng/kg/day from water. The food residue level estimated (15 μg) is higher than the 1 to 6 μg/day intake calculated when the calculations took into consideration dietary consumption by food class.

An alternative approach to estimating human exposure is extrapolation from urine residue data since PCP is primarily eliminated in the urine and at equilibrium excretion equals daily intake. In Hawaii, where exposure for general population may be higher than persons living in colder climates due to differences in use of PCP treated wood in home construction, Bevenue reported an average PCP urine value of 40 μg/l. Assuming a daily urine void of 1.4 liters, the total daily PCP excretion would be 56 μg, an amount equal to the intake. An average of 5.8 μg/l in six general population urine samples and an average of 6.3 μg/l for 416 samples were reported by different investigators. Consequently, location of residence may influence PCP exposure. Based on available data, the exposure for the general population is estimated to range from 1 to 50 μg/person/day.

Exposure will increase sharply if an individual works with the material and inhales vapors and/or experiences dermal absorption. In two subjects studied following a brush application, the urine PCP concentrations peaked at 300 to 500 μg/l.

Occupationally exposed individuals excrete more PCP in the urine than does the general population. Reported urine values include an average of 1.8 mg/l for 130 pest control operators; 1 to 10 mg/l for wood treaters; 2.8 mg/l for dip treaters; 0.98 mg/l for spray treaters and 1.24 mg/l for pressure treaters. Using the same assumption of 1.4 liters of urine per day the estimated occupational exposures would range from 1.37 to 14 mg per person per day.

Special Groups at Risks: Two groups can be expected to encounter the largest exposures. There are a small number of employees involved in the manufacture of PCP. All of these are presently under industrial health surveillance programs.

The second and larger group are the formulators and wood treaters. Exposure, hygiene and industrial health practices can be expected to vary from the small treaters to the larger companies. Health related data in general are not available for this group. Employees of two Hawaiian wood treating companies have been studied for a number of years and although exposures have resulted in blood and urine levels of 1 to 10 mg/l, adverse health effects have been minimal.

Existing Guidelines and Standards: The maximum air PCP concentation established by the American Industrial Hygiene Association as of 1979 is 0.5 mg PCP or 0.5 mg Na-PCP/m^3 for an 8 hr exposure (TLV) and is 1.5 mg/m^3 on a short-term exposure limit (STEL) basis. *The Code of Federal Regulations* allows up to 50 ppm PCP in treated wood intended for use in contact with food. A tolerance for PCP in food has not been established.

A no-adverse-effect level in drinking water of 0.021 mg PCP/l is suggested by the National Research Council (51–2). The recommendation is based on a NOEL of 3 mg/kg in the 90-day to 8-month rat studies. A safety or "uncertainty factor" of 1,000 and a water consumption of 2 l/day were used in arriving at the level. The longer duration study of Schwetz, et al (51–3), the negative results of Innes, et al (51–4) for carcinogenicity and the results of human epidemiology studies were apparently not available or not considered in setting the uncertainty factor.

Summary of Proposed EPA Criteria: *Freshwater Aquatic Life* — For pentachlorophenol the criterion to protect freshwater aquatic life as derived using procedures other than the Guidelines is 6.2 µg/l as a 24 hr average and the concentration should not exceed 14 µg/l at any time.

Saltwater Aquatic Life — For pentachlorophenol the criterion to protect saltwater aquatic life as derived using the Guidelines is 3.7 µg/l as a 24 hr average and the concentration should not exceed 8.5 µg/l at any time.

Human Health — For the protection of human health from the toxic properties of pentachlorophenol ingested through water and through contaminated aquatic organisms, the ambient water quality criterion is determined to be 140 µg/l.

Basis for the Proposed Human Health Criteria — Based on available and cited literature, PCP is not considered to be carcinogenic. A criterion can be calculated using the data from the chronic toxicity studies. Using a NOEL of 3 mg/kg for low nonphenolic PCP and applying a 0.01 animal to human uncertainty factor the upper limit for nonoccupational daily exposure is 0.03 mg/kg or 2.10 mg/70 kg person.

For the purposes of establishing a water quality criterion, human exposure to PCP is considered to be based on ingestion of 2 liters of water and 18.7 g of fish. The amount of water ingested is approximately 100 times greater than the amount of fish consumed. However, fish bioaccumulate PCP from water by a factor of 58 and thus contain about half as much PCP per gram as water. With these considerations in mind, the following equation has been established: $2X + (0.0187 \times 58)X = 2.10$ mg, where 2.10 mg = limit on daily exposure for a 70 kg person (ADI), 2 = liters of drinking water consumed,

0.0187 kg = amount of fish consumed, and 58 = bioaccumulation factor. The solving for X is as follows: X = 0.68 mg/l. Thus, 1.4 mg of the ADI can be obtained from 2 liters of drinking water and 0.7 mg from ingested fish.

The food residues of PCP are reported to be 0 to 10 μg/kg and one report of 0.06 μg/kg in water. These levels are well below the criterion and total daily general population exposures are less than 1% of the calculated maximum value based on toxicologic considerations.

It should be noted that the criterion recommended in this document is based on a NOEL of low nonphenolic PCP, a compound found to be noncarcinogenic at the dosages tested. However, NCI is presently conducting studies on the carcinogenicity of PCP contaminants, hexachloro-p-dioxin, and octachloro-p-dioxin, the results of which are not yet available. The results of these studies should be evaluated before any EPA regulatory standards are established.

References

(51-1)   Wong, A.S., and Crosby, D.G., "Photodecomposition of pentachlorophenol (PCP)," *Proc. Symp. on Pentachlorophenol,* U.S. Environ. Prot. Agency and Univ. West Florida (June 27–29, 1977).

(51-2)   National Research Council, *Drinking Water and Health*, Washington, D.C. (1977).

(51-3)   Schwetz, B.A. et al, "Results of two-year toxicity and reproduction studies of pentachlorophenol in rats" in K.R. Rao, Ed., *Pentachlorophenol: Chemistry, Pharmacology and Environmental Toxicology*, New York, Plenum Press (1978).

(51-4)   Innes, J.R.M. et al, "Bioassay of pesticides and industrial chemicals for tumorigenicity in mice, a preliminary note," *Jour. Nat. Cancer Inst. 42*, 1101 (1969).

PHENANTHRENE

See "Polynuclear Aromatic Hydrocarbons," (55).

PHENOL (#52)

Phenol, C_6H_5OH, is sometimes referred to as carbolic acid.

Occurrence: Phenol is a high volume industrial chemical which is largely used as an intermediate for the manufacture of other chemicals. Phenol is also produced by biological processes and is a by-product of combustion and some industrial processes.

Information concerning the presence and persistence, and fate of phenol in the environment is incomplete or not available. A limited number of studies indicate that phenol does not bioconcentrate appreciably in aquatic organisms.

The widespread use of phenol as an important chemical intermediate, the generation of phenolic wastes by industry and agriculture, and the toxicological and organoleptic properties indicate its importance in potential point source and nonpoint source water contamination.

The National Organic Monitoring Survey in 1977 reported finding unspecified concentrations of phenol in 2 out of 110 raw water supplies by GLC/MS. The survey found no phenol in any finished water supplies. The National Commission on Water Quality in 1975 reported from U.S. Geological Survey data that the annual mean concentration of phenol in the lower Mississippi River was 1.5 μg/l with a maximum of 6.7 μg/l and a minimum of 0.0 μg/l. The International Joint Commission in 1978 reported finding <0.5 to 5 μg/l phenol in the Detroit River between 1972 and 1977.

Phenol is also produced endogenously in the mammalian intestinal tract through the microbial metabolism of 1-tyrosine and p-hydroxybenzoic acid. In addition, exposures to benzene and the ingestion of certain drugs can lead to increased phenol production and excretion.

Physical Properties: Phenol, is a clear, colorless (light pink when impurities are present), hygroscopic, deliquescent, crystalline solid at 25°C. It has the empirical formula C_6H_6O, a molecular weight of 94.11, a specific gravity of 1.071 at 25°C/4°C and a vapor pressure of 0.3513 mm Hg at 25°C. Phenol has a melting point of 43°C and a boiling point of 182°C at 760 mm Hg.

Phenol has a water solubility of 6.7 g/100 ml at 16°C and is soluble at all proportions in water at 66°C. It is also soluble in relatively nonpolar solvents such as benzene, petrolatum, and oils.

Chemical Properties: Due to the electronegative character of the phenyl group, phenol exhibits weakly acidic properties. It possesses a pKa of 9.9 to 10.0 and readily reacts with strong bases to form salts called phenoxides. Phenoxides exist in highly alkaline aqueous solutions and many, particularly the sodium and potassium salts, are readily soluble in water.

Phenol undergoes oxidation to a variety of products, such as the benzenediols, benzenetriols, and derivatives of diphenyl and diphenylene oxide, depending on the oxidizing agent and conditions. However, phenol may be biochemically hydroxylated to ortho- and para-dihydroxybenzenes and readily oxidized to the corresponding benzoquinones. These may in turn react with numerous components of industrial waters or sewage such as mercaptans, amines or the −SH or −NH groups of proteins. In the absence of these compounds, the quinones, especially the ortho-isomers, can be quickly destroyed by hydrolytic oxidizing reactions.

The chlorination of phenol in aqueous solutions to form 2-chloro-, 4-chloro-, or higher chlorophenols has been demonstrated under conditions similar to those used for disinfection of waste water effluents and represents a potential amplification of the organoleptic problems associated with phenol contamination. Synthesis of 2-chlorophenol within one hour in aqueous solutions containing as little as 10 mg/l phenol and 20 mg/l chlorine has been reported (52–1).

The photooxidation of phenol in water at alkaline pH has been studied. Irradiation with a mercury arc lamp produced several intermediate compounds and p-benzosemiquinone as the final product. The photooxidation of phenol with ultraviolet irradiation (253.7 nm) yielded the conclusion that the reaction initially leads to the formation of a complex mixture of tri- and tetrahydroxybiphenyls, quinones and diphenols. Aqueous phenol solutions irradiated with sunlight for seven days were reported to degrade to hydroquinone and pyrocatechol.

Subsequent irradiation of pyrocatechol with sunlight for seven days yielded pyrogallol. The end products of photodecomposition were reported to be humic acids. Conversely, similar studies utilizing natural sunlight as the source of irradiation indicated that phenol concentrations in solutions of pure water remained unchanged after ten days. However, phenol degradation did occur in industrial sewage effluents and led to the conclusion that unidentified microorganisms, not sunlight, were responsible for the destruction of phenol.

The microbiological degradation of phenol has been widely studied. The conversion of phenol to catechol by *Pseudomonas putida* has been reported. The oxidation of phenol by both intact cells and extracts of the microorganism, *Trichosporon cutaneum* has been observed. The thermophilic bacteria, *Bacillus stearothermophilus* has been shown to catabolize phenol. In these studies, the bacteria first converted phenol to catechol and subsequently cleaved the aromatic ring to form 2-hydroxymuconic semialdehyde. In view of the fact that phenol represented the primary carbon source provided to isolated and adapted microorganisms in these studies, the importance of microbiological degradation within the environment remains unclear.

Uses: Phenol has a long history of industrial and medical uses. In 1867, Lister reported on the use of phenol sprays for disinfecting operating rooms. Today its medicinal uses are limited to a few mouth, throat, and skin medications. The industrial capacity for the production of phenol in the United States was 2,885 x 10^6 lb/yr in 1975, about 90% of which was used in the production of phenolic resins, caprolactam, bisphenol-A, alkylphenols, and adipic acid.

Toxic Effects: Although phenol appears to be less toxic than the chlorinated phenols and certain other substituted phenols, its toxicity to microorganisms, plants, aquatic organisms and mammals, including man, has been demonstrated. Phenol also has been reported to exhibit carcinogenic activity in mice. These findings, together with potential pollution from waste sources and the possible chlorination of phenol present in drinking water sources, indicate that phenol is potentially hazardous to aquatic and terrestrial life.

Current Levels of Exposure: The EPA's National Organic Monitoring Survey in 1977 reported finding unspecified concentrations of phenol in 2 out of 110 raw water supplies. The survey found no phenol in any finished water supplies. The National Commission on Water Quality in 1975 reported that the annual mean phenol concentration in the lower Mississippi River was 1.5 μg/l in 1973, with a maximum of 6.7 μg/l.

Endogenously produced phenols in man occur at significantly higher concentration than this. They result in total urinary free and conjugated phenol concentrations ranging from 5 to 55 mg/l.

Occupational exposures at a TLV of 20 mg/m^3 TWA would result in the absorption of 105 mg phenol from the inspired air, assuming moderate to low activity (7 m^3 air breathed per 8 hr), and an adsorption efficiency of 75%. During heavier activity (equivalent to 20 m^3/8 hr) the absorption would rise to 300 mg phenol for an 8 hr shift. The additional skin absorption would be expected to substantially increase these quantities.

Special Groups at Risk: In 1976, NIOSH estimated (52–2) the number of people who may be exposed to phenol at 10,000. This reflects the number of people that are employed in the production of phenol, formulation into products, or distribution of concentrated products. In addition, an uncertain but probably large number of people will have intermittent contact with phenol as components of medications or in the workplace as chemists, pharmacists, biomedical personnel, and other occupations.

Existing Guidelines and Standards: In 1974, the Federal standard for phenol in air in the workplace was 19 mg/m^3 or 5 ppm as the time weighted average (39 *FR* 125). This coincides with the recommendation of the American Council for Governmental Industrial Hygienists as of 1979 which also sets a tentative STEL value of 10 ppm (38 mg/m^3). The NIOSH (52–2) criteria for a recommended standard for occupational exposure to phenol are 20 mg/m^3 in air as a time weighted average for up to a 10 hr work day and a 40 hr work week, with a ceiling concentration of 60 mg/m^3 for any 15 min period.

The U.S. EPA interim drinking water limit for phenol is 0.001 mg/l, which is largely an aesthetic standard based on the objectionable taste and odor produced by chlorinated phenols. In response to a phenol spill in Southern Wisconsin, the U.S. EPA proposed on November 26, 1974 an emergency standard of 0.1 mg phenol per liter as being temporarily acceptable for human consumption (52–3).

Summary of Proposed EPA Criteria: *Freshwater Aquatic Life* — For phenol the criterion to protect freshwater aquatic life as derived using the Guidelines is 600 μg/l as 24 hr average, and the concentration should not exceed 3,400 μg/l at any time.

Saltwater Aquatic Life:– For saltwater aquatic life, no criterion for phenol can be derived using the Guidelines, and there are insufficient data to estimate a criterion using other procedures.

Human Health – For the protection of human health from phenol ingested through water and through contaminated aquatic organisms the concentration in water should not exceed 3.4 mg/l. For the prevention of adverse effects due to the organoleptic properties of chlorinated phenols inadvertently formed during water purification processes, the phenol concentration in water should not exceed 1.0 μg/l.

Basis for the Proposed Human Health Criteria – Heller and Pursell (52-4) reported no significant effects in a multigeneration feeding study in rats at 100, 500 and 1,000 mg/l of phenol in drinking water for five generations and at 3,000 and 5,000 mg/l for three generations. Assuming a daily water intake of 30 ml and an average bodyweight of 300 g, these rats would have received daily doses of 10, 50, 100, 300 and 500 mg/kg/day. The upper range approaches a single LD_{50} dose per day. Deichmann and Oesper (52-5) reported no significant effects in rats receiving approximately 70, 100 or 163 mg/kg/day in their drinking water for 12 months. However, both of these studies did not report detailed pathological or biochemical studies but relied mostly on the weights and the general appearance of the animals for evaluation.

In a more recent study (52-6), 135 dosings by gavage over six months at 100 mg/kg/dose resulted in some liver and kidney damage. At 50 mg/kg/dose the exposure resulted in only slight kidney damage. It must be noted that in the first two studies the phenol is incorporated into the drinking water so that the daily dose is taken gradually. In the Dow study (52-6) the phenol is administered in a single slug. A 500-fold uncertainty factor applied to the 50 mg/kg exposure in the Dow study would provide an estimated acceptable level of 0.1 mg/kg/day for man. In the case of phenol a great deal of information on human exposure exists.

Long term animal data are available as well, however, the detail in these studies is very incomplete. Shorter term studies of sufficient detail provide the lowest dose level in animal studies for which an adverse effect was seen. It was judged that the existing data did not fully satisfy the requirements for the use of a 100X uncertainty factor but were better than the requirements for a 1000X uncertainty factor (Table 75). Consequently, an intermediate 500X uncertainty factor was selected.

When one examines the amount of phenol absorbed through inhalation near the TLV of 20 mg/m³ for occupational exposures by using the Stokinger and Woodward model (52-7), then at a breathing rate of 10 m³ for an 8 hr day with 75% absorption and a body weight of 70 kg, a man would absorb approximately 2.14 mg/kg/working day, assuming no skin absorption. The use of the Stokinger-Woodward model may be applicable to estimate acceptable intake from water.

Table 75: Guidelines for Using Uncertainty Factors (*Drinking Water and Human Health, NAS, 1977*)

Uncertainty Factor	Acceptable Human Ingestion of Drinking Water
10	Valid experimental results from studies on prolonged ingestion by man, with no indication of carcinogenicity.
100	Experimental results of studies of human ingestion not available or scanty (e.g., acute exposure only). Valid results on long-term feeding studies on experimental animals or in the absence of human studies, valid animal studies on one or more species. No indication of carcinogenicity.
1,000	No long term or acute human data. Scanty results on experimental animals. No indication of carcinogenicity.

Source: Reference (52)

It has been established that phenol is absorbed rapidly by all routes and subsequently is distributed rapidly. If a ten-fold safety factor is applied to the projection doses absorbed from inhalation at the TLV (which already incorporates some safety factors), then the projected acceptable level would be 0.2 mg/kg/day. The estimate from animal data is 0.1 mg/kg/day. On the basis of chronic toxicity data in animals and man, an estimated acceptable daily intake for phenol in man should be 0.1 mg/kg/day or 7.0 mg/man, assuming a 70 kg body weight. Therefore, consumption of 2 liters of water daily and 18.7 g of contaminated fish having a bioconcentration factor of 2.3, would result in assuming 100% gastrointestinal absorption of phenol, a maximum permissible concentration of 3.4 mg/l for the ingested water:

$$\frac{7.0 \text{ mg/day}}{2 \text{ liters} + (2.3 \times 0.0187) \times 1.0} = 3.4 \text{ mg/l}$$

The water quality criterion is in the range of reported taste and odor threshold values for phenol which have been reported. It is recognized that when ambient water containing this concentration of phenol is chlorinated, various chlorinated phenols may be produced in sufficient quantities to produce objectional taste and odors. However, the ambient water quality criterion for phenol is based on phenol alone. For the criteria of 2-chlorophenol, 2,4-dichlorophenol and other chlorophenols, reference should be made to their specific criterion documents (20, 28).

In summary, based on the use of chronic toxicologic test data for rats and an uncertainty factor of 500, the criterion for phenol corresponding to the calculated acceptable daily intake of 0.1 mg/kg/day is 3.4 mg/l. Drinking water contributes 98% of the assumed exposure while eating contaminated fish products accounts for 2%. The criterion level could alternatively be expressed as 163 mg/l if exposure is assumed to be from the consumption of fish and shellfish products alone. Based on the potential chlorination of phenol in water, the criterion for phenol is 1.0 μg/l in those instances where such inadvertent chlorination may take place.

References

(52-1)   Barnhart, E.L. and Campbell, G.R., *The effect of chlorination on selected organic chemicals*, U.S. Environ. Prot. Agency, Washington, D.C. (1972).

(52-2)   National Inst. for Occup. Safety and Health, *Criteria for a Recommended Standard: Occupational Exposure to Phenol*, NIOSH Doc. No. 76–196, Washington, D.C. (1976).

(52-3)   Baker, E.L. et al, "Phenol poisoning due to contaminated drinking water," *Arch. Envir. Health 33*, 89 (1978).

(52-4)   Heller, V.G. and Pursell, L., "Phenol-contaminated waters and their physiological action," *Jour. Pharmacol. Exp. Ther. 63*, 99 (1938).

(52-5)   Deichmann, W.B. and Oesper, P., "Ingestion of phenol: effects on the albino rat," *Ind. Med. 9*, 296 (1940).

(52-6)   Dow Chemical Co., "References and Literature Review Pertaining to Toxicological Properties of Phenol," Midland, Mich., Toxicol Res. Lab. (1976).

(52-7)   Stokinger, H.E. and Woodward, R.L., "Toxicological methods for establishing drinking water standards," *Jour. Am. Water Works Assoc. 50*, 517 (1958).

PHTHALATE ESTERS (#53)

The phthalate esters have the general formula:

$$
\begin{array}{c}
\text{(benzene ring)} \\
\end{array}
\quad
\begin{array}{l}
\overset{\displaystyle O}{\overset{\|}{C}}\text{—OR} \\
\underset{\displaystyle O}{\underset{\|}{C}}\text{—OR}'
\end{array}
$$

The alkyl groups, R and R', may be the same or different. The points of attachment to
the ring may be as shown or may be as in terephthalate esters:

$$O=C-OR$$

$$O=C-OR'$$

Occurrence: The extremely large production of phthalates and the variety of uses for these
esters have led to the presence of these esters in water sources, food, consumer products,
air (industrial settings, automobiles having vinyl furnishings), and in medical devices such
as tubings and blood bags. Esters can thus enter the environment and biological species,
including man, through a variety of sources.

Therefore, man is exposed to phthalates from a variety of routes such as: ingestion from
water, ingestion from food, inhalation, dermal, and through parenteral administration (via
blood bags and tubes in which the ester is extracted by a parenteral solution including
blood).

The ease of extraction of phthalate esters and their widespread use in PVC or alone account
for their ubiquity. PAEs have been detected in soil, water, fish, air and animal and human
tissues. Their detection in certain vegetation, animals and minerals, and in areas remote
from industrial sites have raised questions about possible natural origins of PAEs. Esters
detected in the EPA survey were diethyl phthalate, diisobutyl phthalate, and dioctyl phthalate.

Physical Properties: For the most part, the esters are colorless liquids, have low volatility,
and are poorly soluble in water but soluble in organic solvents and oils. Table 76 lists
several of the physical properties of these esters.

Table 76: Physical Properties of Phthalate Esters

Compound	Molecular Weight	Specific Gravity		BP ($^\circ$C)	Solubility in H_2O (g/100 ml)
Dimethyl phthalate	194.18	1.189	(25/25)	282	0.5
Diethyl phthalate	222.23	1.123	(25/4)	296.1	insoluble
Diallyl phthalate	246.27	1.120	(20/20)	290	0.01
Diisobutyl phthalate	278.3	1.040		327	insoluble
Dibutyl phthalate	278.34	1.0465	(21)	340	0.45 (25°C)
Dimethoxyethyl phthalate	282.0	1.171	(20)	190-210	0.85
Dicyclohexyl phthalate	330.0	1.20	(25/25)	220-228	insoluble
Butyl octyl phthalate	334.0	—		340	—
Dihexyl phthalate	334.0	0.990		—	insoluble
Butyl phthalylbutyl glycolate	336.37	1.097	(25/25)	219*	0.012
Dibutoxyethyl phthalate	366.0	1.063		210	0.03
Di(2-ethylhexyl) phthalate	391.0	0.985	(20/20)	386.9*	insoluble
Diisooctyl phthalate	391.0	0.981		239*	insoluble
Di-n-octyl phthalate	391.0	0.978		220*	insoluble
Dinonyl phthalate	419.0	0.965		413	insoluble

*Per 5 mm.

Source: Reference (53)

Chemical Properties: The phthalate esters are quite stable. They may of course be split
by hydrolysis under severe conditions.

Uses: Phthalic acid esters have a large number of commercial uses, the largest being as
plasticizers for specific plastics such as polyvinyl chloride. Other uses for these esters

include: defoaming agents in the production of paper, in cosmetic products as a vehicle (primarily diethyl phthalate) for perfumes, in lubricating oils, and in other industrial and consumer applications.

Dioctyl phthalate (includes di-2-ethylhexyl phthalate and other dioctyl phthalates) accounts for approximately 42% of the esters produced in this country, followed by diisodecyl phthalate. Dioctyl phthalate (DOP) and di-2-ethylhexyl phthalate (DEHP) are often used synonymously even though it should be clear that they are not the same, one being the isomer of the other.

Toxic Effects: PAEs have been reported to be acutely and chronically toxic to freshwater and marine aquatic organisms (53–1, 53–2). Levels of PAE residues detected in fish from ambient waters have not been correlated with adverse biological effects (53–3). Data show that phthalate esters can be chronically toxic to aquatic organisms at low concentrations. DEHP impairs reproduction in *Daphnia magna* by 60% at a concentration as low as 3 μg/l (53–2). Toxicological investigations in mammals show that phthalates have low acute toxicities but induce serious chronic effects including teratogenicity and mutagenicity (53–4).

Current Levels of Exposure: Lack of sufficient data prevents an accurate assessment of levels of exposure of man and animals to phthalate esters. It is, however, well known that man is exposed to these esters through a number of routes such as industrial sites in which the esters are manufactured or used. Esters may also reach man through indirect means such as inhalation of the esters inside vehicles containing PVC or in foods and from water. Direct injection (intravenous) of specific phthalate esters can also occur when PVC blood bags and tubings are used to transfuse blood and blood products to man. The ubiquitous nature of the phthalate ester is apparent since tissues of deceased persons have revealed the presence of phthalic acid esters, even though the individuals were not apparently exposed to these esters.

Even though it is well established that workers in occupations in which phthalate esters are used are exposed to various levels of phthalate esters and thus can absorb these esters through inhalation or through dermal absorption, the lack of sufficient data precludes establishing what are the levels of exposure. Dermal absorption of the low molecular weight esters such as dimethyl phthalate (mosquito repellent) and diethyl phthalate (in cosmetic products) probably is also occurring but the quantity absorbed through the skin is not known.

A survey was conducted by the Bureau of Foods (FDA) in 1974 to determine if phthalate esters were entering the food supply through the processing, packaging, handling and transportation chain. In the study, ten basic and stable food products were analyzed for the presence of these esters. Conclusions reached in the report are presented below.

    (a)   The frequency and levels of phthalate esters reported as well as the possible cumulative intake of phthalates in baked beans in cans or jars, canned whole kernel corn, margarine, cereals, eggs, bread, corn meal, meat, milk, and cheese do not pose a hazard to the consumer.

    (b)   DEHP was the ester most frequently detected in the food commodities. Dibutyl phthalate, dicyclohexyl phthalate and butylphthalylbutyl glycolate were found in comparatively few samples. Diisooctyl and diisodecyl phthalates, although looked for, were not detected.

    (c)   Phthalate ester contamination was found in a higher proportion of milk and cheese samples than in other foods. (However, the findings are uncertain.)

In the above survey, the highest levels of phthalate esters were present in margarine (13.7 and 56.3 ppm on fat basis). In cheese, the highest levels of esters were 22.8 and 24.9 ppm for DNBP and 35 ppm for DEHP but most cheese samples contained less than 5 ppm of phthalates.

In a published study by Tomita et al (53-5), information is presented dealing with phthalate (DEHP and DNBP) residues in various commercial foodstuffs in Japan. They concluded that foods packaged in plastic films with printing are a greater source of contamination to the product with the esters than if the foods were in plastic bottles. They also noted that persons had significantly higher levels of the esters after meals from foods packaged in the film. Extremely high levels of the two esters (combined) were found in tempura powder stored for eight months (up to 454 ppm).

The residue level of the esters from plastic films containing the plasticizers, as would be expected, migrated to fatty foods or fatty-like foods to a greater extent than to foods having low fat content. The authors included in their conclusion the following: "The daily intake of PAEs (phthalic acid esters) from present foodstuffs may not exceed the ADI of DNBP and DEHP but an effort to reduce the PAE levels in foodstuffs should be continuously made."

The Bureau of Foods (FDA) in another survey on fish from a number of locations in the U.S. noted that the highest level of DEHP (7.1 ppm) was present in shark. In most other instances, the fish which were studied were free of the esters.

Patients receiving repeated transfusions with whole blood, packed cells, platelets and plasma stored in PVC may receive up to 70 mg of DEHP and, in some instances, the quantity even exceeds 500 mg. Hemodialysis patients may receive up to 150 mg of DEHP.

Special Groups at Risk: Two groups are at risk in regard to phthalic acid esters. These are workers in the industrial environment in which the phthalates are manufactured or used and patients receiving chronic transfusion of blood and blood products stored in PVC blood bags.

Existing Guidelines and Standards: The Threshold Limit Value for dimethyl, dibutyl and di-2-ethylhexyl phthalate esters established by the American Conference of Governmental and Industrial Hygienists is 5 mg/m^3. The Short Term Exposure Limit is 10 mg/m^3.

The Food and Drug Administration has approved the use of a number of phthalate esters in food packaging materials. Prior to 1959 (before enactment of the food additive amendment), FDA approved five esters; these are diethyl phthalate, diisobutyl phthalate, ethyl phthalyl ethyl glycolate, diisooctyl phthalate and di-2-ethylhexyl phthalate. Since then, 19 additional phthalates used in packaging material for foods of high water content have also been approved. More specific uses and restrictions of phthalic esters are set forth by FDA in its regulations.

Summary of Proposed EPA Criteria: *Freshwater Aquatic Life* — For freshwater aquatic life, no criterion for any phthalate ester can be derived using the Guidelines, and there are insufficient data to estimate a criterion using other procedures.

Saltwater Aquatic Life — For saltwater aquatic life, no criterion for any phthalate ester can be derived using the Guidelines, and there are insufficient data to estimate a criterion using other procedures.

Human Health — For the protection of human health from the toxic properties of phthalate esters ingested through water and through contaminated aquatic organisms, the ambient water criteria for dimethyl phthalate and diethyl phthalate are determined to be 160 mg/l and 60 mg/l, respectively. The water quality criteria for dibutyl phthalate and di-2-ethylhexyl phthalate are determined to be 5 mg/l and 10 mg/l, respectively.

Basis for the Proposed Human Health Criteria: From the available information, the phthalic acid esters have not been found to be carcinogenic in animals or man. At high doses when injected i.p., the esters can act as teratogenic agents and possibly as mutagenic agents in rats. These esters also have an effect upon gonads in rats. Evidence is also on hand to show that the esters may bring about biochemical and pathological changes in the liver of rats when repeatedly administered orally or by i.p. When solubilized in blood components, DEHP has demonstrated liver involvement when these products have been repeatedly administered i.v. to monkeys. Inhalation studies in rats and man suggest that certain phthalates may be responsible for neurological disorders, but these results need further verification since other nonphthalate esters may also have been present leading to the problems.

Since a number of phthalate esters are in the environment or may be present in water, it was thought appropriate to review chronic toxicity data for those esters in which well established chronic toxicity data were reported to establish an allowable daily intake (ADI). In calculating the ADI, an uncertainty factor of 100 was used based upon a 70 kg person.

Table 77, taken from Shibko (53-6), lists eight esters in which the no effect dose was established from chronic toxicity studies in rats or dogs. The table also includes the number of days the animals were fed the specific phthalate esters and the calculated ADI. It will be noted that the ADI ranged from a low of 9.8 mg/day for dicyclohexyl phthalate to a high of 700 mg/day for dimethyl phthalate.

For the sake of establishing water quality criteria, it is assumed that on the average a person ingests 2 liters of water and 18.7 g of fish/day. The amount of water ingested is approximately 100 times greater than the amount of fish consumed. Since fish may biomagnify the esters to various degrees, a biomagnification factor (F) is used in the calculation. Biomagnification factors for dimethyl, diethyl, dibutyl and di-2-ethylhexyl esters were derived by the EPA ecological laboratories, Duluth.

Table 77: Calculated Allowable Daily Intake in Water and Fish for Various Phthalate Esters

Ester	No Effect Dose* (mg/kg/day)	Species	Days	ADI** (mg/day)	Biomagnification Factor (F)	Recommended Criteria (mg/l)
Dimethyl	1,000	rat	104	700.0	130	160
Diethyl	625	dog	52	438.0	270	60
Dibutyl	18	dog	52	12.6	26	5
Dicyclohexyl	14	dog	52	9.8	***	—
Methyl phthalyl ethyl glycolate	750	rat	104	525.0	***	—
Ethyl phthalyl ethyl glycolate	250	rat	104	175.0	***	—
Butyl phthalyl ethyl glycolate	140	dog	104	96.0	***	—
Di-2-ethylhexyl	60	dog	52	42.0	95	10

*From Shibko (53-6).
**Allowable Daily Intake for 70 kg person (100 safety factor).
***Not established.

Source: Reference (53-6)

Due to lack of data, bioconcentration factors could not be derived for dicyclohexyl, methyl phthalyl ethyl glycolate, ethyl phthalyl ethyl glycolate and butyl phthalyl ethyl glycolate. The equation for calculating an acceptable amount of ester in water based on ingestion of 2 liters of water and 18.7 g fish is: $2X + (0.0187 \times F)X = ADI$ where 2 is 2 liters of drinking water consumed; 0.0187 kg is the amount of fish consumed daily; F is biomagnification factor and ADI is the allowable daily intake (mg/day for 70 kg person). For example, consider that the ADI for dimethyl phthalate is 700 mg/day and the biomagnification factor is 130, the above equation can be solved as follows:

$$2X + (0.0187 \times 130)X = 700$$
$$2X + (2.43)X = 700$$
$$4.43X = 700$$
$$X = 158 \ (or \approx 160 \ mg/l)$$

Thus, the recommended water quality criterion is 160 mg/l. Similar calculations were made for each of the esters and are presented below.

Diethyl

$$2X + (0.0187 \times 270)X = 438$$
$$2X + 5.05X = 438$$
$$7.05X = 438$$
$$X = 62 \text{ mg/l (or } \approx 60 \text{ mg/l)}$$

Dibutyl

$$2X + (0.0187 \times 26)X = 12.6$$
$$2X + 0.486X = 12.6$$
$$2.486X = 12.6$$
$$X = 5.07 \text{ mg/l (or } \approx 5 \text{ mg/l)}$$

Di-2-ethylhexyl

$$2X + (0.0187 \times 95)X = 42$$
$$2X + 1.7765X = 42$$
$$3.7765X = 42$$
$$X = 11.12 \text{ mg/l (or } \approx 10 \text{ mg/l)}$$

Thus the recommended water quality criteria for four phthalate esters are: dimethyl, 160 mg/l; diethyl, 60 mg/l; dibutyl, 5 mg/l and di-2-ethylhexyl, 10 mg/l (see Table 77).

It seems clear that exposure from the water route presents no real risk to the population in regard to the phthalate esters. Reported levels of phthalate esters in U.S. surface waters have only been in the parts per billion range; at approximately 1 to 2 μg/l.

Other routes of exposure such as inhalation (industrial sites manufacturing the esters), dermal exposure, consumption of certain fatty or fatty-like foods and certain fish will be the major contributors to the body-load of phthalate esters. Phthalate ester residues in foods such as margarine, cheese and milk may, on some occasions, reach 50 ppm. Also a special group at risk will be patients to whom chronic transfusions of blood and blood products are administered.

Although it is recognized that routes of exposure other than water contribute more to the body burden of phthalate esters, this information will not be considered in forming ambient water quality criteria until additional analysis can be made. Therefore, the criteria presented assumed a risk estimate based only on ambient water exposure.

The need for more accurate residue content of foods, fish and water is still very apparent and, as more data become available, a reevaluation should be made as to the possible hazard to the population by the ingestion of phthalate esters.

In summary, based on the use of chronic toxicologic data and uncertainty factors of 100, the criteria levels for phthalate esters have been established. The percent contribution of drinking water and of ingesting contaminated fish is given in Table 78. Also given are the criteria levels recommended if exposure is assumed to be from fish and shellfish products alone.

Table 78: Contributions of Water and Fish to Phthalate Ester Criteria

Esters	Criteria Level (mg/l)	Contribution of Drinking Water (%)	Contribution of Fish Products (%)	Criteria if Exposure is from Fish Alone (mg/l)
Dimethyl	160	45	56	288
Diethyl	60	29	71	87
Dibutyl	5	81	19	26
Di-2-ethylhexyl	10	53	47	24

Source: Reference (53)

References

(53-1)   U.S. EPA "In-depth studies on health and environmental impacts of selected water pollutants"
         Report on Contract No. 68-01-4646, Washington, D.C. (1978).
(53-2)   Mayer, F.L. Jr., and Sanders, H.O. "Toxicology of phthalic acid esters in aquatic organisms"
         Environ. Health Perspect. 3, 153 (1973).
(53-3)   Johnson, B., et al "Dynamics of phthalic acid esters in aquatic organisms" in I.H. Suffet, ed.,
         Fate of pollutants in air and water environments, Part 2, New York, Wiley-Interscience Pub-
         lishers (1974).
(53-4)   Peakall, D. "Phthalate esters: Occurrence and biological effects", *Residue Rev. 54*, 1 (1975).
(53-5)   Tomita, L., et al, "Phthalic acid esters in various foodstuffs and biological materials," *Ecotoxi-
         cology and Environmental Safety 1*, 275 (1977).
(53-6)   Shibko, S., "Toxicology of phthalic acid esters" in *Environmental Quality and Food Supply* (1974).

POLYCHLORINATED BIPHENYLS (PCBs) (#54)

Polychlorinated biphenyls (PCBs) are the chlorinated derivatives of a class of aromatic organic compounds called biphenyls and are manufactured by the direct chlorination of the
biphenyl ring system. Typically, a PCB formula might be

Occurrence

PCBs have become widespread in the environment since the introduction of their commercial use in 1929. The magnitude of the dispersal of these chemicals is revealed by
their detection in the tissues of plants and animals in all parts of the world. PCB residues
have been observed in wildlife in Sweden, North America, Great Britain, the Netherlands,
and even the Arctic. Because PCBs are not naturally occurring substances, their dissemina-
tion is entirely the result of human activity. Their entry into the environment has occurred by vaporization into the atmosphere, and by spilling or dumping into water or onto
land.

It has been estimated that of the 1970 sales of PCBs in North America only 20% represented a net increase in the total amount in service. Estimated sources of loss for that
year were $1\text{-}2 \times 10^3$ tons for evaporation; $4\text{-}5 \times 10^3$ tons for leaks and disposal of fluids; and
22×10^3 tons from disposal by incineration and burial (54–1). The cumulative input to the
environment between 1930 and 1970 was estimated to be 3×10^4 tons to air, 6×10^4 tons to
fresh and coastal waters, and 3×10^5 tons to dumps and landfills.

In that time, up to $\frac{1}{3}$ of the PCBs released to air and $\frac{1}{2}$ of that released to water were
probably degraded. Degradation in landfills is more difficult to estimate (54–1). PCBs
have been found repeatedly to be widespread in analyses of human tissues. For example,
detectable levels of PCBs have been reported in adipose tissue samples of up to 91% of
individuals sampled in a survey of the United States population. This finding suggests
that environmental contamination may be a significant source of human exposure. Likely
routes of exposure for the general population are water and particularly food while inhalation and dermal contact are likely to be more significant routes in occupational exposure.

Physical Properties: The physical properties of individual chlorinated biphenyls are known
(54–2). Lower chlorinated Aroclors (1221, 1232, 1016, 1242, and 1248) are colorless
mobile oils. Increasing chlorine content results in mixtures taking on the consistency of
viscous liquids (Aroclor 1254) or sticky resins (Aroclors 1260 and 1262). Aroclors 1268

and 1270 are off-white or white powders. With the exception of Aroclors 1221 and 1268, Aroclors do not crystallize upon heating or cooling but at a specific temperature, defined as a pour point, change into a resinous state.

Solubilities of the individual chlorinated biphenyls in water have been studied by several workers and an inverse correlation between solubility and degree of chlorination has been reported. The problem in obtaining true solution equilibria data for PCBs in water has been explained by Schoor (54-3) who has given evidence that solutions of PCBs in water are in fact stable emulsions of PCB aggregates and that the true solubility of Aroclor 1254 is less than 0.1 μg/l in fresh water and 0.04 μg/l in marine water.

Chlorobiphenyls are freely soluble in relatively nonpolar organic solvents and lipids in biological systems. Metcalf, et al (54-4) have reported partition coefficients between octanol and water in the range of 10,000 to 20,000 for representative tri-, tetra-, and pentachlorobiphenyls. Partition coefficients with this biphasic solvent system have been found to correlate well with ecological magnification factors in aquatic organisms.

PCBs are strongly adsorbed on solid surfaces, including glass and metal surfaces in laboratory apparatus and soils, sediments, and particulates in the environment.

Chemical Properties: PCBs are considered to be inert to almost all of the typical chemical reactions. PCBs do not undergo oxidation, reduction, addition, elimination, or electrophilic substitution reactions except under extreme conditions. Chlorines can be replaced by reductive dechlorination with any metal hydride such as lithium aluminum hydride but temperatures of 245°C or greater are required to effect chlorine displacement.

The reactions of environmental importance that PCBs appear to undergo include alkali- and photochemically-catalyzed nucleophilic substitutions and photochemical free radical substitutions, all of which occur with alkali and water.

The creation of free radicals by sunlight allows the environmental replacement of chlorines by hydroxy groups from water without the intervention of alkali. When this occurs at the ortho position (found to be the most preferred for chlorine loss) the resulting 2-hydroxychlorobiphenyl is perfectly positioned to allow oxygen to bond to an ortho position of the other ring. This results in the creation of potentially the most important class of contaminant in commercial mixtures of PCBs, the chlorodibenzofurans (CDFs).

Uses: The commercial products are complex mixtures of chlorobiphenyls and are marketed for various uses according to the percentage of chlorine in the mixture. Currently there is no production of PCBs in the United States but the sole producer of PCBs in the United States previously marketed four mixtures containing 21, 41, 42 and 54% chlorine for use only in closed electrical systems under the trademark Aroclor. Prior to 1971 mixtures containing up to 68% chlorine were used in a number of other applications, including plasticizers, heat transfer fluids, hydraulic fluids, fluids in vacuum pumps and compressors, lubricants, and wax extenders.

In 1974 approximately 65 to 70% of domestic sales were to manufacturers of capacitors and the remainder to manufacturers of transformers while approximately 450,000 lb of PCBs were imported primarily for use in nonclosed systems. U.S. production appeared to be half of the world total.

As a result of the long life of many products containing PCBs, it is believed that a substantial portion of the PCBs manufactured before 1971 are still in service and thus represent potential pollution through possible future discharge into the environment.

Toxic Effects: PCBs have caused profound toxic effects in man and animals, particularly if repeated exposures occur. The skin and liver are major sites of pathology with the gastrointestinal tract and nervous systems also being targets. Polychlorodibenzofurans which contaminate commercial PCB mixtures may contribute significantly to their toxicity.

Several studies in rodents suggest strongly that some PCBs are carcinogenic and that they can enhance the carcinogenicity of other chemicals.

PCBs accumulate in the fatty tissues and skin of man and other mammals. Metabolism occurs by hydroxylation and dihydrodiol formation with arene oxides as probable intermediates. The rate of metabolism and excretion slows dramatically as the chlorination of the biphenyl nucleus increases. Arrangement of chlorines which eliminate adjacent unsubstituted carbons greatly increase resistance to metabolism.

Toxic materials other than chlorinated biphenyls have been found in commercial PCB mixtures. Vos, et al (54-5), Bowes, et al (54-6), Roach and Pomerantz (54-7), Nagayama, et al (54-8), and Kuratsume, et al (54-9) have detected polychlorinated dibenzofurans (PCDFs) in a number of domestic and foreign PCB mixtures at levels of 0.8 to 33 mg/kg. Polychlorinated naphthalenes (PCNs) have also been identified in small quantities.

There appear to be no authenticated reports of polychlorinated dibenzo-p-dioxins (PCDDs) in commercial PCBs (54-6). The presence of potentially toxic compounds other than polychlorinated biphenyls in commercial PCB mixtures complicates both analytical and toxicological evaluation of such mixtures.

Current Levels of Exposure: Human exposure to PCBs in the United States has been broad. Several studies of tissue and plasma levels of PCBs have detected them in a high percentage of randomly chosen subjects; one study detected PCBs in 31.1% of 637 human adipose tissue samples. The National Human Monitoring Program for Pesticides in fiscal years 1973 and 1974 found PCBs in 35.1 and 40.3% of adipose tissues tested.

A study of Canadian human adipose tissue PCB levels found 1 ppm or more in 30% of 172 samples. The eastern provinces, particularly Ontario, had the highest incidences. Average adipose tissue PCB levels were just below 1 mg/kg (ppm) with males having slightly higher accumulations than females. The same study found human breast milk to contain about 1 mg/kg on a fat basis. PCBs were detected in 8 of 40 samples of breast milk in Colorado at levels between 40 and 100 ppb (whole milk). A Japanese study found average levels in 400 milk samples of about 30 ppb. PCB levels in plasma in U.S. populations were detected in 43% of 723 samples. Levels in positive samples ranged from 1.5 to 29 ppb with a mean around 2 to 3 ppb. White populations had higher levels than black populations.

The median water levels of PCBs are around 0.1 to 0.3 μg/l in positive samples with 0 to 20% of samples being positive around the U.S. Average PCB intake in food was estimated in the mid-1970s to be about 9 μg/day with fish being the major dietary source. Ambient air concentrations are around 100 ng/m^3.

Special Groups at Risk: The preceding discussion of human exposure makes clear the fact that a high percentage of the U.S. population has been and is exposed to low levels of PCBs in food, water, and air. Those groups at particular risk for PCB exposure include industrial workers exposed in the workplace, individuals consuming large amounts of contaminated fish, such as sport fisherman, and nursing infants who, per kilogram body weight, may accumulate significant body burdens from the levels in human breast milk. With the cessation of manufacture of PCBs by Monsanto in 1977 and the great decline in its use which should result from the implementation of Section 6(e) of TSCA, industrial exposure should decline substantially. Since many PCB-containing sealed systems can be expected to remain in service for many years, continuing vigilance will be necessary to minimize accidental pollution of waterways or air and to prevent further occupational exposure.

Existing Guidelines and Standards: The Toxic Substances Control Act (TSCA) (P.L. 94-469) was signed into law October 11, 1976. Provisions in Section 6(e) of the law specifically regulate the manufacture, sale, distribution, and disposal of PCBs. Manufacture, sale or distribution of PCBs was restricted to sealed systems as of October 11, 1977. Manufacture was banned as of January 1, 1979 and all processing and distribution in commerce ceased on July 1, 1979. Allowance for certain exemptions is provided in the law. The proposed rules to implement the terms of Section 6(e) of TSCA were released June 7, 1978. Proposed rules on the disposal of PCBs were released February 17, 1978. The Environmental Protection Agency has proposed a water quality criterion for the protection of fresh water and marine life of 0.001 μg/l. The Food and Drug Administration established tolerance levels in foods in 1973 and proposed new tolerance levels further restricting levels in 1977. Both the current allowed levels and the proposed levels are presented in Table 79.

The occupational exposure limits adopted in 1968 are based on the recommendations of the American Conference of Governmental Industrial Hygienists (ACGIH) (1968). They set the time-weighted average 8 hr exposure limits to 1.0 mg/m^3 for mixtures containing 42% chlorine and 0.5 mg/m^3 for mixtures containing 54% chlorine. The newly recommended standard proposed by NIOSH (54-11) is 1.0 μg/m^3 air TWA over a 10 hr day and 40 hr work week.

Table 79: FDA Regulations for PCBs

. . . .(1) Temporary Tolerances . . . .

Commodity	PCB Concentration (ppm)	Proposed Guidelines 1977
Milk (fat basis)	2.5	1.5
Dairy products (fat basis)	2.5	1.5
Poultry (fat basis)	5.0	3.0
Eggs	0.5	0.3
Finished animal feed	0.2	0.2
Animal feed components	2.0	2.0
Fish (edible portion)	5.0	2.0
Infant and junior foods	0.2	pending
Paper food-packaging material without PCB-impermeable barrier	10.0*	–

. . . . (2) Use Prohibited in Food, Feed, Food Packaging Plants. . . . .

*Administrative guideline, pending hearing.

Source: References (54) and (54-10)

Summary of Proposed EPA Criteria: *Freshwater Aquatic Life* — For polychlorinated biphenyls the criterion to protect freshwater aquatic life as derived using the Guidelines is 0.0015 μg/l as a 24 hr average and the concentration should not exceed 6.2 μg/l at any time.

Saltwater Aquatic Life — For polychlorinated biphenyls the criterion to protect saltwater aquatic life as derived using the Guidelines is 0.024 μg/l as a 24 hr average and the concentration should not exceed 0.20 μg/l at any time.

Human Health — For the maximum protection of human health from the potential carcinogenic effects of exposure to PCBs through ingestion of water and contaminated aquatic organisms, the ambient water concentration is zero. Concentrations of PCBs estimated to result in additional lifetime cancer risks ranging from no additional risk to an additional risk of 1 to 100,000 are presented in the Criterion Formulation section of this document. The EPA is considering setting criteria at an interim target risk level in the range of 10^{-5}, 10^{-6}, or 10^{-7} with corresponding criteria of 0.26 ng/l, 0.026 ng/l and 0.0026 ng/l respectively.

Basis for the Proposed Human Health Criteria: An assessment of carcinogenic risk will be made by extrapolation from animal data using a linear (nonthreshold) model. The model used takes into account the bioaccumulation of PCBs in fish and shellfish. It is assumed that an average of 2 l/day of water are consumed along with 18.7 g of fish taken from a water source. Exposures from other food sources, air or occupational exposure are not included in the risk assessment.

Among the studies reviewed by this document, only one appears suitable for use in the cancer risk assessment. None of the mouse studies involved feeding for most or all of a lifetime and are, therefore, unsuitable. Of the rat studies, the only one involving long term exposure and adequate numbers of animals is the study in Sherman rats by Kimbrough, et al (54-12).

This study has some drawbacks in that it lacks any evidence of a dose-response (due to the use of only one dose level), it tests only one sex of the species, and only one commercial mixture of PCBs was tested. Yet the experimental design is a good one in many ways; the treatment was given over a good proportion of the lifespan, there was an appropriate route (food) and distribution of exposure (uniform dose over time), the authors provided good documentation of the actual intake dose, a sufficiently large number of experimental and control animals were used to detect a statistically significant increase in tumors and there was a thorough and well documented description of the pathology (hepatocellular carcinoma).

The NCI study (54-13) was the only other study involving a long term exposure and was suggestive of a carcinogenic effect, however, the lack of an adequate number of animals renders it unsuitable as a study upon which to base an estimate of carcinogenic risk.

Under the Consent Decree in NRDC vs Train, criteria are to state, "recommended maximum permissible concentrations (including where appropriate, zero) consistent with the protection of aquatic organisms, human health, and recreational activities." PCBs are suspected of being human carcinogens. Because there is no recognized safe concentration for a human carcinogen, the recommended concentration of PCBs in water for maximum protection of human health is zero.

Because attaining a zero concentration level may be infeasible in some cases and in order to assist the EPA and States in the possible future development of water quality regulations, the concentration of PCBs corresponding to several incremental lifetime cancer risk levels have been estimated. A cancer risk level provides an estimate of the additional incidence of cancer that may be expected in an exposed population. A risk of 10^{-5} for example, indicates a probability of one additional case of cancer for every 100,000 people exposed, a risk of 10^{-6} indicates one additional case of cancer for every million people exposed, and so forth.

In the *Federal Register* notice of availability of draft ambient water quality criteria, EPA stated that it is considering setting criteria at an interim target risk level of 10^{-5}, 10^{-6} or 10^{-7} as shown in Table 80.

Table 80: Possible Alternative Criteria for Polychlorinated Biphenyls

Exposure Assumptions (per day)	Risk Levels and Corresponding Criteria			
	0	10^{-7}	10^{-6}	10^{-5}
	. . . . .ng/l			
2 liters of drinking water and consumption of 18.7 grams fish and shellfish*	0	0.0026	0.026	0.26
Consumption of fish and shellfish only	0	0.0026	0.026	0.26

*Approximately 99.8% of the PCB exposure results from the consumption of aquatic organisms which exhibit an average bioconcentration potential of 46,000-fold. The remaining 0.2% of PCB exposure results from drinking water.

Source: Reference (54)

In Table 80, the risk levels and corresponding criteria are calculated by applying a modified one-hit extrapolation model described in *FR* 15926 (1979). Since the extrapolation model is linear at low doses, the additional lifetime risk is directly proportional to the water concentration. Therefore, water concentrations corresponding to other risk levels can be derived by multiplying or dividing one of the risk levels and corresponding water concentrations shown in the table by factors such as 10, 100, 1,000 and so forth.

Concentration levels were derived assuming a lifetime exposure to various amounts of PCBs, occurring from the consumption of both drinking water and aquatic life grown in waters containing the corresponding PCB concentrations and, occurring solely from consumption of aquatic life grown in the waters containing the corresponding PCB concentrations. Although total exposure information for PCBs is discussed and an estimate of the contribution from other sources of exposure can be made, this data will not be factored into ambient water quality criteria formulation until additional analysis can be made. The criteria presented, therefore, assume an incremental risk from ambient water exposure only.

The very low limits suggested by this risk estimate are due in large part to the very large bioaccumulation factor in fish (46,000). This figure is an average for a wide variety of saltwater and freshwater organisms.

As possible strategies to reduce human exposures to PCBs are considered, the relative contributions of ingested water and fish should be kept in mind. At the assumed consumption rate of 2 liters of drinking water and 18.7 g of fish per day, over 99% of the dietary PCBs will be obtained from fish. Strategies which focus separately on the reduction of PCB levels in water and fish for consumption might be more practical and productive than a single standard for water which takes bioaccumulation in fish into account.

A final comment about the risk level derived from this study is that it is based on animal data which are statistically weak. The weight of evidence indicates that PCBs are carcinogenic in rodents. However, the carcinogenic activities of these compounds are not great. An acceptable noncarcinogenic level could be established with greater certainty if better quantitative data on carcinogenicity were available. Studies with larger numbers of animals designed to measure relatively small effects are needed. Also, the rats appear to be much less sensitive to the acute and subacute effects of PCBs than man or nonhuman primates. Further investigation of the effects of PCBs in rhesus monkeys, particularly with reference to the gastric lesions produced, would be useful.

Summary of Pertinent Data — The water quality criterion for PCBs is derived from the hepatocellular carcinoma and neoplastic nodule response of Sherman strain female rats fed 100 ppm Aroclor 1260 (54–12). A time-weighted average dose of 88.4 ppm was administered for approximately 21.5 months and the animals were observed for an additional six weeks before terminal sacrifice. The incidence of hepatocellular carcinoma and neoplastic nodules was 170/184 in the treated group and 1/173 in the control group. Assuming a fish bioaccumulation factor of 46,000, the criterion is calculated from the following parameters: n_t is 170, N_t is 184, n_c is 1, N_c is 173, Le is 730 days, le is 645 days, d is 88.4 x 0.05 = 4.42 mg/kg/day, w is 0.4 kg, L is 730 days, R is 46,000 and F is 0.0187 kg/day.

Based on these parameters, the one-hit slope B_H is 3.25 $(mg/kg/day)^{-1}$. The resulting water concentration of PCBs calculated to keep the individual lifetime cancer risk below 10^{-5} is 0.26 ng/l.

References

(54-1)   Nisbet, L.C. and Sarofim, A.F., "Rates and routes of transport of PCBs in the environment," *Envir. Health Perspect. 1*, 21 (1972).

(54-2)   Cook, J.W. "Some chemical aspects of polychlorinated biphenyls (PCBs)" *Environ. Health Perspect. 1*, 1 (1972).

(54-3)   Schoor, W.P. "Problems associated with low-solubility compounds in aquatic toxicity tests: theoretical model and solubility characteristics of Aroclor 1254 in water" *Water Res. 9*, 937 (1975).

(54-4)   Metcalf, R.L., et al, "Laboratory model ecosystem studies of the degradation and fate of radiolabeled
          tri, tetra-, and pentachlorobiphenyl compared with DDE," *Arch. Environ. Contam. Toxicol. 3*, 151
          (1975).

(54-5)   Vos, J.G.,and Koeman, J.H., "Comparative toxicologic study with polychlorinated biphenyls in
          chickens with special reference to porphyria, edema formation, liver necrosis, and tissue residues,"
          Toxicol. Appl. Pharm. 17, 656 (1970).

(54-6)   Bowes, G.W., et al, "Identification of chlorinated dibenzofurans in American polychlorinated bi-
          phenyls", *Nature 256*, 305 (1975).

(54-7)   Roach, J.A.G. and Pomerantz, I.H., "The finding of chlorinated dibenzofurans in a Japanese poly-
          chlorinated biphenyl sample," *Bull. Environ. Contam. Toxicol. 12*, 338 (1974).

(54-8)   Nagayama, J,, et al, "Determination of chlorinated dibenzofurans in Kanechlors and 'Yusho Oil',"
          Bull. Environ. Contam. Toxicol. 15, 9 (1976).

(54-9)   Kuratsume, M. et al, "Some of the recent findings concerning Yusho," *Proc. Nat. Conf. on Poly-
          chlorinated Biphenyls*, Chicago, Ill. (Nov. 19–21, 1975), reported in EPA Report 560/6–75–004,
          Washington, D.C., U.S. Envir. Protect. Agency (1976).

(54-10)   Jelinek, C.F. and Corneliussen, P.E., *Levels of PCBs in the U.S. Food Supply* in EPA Report 560/
          6–75–004, Washington, D.C., U.S. Envir. Protect. Agency (1976).

(54-11)   Nat. Inst. for Occup. Safety and Health, *Criteria for a Recommended Standard: Occupational Ex-
          posure to PCBs*, NIOSH Doc. No. 77–225 (1977).

(54-12)   Kimbrough, R.D., et al, "Induction of liver tumors in Sherman strain female rats by polychlorinated
          biphenyl Aroclor 1260, *Jour. Natl. Cancer Inst. 55*, 1453 (1975).

(54-13)   National Cancer Institute, *Bioassay of Aroclor 1254 for possible carcinogenicity*, Carcinogenesis
          Technical Report Series No. 38, DHEW Publ. No. (NIH) 78–838, Washington, D.C. (1978).

POLYNUCLEAR AROMATIC HYDROCARBONS (PAH)(#55)

Polynuclear aromatic hydrocarbons (PAH) are a diverse class of compounds consisting of substituted and unsubstituted polycyclic and heterocyclic aromatic rings.

Among these PAH are compounds such as benzo[a] pyrene and benzo[a] anthracene, which are
well-known for their ubiquitous presence in nature and carcinogenic effects in experimental
animals.

Other polynuclear aromatics among the 65 categories of priority pollutants which are discussed in separate sections in this volume are as follows:

> Acenaphthene (1)
> Fluoranthene (36)
> Naphthalene (46)

The polynuclear aromatic hydrocarbons specifically listed in the expansion of the original
65 priority pollutants and classes of pollutants to 129 specific chemical entities were as
follows:

> Acenaphthylene
> Anthracene
> Benzo[a] anthracene (1,2-benzanthracene)
> 3,4-Benzofluoranthene
> Benzo[k] fluoranthene (11,12-benzofluoranthene)
> Benzo[ghi] perylene (1,12-benzoperylene)
> Benzo[a] pyrene (3,4-benzopyrene)
> Chrysene
> Dibenzo[ah] anthracene (1,2,5,6-benzanthracene)
> Fluorene
> Indeno[1,2,3-cd] pyrene
> Phenanthrene
> Pyrene

A variety of abbreviations are in common use for the polynuclear aromatics and they are
listed in Table 81 as a guide to the text which follows.

Table 81: Some Abbreviations for Polynuclear Aromatics

Abbreviation	Compound Designated
A	Anthracene
BaA	Benzo[a]anthracene (1,2-benzanthracene)
BaP (also BP)	Benzo[a]pyrene (3,4-benzopyrene)
BbFL (also BbF)	Benzo[b]fluoranthene
BeP	Benzo[e]pyrene
BjFL (also BjF)	Benzo[j]fluoranthene
BkFL (also BkF)	Benzo[k]fluoranthene (11,12-benzofluoranthene)
BPR	Benzo[ghi]perylene (1,12-benzoperylene)
CH (also CR)	Chrysene
DBA	Dibenzo[a,h]anthracene (1,2,5,6-benzanthracene)
F	Fluorene
FL (also F)	Fluoranthene
IP	Indeno[1,2,3-cd]pyrene
P	Pyrene
PA (also Phen)	Phenanthrene
PR (also Per)	Perylene

Note: These abbreviations are not endorsed by any body such as the
International Union of Chemistry; rather they are a form of
shorthand used by authors for convenience, and they vary
with the author.

Occurrence: PAH are formed as a result of incomplete combustion of organic compounds
with insufficient oxygen. This leads to the formation of C–H free radicals which can polymerize to form various PAH which are also referred to as PNAs.

PNAs can be formed in any hydrocarbon combustion process and may be released from oil
spills. The less efficient the combustion process, the higher the PNA emission factor is
likely to be. The major sources are stationary sources, such as heat and power generation,
refuse burning, industrial activity, such as coke ovens, and coal refuse heaps. While PNAs
can be formed naturally (lightning-ignited forest fires), impact of these sources appears to
be minimal. It should be noted, however, that while transportation sources account for
only about 1% of emitted PNAs on a national inventory basis, transportation-generated
PNAs may approach 50% of the urban resident exposures.

Because of the large number of sources, most people are exposed to very low levels of
PNAs. BaP has been detected in a variety of foods throughout the world. A possible
source is mineral oils and petroleum waxes used in food containers and as release agents
for food containers. FDA studies have indicated no health hazard from these sources.

Physical Properties: Benzo[a]pyrene, $C_{20}H_{12}$, is a yellowish crystalline solid, melting at
179°C. It consists of five benzene rings joined together.

Chemical Properties: The polynuclear aromatic hydrocarbons generally exhibit the properties characteristic of simpler aromatic hydrocarbons, e.g., oxidation to quinones and carboxylic acids. They are in general quite stable, however, and resistant to environmental
degradation.

Uses: The polynuclear aromatics have uses only in the case of the simpler molecules.
Thus, naphthalene (46), the simplest polynuclear aromatic, has the most uses.

Going from 2-ring condensed aromatics to 2-ring compounds with external methylene
bridges, one encounters acenaphthene (1) with a few uses as an intermediate in dyestuff,
plastics and pesticide manufacture. Fluorene, another methylene-bridged 2-ring aromatic,
has few uses.

Then going to 3-ring compounds, anthracene is the first polynuclear aromatic encountered.
Phenanthrene, an isomer of anthracene, is another. These have limited uses as chemical
intermediates.

When one goes to 4-ring condensed aromatics (chrysene, pyrene, benzanthracene) and on to 5-ring compounds (dibenzanthracene, benzopyrene, perylene) and to higher compounds yet, one finds no uses.

Toxic Effects: Under the Consent Decree in NRDC vs Train maximum permissible concentrations are to be recommended for the following PAH: benzopyrene, benzanthracene, chrysenes, benzofluoranthrenes, and indenopyrenes.

There are no published studies available which adequately compare the carcinogenic activities of all ten of the specified PAH under similar experimental conditions. Likewise, there are no data available concerning human responses to individual compounds in the PAH class, since environmental exposures to PAH invariably involve contact with complex, and usually undefined, PAH mixtures.

Certain PNAs which have been demonstrated as carcinogenic in test animals at relatively high exposure levels are being found in urban air at very low levels. Various environmental fate tests suggest that PNAs are photo-oxidized, and react with oxidants and oxides of sulfur. Because PNAs are adsorbed on particulate matter, chemical half-lives may vary greatly, from a matter of a few hours to several days. One researcher reports that photo-oxidized PNA fractions of air extracts also appear to be carcinogenic. Environmental behavior/fate data have not been developed for the class as a whole.

It has been observed that PNAs are highly soluble in adipose tissue and lipids. Most of the PNAs taken in by mammals are oxidized and the metabolites excreted. Effects of that portion remaining in the body at low levels have not been documented.

Benzo[a]pyrene (BaP), one of the most commonly found and hazardous of the PNAs has been the subject of a variety of toxicological tests, which have been summarized by the International Agency for Research on Cancer. 50 to 100 ppm administered in the diet for 122 to 197 days produced stomach tumors in 70% of the mice studied. 250 ppm produced tumors in the forestomach of 100% of the mice after 30 days. A single oral administration of 100 mg to nine rats produced mammary tumors in eight of them. Skin cancers have been induced in a variety of animals at very low levels, and using a variety of solvents (length of application was not specified).

Long cancer developed in 2 of 21 rats exposed to 10 mg/m^3 BaP and 3.5 ppm SO_2 for 1 hr/day, five days a week, for more than one year. Five of 21 rats receiving 10 ppm SO_2 for 6 hr/day, in addition to the foregoing dosage, developed similar carcinomas. No carcinomas were noted in rats receiving only SO_2. No animals were exposed only to BaP. Transplacental migration of BaP has been demonstrated in mice. Most other PNAs have not been subjected to such testing.

Current Levels of Exposure: The Criteria Document (55) presents considerable data which may be used to calculate an estimate of human exposure to PAH by all routes of entry to the body. However, quantitative estimates of human exposure to PAH require numerous assumptions concerning principal routes of exposure, extent of absorption, conformity of human lifestyle, and lack of geographic-, sex-, and age-specific variables. Nevertheless, by working with estimates developed for PAH as a class, it is possible through certain extrapolations to arrive at an admittedly crude estimate of PAH exposure.

Unfortunately, there are no environmental monitoring data available for most of the PAH which are specified under the Consent Decree in NRDC vs Train. By far the most widely monitored PAH in the environment is BaP; data on BaP levels in food, air and water are often used as a measure of total PAH. Among the PAH routinely monitored in water, four compounds are included in the Consent Decree list: BaP, IP, BbFL and BjFL. In addition, levels of FL and BPR have been routinely determined in water, as recommended by the World Health Organization.

The reported estimated average concentrations of BaP, carcinogenic PAH (BaP, BjFL, and IP), and total PAH in drinking water are 0.55 ng/l, 2.1 ng/l, and 13.5 ng/l, respectively.

Thus, assuming that a human consumes 2 liters of water per day, the daily intake of PAH via drinking water would be: 0.55 ng/l x 2 l/day = 1.1 ng/day (BaP); 2.1 ng/l x 2 l/day = 4.2 ng/day (carcinogenic PAH); and 13.5 ng/l x 2 l/day = 27.0 ng/day (total PAH).

It has been estimated that the daily dietary intake of PAH is about 8 to 11 μg/day. As a check on this estimate, PAH intake may be calculated based on reported concentrations in various foods and the per capita estimates of food consumption by the International Commission on Radiological Protection. Taking a range of 1.0 to 10.0 ppb as a typical concentration for PAH in various foods, and 1,600 g/day as the total daily food consumption by man from all types of foods (i.e., fruits, vegetables, cereals, dairy products, etc.), the intake of PAH from the diet would be in the range of 1.6 to 16.0 μg/day. An estimate of BaP ingestion from the diet may be similarly derived. Using 0.1 to 1.0 ppb as the range of BaP concentration in varous foods, total daily BaP intake would be .16 to 1.6 μg/day.

Ambient air is reported to contain average levels of 0.5 ng/m^3, 2.0 ng/m^3, and 10.9 ng/m^3 for BaP, carcinogenic PAH, and total PAH, respectively. Taking the range of 15 to 23 m^3 as the average amount of air inhaled by a human each day results in an estimated intake of 0.008 to 0.0115 μg/day, 0.03 to 0.046 μg/day, and 0.164 to 0.251 μg/day for BaP, carcinogenic PAH, and total PAH, respectively. In summary, a crude estimate of total daily exposure to PAH would be as shown in Table 82.

Two important factors are not taken into account in this estimate. First, it is known that tobacco smoking can contribute greatly to PAH exposure in man. Exposure to BaP from smoking one pack of cigarettes per day was shown to be 0.4 μg/day (55-1). Second, the possibility for dermal absorption of PAH is assumed to contribute only a negligible amount to the total exposure. Only in certain occupational situations is dermal exposure expected to be quantitatively important.

Table 82: Estimate of Human Exposure to PAH from Various Media

Source	BaP	Carcinogenic PAH*	Total PAH
	. . . . .μg/day		
Water	0.0011	0.0042	0.027
Food	0.16-1.6	-	1.6-16.0
Air	0.008-0.0115	0.03-0.046	0.164-0.251
Total	0.169-1.6	-	1.8-16.3

*Total of BaP, BjFl and IP; no data are available for food.

Special Groups at Risk: An area of considerable uncertainty with regard to the carcinogenic hazard of PAH to man involves the relationship between aryl hydrocarbon hydroxylase (AHH) activity and cancer risk. Genetic variation in AHH inducibility has been implicated as a determining factor for susceptibility to lung and laryngeal cancer (55-2,55-3). It was suggested that the extent of AHH inducibility in lymphocytes was correlated with increasing susceptibility to lung cancer formation.

One must consider the total exposure of all environmental agents and their possible effect on critical enzymatic processes before attempting to assess the toxicologic impact of exposure to a specific PAH. There is a need to further explore the relative effects of enzyme induction on the metabolic activation of chemicals to toxic products, versus metabolism of chemicals via detoxification pathways, when considering the possibility of special groups at risk.

Existing Guidelines and Standards: There have been few attempts to develop exposure standards for PAHs, either individually or as a class. In the occupational setting, a Federal standard has been promulgated for coke oven emissions, based primarily on the presumed effects of the carcinogenic PAH contained in the mixture as measured by the benzene soluble fraction of total particulate matter. Similarly, the American Conference of Governmental Industrial Hygienists recommends a workplace exposure limit for coal tar pitch volatiles, based on the benzene-soluble fraction containing carcinogenic PAH. The National Institute for Occupational Safety and Haalth has also recommended a workplace standard for coal tar products (coal tar, creosote, and coal tar pitch), based on measurements of the cyclohexane extractable fraction. These standards are summarized below:

Substance	Exposure Limit	Agency
Coke oven emissions	150 $\mu g/m^3$, 8 hr time-weighted average	U.S. Occupational Safety and Health Administration (55-4)
Coal tar products	0.1 mg/m^3, 10 hr time-weighted average	U.S. National Institute for Occupational Safety and Health (55-5)
Coal tar pitch and volatiles	0.2 mg/m^3 (benzene soluble fraction) 8 hr time-weighted average	American Conference of Governmental Industrial Hygienists (55-6)

A drinking water standard for PAH as a class has been developed. The 1970 World Health Organization European Standards for Drinking Water recommends a concentration of PAH not to exceed 0.2 $\mu g/l$. This recommended standard is based on the composite analysis of six PAH in drinking water:

(1) Fluoranthene,
(2) Benzo[a] pyrene,
(3) Benzo[g,h,i] perylene,
(4) Benzo[b] fluoranthene,
(5) Benzo[k] fluoranthene, and
(6) Indeno[1,2,3-cd] pyrene.

The designation of these six PAH for analytical monitoring of drinking water was not made on the basis of potential health effects or bioassay data on these compounds (Borneff and Kunte, 1969). Thus, it should not be assumed that these six compounds have special significance in determining the likelihood of adverse health effects resulting from absorption of any particular PAH. They are, instead, considered to be useful indicators for the presence of PAH pollutants. Borneff and Kunte (55-7) found that PAH were present in ground water at concentrations up to 50 ng/l, and in drinking water at concentrations up to 100 ng/l. Based on these data they suggested that water containing more than 200 ng/l should be rejected. However, as data from a number of U.S. cities indicate, levels of PAH in raw and finished waters are typically much less than the 0.2 $\mu g/l$ criterion. As an aid to standard setting, EPA has published two reports on polycyclic aromatics (55-8, 55-9).

Summary of Proposed EPA Criteria: *Freshwater Aquatic Life* — For freshwater aquatic life, no criterion for any polynuclear aromatic hydrocarbon can be derived using the Guidelines, and there are insufficient data to estimate a criterion using other procedures.

Saltwater Aquatic Life — For saltwater aquatic life, no criterion for any polynuclear aromatic hydrocarbon can be derived using the Guidelines, and there are insufficient data to estimate a criterion using other procedures.

Human Health — For the maximum protection of human health from the potential carcinogenic effects of exposure to polynuclear aromatic hydrocarbons (PAH) through ingestion of water and contaminated aquatic organisms, the ambient water concentration is zero. Concentrations of PAH estimated to result in additional lifetime cancer risks ranging from no additional risk to an additional risk of 1 in 100,000 are presented in the Criterion document. The EPA is considering setting criteria at an interim target risk level in the range of 10^{-5}, 10^{-6}, or 10^{-7} with corresponding criteria of 9.7 ng/l, 0.97 ng/l and 0.097 ng/l, respectively.

Basis for the Proposed Human Health Criteria: The presently available data base is inadequate to support the derivation of individual criteria for each of the PAH as specified under the Consent Decree. This problem arises primarily from the diversity of test systems and bioassay conditions employed for determining carcinogenic potential of individual PAH in experimental animals. Furthermore, it is not possible to estimate the intake via water of individual PAH except for those compounds which have been selected by the World Health

Organization for environmental monitoring. Therefore, an approach to criterion development is adopted in this report with the objective of deriving a single criterion to encompass the entire PAH class. This approach is attractive in that it recognizes the fact that environmental exposure to PAH invariably occurs by contact with complex undefined PAH mixtures.

The attempt to develop a drinking water criterion for PAH as a class is hindered by several gaps in the scientific data base:

(1) The PAH class is composed of numerous compounds having diverse biological effects and varying carcinogenic potential. A representative PAH mixture has not been defined.

(2) The common practice of using data derived from studies with BaP to make generalizations concerning the effects of environmental PAH may not be scientifically sound.

(3) No chronic animal toxicity studies exist involving oral exposure to PAH mixtures.

(4) No direct human data exist concerning the effects of exposure to defined PAH mixtures.

However, assuming that the development of a criterion must proceed despite these obstacles certain approaches may be taken to circumvent deficiencies in the data base. The choice of an appropriate animal bioassay from which to derive data for application to the linear nonthreshold model for human cancer risk assessment should be guided by several considerations. Primary emphasis must be placed on appropriate animal studies which include sufficient numbers of animals for statistically reliable results; involve long-term low-level exposures to PAH; include a proper control group; and achieve positive dose-related carcinogenic response.

Because there are no studies available regarding chronic oral exposure to PAH mixtures, it is necessary to derive a criterion based upon data involving exposure to a single compound. Even when considering single chemicals, almost no studies are available which involved oral exposure at more than one dose level to a reasonable number of animals. Two studies have been selected, one involving BaP ingestion (55-10) and one involving DBA ingestion (55-11). Both compounds are recognized as animal carcinogens, and both are known to be environmental contaminants to which humans are exposed.

In the strictest sense it can be argued that a criterion for a chemical class derived from experiments involving a single component of that class is invalid. On the other hand, selection of those components (e.g., BaP and DBA) which are among the more potent carcinogens in the PAH class should lead to a conservative criterion approach. It must be assumed that interactions among the various PAH components resulting in either an enhancement or inhibition of biological effect will cancel each other out in the environment. Presently, there is no way to quantitate the potential human health risks incurred by the interaction of PAH, either among themselves or with other agents (e.g., tumor initiators, promoters, or inhibitors) in the environment.

In addition, it is known that PAH commonly produce tumors at the site of contact (i.e., forestomach tumors by oral exposure to BaP; lung tumors by intratracheal administration, or skin tumors by dermal application). Thus, consideration of the extent of absorption may not always be necessary in the case of carcinogenic PAH, and will in fact result in underestimation of actual risk if only distant target sites are considered. Calculations of water quality criteria for PAH based upon bioassay data for BaP and DBA are presented in the summary of pertinent data.

The water quality criteria for BaP and DBA derived using the linear nonthreshold model as described in Chapter One are 27.5 ng/l and 43 ng/l, respectively. For the sake of comparison, a water quality criterion for DBA was calculated using the procedure developed by Mantel and Bryan (55-12). As opposed to the linear nonthreshold model, which is logistic and defines acceptable risk as 1/100,000, the Mantel and Bryan model is probabilistic and defines acceptable risk as 1/100,000,000. Furthermore, the Mantel and Bryan approach is concerned with the maximum tumor incidence in treated animals in the 99% assurance level. Using the Mantel and Bryan approach with DBA, the resultant water quality criterion is 13.3 ng/l.

Under the Consent Decree in NRDC vs Train, criteria are to state, "recommended maximum permissible concentrations (including where appropriate, zero) consistent with the protection of aquatic organisms, human health, and recreational activities." BaP and DBA are known animal carcinogens. Because there is no recognized safe concentration for a human carcinogen, the recommended concentration in water for maximum protection of human health is zero.

Because attaining a zero concentration level may be infeasible in some cases and in order to assist the EPA and States in the possible future development of water quality regulations, the concentrations of BaP and DBA corresponding to several incremental lifetime cancer risk levels have been estimated. A cancer risk level provides an estimate of the additional incidence of cancer that may be expected in an exposed population. A risk of 10^{-5}, for example, indicates a probability of one additional case of cancer for every 100,000 people exposed, a risk of 10^{-6} indicates one additional case of cancer for every million people exposed, and so forth.

PAH are widely distributed in the environment as evidenced by their detection in sediments, soils, air, surface waters, and plant and animal tissues. The ecological impact of these chemicals, however, is uncertain. Numerous studies show that despite their high lipid solubility, PAHs show little tendency for bioaccumulation in the fatty tissues of animals or man. This observation is not unexpected, in light of convincing evidence to show that PAH are rapidly and extensively metabolized.

Lu, et al (55-13) have published the only available study regarding the bioconcentration and biomagnification of a PAH in model ecosystem environments. They reported that the bioconcentration of BaP, expressed as concentration in mosquitofish/concentration in water was zero. This was apparently due to the fact that the fish metabolized the BaP about as rapidly as it was absorbed. On the other hand, in a 33 day terrestrial-aquatic model ecosystem study, BaP showed a small degree of biomagnification which probably resulted from food chain transfer.

In this case the biomagnification factor for mosquitofish was 30. Based on the results of Lu, et al (55-13) a bioconcentration (BCF) factor of 30 was employed for the purpose of calculating a water quality criterion. In contrast, as can be noted in the criterion document, the Cancer Assessment Group applied the BCF of 6,800, a value derived from octanol-water partition coefficients, in its calculation of the water quality criterion for PAH.

In the *Federal Register* notice of availability of draft ambient water quality criteria, EPA stated that it is considering setting criteria for BaP and DBA at an interim target risk level of 10^{-5}, 10^{-6} or 10^{-7} as shown in Table 83.

Summary of Pertinent Data — The water quality criterion for PAH is based on the experiment reported by Neal and Rigdon (55-10) in which benzo[a]pyrene at doses ranging between 1 and 250 ppm in the diet was fed to strain CFW mice for approximately 110 days. Stomach tumors, which were mostly squamous cell papillomas but some carcinomas, appeared with an incidence statistically higher than controls at doses of 45 ppm and above. At 45 ppm the incidence in controls and treated groups was 0/289 and 4/40, respectively. The one-hit model has the following parameters: $n_t = 4$, $N_t = 40$, $n_c = 0$, $N_c = 289$, Le = 110 days, le = 110 days, d = 45 ppm x 0.13 = 5.85 mg/kg/day, w = 0.034 kg, L = 78 weeks x 7 days/wk = 546 days, R = 30 and F = 0.0187 kg/day.

With these values, the one-hit slope parameter is $B_H = 28.020$ $(mg/kg/day)^{-1}$. The result is that the water concentration of BaP should be less than 9.7 ng/l in order to keep the individual lifetime risk below 10^{-5}. On the conservative assumption that all carcinogenic PAH compounds are as potent as BaP, that the effect of a mixture of carcinogenic PAH compounds depends on the sum of their concentrations, and that the noncarcinogenic PAH compounds have no effect on the response of the carcinogenic PAH, it follows that the sum of the concentrations of all carcinogenic PAH compounds should be less than 9.7 ng/l in order to keep the lifetime risk less than 10^{-5}.

Table 83: Possible Alternative Criteria for Polynuclear Aromatics

Exposure Assumptions (per day)	Risk Levels and Corresponding Criteria			
	0	10^{-7}	10^{-6}	10^{-5}
	. . . . (ng/l)			
Benzo[a]pyrene (BaP)				
2 liters of drinking water and consumption of 18.7 grams fish and shellfish	0	0.097	0.97	9.7
Consumption of fish and shellfish only	0	0.44	4.45	44.46
Dibenzo[a,h]anthracene (DBA)				
2 liters of drinking water and consumption of 18.7 grams fish and shellfish	0	0.043	0.43	4.30
Consumption of fish and shellfish only	0	0.196	1.96	19.63

Source: Reference (55)

References

(55-1)   National Academy of Sciences, *Biological Effects of Atmospheric Pollutants: Particulate Polyclic Organic Matter*, Washington, D.C. (1972).

(55-2)   Kellerman, G., et al, "Aryl hydroxylase inducibility and bronchogenic carcinoma," *New England Jour. Med. 289*, 934 (1973).

(55-3)   Kellerman, G., et al, "Genetic variation of aryl hydrocarbon hydroxylase in human lymphocytes," *Am. Jour. Hum. Genet. 25*, 327 (A73).

(55-4)   National Inst. for Occup. Safety and Health, *Criteria for a Recommended Standard: Occupational Exposure to Coke Oven Emissions*, NIOSH Doc. No. 73-11016 (1973).

(55-5)   National Inst. for Occup. Safety and Health, *Criteria for a Recommended Standard: Occupational Exposure to Coal Tar Products*, NIOSH Doc. No. 78-107 (Sept. 1977).

(55-6)   Am. Conf. of Govt. Ind. Hygienists, *Threshold Limit Values for Chemical Substances in Workroom Air*, Cincinnati, Ohio (1979).

(55-7)   Borneff, J. and Kunte, H. "Carcinogenic substances in water and soil, XXVI, a routine method for the determination of PAH in water," *Arch. Hyg. (Berl) 153*, 220 (1969).

(55-8)   U.S. Environmental Protection Agency, *Scientific and Technical Assessment Report on Particulate Polycyclic Organic Matter (PPOM)*, Publ. No. EPA-600/6-75-001, Washington, D.C. (1975).

(55-9)   Santodonato, J, et al, *Health Assessment Document for Polycyclic Organic Matter*, Washington, D.C., U.S. Environmental Protection Agency (1978).

(55-10)   Rigdon, R.H. and Neal, J., "Effects of feeding benzo[a]pyrene on fertility, embryos and young mice," *Jour. Nat. Cancer Inst. 34*, 297 (1965).

(55-11)   Snell, K.C. and Stewart, H.L., "Induction of pulmonary adenomatosis in DBA/Z mice by the oral administration of dibenz[a,h]anthracene", *Acta Un. Int. Canc. 19*, 692 (1962).

(55-12)   Mantel, N. and Bryan, R.W., "Safety testing of carcinogenic agents," *Jour. Nat. Cancer Inst. 27*, 455 (1961).

(55-13)   Lu, P.Y., et al, "The environmental fate of three carcinogens:benzo[a]pyrene, benzidine and vinyl chloride evaluated in laboratory model ecosystems," *Arch. Environ. Contam. Toxicol. 6*, 129 (1977).

PYRENE

See "Polynuclear Aromatic Hydrocarbons" (55).

S

SELENIUM (#56)

Selenium, symbol Se, is an element in group VI-A of the Periodic Table. It has an atomic number of 34 and an atomic weight of 78.96.

Occurrence: Selenium is a naturally occurring element. The major source of selenium in the environment is the weathering of rocks and soils (56-1), but human activities contribute about 3,500 metric tons per year (56-2).

Physical Properties: Solubilities of selenium compounds in water range from very high (e.g., greater than 40% by weight for sodium selenate) to very low (e.g., 16,000 to 33,000 μg/l for the silver selenates). Heavy metal selenides are very insoluble (56-3).

Chemical Properties: Selenium reacts with metals to form ionic selenides with a valence of -2 and with most other chemicals to form covalent compounds. It may assume any of several valence states ranging from -2 to $+6$. Depending on its oxidation state, selenium may act as either an oxidizing agent or a reducing agent (56-3). Inorganic selenium may be converted to organic forms by biological action. Biological systems may also convert nonvolatile selenium compounds to volatile ones which might escape to air (56-4).

Uses: Selenium is used in photocopying, the manufacture of glass, electronic devices, pigments, dyes and insecticides. It is also used in veterinary medicine and antidandruff shampoos.

Toxic Effects: Selenium is acutely toxic to aquatic invertebrates and to fishes. Normal human selenium intake has been estimated at 50 to 150 μg per day (56-5). While selenium is an essential nutrient for humans and other species (56-6) it is toxic in excessive amounts (56-1, 56-7). Selenium poisoning produces symptoms in man similar to those of arsenic (56-8, 56-9). It has been shown to produce tumors in animals (56-10, 56-11) and is among the list of cancer-producing agents prohibited by the Delaney Clause (56-6).

Current Levels of Exposure: It is estimated that the average adult intake of selenium is roughly 130 to 150 μg of selenium each day from food. However, it is well known that the level of selenium in food is very dependent on the amounts in the soil and water where the food is grown or in the feeds that the livestock eat. The range of levels for specific vegetables grown in nonseleniferous versus seleniferous areas are: potato (0.005 to 0.940 μg/gram), tomato (0.005 to 1.22 μg/gram), carrots (0.022 to 1.30 μg/gram), cabbage (0.022 to 4.52 μg/gram), and onion (0.015 to 17.8 μg/gram). Hence, persons living in areas where the selenium content of the soils is high will likely be exposed to daily dietary levels above 150 μg. It has been estimated that an average 6-month-old infant consumes 28 μg of selenium per day from food.

Levels of air selenium in municipalities and communities range from 0.0025 μg/m^3 to 0.0097 μg/m^3. Assuming average total daily inhaled volumes of 21.2, 11.1, and 1.4 m^3 for men, women and infants (0 to 11 weeks of age), the estimated ranges of daily selenium exposures from ambient air are 0.053 to 0.206 μg, 0.028 to 0.108 μg, 0.004 to 0.014 μg, respectively; estimated volumes of inhaled air are based on time-weighted averages of volumes and respiratory frequencies. Clearly, selenium in ambient air does not contribute significantly to the overall selenium exposure level of the general population. Levels of exposure from use of selenium based shampoos are unknown.

Special Groups at Risk: Since selenium toxicity depends on levels of nutrition and exposure to other synergistic and antagonistic elements, it would be expected that some individuals are at greater risk than others due to dietary differences.

Existing Guidelines and Standards: In 1942, the U.S. Public Health Service established 50 μg/l as the maximum level of selenium permissible in the finished water of Interstate Carrier water supply systems. When the standards were reevaluated and revised in 1962, the maximum permissible level was reduced to 10 μg/l. The U.S. Environmental Protection Agency has established a 0.01 mg/l limit as part of the U.S. Environmental Protection Agency National Interim Primary Drinking Water Regulations that went into effect in June of 1977. According to the Safe Drinking Water Act this level now applies to all utilities that serve 25 persons and/or have 15 service connections.

The Threshold Limit Value (TLV) set for the time-weighted average concentrations of selenium in air for a normal 8-hour work day or 40-hour work week is 0.2 mg/m^3.

The Food and Drug Administration ruled in 1973 that sodium selenite or sodium selenate may be added to the complete feed for swine and chickens up to 16 weeks of age at a level not to exceed 0.1 μg/g, and for turkeys not to exceed 0.2 μg/g.

Summary of Proposed EPA Criteria: *Freshwater Aquatic Life* — For selenium the criterion to protect freshwater aquatic life, as derived using procedures other than the Guidelines, is 9.7 μg/l as a 24-hour average and the concentration should never exceed 22 μg/l at any time.

Saltwater Aquatic Life — For selenium the criterion to protect saltwater aquatic life as derived using the Guidelines is 4.4 μg/l as a 24-hour average and the concentration should not exceed 10 μg/l at any time.

Human Health — For the protection of human health from the toxic properties of selenium ingested through water and through contaminated aquatic organisms, the ambient water criterion is determined to be 10 μg/l.

Bases for the Proposed Human Health Criteria: The question of the carcinogenic potential for ingested selenium has been reviewed in recent years by the National Academy of Sciences (56-3), while studies by the National Cancer Institute (56-12) have added new but inconclusive evidence to the issue. The Academy states that although the 1962 drinking water standard was recommended at 10 μg/l because of evidence that selenium was carcinogenic in animal studies, "a current literature review of animal studies does not support this contention."

An NCI bioassay of selenium disulfide (56-12) at 100 mg/kg (equivalent to 400 ppm of selenium alone) has reported the induction of hepatocellular carcinomas in female mice. This is consistent with an earlier report by Nelson, et al, that seleniferous grains and ammonium potassium selenide at 10 ppm induced liver tumors in rats. However, several inconclusive and negative carcinogenesis studies of selenite and selenate compounds ranging from 2 to 15 ppm have been reported since Nelson's work (56-10).

The carcinogenicity of selenium compounds is a complex issue because: (1) There is evidence that selenates, selenites, and selenides at nontoxic levels inhibit the development of spontaneous tumors, protect against the induction of tumors by known carcinogens, counteract the promotion of tumors in mouse skin initiator-promotor experiments, and inhibit the mutagenic action of chemicals in bacteria; (2) human cancer mortality at several organ sites appears to be negatively correlated with estimated selenium dietary intake and blood selenium levels, according to a tabulation of data from several countries; (3) even at moderate concentrations (5 to 10 ppm) of selenates and selenites the chronic toxicity is high, and this toxicity interferes with the development of tumors because of early deaths; (4) the aqueous solubility and therefore the availability of different selenium compounds for absorption from the GI tract is markedly variable; (5) low concentrations of selenium (0.01 to 0.1 ppm in the diet) appear to be nutritionally essential; and (6) the reports of the chronic toxicity studies are difficult to compare because of the large number of different selenium compounds studies, the dependence of tumor induction on changes in protein and selenium levels in the diet and the incomplete histopathological examination performed in many of the available studies.

For these reasons it does not seem reasonable to use carcinogenic toxicity and risk as a basis for health criteria without additional research.

Obviously, one of the major factors involved in estimation of the minimum dose of selenium required to produce chronic toxicity in man or animals is the criteria, or definition, of chronic toxicity. The National Research Council (56-3) has reviewed the literature in an attempt to establish a "no-effect" dose level for selenium and thus arrive at some conclusion concerning the level in water that can be expected to injure man.

From this review, they found that the growth rate for rats fed a normal diet was inhibited if exposed to 4 to 5 μg/g of selenium in the diet. Only 1 μg/g of selenium in the diet was required to reduce growth in rats fed a diet severely deficient in vitamin E. Hadjimarkos (56-13) has demonstrated in rats that selenium added to drinking water at a level as low as 2.3 mg/l during tooth development increases the incidence of caries. The National Research Council suggests that if histopathologic observations are used as the criteria for chronic toxicity that 1 μg/g of selenium in the diet or 1 mg/l of selenium in drinking water may be shown to be sufficient to produce toxicity. However, it is recognized that the physiologic significance of the findings may not be clear, and the same may be said for biochemical parameters indicating that even lower levels can be toxic.

The amount of selenium needed to prevent deficiency diseases in animals is very small; 0.1 μg/g in the diet is a nutritionally adequate level for most species. Such a level translates into a human requirement of about 60 to 120 micrograms per day depending on the biologic availability in the diet, a person's physiologic status with regard to other nutrients, and other factors.

It is estimated that on the average, adults intake roughly 130 to 150 μg of selenium per day from food. Levander (56-14) has estimated that an average six month old infant consumes 28 μg of selenium per day from food.

The uneven distribution of selenium in the soils of the United States could conceivably cause persons living in low-selenium areas and consuming only locally produced foods to develop a low-selenium state, just as some who live in high-selenium areas may ingest excess selenium. However, most nutrition authorities agree that there is currently no evidence of selenium deficiency in human populations in the United States, probably because of interregional food shipment that characterizes our present-day food supply.

Hence, there is no need to use water as a vehicle for supplementing the diets of the general population.

In consideration of the probable importance selenium plays in the human diet, and the varied but definite exposure potential from food intake, drinking water and other sources, the strategy for identifying a criterion level for ambient waters must be based on minimizing the likelihood of contributing a sufficient amount of selenium that would increase an average total exposure above a selected toxic level.

The growth inhibition with vitamin E deficiency would be the candidate of first choice for toxicity effect and extrapolation into human effects. However, the vitamin E circumstance would be a special situation for the average population and therefore the increased incidence of dental caries at 2.3 mg/l becomes the targeted effect for extrapolation to humans.

If it is assumed that rats consume 10% of their body weight per day during their growth period, the toxic effect (incidence of dental caries) is demonstrated at levels of selenium as low as 16 mg selenium intake per day.

2.3 mg/l Se = 2.3 mg/kg feed

Assuming 300 g rat:

Feed intake = 2.3 mg/kg x 10% (300g) = 69 x 10^{-3} mg Se/day

Animal dose = $\dfrac{69 \times 10^{-3} \text{ mg/day}}{300 \text{ g}}$ = 0.23 mg Se/kg body weight

Equivalent human dose = 0.23 mg Se/kg body weight x 70 kg man = 16.1 mg Se

Thus, the equivalent human dose for incidence of dental caries is 16.1 mg Se/day. For comparison purposes a similar calculation for the growth inhibition under vitamin E deficiency is 7 mg Se/day.

Summary of Pertinent Data — In summary, the minimum toxic daily dose is 16,100 micrograms and the average daily dietary intake is 130 to 150 μg leaving a difference of 15,950 μg. Populations living in seleniferous areas may be exposed to much higher levels of selenium both in the food and water. Since little is known concerning the minimum toxic dose in humans and there is uncertainty about the carcinogenic potential of Se, it does not seem reasonable to permit the level in water to be more than 10 to 20% of the dietary level. If the maximum water contribution is set at 13 to 30.0 μg/day, the total level (dietary and water) will be well below the estimated minimum toxic dose. Assuming that the average individual consumes 2 liters of drinking water per day, 18.7 g of fish, and that the bio-accumulation factor for fish is 18, the estimated level for water is calculated as follows:

$$\text{Criterion Level} = \frac{13}{2 + (0.0187)18} = 5.56 \ \mu\text{g/l}$$

$$\text{or} = \frac{30.0}{2 + (0.0187)18} = 12.84 \ \mu\text{g/l}$$

Based on these calculations it appears that the U.S. Environmental Protection Agency Drinking Water Standard of 10 μg/l is probably an appropriate ambient criterion level to protect the health of the U.S. population.

References

(56-1) Rosenfeld, I., and O.A. Beath. *Selenium; geobotany, biochemistry, toxicology and nutrition.* New York, Academic Press, (1964).

(56-2) U.S. EPA. *Preliminary investigation of effects on the environment of boron, indium, nickel, selenium, tin, vanadium and their compounds. Selenium.* Washington, D.C., (1975).

(56-3) National Academy of Sciences. *Selenium.* Washington, D.C. (1976). (Also issued by EPA Health Effects Res. Lab. as Report EPA-600/1-76-014, Research Triangle Park, N.C.)

(56-4) Chan, Y.K., et al. "Methylation of selenium in the aquatic environment." *Science* 192, 1130 (1976).

(56-5) Sakurai, H., and T. Tsuchiya. "A tentative recommendation for the maximum daily intake of selenium." *Environ. Physical Biochem.* 5, 107. (1975)

(56-6) Schroeder, H.A. "Selenium." *The poisons around us.* Indiana University Press, Bloomington. (1974).

(56-7) Halverson, A.W., et al. "Toxicology of selenium to postweaning rats." *Toxicol. Appl. Pharmacol.* 9, 477. (1966).

(56-8) Keboe, R.H., et al. "The hygienic significance of the contamination of water with certain mineral constituents." *Jour. Am. Water Works Assoc.* 36, 645. (1944).

(56-9) Fairhill, L.T. "Toxic contaminants in drinking water." *Jour. New England Water Works Assoc.* 55, 400. (1941).

(56-10) Nelson, A.A., et al. "Liver tumors following cirrhosis caused by selenium in rats." *Cancer Res.* 3, 230. (1943).

(56-11) Innes, J.R.M., et al. "Bioassay of pesticides and industrial chemicals for tumorigenicity in mice: a preliminary note." *Jour. Natl. Cancer Inst.* 42, 1101. (1969).

(56-12) National Cancer Institute, *NCI Carcinogenesis Bioassay Experimental Design Status Report for Selenium Disulfide,* Washington D.C. (1978).

(56-13) Hadjimarkos, D.M., *The Role of Selenium in Dental Caries. Trace Substances in Environmental Health,* Columbia, Univ. of Missouri (1971).

(56-14) Levander, O.A., "Selenium in Foods." *Proc. of Symp. on Selenium-Tellurium in the Environment,* Ind. Health Fdn., Inc. (1976).

SILVER (#57)

Silver, symbol Ag, is an element in Group I-B of the Periodic Table. Its atomic number is 47 and its atomic weight is 107.88.

Occurrence: Silver is a white ductile metal occurring naturally in the pure form and in ores. Silver concentrations in samples of well and surface water in the U.S. range from 0.1 to 38 μg/l with a median of 2.6 μg/l. Silver can be easily removed from water supply sources by conventional coagulation and lime softening treatment methods.

Physical Properties: Silver is a white metal that can exist in two valence states, Ag+ and Ag++. It has an atomic weight of 107.87. Solubilities of a few common silver salts in water are: AgCl, 1,930 μg/l; $AgNO_3$, 2.5 x 10^9 μg/l; and AgI, 30 μg/l. Many silver salts are light-sensitive.

Chemical Properties: Water or atmospheric oxygen have no effect on metallic silver; however, ozone, hydrogen sulfide, or sulfur will blacken it.

Uses: Principal uses of silver are in photographic materials, electroplating, as a conductor, in dental alloys, solder and brazing alloys, paints, jewelry, silverware, coinage, and mirror production.

Toxic Effects: While metallic silver in the zero valence state is not considered to be toxic, most of its salts are toxic to a large number of organisms. Silver salts can combine with certain biological molecules and subsequently alter their properties. Silver is of some use as an antibacterial agent and has been shown to be bactericidal even in concentrations that are not great enough to precipitate proteins; the assumption is that silver is capable of interfering with essential metabolic processes in the bacterial cell (57-1).

Concentrations from 0.001 to 500 μg/l of silver have been reported sufficient to sterilize water (57-2). Upon ingestion, many silver salts are absorbed in the human circulatory system and deposited in various body tissues, resulting in generalized or sometimes localized gray pigmentation of the skin and mucous membranes known as argyria. There is no known method for removing silver from the tissues once deposited, and the effect is cumulative. This discoloration is due either to silver sulfide or metallic silver from the reduction of silver in tissue (57-1).

Toxic effects in aquatic organisms have been demonstrated for silver at very low concentrations. In freshwater fish, silver toxicity has been associated with changes in swimming behavior, decreased growth, and certain nervous system damage leading to mortality. Silver compounds have also been shown to cause ovarian cytopathic effects when administered orally to mice (57-3). Overall effects of silver in nonhuman mammals include cytopathic, ventricular hypertrophy and pigmentation of body tissues (57-4).

Current Levels of Exposure: Estimates of silver in human diets have varied widely, from an average of 0.4 μg/day for three Italian populations to 27 ± 17 μg/day (excluding water); in the United Kingdom from 35 μg/day (per man) and 40 μg/day (per woman) to 88 μg/day. The average intake of silver by man has been estimated to be 70 μg/day based on a review of the literature. Some of these estimates were based on intake of both food and water. An estimate of 30 μg/day for the average human intake in food is reasonable.

Ambient air levels of silver up to 10.5 ng/m^3 would lead to intake of up to 0.24 μg silver per day (at 23 m^3 respired air per 24 hour period.) Exposure from cigarettes is negligible.

An average value for silver ingestion by water intake cannot be made. Silver was detected in only 6.1% of 380 finished waters (and in only 6.6% of U.S. surface waters.) Because of the recent increase of interest in water purification by silver in the United States, many people are probably ingesting water from nonpublic potable water sources at the 1962 drinking water limit of 0.05 mg/l. Shorter exposure of the U.S. population to European limits might occur during travel by plane or ship.

A diet high in seafood taken from silver-polluted water may increase daily silver consumption. Organisms serving as food for high trophic level aquatic species concentrate silver by a factor of about 200 (brown algae, 240; diatoms, 210.) Other concentration factors in higher organisms of the food chain are mussels, 330; scallops, 2,300; oysters, 18,700; and North Sea marine organisms, average 22,000. Thus, regular ingestion of fish, etc., from contaminated water might significantly increase silver dietary intake.

In the workplace, daily intake in the United States is limited to 100 μg/day (0.01 mg/m^3 x 10 m^3 per workday.) Ground-based cloud-seeding generator operators, however, are exposed to air concentrations exceeding the maximum permissible concentration for several hours at a time.

Special Groups at Risk: People treated with silver-containing medicinals are most at risk of developing argyria, as demonstrated by Hill and Pillsbury (57-5) who summarized 357 recorded cases of argyria, 89% of which were due to therapeutic use of silver. In the period 1931 to 1939, when more people were exposed to therapeutic forms of silver than in any previous period, 92% of the cases were due to medicinals. Cases of occupationally-caused argyria are seldom encountered in the recent literature and were usually diagnosed at least 30 years ago. Hobbyists (e.g., jewelry makers, photograph developers) may not be aware of the precautions needed with silver and may be more at risk of argyria.

There are large individual variations in silver absorption, retention, eliminations, and/or susceptibility to argyria. Although intravenous administration of a total of 0.91 to 7.6 g (average 2.3 g) silver as silver arsphenamine for 2 to 10 years has caused argyria, hundreds of patients have received up to 1.7 g silver intravenously as arsphenamine without developing argyria (57-5,57-6).

Over 10,000 cases of burn and leg ulcer patients have been treated with silver medicinals. No cases of argyria have been reported, even when 0.5% silver nitrate was used and systemic absorption was shown.

Aside from argyria, more subtle effects may be due to silver ingestion. On the basis of animal experiments, people marginally deficient or deficient in copper, selenium, or vitamin E may have their deficiency symptoms exacerbated. But rat studies did not support this suggestion. The possibility that silver might render iodine unavailable in regions that otherwise might have just enough iodine to prevent goiter is another suggested consequence of silver in drinking water. To support the contention, however, elevated silver concentrations had been found in the water of endemic goiter regions such as the western slopes of the Colorado mountains.

Existing Guidelines and Standards: Both of the U.S. standards for silver in drinking water and in workplace air have been based on a presumed 1 g minimum dose of silver that has caused argyria. (See Table 84 on existing standards for silver.) It should be pointed out how the minimum 1 g silver needed to produce argyria was determined. Hill and Pillsbury (57-5) stated that only intravenous doses of silver could be used to determine accurately the amount of silver actually taken into the body since the extent of gastrointestinal or mucous membrane absorption was unknown. Silver arsphenamine had been administered intravenously to human patients suffering from syphilis; 19 of them (14 had advanced symptoms of syphilis; 11 had received other heavy metal treatment) developed argyria. Those patients developing argyria had received total doses of silver ranging from 0.91 g to 7.6 g within 2 to 10 years. The average total dose was 2.3 g silver. (Fourteen of the patients developing argyria were males.) The total number of patients that had been treated with silver arsphenamine was not estimated, but they were probably quite numerous.

Table 84: Existing Standards Regarding Silver

Medium	Silver Concentration	Authority
Drinking water	50 μg/l	U.S. EPA, (57-7); National Academy of Sciences (57-8)
Drinking water	0.5 μg/l	State of Illinois (cited in National Academy of Sciences) (57-8)
Drinking water	10 μg/l	State of California (cited in National Academy of Sciences) (57-8)
Workplace air, threshold limit value, 8 hour time-weighted	0.01 mg/m^3	Occupational Safety and Health Administration (1974) (57-9)

Source: Reference (57)

Until the U.S. Public Health Service Drinking Water Standards of 1962, there were no restrictions on silver in drinking water. Neither the World Health Organization International Standards of 1958 nor the European Standards of 1961 set a limit for silver in drinking water.

The 1976 National Interim Primary Drinking Water Regulations (57-7) included a section on silver that is practically identical to the 1962 Drinking Water Standards. Both begin, "The need to set a water standard for silver (Ag) arises from its intentional addition to waters for disinfection." Both state, ". . . the amount of silver from injected Ag-arsphenamine, which produces argyria, is precisely known. This value is any amount greater than 1 g of silver, 8 g Ag-arsphenamine." The condition to be avoided was argyria. The phraseology "any amount" is misleading, since probably hundreds of patients over at least 2 decades of this treatment for syphilis had received total doses of silver greater than 0.91 g (57-5).

The two documents acknowledge, however, that there is "considerable variability in predisposition to argyria", which is clearly seen upon examination of Hill and Pillsbury's report (57-5) of a few hundred case histories from the literature.

The 1976 document omits the calculations from the 1962 document: "Assuming that all silver ingested is deposited in the integument, it is readily calculated that 10 μg/l could be ingested for a lifetime before 1 g silver is attained from 2 liters water intake per day; 50 μg/l silver could be ingested approximately 27 years without exceeding silver deposition of 1 g." Yet, both also consider that intake from foods is 60 to 80 μg/day, and that silver would be increased in sulfur-containing foods by combination with silver in the cooking water.

The National Academy of Sciences (57-8) in *Drinking Water and Health* made a somewhat different calculation: "the interim drinking water level of 50 μg/l would be equivalent to a retention of 50 μg of silver per day (on the assumption that 50% of the intake is retained in the body), and would result in an accumulation of 1 g in 55 years, to give a probable borderline argyria."

The U.S. National Aeronautics and Space Administration recommended silver at 100 μg/l for safely providing pure drinking water on space flights; Swiss health officials, 200 μg/l; and German health officials, 100 μg/l (57-10).

Maximum contaminant levels for inorganic chemicals in the 1975 National Interim Primary Drinking Water Regulations are based on an average consumption of 2 liters of water per day.

Summary of Proposed EPA Criteria: *Freshwater Aquatic Life* — For silver, the criterion to protect freshwater aquatic life derived using the Guidelines, is 0.0090 µg/l as a 24-hour average and the concentration should not exceed 1.9 µg/l at any time.

Saltwater Aquatic Life — For silver, the criterion to protect saltwater aquatic life as derived using the Guidelines is 0.26 µg/l as a 24-hour average and the concentration should not exceed 0.58 µg/l at any time.

Human Health — For silver, the criterion to protect human health from the toxic properties of silver ingested through water and through contaminated aquatic organisms is 10 µg/l.

Bases for the Proposed Human Health Criteria: None of the carcinogenicity studies mentioned in the criteria document (57) are acceptable for extrapolation to drinking water by use of the linear nonthreshold model. No study demonstrating carcinogenicity of silver has met all of the criteria described regarding appropriate route, chemical form, number of animals, histologic examination of organs and all obvious lesions, concurrently run control group, etc.

Although numerous references to the health effects of silver on humans are available, relatively little toxicological or epidemiological data have been reported in the past 30 years. The primary health effect reported is argyria, the unsightly blue-gray discoloration of the skin (and other organs) that develops after repeated exposures to silver compounds. (It is rarely seen today.) The current drinking water standard of 50 µg/l was designed to protect against argyria.

In ten experiments on chronic ingestion by a limited number of rats (rabbits included in one study) of drinking water containing 50 to 20,000 µg/l silver ions, effects were not observed in rats ingesting silver at less than 400 µg/l. However, in four studies, some physiological effect was noted at 400 or 500 µg/l of silver. Thus, for the purpose of developing a criterion for silver based on animal studies of reasonable quality, the following calculation may be made:

$$\frac{(0.2 \text{ mg/liter}) \ (0.035 \text{ liter/day}^{*})}{0.3 \text{ kg}^{**}} = 0.023 \text{ mg/kg/day}$$

0.023 mg/kg/day x 70 kg/adult human male = 1.6 mg/day

[*]Estimated volume of water consumed by rats.
[**]Estimated weight of one rat.

A safety factor of 10 to 100 is indicated here, based on several factors. The National Academy of Sciences Guidelines (57-8) state the following: Some valid experimental results are available for prolonged human ingestion with no indication of carcinogenicity, but data are less than complete.

The water consumption rate for rats is considerably higher than that for humans on equivalent body weight basis. The retention rate of silver in humans versus that in rats is uncertain. While silver had not been found to be carcinogenic by normal intake routes, some evidence exists that it may have carcinogenic activity when implanted as a solid or have activity as a promoter for other carcinogens.

Application of a safety factor of 100 yields a concentration of 8 µg/l, i.e.

$$\frac{1.6 \text{ mg/day}}{(100)2 \text{ liters}} = \frac{0.016 \text{ mg/day}}{2 \text{ liters}} = 0.008 \text{ mg/l} = 8 \text{ µg/l}$$

Because of the inherent uncertainties in such a calculation, a value of 10 µg/l silver in water is chosen as the criterion level for protection of human health.

References

(57-1) Goodman, L.S. and A. Gilman, eds. *The pharmacological basis of therapeutics.* 5th ed. New York, Macmillan Publishing Co. Inc., (1975).

(57-2) McKee, J.E., and H.W. Wolf. *Water quality.* Publ. 3-A. Sacramento, Calif. State Water Resour. Control Board. (1963).

(57-3) Hadek, R. "Preliminary report on the cellular effect of intravital silver in the mouse ovary." *Jour. Ultrastruct. Res.* 15, 66 (1966).

(57-4) Olcott, C.T. "Experimental argyrosis. IV. Morphologic changes in the experimental animal." *Am. Jour. Pathol.* 24, 813 (1948).

(57-5) Hill, W.R. and Pillsbury, D.M., *Argyria, the Pharmacology of Silver,* Baltimore, The Williams and Wilkins Co. (1939).

(57-6) Cooper, C.F. and Jolly, W.C., *Ecological Effects of Weather Modification: A Problem Analysis,* Ann Arbor, Mich., School of Nat. Resources, Univ. of Mich. (1969).

(57-7) U.S. Environmental Protection Agency, *National Interim Primary Drinking Water Regulations* Report EPA-560/9-76-003, Wash., D.C., Office of Water Supply (1976).

(57-8) National Academy of Sciences, *Drinking Water and Health,* Washington, D.C. (1977).

(57-9) 39 *FR* 23541 (1974).

(57-10) Silver Institute, "Silver Guards Good Health", *Silver Inst. Letter* 5, no. 5, 1 (1975).

T

TETRACHLOROBENZENE

See "Chlorinated Benzenes" (14).

2,3,7,8-TETRACHLORODIBENZO-p-DIOXIN (TCDD) (#58)

TCDD is a symmetrical, nearly planar molecule with the empirical formula $C_{12}H_4Cl_4O_2$ and the structural formula:

Occurrence: 2,3,7,8-Tetrachlorodibenzo-p-dioxin (TCDD) is a contaminant inadvertently formed during the production of 2,4,5-trichlorophenol (2,4,5-TCP) from 1,2,4,5-tetrachlorobenzene (58-1)(58-2). 2,4,5-TCP represents the major chemical feedstock for the production of numerous herbicides and TCDD has been reported to be a contaminant of 2,4,5-trichlorophenoxyacetic acid (2,4,5-T), 2,4,5-T esters, silvex, 2,4-dichlorophenoxyacetic acid (2,4-D), and clophen. It has also been reported that TCDD may be formed during the burning of vegetation treated with 2,4,5-T.

Physical Properties: TCDD is a white crystalline solid with a melting point range of 302° to 305°C. Decomposition begins at 500°C and is virtually complete within 21 seconds at a temperature of 800°C. TCDD has a molecular weight of 321.98 and is not volatile. TCDD is lipophilic, exhibiting a high degree of solubility in fats, oils, and other relatively nonpolar solvents, and is only slightly soluble in water (0.2 to 0.6 μg/l). The partition coefficient of TCDD in a water:hexane system has been reported to be 1,000.

Chemical Properties: TCDD is considered to be a highly stable compound which can be degraded only by temperatures in excess of 500°C or by irradiation with UV light under certain conditions.

Uses: TCDD has no uses as such. As noted above, TCDD is an inadvertent contaminant in herbicide precursors and thus in the herbicides themselves. Thus, it is applied in herbicide formulations, but is not used per se. It has been estimated that approximately 2 million acres in the United States have been treated for weed control on one or more occasions with approximately 15 million pounds of TCDD contaminated 2,4,5-T, 2,4-D, or combinations of the two.

Toxic Effects: TCDD is one of the most toxic substances known (58-3). It exhibits a delayed biological response in many species and is highly lethal at low doses to aquatic organisms, birds, and mammals, including man. It has been shown to be acnegenic, embryolethal, teratogenic, mutagenic (in certain organisms), carcinogenic, and to affect the immune responses in mammals. TCDD has also been shown to persist for 10 years after application to soils and to bioaccumulate in aquatic organisms by factors as high as 8,000-fold. These findings in conjunction with the wide distribution of contaminated products, lead to the conclusion that TCDD represents a potential hazard to both aquatic and terrestrial life.

Current Levels of Exposure: The amount of human exposure to TCDD that can be directly attributed to water cannot be determined. TCDD is believed not to occur naturally in the environment. However, a recent study by the Dow Chemical Co.-organized "chlorinated dioxin task force" reported that chlorinated dioxins, including TCDD, "were found in every sample of particulate matter taken from the air emissions of a wide variety of commercial and domestic combustion processes." The solubility of TCDD and its inability to vertically migrate through soil indicate that ground water would probably not be contaminated although run-off from soil treated with TCDD containing herbicides is not precluded.

The several reported incidents of toxic manifestations of exposure to TCDD in factories and from accidental contamination via inhalation and/or dermal routes illustrate the toxicity of the compound. The levels and duration of exposure were not determinable in most cases.

Special Groups at Risk: A special group at risk would be workers in an industrial environment where exposure to TCDD-contaminated products is a possibility. A special subgroup at risk are women of childbearing age and children.

Existing Guidelines and Standards: There are no existing guidelines or standards other than a calculated acceptable daily intake (ADI) of 10^{-4} μg/kg/day for 2,3,7,8-tetrachlorodibenzo-p-dioxin (TCDD). The data base for the calculation did not consider TCDD to be a known or suspect carcinogen (58-4). Although TCDD is a contaminant of some chlorinated herbicides, there are no tolerances for TCDD in or on food crops. 40 *CFR* 180.302 does, however, establish a tolerance of 0.05 ppm hexachlorophene in or on cotton seed (a non-human dietary food item) and states that technical grade hexachlorophene shall not contain more than 0.1 ppm TCDD.

Summary of Proposed EPA Criteria: *Freshwater Aquatic Life* — For freshwater aquatic life, no criterion for 2,3,7,8-tetrachlorodibenzo-p-dioxin can be derived using the Guidelines, and there are insufficient data to estimate a criterion using other procedures.

Saltwater Aquatic Life — For saltwater aquatic life, no criterion for 2,3,7,8-tetrachlorodibenzo-p-dioxin can be derived using the Guidelines, and there are insufficient data to estimate a criterion using other procedures.

Human Health — For the maximum protection of human health from the potential carcinogenic effects of exposure to TCDD through ingestion of water and contaminated aquatic organisms, the ambient water concentration is zero. Concentrations of TCDD estimated to result in additional lifetime cancer risks ranging from no additional risk to an additional risk of 1 in 100,000 are presented in the Criterion Formulation section of this document. The EPA is considering setting criteria at an interim target risk level in the range of 10^{-5}, 10^{-6}, or 10^{-7} with corresponding criteria of 4.55×10^{-7} μg/l, 4.55×10^{-8} μg/l, and 4.55×10^{-9} μg/l, respectively.

Basis for the Proposed Human Health Criteria: TCDD is an extremely toxic compound exhibiting acute, subchronic and chronic effects in animals and humans. The liver appears to be the target organ of acute exposure. Retention of TCDD by the liver indicates that it apparently undergoes little or no metabolism.

Acute effects of exposure include chloracne, porphyria cutanea tarda, hepatotoxicity, psychological alterations, weight loss, thymic atrophy, thrombocytopenia, suppression of cellular immunity and death. TCDD is teratogenic and fetotoxic. Oral exposure of pregnant rats to 0.125 to 2.0 μg TCDD/kg/day produced fetal mortality, fetal intestinal hemorrhage and both early and late resorptions. There was found an increased incidence of cleft palate when pregnant mice were given TCDD doses of 1.0 μg/kg/day for 10 days during gestation. TCDD has been shown to be mutagenic in three bacterial systems and a potent inducer of hepatic and renal microsomal drug metabolizing enzymes.

The carcinogenic potential of tetrachlorodibenzo-p-dioxin has been established by the findings of two feeding studies. One study found that Sprague-Dawley rats fed dose levels of 5 ppt to ppb TCDD had a significant excess of tumors as compared to the controls. Another feeding study, conducted by Kociba, et al (58-5) using the same strain of rats given 0.1, 0.01, 0.001 μg TCDD/kg/day, induced a statistically significant excess of hepatocellular carcinoma in treated rats. Based on these two studies, tetrachlorodibenzo-p-dioxin is likely to be a human carcinogen.

Under the Consent Decree in NRDC vs Train, criteria are to state "recommended maximum permissible concentrations (including where appropriate, zero) consistent with the protection of aquatic organisms, human health, and recreational activities." TCDD is suspected of being a human carcinogen. Because there is no recognized safe concentration for a human carcinogen, the recommended concentration of TCDD in water for maximum protection of human health is zero.

Because attaining a zero concentration level may be infeasible in some cases and in order to assist the EPA and States in the possible future development of water quality regulations, the concentrations of TCDD corresponding to several incremental lifetime cancer risk levels have been estimated. A cancer risk level provides an estimate of the additional incidence of cancer that may be expected in an exposed population. A risk of 10^{-5} for example, indicates a probability of one additional case of cancer for every 100,000 people exposed, risk of 10^{-6} indicates one additional case of cancer for every million people exposed, and so forth.

In the *Federal Register* notice of availability of draft ambient water quality criteria, EPA stated that it is considering setting criteria at an interim target risk level of 10^{-5}, 10^{-6} or 10^{-7} as shown in Table 85. In Table 85, the risk levels and corresponding criteria are calculated by applying a modified "one hit" extrapolation model.

Since the extrapolation model is linear at low doses, the additional lifetime risk is directly proportional to the water concentration. Therefore, water concentrations corresponding to other risk levels can be derived by multiplying or dividing one of the risk levels and corresponding water concentrations shown in the table by factors such as 10, 100, 1,000, and so forth.

Table 85: Possible Alternative Criteria for TCDD

Exposure Assumptions (per day)	Risk Levels and Corresponding Criteria, (μg/l)			
	0	10^{-7}	10^{-6}	10^{-5}
2 liters drinking water and consumption of 18.7 grams fish and shellfish*	0	4.55×10^{-9}	4.55×10^{-8}	4.55×10^{-7}
Consumption of fish and shellfish only	0	4.63×10^{-9}	4.63×10^{-8}	4.63×10^{-7}

*Approximately 98% of the TCDD exposure results from the consumption of aquatic organisms which exhibit an average bioconcentration potential of 5,800-fold. The remaining 2% of TCDD exposure results from drinking water.

Source: Reference (58)

Concentration levels were derived assuming a lifetime exposure to various amounts of TCDD, (1) occurring from the consumption of both drinking water and aquatic life grown in waters containing the corresponding TCDD concentrations and, (2) occurring solely from consumption of aquatic life grown in the waters containing the corresponding TCDD concentrations.

Because data indicating other sources of TCDD exposure and their contributions to total body burden are inadequate for quantitative use, the figures reflect the incremental risks associated with the indicated routes only.

Summary of Pertinent Data — The Kociba, et al study (58-5) of Sprague-Dawley rats in which dioxin was added to the diet at a concentration of 0.1 μg/kg/day for 2 years resulted in hepatocellular carcinoma in 11 of 49 treated females whereas only 1 of 86 controls had hepatocellular carcinoma. Using a bioaccumulation factor 5,800 the parameters of the extrapolation model are:

$$
\begin{aligned}
n_t &= 11 \\
N_t &= 49 \\
n_c &= 1 \\
N_c &= 86 \\
Le &= 24 \text{ months} \\
le &= 24 \text{ months} \\
d &= 10^{-4} \text{ mg/kg/day} \\
w &= 0.37 \text{ kg} \\
L &= 24 \text{ months} \\
R &= 5,800
\end{aligned}
$$

The result is that the water concentration should be less than 4.55×10^{-7} micrograms per liter in order to keep the individual lifetime risk below 10^{-5}.

References

(58-1)   Milnes, M.H. "Formation of 2,3,7,8-tetrachlorodibenzo-p-dioxin by thermal decomposition of sodium 2,4,5-trichlorophenate." *Nature* 232, 395 (1971).

(58-2)   Firestone, D., et al "Determination of polychlorodibenzo-p-dioxin and related compounds in chemical chlorophenols." *Jour. Assoc. Off. Anal. Pharm.* 55, 85 (1972).

(58-3)   Kimbrough, R.D. "The toxicity of polychlorinated polycyclic chemicals and related compounds." *Crit. Rev. Toxicol.* 2, 445 (1974).

(58-4)   National Research Council, *Drinking Water and Health,* Wash., D.C. (1977).

(58-5)   Kociba, R.J. et al, *Toxic and Applied Phar.* (In Press -1979).

1,1,2,2-TETRACHLOROETHANE

See "Chlorinated Ethanes" (15).

TETRACHLOROETHYLENE (#59)

Tetrachloroethylene (1,1,2,2-tetrachloroethylene) is also known as perchloroethylene and PCE.

Occurrence: Perchloroethylene is widespread in the environment, and is found in trace amounts in water, aquatic organisms, air, foodstuffs, and human tissue (59-1). The highest environmental levels of PCE are found in the commercial dry cleaning and metal degreasing industries [Natl. Inst. Occup. Safety Health (59-2)]. The current level of PCE permissible in U.S. working environments is 670 mg/m^3 (100 ppm). Although PCE is released into water via aqueous effluents from production plants, consumer industries, and household sewage, its level in ambient water is reported to be minimal due to its high volatility. PCE has been detected at levels below 1 μg/l in waters surrounding chlorinated hydrocarbon production plants in England and in U.S. surface waters.

Physical Properties: PCE is a colorless, nonflammable liquid which has the molecular formula C_2Cl_4 and a molecular weight of 165.85. Other physical properties of PCE include a melting point of -23.25°C, a density of 1.623 g/ml, a vapor pressure of 19 mm Hg, a water solubility of 150 μg/ml and an octanol/water partition coefficient of 339 (log P = 2.53). The log P value indicates that PCE has a high affinity for lipid material and may bioaccumulate in animals.

Chemical Properties: Tetrachloroethylene is quite stable. However it reacts violently with concentrated nitric acid to give carbon dioxide as a primary product. With formaldehyde and sulfuric acid, tetrachloroethylene reacts to form $HOCH_2CCl_2COOH$ by a peculiar combination of condensation, hydrolysis and dehydration.

Uses: Tetrachloroethylene is used primarily as a solvent in the dry cleaning industries. It is used to a lesser extent as a degreasing solvent in metal industries.

Toxic Effects: In the laboratory, PCE has been demonstrated to be toxic to aquatic organisms (59-3)(59-4). The primary toxic effect observed in human and nonhuman mammals after acute or chronic inhalation of PCE is central nervous system depression (59-2)(59-5). PCE has also been reported to be hepatotoxic to mammals (59-6)(59-7) and carcinogenic in mice (59-8); thus, there is concern about its toxicity to humans (59-9).

Current Levels of Exposure: The National Organics Monitoring Survey detected tetrachloroethylene (perchloroethylene, PCE) in 9 of 105 drinking waters sampled between November 1976 and January 1977 (range, <0.2 to 3.1 μg/l; median <0.2 μg/l). The mean concentration of the nine positive samples was 0.81 μg/l. PCE was one of two halogenated compounds indentified both in the drinking water and in the plasma of individuals living in New Orleans.

No data were found on levels of PCE in United States food. In England, PCE concentrations in foods ranged from nondetectable amounts (<0.01 μg/kg) in orange juice to 13 μg/kg in English butter. General environmental PCE concentrations tend to be low. Surveys at eight locations in the U.S. found concentrations of up to 6.7 μg/m^3 in urban areas and less than 0.013 μg/m^3 in rural areas.

Special Groups at Risk: By far the most significant exposure to PCE occurs in industrial environments (59-10). The major uses of PCE are in textile and dry cleaning industries (69%), metal cleaning (16%), and as a chemical intermediate (12%). As with inhalation exposures, dermal exposures of significance would be primarily confined to occupational exposure.

Existing Guidelines and Standards: Existing tetrachloroethylene (PCE) standards are primarily applicable to occupational exposures. The present American Governmental Conference on Industrial Hygiene threshold limit value (TLV) listed in Table 86, has been established primarily on the basis of measurable deficits in central nervous system function resulting from short-term exposures of healthy male volunteers. As Stewart, et al (59-11) point out this figure incorporates a negligible factor of safety even for this group. Thus, sensitive populations or the possibility of other environmental conditions which might synergize with PCE toxicity have not been considered. Additionally, it does not yet incorporate consideration of PCE carcinogenicity (59-8). The NIOSH (59-9) has called attention to carcinogenic problems in a follow-up to its original criteria document (59-2).

Table 86: Industrial Hygiene Standards for Tetrachloroethylene in Various Countries

		Calculated Allowable Daily Exposure (mg/day)
U.S.A.	670 mg/m^3	4,793
German Democratic Republic	250 mg/m^3	1,786
U.S.S.R.	1 mg/m^3	7

Source: Reference (59-10).

Summary of Proposed EPA Criteria: *Freshwater Aquatic Life* — For tetrachloroethylene, the criterion to protect freshwater aquatic life, as derived using procedures other than the Guideline, is 310 μg/l as a 24-hour average and the concentration should not exceed 700 μg/l at any time.

Saltwater Aquatic Life — For tetrachloroethylene the criterion to protect saltwater aquatic life as derived using the Guidelines is 79 μg/l as a 24-hour average and the concentration would not exceed 180 μg/l at any time.

Human Health — For the maximum protection of human health from the potential carcinogenic effects of exposure to tetrachloroethylene through ingestion of water and contaminated aquatic organisms, the ambient water concentration is zero. Concentrations of tetrachloroethylene estimated to result in additional lifetime cancer risks ranging from no additional risk to an additional risk of 1 in 100,000 are presented in the Criterion Formulation section of this document. The EPA is considering setting criteria at an interim target risk level in the range of 10^{-5}, 10^{-6} or 10^{-7} with corresponding criteria of 2.0 μg/l, 0.20 μg/l, 0.020 μg/l respectively.

Basis for the Proposed Human Health Criteria: Under the Consent Decree in NRDC vs Train, criteria are to state "recommended maximum permissible concentrations (including where appropriate, zero) consistent with the protection of aquatic organisms, human health, and recreational activities." Tetrachloroethylene is suspected of being a human carcinogen. Because there is no recognized safe concentration for a human carcinogen, the recommended concentration of tetrachloroethylene in water for maximum protection of human health is zero.

Because attaining a zero concentration level may be infeasible in some cases and in order to assist the EPA and States in the possible future development of water quality regulations, the concentrations of tetrachloroethylene corresponding to several incremental lifetime cancer risk levels have been estimated. A cancer risk level provides an estimate of the additional incidence of cancer that may be expected in an exposed population. A risk of 10^{-5} for example, indicates a probability of one additional case of cancer for every 100,000 people exposed; a risk of 10^{-6} indicates one additional case of cancer for every million people exposed, and so forth.

In the *Federal Register* notice of availability of draft ambient water quality criteria, EPA stated that it is considering setting criteria at an interim target risk level of 10^{-5}, 10^{-6} or 10^{-7} as shown in Table 87. In the table risk levels and corresponding criteria are calculated by applying a modified "one hit" extrapolation model described in the Methodology Document to the animal bioassay data presented in Summary of Pertinent Data. Since the extrapolation model is linear at low doses, the additional lifetime risk is directly proportional to the water concentration. Therefore, water concentrations corresponding to other risk levels can be derived by multiplying or dividing one of the risk levels and corresponding water concentrations shown in the table by factors such as 10, 100, 1,000, and so forth.

Table 87: Possible Alternative Criteria for Tetrachloroethylene

Exposure Assumptions (per day)	Risk Levels and Corresponding Criteria			
	0	10^{-7}	10^{-6}	10^{-5}
	. . . . (μg/l)			
2 liters of drinking water and consumption of 18.7 grams fish and shellfish*	0	0.020	0.20	2.0
Consumption of fish and shellfish only	0	0.040	0.40	4.0

*Approximately 51% of the tetrachloroethylene exposure results from the consumption of aquatic organisms which exhibit an average bioconcentration potential of 110-fold. The remaining 49% of tetrachloroethylene exposure results from drinking water.

Source: Reference (59)

Concentration levels were derived assuming a lifetime exposure to various amounts of tetrachloroethylene, (1) occurring from the consumption of both drinking water and aquatic life grown in waters containing the corresponding tetrachloroethylene concentrations and, (2) occurring solely from consumption of aquatic life grown in the waters containing the corresponding tetrachloroethylene concentrations. Because data indicating other sources of tetrachloroethylene exposure and their contributions to total body burden are inadequate for quantitative use, the figures reflect the incremental risks associated with the indicated routes only.

Tetrachloroethylene administered by gavage to mice caused hepatocellular carcinomas in both males and females in the NCI bioassay (59-8) at both the high and low dose levels. The females were treated at 772 and 386 mg/kg five times per week for 78 weeks and held until 90 weeks for observation. In females of the high dose group the lifetime probability of dying of hepatocellular carcinoma was 0.938, whereas the matched vehicle and matched untreated controls had an incidence of hepatocellular carcinoma indistinguishable from that of pooled controls, which was 6/196. The lifetime probability given in the NCI report is used for the water criteria documents rather than the actual incidence because a correction is needed for the excess early deaths in the treated groups due to kidney toxicity. With a fish bioaccumulation factor of 110, the parameters of the extrapolation model are:

$$
\begin{aligned}
n_t/N_t &= 0.938 \\
n_c &= 6 \\
N_c &= 196 \\
Le &= 90 \text{ weeks} \\
le &= 78 \text{ weeks} \\
d &= 772 \times {}^5\!/_7 = 551 \text{ mg/kg/day} \\
w &= 0.026 \text{ kg} \\
L &= 90 \text{ weeks} \\
R &= 110
\end{aligned}
$$

The result is that the water concentration should be less than 2.0 micrograms per liter in order to keep the individual lifetime risk below 10^{-5}.

References

(59-1) McConnell, G., et al, "Chlorinated hydrocarbons and the environment." *Endeavour* 34, 13 (1975).

(59-2) National Institute of Occupational Safety and Health. *Criteria for a Recommended Standard: Occupational Exposure to Tetrachloroethylene (Perchloroethylene)*, NIOSH Doc No. 76-185 Washington, D.C. (1976).

(59-3) Alexander, H., et al, "Toxicity of perchloroethylene, trichloroethylene, 1,1,1-trichloroethane, and methylene chloride to fathead minnows." *Bull. Environ. Contam. Toxicol.* 20, 344 (1978).

(59-4) Pearson, C., and G. McConnell. "Chlorinated C_1 and C_2 hydrocarbons in the marine environment." *Proc. R. Soc. London* 189, 305 (1975).

(59-5) Patty, F. "Aliphatic halogenated hydrocarbons," *Ind. Hyg. Toxicol.* 2, 1314 (1963).

(59-6) Kylin, B., et al, "Hepatotoxicity of inhaled trichloroethylene and tetrachloroethylene. Long term exposure." *Acta Pharmacol. Toxicol.* 22, 379 (1965).

(59-7) Rowe, V., et al, "Vapor toxicity of tetrachloroethylene for laboratory animals and human subjects." *Arch. Ind. Hyg. Occup. Med.* 5, 566 (1952).

(59-8) National Cancer Institute. *Bioassay of tetrachloroethylene for possible carcinogenicity.* DHEW Publ. No. (NIH) 77-813, Washington, D.C. (Oct. 1977).

(59-9) Nat Inst. for Occup. Safety and Health, *Current Intelligence Bulletin No. 20: Tetrachloroethylene,* Wash., D.C. (Jan. 20, 1978).

(59-10) Fishbein, L., "Industrial mutagens and potential mutagens, I, halogenated aliphatic hydrocarbons," *Mutat. Res.* 32, 267 (1976).

(59-11) Stewart, R.D. et al, "Experimental human exposure to tetrachloroethylene," *Arch. Envir. Health* 20, 225 (1970).

TETRACHLORONAPHTHALENES

See "Chlorinated Naphthalenes" (17).

TETRACHLOROPHENOLS

See "Chlorinated Phenols" (18).

THALLIUM (#60)

Thallium is an element in Group III—A of the Periodic Table having the chemical symbol Tl and is a soft, malleable, heavy metal with a silver-white luster (60-1). It has an atomic number of 81 and an atomic weight of 204.37.

Occurrence: The average concentration of thallium in seawater has been reported to be 10 ng/l. Analyses of U.S. river water during 1958 and 1959 reported no thallium at detection limits. More recent analyses of household tap water samples have detected thallium at an average concentration of less than 1 μg/l in less than one percent of all samples.

Physical Properties: Thallium has an atomic weight of 204.37, a melting point of 303.5°C, a boiling point of 1,457 ± 10°C, and a specific gravity of 11.85 at 20°C. Thallium metal closely resembles lead in a number of its physical properties.

Thallium exists in either the monovalent (thallous) or trivalent (thallic) form, the former being the more common and stable and therefore forming more numerous and stable salts. Thallic salts are readily reduced by common reducing agents to the thallous salts. While thallium itself is relatively insoluble in water, thallium compounds exhibit a wide range of solubilities.

Chemical Properties: Thallium is chemically reactive with air and moisture, oxidizing slowly in air at 20°C and more rapidly as the temperature increases, with the presence of moisture enhancing this reaction. Thallous oxide, formed by oxidizing the metal at low temperatures, is easily oxidized to thallic oxide or reduced to thallium. Thallous oxide is a very hygroscopic compound and has a vapor pressure of 1 mm Hg at 580°C. Thallous hydroxide is formed when thallium contacts water containing oxygen.

Uses: Industrial uses of thallium include the manufacture of alloys, electronic devices, and special glass. Many thallium-containing catalysts have been patented for industrial organic reactions (60-2). Production and use of thallium and its compounds approximated 680 kg in 1976. The first important application of thallium was in 1920 when a German producer introduced a rat poison whose principal constituent was thallium sulfate. It is still used in rat poison and ant bait.

Toxic Effects: Thallium is harmful to a wide variety of organisms at low concentrations. In the aquatic environment, thallium has been demonstrated to be chronically toxic to fish at concentrations as low as 20 μg/l and to bioconcentrate by a factor of up to 130. In nonaquatic organisms, including humans, symptoms of acute exposure to thallium include alopecia, ataxia, and tremors (60-3), occasionally leading to irreversible coma and death (60-4).

Current Levels of Exposure: It is extremely difficult to specify current levels of exposure for either man or animals because of the scarcity of good data. This is due to the fact that analytical methods which have been applied to the problem have generally not been sufficiently sensitive for determination of thallium in major media (air, food, water) or in normal man. This is not to say that adequate methods do not exist. For example, the mass spectroscopic-isotope dilution procedure could detect thallium in urine in the range of 0.01-0.1 ng/g. There probably has not been sufficient motivation to develop alternate adequately sensitive methodology to define human exposure adequately in the normal range.

Certain approximations as to usual human exposure are possible. Thus, based on one extensive study it seems that tap water seldom exceeds 0.3 μg Tl/l. Assuming that the average adult consumes 2 liters of water per day, total input would be somewhat less than 1 μg/d.

Even in the worst conditions of water pollution, the concentration of thallium probably seldom exceeds 30 μg/l. These conditions occur in the immediate vicinity of ore processing operations and possibly in streams draining ore-rich soils. e.g., the Colorado River as it courses through western Arizona.

Limited data on thallium in vegetables suggest that these, as a class of food, may have considerably higher concentrations of thallium, perhaps 10 μg/kg wet weight, than other classes of foods. Bread and muscle, for example, contain 1 μg/kg or less. This may explain the observation that vegetarians excrete considerably more thallium in the urine than nonvegetarians. Assuming that total food consumption is 1.6 kg/d, that 0.38 kg is in the form of vegetables, and that the remainder has a concentration of only 1 μg/kg, total thallium intake would be $(0.38)(10) + (1.2)(1) = 5$ μg. This estimate probably is on the high side since prepared vegetables would likely have less thallium than raw vegetables due to leaching of thallium into water during cooking.

So far as ambient air as a source is concerned, the single largest anthropogenic source of thallium is considered to be stack emissions from coal-fired plants. It has been estimated that flue gas would contain about 0.7 mg/m^3, with a likely ground level concentration of 0.7 μg/m^3. Given that a large factor of dilution would result by dispersion from the base of a stack, it seems unlikely that the contribution of coal combustion to thallium in ambient air would be significant. The highest measurement of thallium reported in ambient air indicated a range of 0.04-0.48 ng/m^3.

Inhalation of thallium in cigarette smoke may, on the other hand, be a very significant source. The urinary excretion of thallium in smokers is about twice that in nonsmokers and the concentration in cigar stubs has been shown to be 57-170 ng/g, about 20 times the concentration estimated for the diet.

Total intake in the general nonsmoking adult population calculated on the basis of exposure data thus would consist of no more than 1.0 μg/d from water and no more than 5 μg/d from food, even assuming that virtually all ingested thallium likely is absorbed.

The total daily assimilation of thallium by adults in the general population has been also arrived at by consideration of excretion data and estimated body burden. The estimated daily intake arrived at by consideration of food and water exposure and by these other two methods is as follows:

Basis	Estimated Daily Adult Intake (μg/d)
Food, air and water exposure	$\leqslant 6$
Excretion data	1.64
Body burden data	2.3

Special Groups at Risk: From the standpoint of age, there is no basis for believing that children are more susceptible to thallium intoxication than adults. Children, however, experience neurological sequelae, while adults do not. There is no reason for suspecting either that the fetus is unusually sensitive. Essentially nothing is known regarding sex differences in susceptibility. One study in rats indicated that females are more resistant to subchronic toxicity than males.

From the standpoint of exposure hazard, it would seem that smokers may have twice as great a level of thallium intake as nonsmokers. This suggestion is based solely on data concerning urinary thallium excretion in six people and on very limited information concerning thallium in cigars. Obviously, people occupationally exposed to thallium may constitute a special risk category, but this matter has received little attention, largely because total annual industrial production of thallium is so small, probably about 0.5 tons. In the U.S., the main source of poisoning, thallium-containing rodenticides and insecticides, has been terminated. The manufacture and distribution of these products is no longer permitted.

Existing Guidelines and Standards: There is a threshold limit value of 0.1 mg/m^3 for thallium in workplace air. This value is based on analogy to other highly toxic metals. This standard which has been adopted by the Occupational Safety and Health Administration (OSHA), is the same as for East Germany and West Germany (60-5). The U.S.S.R. standard is 0.01 mg/m^3. No criteria have been developed for irrigation water, drinking water, fresh water or other media.

Summary of Proposed EPA Criteria: *Freshwater Aquatic Life* — For freshwater aquatic life, no criterion for thallium can be derived using the Guidelines, and there are insufficient data to estimate a criterion using other procedures.

Saltwater Aquatic Life — For saltwater aquatic life, no criterion for thallium can be derived using the Guidelines, and there are insufficient data to estimate a criterion using other procedures.

Human Health — For the protection of human health from the toxic properties of thallium ingested through water and contaminated aquatic organisms, the ambient water criterion is 4 μg/l.

Basis for the Proposed Human Health Criteria: The proposed criterion for thallium in water is derived from (1) estimated least toxic level on chronic intake in man (2) introduction of a margin of safety and (3) relative contribution of water and other media to total daily intake in the general population.

In estimating the least toxic level of intake, the effect to which man is most sensitive probably is alopecia. Loss of scalp hair in man and of body fur in animals seems to occur at somewhat lower levels of intake than any other known effects. This is not so clearly the case in adults as in children and animals. There is, however, no great difference between the acute or chronic dose causing alopecia and the dose causing neurologic effects. The least daily amount of thallium which, when taken for a lifetime, will cause alopecia can only be estimated on the basis of subchronic animal exposure data combined with some kinetic considerations. It is estimated that the least toxic subchronic level of intake in rats was 1.6 mg Tl/kg/d. Alopecia occurred in 2 weeks as a result of the administration of thallium at 12 ppm in the diet. In the following the average weight of rats is derived from inspection of the authors' report; the average food was assumed to be 10 g at that weight:

(1) least toxic dietary level = 15 ppm thallous acetate = 12 ppm thallium (12 μg/g),

(2) average weight of rats = 0.075 kg,

(3) average diet consumption = 10 g/d,
(12 μg/g)(10 g/d) = 120 μg Tl/d/0.075 kg = 1.6 mg/kg/d.

In spite of continuous intake for 105 days, animals receiving a modestly lower level (one-third) showed no alopecia or other effects. At the least toxic dose level effects occurred within two weeks or they did not occur with continued intake. This is consistent with the rapid turnover of thallium in rats and the consequently rapid attainment of a steady state level of thallium in the body. Within two weeks, a steady state is virtually achieved since 14 days represents more than three half-lives for thallium clearance from the body. Thus, steady state for input vs output:

$$A = \frac{1.6 \text{ mg/kg/d}}{0.18 \text{ day}^{-1}}$$

$$A = 8.9 \text{ mg/kg}$$

where: A is the amount in 1 kg body weight.

At 14 days, A is 8.1 mg/kg (compared to 8.9 above).

$$A = \frac{1.6 \text{ mg/kg/d}}{0.18 \text{ day}^{-1}} \cdot (1 - e^{-0.17 \cdot 14}) = \frac{1.6}{0.18} \cdot (1 - 0.09)$$

Extrapolation of this minimal toxic level of 1.6 mg/kg/d to man requires one assumption, that man and rat are about equally sensitive to the toxic effects of thallium. This seems reasonable. A comparison of minimal acute lethal doses is possible; 13 to 20 mg/kg in rats and 8 to 10 mg/kg in man. However, in order for man to attain the same toxic level in the body as the rat, the required intake is much smaller because the turnover of thallium in the body is much slower ($k = 0.18$ in the rat vs $k = 0.023$ in man). Thus, in man, the dose required to attain a minimally toxic steady state whole body concentration of thallium would be only 0.20 mg/kg/d from the relationship: k (man)/k (rat) equals A_D (man)/A_D (rat), where A_D = mg Tl/kg/d = 1.6 mg/kg (rat) and k = constant for rate of excretion.

Because of the tenuous nature of the data on which these calculations are based, it must be accepted that the minimal toxic level of chronic exposure may be lower than estimated here. Even assuming that the minimal toxic dose is actually lower than estimated, the spread between toxic intake and man's current level of intake is considerable. It is estimated that the usual input from drinking water, food and air is no more than 6 μg/d for an adult weighing 70 kg. This is in contrast to a minimal toxic level of 15.4 mg/day for a person weighing 70 kg. The safety factor is thus approximately 2,500.

So far as a safe level of thallium in drinking water is concerned, there does not seem to be any reasonable possibility that even the most thallium-polluted waters would have a toxic effect. In the worst case identified by Zitko et al (60-6) the concentration of thallium was 88 μg/l. Assuming that this were a human water supply, the daily input at 2 l/d would be only 176 μg Tl, 0.011 times the minimally toxic input calculated in this document.

Since there is a paucity of chronic data, including mutagenicity, teratogenicity and carcinogenicity, it seems prudent to keep exposure at or below their present levels. From the data, it would seem that few if any public water supplies would ever contain more than 4 μg/l. This seems a reasonable standard which would protect against gross excursions beyond the usual range of thallium in water, (0.1-1 μg/l). This also provides a safety factor of three orders of magnitude. Consumption of 2 l/d H_2O and 18.7 g of fish and shellfish products per day with an average BCF of 61 from ambient waters-containing 4 μg/l of thallium results in an intake of 12.56 μg Tl/day, compared to the estimated minimal toxic dose of 15,400 μg/d. In summary form, the dose-response scale for man is estimated to be as follows:

Dose

8 to 10 mg/kg	minimally lethal single dose
220 μg/kg/d	minimally toxic dose over a lifetime
1,000 μg/kg/d	category 3 safety factor recommended by NAS according to available data
4 μg/l H_2O	recommended standard
20 μg/70kg/d	thallium consumption @ 10 μg/l
1 μg/l	probable limit for >99% of U.S. tap waters
$\leq$ 1 μg/d	probable current level of daily adult thallium comsumption from drinking water
15.4 mg/d	acceptable total daily intake of thallium from air, water, and food

References

(60-1)   Lee, A.G., *The chemistry of thallium,* Amsterdam, Elsevier Publishing Co., (1971).

(60-2)   Zitko, V., "Toxicity and pollution potential of thallium." *Sci. Total Environ.* 4, 185 (1975).

(60-3)   Reed, D., et al, "Thallotoxicosis: acute manifestations and sequelae." *Jour. Am. Med. Assoc.* 188, 516 (1963).

(60-4)   Bank, W.J., et al, "Thallium poisoning." *Arch. Neurol.*, 26, 456 (1972).

(60-5)   Winel, M., "An international comparison of hygienic standards for chemicals in the work environ-
         ment," *Ambio,* 4, 34 (1975).

(60-6)   Zitko, V. et al, "Thallium: occurrence in the environment and toxicity to fish," *Bull. Environ.
         Contam. Toxicol.* 13, 23 (1975).

TOLUENE (#61)

Toluene C_7H_8 or $C_6H_5CH_3$, also referred to as toluol, methylbenzene, Methacide, and phenyl-
methane, is an aromatic hydrocarbon which is both volatile and flammable. The molecular
structure is distinguished from that of benzene by the substitution of a methyl group for
one hydrogen atom.

Occurrence: Although toluene is a volatile compound and has been shown to be readily
transferred from water surfaces to the atmosphere under ideal conditions, its transport and
persistence under environmental conditions is not well known. In the atmosphere, toluene
is subject to photochemical degradation to benzaldehyde and traces of peroxybenzoyl nitrate. It is known also that toluene can reenter the hydrosphere in rain.

Toluene has been detected in municipal finished water supplies at levels ranging from 0.1
$\mu g/l$ to 11 $\mu g/l$. The toluene metabolites benzaldehyde and benzoic acid, were also found
in finished water at concentrations up to 19 $\mu g/l$. Toluene is produced primarily from petroleum or petrochemical processes (96%), and on a small scale from metallurgical coke
manufacturing.

The total annual discharge of toluene to the environment by industry is estimated at
691,800 metric tons; 99.3% (686,960 kkg) is in the form of atmospheric emissions and
0.7% (4,840 kkg) as a constituent in wastewater.

Physical Properties: Toluene has a molecular weight of 92.13, a boiling point of 110.625°C,
freezing point of -94.9°C, specific gravity of 0.86694 at 20°C, vapor pressure of 30 mm Hg at
26.03°C, and a refractive index of 1.4893 at 24°C. Toluene is only slightly soluble in water,
534.8±4.9 mg/l in freshwater and 379.3±2.8 mg/l in seawater. It is miscible with alcohol,
chloroform, ether, acetone, glacial acetic acid, carbon disulfide and other organic solvents.

Chemical Properties: The nucleus of toluene, like that of benzene, undergoes substitution
reactions. Substitution occurs almost exclusively in the orthro (2) and para (4) positions
and occurs faster with toluene than with benzene. The presence of a methyl group offers
additional possibilities for reaction; the most important is dealkylation to produce benzene.
Hydrogenation of toluene takes place readily to form methylcyclohexane. Toluene may be
oxidized with air in the presence of manganese or cobalt naphthenates to form benzoic acid;
controlled chlorination of toluene yields benzyl dichloride which may be hydrolized to
benzaldehyde. Most reactions, however, require specialized conditions and are carried out
commercially.

Uses: The production of toluene in the United States has increased steadily since 1940
when approximately 31 million gallons were produced: in 1970, production was 694
million gallons. Approximately 70% of the toluene produced is converted to benzene, another 15% is used to produce chemicals, and the remainder is used as a solvent for paints
and as a gasoline component.

Toxic Effects: Freshwater aquatic studies indicate that toluene is toxic to goldfish, *Caras-
sius auratus,* fatheads, *Pimephales promelas,* bluegill, *Lepomis macrochirus,* and guppies,
Poecilia reticulata. Toxicity data for several species of freshwater algae have demonstrated
that they are more resistant to toluene than fish. Several marine studies indicate that
toluene is toxic to marine bacteria (interfering with chemoreception and chemotaxis), phy-
toplankton, *Artemia,* and marine fish (coho salmon, *Oncorhyncus kisutch).*

The effect of inhaled toluene on workers who had been subjected to chronic exposure
to toluene vapor in numerous industrial plants has been reported. The effects of toluene
inhalation include decreased phagocytic activity of leukocytes, depression of the central
nervous system, narcosis, addiction and even death at high levels. Animal studies have
demonstrated similar effects.

Current Levels of Exposure: Toluene has been detected in raw water and in finished water
supplies of several communities in the United States. Levels of up to 11 μg/l were found
in finished water from the New Orleans area. In a nationwide survey of water supplies from
ten cities in 1975, six were discovered to be contaminated with toluene.

Concentrations of 0.1 and 0.7 μg/l were measured in two of these water supplies. Toluene
was detected in 1 of 111 communities' finished drinking waters during a second nationwide
survey. In a subsequent phase of this survey in 1977, toluene was found in one raw water
and three finished waters out of 11 surveyed. A level of 19 μg/l measured by gas chroma-
tography/mass spectrometry, was found in one of these finished waters, and 0.5 μg/l was
found in another.

There is a paucity of data available on levels of toluene in foods. Toluene has been detected
in fish caught from polluted waters in the proximity of petroleum and petrochemical plants
in Japan. A concentration of 5 μg/g was measured in the muscle of one such fish. Two
major metabolites of toluene, benzaldehyde and benzoic acid, naturally occur in foods or
are intentionally added. Benzaldehyde is a flavoring agent, while benzoic acid is a preservative. Benzoic acid is also given in large oral doses to humans as a clinical method for
measuring liver function.

Although toluene has been detected in the atmosphere, concentrations are many times
lower than vapor levels considered to be potentially harmful in occupational settings. An
atmospheric concentration of 39 ppb toluene was measured in Zurich, Switzerland. An
average level of 37 ppb toluene was observed in Los Angeles air in 1966. The maximum
amount detected there was 129 ppb. Comparable levels were found upon evaluation of
air in Toronto, Canada. The maximum concentration of toluene measured in Toronto was
188 ppb, while the average concentration was 30 ppb. The atmospheric levels of toluene
in both Toronto and Los Angeles varied considerably according to the time of day and
sampling location. Thus, it appears that atmospheric toluene in urban areas arises primarily
from automotive emissions, with solvent losses as a secondary source.

The most significant toluene inhalation exposures occur in occupational and inhalant abuse
settings. Occupational exposure levels are generally lower than the current standard of
100 ppm, although short exposures to higher vapor concentrations occur. Purposeful inhalation of toluene vapors in order to inebriate oneself is a quite different situation, since
the participant may inhale extremely high concentrations repeatedly for months or years.
Toluene concentrations as high as 20,000 to 30,000 ppm can produce intoxication within
minutes under such circumstances.

Special Groups at Risk: At present levels of exposure to toluene in the environment, available toxicological data do not suggest that any special group in the general population
would be at risk. Exposure to levels of the chemical necessary to produce physiological or
toxicological effects would be anticipated primarily in occupational or solvent abuse situations. Environmental contribution of toluene in such settings should be minimal.

Existing Guidelines and Standards: The only current guideline for toluene exposure has
been established to prevent adverse health effects from the chemical in occupational settings.
The present standard is 100 ppm (375 mg/m^3), determined as a time-weighted average exposure for an eight hour workday, with a ceiling of 200 ppm (61-1). Skin and eye exposure is to be minimized. This standard was set primarily on the basis of subjective and
objective signs of mucus membrane irritation and deficits in central nervous system function upon acute inhalation exposure of human subjects to 200 ppm toluene. Short-term
inhalation of 100 ppm was apparently without demonstrable effect in humans. Reports

reviewed by the National Institute for Occupational Safety and Health (61-1) also have failed to indicate adverse effects on the hematopoietic, hepatorenal, or other systems of workers routinely inhaling approximately 100 ppm toluene.

A review of potentially harmful effects of chemical contaminants of drinking water was undertaken by the Committee on Safe Drinking Water of the National Academy of Sciences (61-2). The recommendations of this committee were to be used by the U.S. EPA as the scientific basis for revision or ratification of the Interim Primary Drinking Water Regulations promulgated under the Safe Drinking Water Act of 1974. Toluene was one of the organic chemicals considered here.

Although it was concluded that toluene and its major metabolite, benzoic acid, were relatively nontoxic, the committee felt there was insufficient toxicological data available to serve as a basis for setting a long-term ingestion standard. It was recommended that studies be conducted to produce relevant information. Toluene has recently been considered for a second time by a reorganized Toxicology Subcommittee of the Safe Drinking Water Committee of the National Academy of Sciences. Results of the deliberations of this group have not yet been made public. There are no Federal or State guidelines, nor standards for general atmospheric pollution by toluene.

Summary of Proposed EPA Criteria: *Freshwater Aquatic Life* — The data base for freshwater aquatic life is insufficient to allow use of the Guidelines. The following recommendation is inferred from toxicity data for saltwater organisms.

For toluene the criterion to protect freshwater aquatic life as derived using procedures other than the Guidelines is 2,300 μg/l as a 24 hr average and the concentration should not exceed 5,200 μg/l at any time.

Saltwater Aquatic Life — For toluene the criterion to protect saltwater aquatic life as derived using the Guidelines is 100 μg/l as a 24 hr average and the concentration should not exceed 230 μg/l at any time.

Human Health — For the protection of human health from the toxic properties of toluene ingested through water and through contaminated aquatic organisms, the ambient water criterion is determined to be 12.4 mg/l.

Basis for the Proposed Human Health Criteria: Although acute exposure to high levels of toluene can result in marked central nervous system depression, this action is rapidly reversible upon cessation of exposure in both laboratory animals (61-3) and in man (61-4). When administered acutely in quite large doses to animals, toluene can alter the metabolism and bioactivity of certain chemicals which are degraded by the mixed function oxidase system. Toluene appears to have little capacity to cause residual tissue injury.

There is no conclusive evidence that the parent compound or its metabolites are mutagenic, although they have apparently not been tested in an *in vitro* mutagenicity assay (61-5). Toluene has not been found to be teratogenic in laboratory animals (61-6)(61-7).

Toluene has not been demonstrated to be carcinogenic when applied to the skin of mice (61-8)(61-9) or when administered by inhalation at concentrations of up to 300 ppm for as long as 18 months to male and female rats. There are no accounts in the literature in which cancer in a human population is attributed specifically to toluene.

A number of investigations of the subacute and chronic toxicity of toluene have been carried out. Although the majority of emphasis has been placed upon inhalation exposure, Wolf, et al (61-11) did conduct a long-term, oral dosing study in which female rats were given 118, 354, and 590 mg/kg of toluene in olive oil by stomach tube 5 times weekly for 193 days. No adverse effects on growth, appearance and behavior, mortality, organ/body weights, blood urea nitrogen levels, bone marrow counts, peripheral blood counts, or morphology of major organs were observed at any dose level. The lack of toxicity reported here is supported by findings of other groups of investigators who found no evidence of residual injury in a variety of animal species subjected to toluene vapors for varying times over periods as long as 18 months (61-10)(61-12)(61-13)(61-14)(61-15).

Therefore, if seems reasonable that the highest dose utilized by Wolf, et al (61-11), namely 590 mg/kg, might serve as the basis for calculating an "Acceptable Daily Intake" for toluene. Although 590 mg/kg will be considered here as a "maximum-no-effect" dose, it should be recognized that the actual "maximum-no-effect" dose may be higher, since Wolf, et al (61-11) did not determine a "minimum-toxic-dose." Reynolds and Yee (61-16) saw no effect on several parameters of hepatotoxicity in rats given a single oral dose of 2.4 g/kg toluene. The oral, acute LD_{50} for toluene in young, adult rats is reported to be 7.0 g/kg (61-11).

It is possible that the actual "maximum-no-effect" dose may be lower than 590 mg/kg, should alternative indices for toxicity be evaluated. Man may prove to be more sensitive to toluene than experimental animals. Thus, assuming a 70 kg body weight, it seems appropriate that a safety factor of 1,000 be applied in the following calculation.

$$\frac{590 \text{ mg/kg} \times 70 \text{ kg} \times {}^{5/7} \text{ day}}{1,000} = 29.5 \text{ mg/day}$$

Therefore, consumption of 2 liters of water daily and 18.7 g of contaminated fish having a bio-concentration factor of 20, would result in, assuming 100% gastrointestinal absorption of toluene, a maximum permissible concentration of 12.4 mg/l for the ingested water:

$$\frac{29.5 \text{ mg/day}}{2 \text{ liters} + (20 \times 0.0187) \times 1.0} = 12.4 \text{ mg/l}$$

References

(61-1) National Inst. for Occup. Safety and Health, *Criteria for a Recommended Standard: Occupational Exposure to Toluene,* NIOSH Doc. No. 73-11023 (1973).

(61-2) National Academy of Sciences, *Drinking Waters and Health,* Wash., D.C. (1977).

(61-3) Peterson, R.G. and Bruckner, J.V., "Measurement of toluene levels in animal tissues," *Proc. Int. Symp. Deliberate Inhalation of Industrial Solvents,* Mexico City (1976).

(61-4) Longley, E.O. et al, "Two acute toluene episodes in merchant ships," *Arch. Environ. Health* 14, 481 (1967).

(61-5) Dean, B.J., "Genetic toxicology of benzene, toluene, xylenes and phenols," *Mutat. Res.* 47, 75 (1978).

(61-6) Roche, S.M. and Hine, C.H., "The teratogenicity of source industrial chemicals," *Toxicol. Appl. Pharmacol,* 12, 327 (1968).

(61-7) Hudak, A. and Ungvary, G., "Embryotoxic effects of benzene and its methyl derivatives: toluene and xylene," *Toxicology* 11, 55 (1978).

(61-8) Poel, W.E., *Skin as a Test Site for the Bioassay of Carcinogens and Carcinogen Precursors,* Nat. Cancer Inst. Monographs 10, 611 (1963).

(61-9) Doak, S.M.A. et al, "The carcinogenic response in mice to the topical application of propane sultone to the skin," *Toxicology* 6, 139 (1976).

(61-10) Gibson, J.E., *Two-Year Vapor Inhalation Toxicity Study With Toluene in Fischer-344 Albino Rats: 18 Month Status Summary,* Research Triangle Park, N.C., Chemical Industry Institute of Technology (1979).

(61-11) Wolf, M.A. et al, "Toxicological studies of certain alkylated benzenes and benzene," *Arch. Ind. Health,* 14, 387 (1956).

(61-12) Jenkins, L.J., Jr. et al, "Long-term inhalation screening studies of benzene, toluene, o-xylene and cumene on experimental animals," *Toxicol. Appl. Pharmacol.* 16, 818 (1970).

(61-13) Carpenter, C.P. et al, "Petroleum hydrocarbon toxicity studies, XIII, animal and human response to vapors of toluene concentrate," *Toxicol. Appl. Pharmacol.* 36, 473 (1976).

(61-14) Bruckner, J.V. and Peterson, R.G., "Evaluation of toluene toxicity utilizing the mouse as an animal model of solvent abuse," *Pharmacologist* 18, 244 (1976).

(61-15) Rhudy, R.L. et al, "Ninety-day subacute inhalation study with toluene in albino rats," *Toxicol. Appl. Phamacol.* 45, 284 (1978).

(61-16) Reynolds, E.S. and Yee, A.G., "Liver parenchymal cell injury, VI, significance of early glucose-6-phosphatase suppression and transient calcium influx following poisoning," *Lab. Invest.* 19, 273 (1968).

TOXAPHENE (#62)

Toxaphene is a chlorinated camphene insecticide which has a formula which approximates $C_{10}H_{10}Cl_8$ and which has a structure of the following type:

$$
\begin{array}{c}
\text{Cl} \\
\text{Cl} \quad \text{Cl} \\
\text{Cl--} \quad \quad \text{--CH}_2\text{Cl} \\
\text{CHCl} \\
\text{Cl--} \quad \quad \text{--CH}_2\text{Cl} \\
\text{CH}_3 \\
\text{Cl}
\end{array}
$$

Occurrence: Toxaphene is commercially produced by reacting camphene with chlorine in the presence of ultraviolet radiation and certain catalysts to yield chlorinated camphene with a chlorine content of 67 to 69%. The chlorine content of the commercial product is limited to this narrow range since the insecticidal activity peaks sharply at those percentage levels. Toxaphene is available in various formulations as an emulsifiable concentrate, wettable powder, or dust.

When dispersed in natural water systems, toxaphene tends to be adsorbed by the particulates present or to be taken up by living organisms and bioconcentrated. Thus, it is seldom found at high levels as a soluble component in receiving waters but can persist in sediments or remain adsorbed on suspended solids for prolonged periods.

Physical Properties: Toxaphene is an amber, waxy solid with a mild terpene odor, a melting point range of 65° to 90°C, a vapor pressure 0.17 to 0.40 mm Hg at 25°C, and a density of 1.64 at 25°C. Toxaphene has a solubility in water of approximately 0.4 to 3.0 mg/l and is readily soluble in relatively nonpolar solvents, with an octanol/water partition coefficient of 825. Others have reported a toxaphene partition coefficient value of 3,300. Gas chromatographic analysis suggests the presence of approximately 177 components in technical toxaphene. Infrared absorptivity at 7.2 microns aids in distinguishing toxaphene from other chlorinated terpene products such as Strobane. Althrough tricyclene may accompany the camphene, the commercial mixture contains less than 5% of other terpenes.

Chemical Properties: The commercial product is relatively stable but may dehydrochlorinate upon prolonged exposure to sunlight, alkali, or temperatures above 120°C.

Uses: Toxaphene is a commercially produced, broad spectrum, chlorinated hydrocarbon pesticide. It was introduced in the United States in 1948 as a contact insecticide under various trade names and is currently the most heavily used insecticide in the United States, having replaced many of the agricultural applications of DDT, for which registration has been cancelled. Annual production of toxaphene exceeds 100 million pounds, with primary usage in agricultural crop application, mainly cotton.

Toxic Effects: Toxaphene has demonstrated carcinogenic effects in laboratory animals. In addition, toxaphene is highly toxic to many aquatic invertebrate and vertebrate species and has been shown to cause the "broken back syndrome" in fish fry. These observations, together with reported bioconcentration factors as high as 91,000 indicate that toxaphene poses a threat to living organisms, particularly in the aquatic environment. On May 25, 1977, the U.S. EPA issued a notice of rebuttable presumption against registration and continued registration of pesticide products containing toxaphene.

Current Levels of Exposure: Quantitative estimates of human exposure to toxaphene are extremely difficult to make based on the data available. The three major obstacles are: (1) the wide variation in toxaphene concentrations noted in food, water, and air; (2) conflicting information concerning the trend of toxaphene residues in food; and (3) the marked seasonal and geographic difference in toxaphene concentrations found in air and food. Given these problems, a conservative approach in estimating exposure to toxaphene is necessary.

The best available estimate of dietary intake is 0.021 μg/kg/day, based on the U.S. Food and Drug Administration market basket surveys between 1964 and 1970 (62-1). Although more recent market basket surveys indicate a decrease in the incidence of toxaphene contamination and the U.S. Department of Agriculture survey suggests that the incidence of toxaphene contamination of raw meat has remained relatively stable since 1969, the U.S. Food and Drug Administration survey of unprocessed food samples shows an almost two-fold increase in the incidence of toxaphene contamination between 1972 and 1976. Given this conflicting information, the current dietary intake is estimated to be 0.042 μg/kg/day, twice that noted by Duggan and Corneliussen (62-1).

No satisfactory estimate can be made of average national inhalation exposures. In areas where toxaphene is not used, inhalation exposure may be negligible. Even in areas of high use, the apparent low absorption of toxaphene across the lungs suggests that inhalation may not be a significant source of exposure. These admittedly tenuous exposure estimates are summarized as follows:

Source	Estimate Intake
Water	no estimate
Food	0 042 μg/kg/day
Air	0

Special Groups at Risk: Individuals working with toxaphene or living in areas where toxaphene is used or produced would seem to be at higher risk than the general population. However, an increased incidence of chromosomal aberration has not been noted in groups with occupational exposure to toxaphene (U.S. EPA, 1978). Further, of 32 samples of human adipose tissue obtained from autopsy or surgery cases in areas of high toxaphene usage, only one sample contained detectable levels of toxaphene (0.13 ppm). This sample was from an individual who lived in the Mississippi Delta, an area of high toxaphene use, and who therefore potentially was exposed to toxaphene through agricultural use (62-2). Thus, there is no firm data to support the assumption that individuals living in high use areas or individuals with occupational exposure to toxaphene are at greater risk than the general population.

Existing Guidelines and Standards: Standards for toxaphene in air, water, and food have been established or recommended by groups within the United States, international agencies, and agencies of other governments. All these standards were set before the results of the National Cancer Institute bioassay of toxaphene for carcinogenicity (62-3) were available.

Both the Occupational Safety and Health Administration and the American Conference of Governmental Industrial Hygienists have established a time-weighted average value of 500 μg/m^3 for toxaphene in the air of the working environment. The American Conference of Governmental Industrial Hygienists based this standard on unpublished acute and chronic toxicity studies conducted in the 1950's and on comparisons of the toxicity of toxaphene with DDT and lindane. A tentative short-term exposure limit for toxaphene has been set at 2.0 mg/m^3 as of 1979.

The national interim primary drinking water standard for toxaphene is 5 μg/l. This standard is based on the reported organoleptic effects of toxaphene at concentrations above 5 μg/l. A standard of 25 μg/l was also calculated based on a concentration of 10 mg/kg in the diet, which was estimated to give an average daily dose of 1 mg/kg body weight, as the lowest long-term level with minimal or no effects in rats. This standard was calculated using the following assumptions:

Weight of rat	300 g
Daily food consumption of rat	50 g
Weight of average human adult	70 kg
Average daily water intake for man	2 l
Safety factor	1/500
Dietary intake, trace	

From these assumptions, the maximum safe daily dose for humans was estimated to be 3.4 μg/kg body weight. It should be noted, however, that the assumption of 50 g daily food consumption for a 300 g rat is probably excessively high.

Based on a study by Fitzhugh and Nelson (62-4), in which rats evidenced increased liver weight and hepatic cell enlargement after exposure to toxaphene at 25 mg/kg diet for two years, the acceptable daily intake for man has been estimated at 1.25 μg/kg (62-5). This is based on (1) the estimate that the daily dose in rats during the Fitzhugh and Nelson study was equivalent to 1.25 mg/kg body weight and (2) the application of a safety factor of 1,000. Assuming a human body weight of 70 kg and a daily water consumption of 2 liters, the suggested no-adverse effect level from water was set at 8.75 μg/l (assigning 20% of the total ADI to water) or 0.44 μg/l (assigning 1% of the total ADI to water). Effluent standards for toxaphene manufacturers have been set at 1.5 μg/l for existing facilities and 0.1 μg/l for new facilities by the EPA in 1976.

Tolerances established by the U.S. Food and Drug Administration for toxaphene residues in various agricultural products are as follows:

Product	Residue Level (mg/kg)
Fat of meat from cattle, goats, and sheep	7
Fat of meat from hogs	7
Fat of meat from horses	7
Cranberries, hazelnuts, hickory nuts, horseradish, parsnips, pecans, peppers, pimentos, rutabagas, walnuts	7
Collards, kale, spinach	7
Crude soybean oil	6
Barley, oats, rice, rye, and wheat	5
Sorghum grain	5
Cottonseed	5
Pineapple and bananas*	3
Soybeans, dry form	2
Sunflower seeds	0 1

*of which not more than 0.3 mg/kg shall be in pulp after the peel is removed and discarded.

In Canada, the tolerance for toxaphene in citrus fruits is 7.0 mg/kg. In both the Netherlands and West Germany, the corresponding standard is 0.4 mg/kg. The World Health Organization has not yet established an acceptable daily intake level for toxaphene. The following information is considered necessary by WHO before an acceptable daily intake can be established:

(1) Adequate toxicological information on camphechlor (toxaphene) as currently marketed, including a carcinogenicity study.

(2) Comparative studies evaluating the toxicological hazard associated with polychlorinated camphene of different manufacture used in worldwide agriculture.

(3) Before recommendations can be made concerning residues from the use of camphechlor, other than that conforming to FAO specifications, information is needed on the composition, uses, and residues arising from such products.

The following guideline levels for toxaphene in specified foods have been recommended by WHO (62-6).

Food	Toxaphene Level (mg/kg)
Fat of meat of cattle, sheep, goats, and pigs	5

(continued)

Food	Toxaphene Level (mg/kg)
Broccoli, brussels sprouts, cabbage, celery, collards, eggplant, kale, kohlrabi, lettuce, okra, peppers, pimentos, spinach, tomatoes, barley, rice (rough), rye, sorghum, bananas (whole), pineapple, beans (snap, dry, lima), peas, cauliflower, oats, wheat, shelled nuts, carrots, onions, parsnips, radishes, rutabagas	2
Soybeans, peanuts (ground-nut), cottonseed oil (refined), rapeseed oil (refined), soybean oil (refined), peanut oil (refined), maize, rice (finished)	0.5
Milk and milk products (fat basis)	0.5

These recommendations are based on levels which might be expected if good application practices are followed and do not reflect a judgement concerning potential human hazard.

The International Joint Commission of the United States and Canada has recommended a water standard of 0.008 μg/l for the protection of aquatic life. This standard is based on a study which found that toxaphene at 0.039 μg/l caused a significant increase in mortality and a significant decrease in growth in brook trout fry over a 90 day period. The standard of 0.008 μg/l is obtained by applying a safety factor of 0.2.

Summary of Proposed EPA Criteria: *Freshwater Aquatic Life* – For toxaphene the criterion to protect freshwater aquatic life as derived using the Guidelines is 0.007 μg/l as a 24 hr average and the concentration should not exceed 0.47 μg/l at any time.

Saltwater Aquatic Life – For toxaphene the criterion to protect saltwater aquatic life as derived using the Guidelines is 0.019 μg/l as a 24 hr average and the concentration should not exceed 0.12 μg/l at any time.

Human Health – For the maximum protection of human health from the potential carcinogenic effects of exposure to toxaphene through ingestion of water and contaminated aquatic organisms, the ambient water concentration is zero. Concentrations of toxaphene estimated to result in additional lifetime cancer risks ranging from no additional risk to an additional risk of 1 in 100,000 are presented in the Criterion Formulation section of this document. The EPA is considering setting criteria at an interim target risk level in the range of 10^{-5}, 10^{-6}, or 10^{-7}, with corresponding criteria of 4.7×10^{-4} μg/l, 4.7×10^{-5} μg/l, or 4.7×10^{-6} μg/l respectively.

Basis for the Proposed Human Health Criteria: Various water concentrations of toxaphene have been recommended to protect man and aquatic organisms from the organoleptic or toxic properties of this compound. These concentrations with the accompanying rationale are summarized below:

Rationale	Level (μg/l)
Organoleptic effects	5.0
Noncarcinogenic mammalian toxicity	2.5
Noncarcinogenic mammalian toxicity	8.75
Noncarcinogenic mammalian toxicity	0.44
Aquatic toxicity data	0.008

Additionally, carcinogenic responses have been induced in mice and rats by toxaphene (62-3). These results, together with the positive mutagenic response, constitute substantial evidence that toxaphene is likely to be a human carcinogen.

Estimated criterion levels for toxaphene in water can be calculated using the linear, non-threshold model and the results of the National Cancer Institute bioassay of toxaphene for carcinogenicity.

Under the Consent Decree in *NRDC vs Train,* criteria are to state "recommended maximum permissible concentrations (including where appropriate, zero) consistent with the protection of aquatic organisms, human health, and recreational activities." Toxaphene is suspected of being a human carcinogen. Because there is no recognized safe concentration for human carcinogens, the recommended concentration of toxaphene in water for maximum protection of human health is zero.

Because attaining a zero concentration level may be infeasible in some cases and in order to assist the EPA and States in the possible future development of water quality regulations, the concentrations of toxaphene corresponding to several incremental lifetime cancer risk levels have been estimated. A cancer risk level provides an estimate of the additional incidence of cancer that may be expected in an exposed population. A risk of 10^{-5} for example, indicates a probability of one additional case of cancer for every 100,000 people exposed, a risk of 10^{-6} indicates one additional case of cancer for every million people exposed, and so forth.

In the *Federal Register* notice of availability of draft ambient water quality criteria, EPA stated that it is considering setting criteria at an interim target risk level of 10^{-5}, 10^{-6} or 10^{-7} as shown in Table 88. In the table below risk levels and corresponding criteria are calculated by applying a modified "one hit" extrapolation model described in the *FR* 15926, 1979. Since the extrapolation model is linear at low doses, the additional lifetime risk is directly proportional to the water concentration. Therefore, water concentrations corresponding to other risk levels can be derived by multiplying or dividing one of the risk levels and corresponding water concentrations shown in the table by factors such as 10, 100, 1,000, and so forth.

Table 88: Possible Alternative Criteria for Toxaphene

Exposure Assumptions (per Day)	Risk Levels and Corresponding Criteria			
	0	10^{-7}	10^{-6}	10^{-5}
	. . . . (ng/l)			
2 liters of drinking water and consumption of 18.7 grams fish and shellfish*	0	0.005	0.05	0.5
Consumption of fish and shellfish only	0	0.005	0.05	0.5

*99% of the toxaphene exposure results from the consumption of aquatic organisms which exhibit an average bioconcentration potential of 18,000 fold. The remaining percent of toxaphene exposure results from drinking water.

Source: Reference (62)

Concentration levels were derived assuming a lifetime exposure to various amounts of toxaphene, (1) occurring from the consumption of both drinking water and aquatic life grown in water containing the corresponding toxaphene concentrations and (2) occurring solely from consumption of aquatic life grown in the waters containing the corresponding toxaphene concentrations.

Although total exposure information for toxaphene is discussed and an estimate of the contributions from other sources of exposure can be made, this data will not be factored into ambient water quality criteria formulation because of the tenuous estimates and the conflicting information regarding the trend of toxaphene residues in food until additional analysis can be made. The criteria presented, therefore, assume an incremental risk from ambient water exposure only.

Summary of Pertinent Data — The water quality criterion for toxaphene is derived from the development of hepatocellular carcinomas and neoplastic nodules in the BCF male mice given the low dose of toxaphene in the NCI bioassay study. In that group, a time-weighted average dose of 99 ppm was administered in the diet for 80 weeks and the animals were observed for additional 10 weeks before terminal sacrifice. The incidence of hepatocellular carcinomas and neoplastic nodules was 7/48 and 40/49 in the pooled control and treated groups, respectively. Assuming a fish bioconcentration factor of 18,000, the criterion is calculated from the following parameters:

$$
\begin{aligned}
nt &= 40 \\
Nt &= 49 \\
nc &= 7 \\
Nc &= 48 \\
Le &= 900 \text{ days} \\
le &= 665 \text{ days} \\
d &= 99 \text{ ppm} \times 0.136 = 13.50 \text{ mg/kg/day} \\
w &= 0.033 \text{ kg} \\
L &= 900 \text{ days} \\
R &= 18,000 \\
F &= 0.0187 \text{ kg/day}
\end{aligned}
$$

Based on these parameters, the one-hit slope (B_H) is 4.42 (mg/kg/day). The resulting water concentrations of toxaphene calculated to keep the individual risk below 10^{-5}, is 4.7×10^{-4} micrograms/liter.

References

(62-1)   Duggan, R.E. and Corneliussen, P.E., "Dietary intake of pesticide chemicals in the United States (III) June 1968-April 1970 (with summary of 1965-1970)." *Pestic. Monitor Jour.* 5, 331 (1972)

(62-2)   U.S. Environmental Protection Agency, *Occupational Exposure to Toxaphene,* Final Report by The Epidemiological Study Program, Wash., D.C., Office of Toxic Substances (1978).

(62-3)   National Cancer Institute, *Bioassay of Toxaphene for Possible Carcinogenicity,* DHEW Publ. No. (NIH) 73-837 (1979).

(62-4)   Fitzhugh, O.G. and Nelson, A.A., "Comparison of chronic effects produced in rats by several chlorinated hydrocarbon insecticides," *Fed. Proc.* 10, 295 (1951).

(62-5)   National Academy of Sciences, *Drinking Water and Health,* Wash., D.C. (1977).

(62-6)   World Health Organization, *Evaluation of Some Pesticide Residues in Foods: Camphechlor.,* Pesticide Residue Series, No. 3 (1974).

1,2-TRANS-DICHLOROETHYLENE

See "Dichloroethylenes" (27).

1,2,4-TRICHLOROBENZENE

See "Chlorinated Benzenes" (14).

1,1,1-TRICHLOROETHANE

See "Chlorinated Ethanes" (15).

1,1,2-TRICHLOROETHANE

See "Chlorinated Ethanes" (15).

TRICHLOROETHYLENE (#63)

Trichloroethylene (1,1,2-trichloroethylene; TCE) is a clear colorless liquid, characterized by the formula C_2HCl_3, or $Cl_2C{=}CHCl$.

Occurrence: Annual production of TCE in the United States approximates 234,000 metric tons. The volatilization of TCE during production and use is the major source of environmental levels of this compound. TCE has been detected in air, in food, and in human tissues (63-1). Its detection in rivers, municipal water supplies, the sea, and aquatic organisms indicates that TCE is widely distributed in the aquatic environment (63-1)(63-2).

Physical Properties: TCE has a molecular weight of 131.4; a water solubility of 1,000 $\mu g/ml$; a vapor pressure of 77 mm Hg at 25°C and a melting point of −83°C. The experimentally determined logarithm of the octanol/water partition coefficient (log P) for TCE is 2.29, which indicates that it may bioaccumulate. Its relative chemical stability, non-flammability, volatility and poor water solubility make TCE a very useful solvent.

Chemical Properties: TCE is not expected to persist in the environment because of its rapid photooxidation in air, its low water solubility and its volatility. Decomposition of trichloroethylene, due to contact with hot metal or ultraviolet radiation, forms products including chlorine gas, hydrogen chloride, and phosgene. Dichloroacetylene may be formed from the reaction of alkali with trichloroethylene.

Uses: TCE is used mainly as a degreasing solvent in metal industries. It also has been used as a household and industrial drycleaning solvent, an extractive solvent in foods, (in extraction of caffeine from coffee) and as an inhalation anesthetic during certain short-term surgical procedures.

Toxic Effects: Under laboratory conditions, TCE has been shown to be toxic to fish (63-1) (63-3)(63-4). The acute toxicity of TCE in mammals is manifested primarily by depression of the central nervous system (63-5). In addition to the neurological effects in humans and experimental animals, TCE produces liver damage. Severe and persistent toxicity to the liver was recently demonstrated when TCE was shown to produce carcinoma of the liver in mouse strain B6C3FI (63-6). This finding has created additional concern about the toxicity of TCE.

Current Levels of Exposure: It was estimated by NIOSH in 1973 (63-8) that 200,000 workers are potentially exposed to trichloroethylene and that many of these exposures are in small workplaces. In 1978, this estimate was revised to 100,000 full-time exposures to TCE with up to 3.5 million more workers subjected to continuous low levels or to brief exposures of various levels.

Special Groups at Risk: The most serious known exposures of humans to TCE occur in the industrial populations that manufacture or use the compound. A partial list of occupations in which exposure may occur includes:

Anesthetic makers	Metal cleaners
Caffeine processors	Oil processors
Cleaners	Perfume makers
Disinfectant makers	Printers
Degreasers	Resin workers
Drug makers	Rubber cementers
Drycleaners	Shoe makers
Dye makers	Soap makers
Electronic equipment cleaners	Solvent workers
Fat processors	Textile cleaners
Glass cleaners	Tobacco denicotinizers
Mechanics	Varnish workers

Existing Guidelines and Standards: Trichloroethylene has been regulated primarily from the industrial health standpoint. Concentrations allowed in the working environment vary widely in different countries (Table 89). Because of use of TCE in decaffeinating coffee and the extraction of spice oleoresins, the Food and Drug Administration has limited concentrations of TCE that may be allowed in the final product. These limits are 10 mg/kg in spice extracts.

The presently established (1978) American Conference of Governmental Industrial Hygienists (ACGIH) TLV has been established entirely on the basis of short-term exposures of healthy male volunteers. This level has not taken into account the possibility of potential synergists present in the general environment or the possibility of sensitive populations. It has not yet incorporated consideration of TCE carcinogenicity indicated by recent NCI data (63-6). As can be seen in Table 89, industrial hygiene standards established by European countries are less than one-half that allowed in the U.S. The ACGIH (63-10) has in 1979 noted an intended change in TLV value from 100 ppm (535 mg/m^3) to 50 ppm (270 mg/m^3) however.

Table 89: Industrial Hygiene Standards for Trichloroethylene in Various Countries

	mg/m^3	Calculated Allowable Daily Exposure mg/day
USA	535	3,821
Sweden	160	1,143
Czechoslovakia	250	1,786
Federal Republic of Germany	260	1,857
German Democratic Republic	250	1,768
USSR	1	7

Source: Reference (63-7)

The National Inst. for Occup. Safety and Health in 1973 (63-8) cited a 100 ppm TWA value, together with a 200 ppm ceiling value and a 300 ppm maximum ceiling (for 5 min in any 2 hr). Then in 1978 (63-9), NIOSH issued a recommendation for a 25 ppm TWA value.

Summary of Proposed EPA Criteria: *Freshwater Aquatic Life* — For trichloroethylene the criterion to protect freshwater aquatic life (as derived using the Guidelines), is 1,500 µg/l at any time.

Saltwater Aquatic Life — For saltwater aquatic life, no criterion for trichloroethylene can be derived using the Guidelines, and there are insufficient data to estimate a criterion using other procedures.

Human Health — For the maximum protection of human health from the potential carcinogenic effects of exposure to trichloroethylene through ingestion of water and contaminated aquatic organisms, the ambient water concentration is zero. Concentrations of trichloroethylene estimated to result in additional lifetime cancer risks ranging from no additional risk to an additional risk of 1 in 100,000 are presented in the Criterion Formulation section of this document. The EPA is considering setting criteria at an interim target risk level in the range of 10^{-5}, 10^{-6}, or 10^{-7} with corresponding criteria of 21 µg/l, 2.1 µg/l, and 0.21 µg/l, respectively.

Basis for the Proposed Human Health Criteria: Under the Consent Decree in *NRDC vs Train,* criteria are to state "recommended maximum permissible concentrations (including where appropriate, zero) consistent with the protection of aquatic organisms, human health, and recreational activities." Trichloroethylene is suspected of being a human carcinogen. Because there is no recognized safe concentration for a human carcinogen, the recommended concentration of trichloroethylene in water for maximum protection of human health is zero.

Because attaining a zero concentration level may be infeasible in some cases and in order to assist the EPA and States in the possible future development of water quality regulations, the concentrations of trichloroethylene corresponding to several incremental lifetime cancer risk levels have been estimated. A cancer risk level provides an estimate of the additional incidence of cancer that may be expected in an exposed population. A risk of 10^{-5} for example, indicates a probability of one additional case of cancer for every 100,000 people exposed, a risk of 10^{-6} indicates one additional case of cancer for every million people exposed, and so forth.

In the *Federal Register* notice of availability of draft ambient water quality criteria, EPA stated that it is considering setting criteria at an interim target risk level of 10^{-5}, 10^{-6}, or 10^{-7} as shown in Table 90. In the table below risk levels and corresponding criteria are calculated by applying a modified "one-hit" extrapolation model described in the methodology section to the animal bioassay data presented in Summary of Pertinent Data. Since the extrapolation model is linear at low doses, the additional lifetime risk is directly proportional to the water concentration. Therefore, water concentrations corresponding to other risk levels can be derived by multiplying or dividing one of the risk levels and corresponding water concentrations shown in the table by factors such as 10, 100, 1,000, and so forth.

Table 90: Possible Alternative Criteria for Trichloroethylene

Exposure Assumption (per day)	Risk Levels and Corresponding Criteria			
	0	10^{-7}	10^{-6}	10^{-5}
			(μg/l)		
2 liters of drinking water and consumption of 18.7 g fish and shellfish*	0	0.21	2.1	21
Consumption of fish and shellfish only	0	0.78	7.8	78

*Approximately 27% of the trichloroethylene exposure results from the consumption of aquatic organisms which exhibit an average bioconcentration potential of 39-fold. The remaining 73% of trichloroethylene exposure results from drinking water.

Source: Reference (63)

Concentration levels were derived assuming a lifetime exposure to various amounts of trichloroethylene, (1) occurring from the consumption of both drinking water and aquatic life grown in waters containing the corresponding trichloroethylene concentrations and, (2) occurring solely from consumption of aquatic life grown in the waters containing the corresponding trichloroethylene concentrations. Because data indicating other sources of trichloroethylene exposure and their contributions to total body burden are inadequate for quantitative use, the figures reflect the incremental risks associated with the indicated routes only.

Summary of Pertinent Data — The NCI bioassay (63-6) with male mice at an average dose, administered by stomach tube of 1,169 mg/kg administered five times per week for 78 weeks is used. The experiment was terminated after 90 weeks. In matched control animals the incidence of hepatocellular carcinoma was $^{1}/_{20}$ and in treated animals it was $^{26}/_{50}$. The fish bioaccumulation factor is 39. The parameters of the extrapolation model are:

$$
\begin{aligned}
nt &= 26 \\
NT &= 50 \\
nc &= 1 \\
NC &= 20 \\
Le &= 90 \text{ weeks} \\
le &= 78 \text{ weeks} \\
d &= 1{,}169 \times {}^{5}/_{7} = 835 \text{ mg/kg/day} \\
w &= 0.034 \text{ kg} \\
L &= 90 \text{ weeks} \\
R &= 39
\end{aligned}
$$

The result is that the water concentration should be less than 21 μg/l in order to keep the individual lifetime risk below 10^{-5}.

References

(63-1) Pearson, C., and G. McConnell, "Chlorinated C_1 and C_2 hydrocarbons in the marine environment."
        Proc. R. Soc. London, B.-189, 305 (1975).

(63-2) McConnell, G., et al, "Chlorinated hydrocarbons and the environment." *Endeavour* 34, 13 (1975).

(63-3) Alexander, H., et al, "Toxicity of perchloroethylene, trichloroethylene, 1,1,1-trichloroethane, and
        methylene chloride to fathead minnows." *Bull. Environ. Contam. Toxicol.* 20:344, (1978).

(63-4) U.S. EPA, *In-depth studies on health and environmental impacts of selected water pollutants,*
        Report on Contract No. 68-01-4646, Wash, D.C. (1978).

(63-5) Stewart, R.D., et al, "Experimental human exposure to trichloroethylene." *Arch. Environ. Health*
        20, 64 (1970).

(63-6) National Cancer Institute, *Carcinogenesis bioassay of trichloroethylene.* CAS No. 79-01-6, NCI-
        CG-TR-2, Wash. D.C. (1976).

(63-7) Fishbein, L., "Industrial mutagens and potential mutagens; I, halogenated aliphatic derivatives,"
        Mut. Res. 32, 267 (1976).

(63-8) National Inst. for Occup. Safety and Health, *Criteria for a Recommended Standard: Occupational
        Exposure to Trichloroethylene,* NIOSH Doc. No. 73-11025, Wash, D.C. (1973).

(63-9) National Inst. for Occup. Safety and Health, *Special Occupational Hazard Review with Control
        Recommendations: Trichloroethylene,* NIOSH Doc. No. 78-130, Wash, D.C. (1978).

(63-10) Am. Conf. of Govt. Ind. Hygienists, *Threshold Limit Values for Chemical Substances in Workroom
        Air,* Cincinnati, Ohio (1979).

TRICHLOROFLUOROMETHANE

See "Halomethanes" (38).

TRICHLORONAPHTHALENES

See "Chlorinated Naphthalenes" (17).

2,4,6-TRICHLOROPHENOL

See "Chlorinated Phenols" (18).

TRINITROPHENOLS

See "Nitrophenols" (49).

V

VINYL CHLORIDE (#64)

Vinyl chloride, $CH_2=CHCl$, is one of the most important monomers. It is used worldwide for the production of polymers and copolymers containing polyvinyl chloride (PVC).

Occurrence: Vinyl chloride is not found in nature. It is synthesized as chlorinated olefinic hydrocarbon monomer derived from petrochemical feedstock and chlorine. As of 1974, approximately fifteen plants synthesized the vinyl chloride monomer, forty-three facilities were engaged in the polymerization of PVC and over 7,500 plants fabricated products from PVC. About 1,500 workers were employed in monomer synthesis and an additional 5,000 in polymerization operations (64-1). As many as 350,000 workers were estimated to be associated with fabrication plants. By 1976 it was estimated that nearly one million persons were associated with manufacturing goods derived from PVC (64-2).

Vinyl chloride levels ranging from barely detectable to high concentrations have been found in drinking water, beverages, food, cosmetics, and other consumer products. Aerosol products containing vinyl chloride as a propellant have been discontinued. However, inciner ators may be an additional source of vinyl chloride emissions since the entrapped monomer escapes following incomplete combustion of PVC products. Insufficient published data are available on exposure levels of persons living in the vicinity of PVC fabricating plants, or on the release of the monomer from various plastic products. However, all of these routes represent additional potential sources of population exposure (64-3).

The large quantities and widespread use of vinyl chloride in the production of PVC, together with recent evidence of occupational hazards resulting from polymerization operations has caused concern for the protection of workers and the environment. Thus far, the principal route of exposure to people working in or living near vinyl chloride industries is thought to be air inhalation. However, the discharge of water used in the polymerization process has become of increased importance as a source of contamination to the aquatic environment and exposure to the public in general. Additional exposure can occur via ingestion of contaminated food and through the skin.

Physical Properties: Vinyl chloride is a highly flammable chloroolefinic hydrocarbon which emits a sweet or pleasant odor and has a vapor density slightly more than twice that of air. It has a boiling point of $-13.9°C$ and a melting point of $-153.8°C$. Its solubility in water at $28°C$ is 0.11 g/100 g water and it is soluble in alcohol and very soluble in ether and carbon tetrachloride. Vinyl chloride is volatile and readily passes from solution into the gas phase under most laboratory and ecological conditions. Many salts such as soluble silver and copper salts, ferrous chloride, platinous chloride, iridium dichloride, and mercurous chloride to name a few, have the ability to form complexes with vinyl chloride which results in its increased solubility in water. Conversely, alkali metal salts such as sodium or potassium chloride may decrease the solubility of vinyl chloride in aqueous ionic strength of the solution. Therefore, the amounts of vinyl chloride in water could be influenced significantly by the presence of salts.

Chemical Properties: The primary reaction of consequence is the polymerization of vinyl chloride monomer which may be carried out in solution in organic solvent, suspension or emulsion in water, or in mass.

Uses: Vinyl chloride has been used for over forty years in producing polyvinyl chloride (PVC) which in turn is the most widely used material in the manufacture of plastics throughout the world. Of the estimated 18 billion pounds of vinyl chloride produced worldwide in 1972, about 25% was manufactured in the United States. Production of vinyl chloride in the United States reached slightly over 5 billion pounds in 1977. Production of vinyl chloride has risen nearly 14% annually between 1968 and 1973 as evidenced by the broad dependence of nearly every branch of industry and commercial activity upon products and components fabricated from polyvinyl chloride.

Vinyl chloride and polyvinyl chloride are used in the manufacture of numerous products in building and construction, the automotive industry, for electrical wire insulation and cables, piping, industrial and household equipment, packaging for food products, medical supplies, and is depended upon heavily by the rubber, paper and glass industries. Polyvinyl chloride and vinyl chloride copolymers are distributed and processed in a variety of forms including dry resins, plastisols (dispersions in plasticizers), organosols (dispersions in plasticizers plus volatile solvent), and latex (colloidal dispersion in water). Latexes are used to coat or impregnate paper, fabric, or leather.

Toxic Effects: There are no aquatic toxicity data available in the scientific literature at the present time. A combination of vinyl chloride's known toxicity via inhalation and its low water solubility makes testing this compound extremely dangerous and difficult. Vinyl chloride has been shown to be toxic to experimental animals and numerous studies have reported its carcinogenic effects in rats, mice, hamsters and rabbits. Vinyl chloride has been shown only recently to be an occupational hazard, resulting in the development of vinyl chloride disease. The disease represents a multisystem disorder incorporating acroosteolysis, a skin disorder characterized by Raynaud's phenomenon, thrombocytopenia, portal fibrosis, and hepatic and pulmonary dysfunction. In addition, there is evidence that workers involved in the polymerization of vinyl chloride monomer show a higher incidence of angiosarcoma, one of the rarest human malignant neoplasms (64-4).

Current Levels of Exposure: Insufficient information is available on the exposure levels and associated risk to man from vinyl chloride-contaminated water supplies. Toxicologic or epidemiologic data are not available in the up-to-date literature. From the available data, it is thought that the hazard is small in comparison to inhalation route of exposure.

Special Groups at Risk: In support of the proposed regulations, the U.S. EPA evaluated the risk to populations living in the vicinity of vinyl chloride and PVC plants in 1975 (64-5). A number of factors influenced the estimate of risk to this population, i.e., the number of persons living at distances up to five miles from vinyl chloride and PVC plants, published by the American Public Health Association (64-6), Table 91.

Table 91: Estimate of Exposed Population in the Vicinity of Vinyl Chloride and PVC Plants

Distance (miles)	Population
0–½	47,000
½–1	203,000
1–3	1,491,000
3–5	2,838,000
Total	4,579,000

Source: Reference (64-6) quoted in Reference (64)

The average exposure of a person chosen at random living in the 5-mile radius was calculated to be 17 ppb. The total number of persons at risk was estimated at 4.6 million. Using standard diffusion models, the annual average ambient concentrations of vinyl chloride were calculated for distances 0 to 0.5; 0.5 to 1.0; 1.0 to 3.0; and 3.0 to 5.0 miles from the plants (Table 92). Quantitative estimates of potential effects which may result from this exposure level were performed using animal data fitted by two different models, the "linear" and "probit" models.

Table 92: Annual Average Concentrations of Vinyl Chloride in the Vicinity of a Vinyl Chloride and PVC Plant

Distance (miles)	Vinyl Chloride Concentration (ppb)	
	PVC Plant	VC Plant
0-½	323	113
½-1	57	20
1-3	15	5.2
3-5	5.7	2.0

Source: Reference (64-5) quoted in Reference (64)

Data published by Maltoni and Lefemine in 1975 (64-7) which reported liver hemangio-sarcoma induction in rats due to vinyl chloride inhalation, were used for calculation of the probability of angiosarcoma cases in highly exposed populations of workers. This predic-tion was tested using epidemiological studies of workers and projecting the results to am-bient air concentrations of vinyl chloride in the vicinity of the plants. Incidence rates of hemangiosarcoma in rats were compared to incidence rates in exposed workers with the assumption that a long-term exposure of rats would produce the same incidence of effects as a long-term exposure of humans. In this instance, the incidence rate following one-year exposure of rats would compare to the incidence of thirty years of human exposure.

In treatment of experimental animal dose-response data, two mathematical models are quoted most often in literature reports: the "linear" or "one-hit" model and the "log-probit" model which is closely related to the Mantel-Bryan proposed data treatment (64-5).

The "linear" model assumes that there is no threshold effect level, i.e., it represents a straight line extrapolation to "zero" level. It is called also a "one-hit" model under the assumption that each small increase of an exposure to a carcinogen has identical probability to cause cancer, notwithstanding the dose level. This model has been widely used in the radiation carcinogenesis evaluation process. In mathematical evaluation of carcinogenic risk due to chemical substances, it is thought that it represents the most sensitive probabil-ity, i.e., the upper limit to low dose-related carcinogenic effect because of the detoxifying mechanisms of the body. Yet, it provides the mathematical analysis of effect data which appears to be the most prudent to use in extrapolating from high dose level animal data to the rather minute quantities of chemicals found in the environment.

The "log-probit" model analysis of biological data results in a straight line when the loga-rithms of the doses are plotted against response, in this case animals with liver angiosarcoma, expressed in probits (probability units). The assumption here is that the observed effects corresponding to dose are related to the variations in susceptibility of the subjects which are assumed to have a log-normal distribution with dose.

Maltoni's liver angiosarcoma data (Experiment BT-1) were analyzed using a linear-dose re-sponse model to calculate the probability of incidence of liver angiosarcoma in high-level-exposed workers during each year of continuous exposure to vinyl chloride. Such treat-ment of the data resulted in an estimate of seventy-one cases per year of uninterrupted exposure to 1 ppm of vinyl chloride per million persons exposed. Using the same tech-nique, the probability of cancer in all body organs was approximately doubled, i.e., 150 cases per year of continuous exposure to 1 ppm of vinyl chloride per million persons (64-5).

Four epidemiological studies in workers (64-8)(64-9)(64-10)(64-11) were used to estimate the hemangiosarcoma incidence rate based on human experience, and to compare the re-sults with the incidence rates derived from animal data. From the epidemiological data the probability that a vinyl chloride worker would suffer from angiosarcoma of the liver at some point in his life was calculated to be 0.0031 per year of exposure. If the animal-derived data are converted to a standard work exposure time (7 hr, 5 days/wk, an exposure to 350 ppm of vinyl chloride), the probability was calculated to be 0.0052. Since such estimates contain a number of inherent errors, the authors concluded that "the slope of the linear animal dose-response relationship for angiosarcomas is consistent with human data."

The results of this analysis were used in estimating the risk to the 4.6 million persons living in the vicinity of the vinyl chloride and PVC plants employing the animal dose-response estimates, which were applied to the 17 ppb of vinyl chloride (average estimated concentration in the 5-mile radius of the plants). Both mathematical probability models were used. The results are tabulated in Table 93.

Table 93: Incidence of Cancer in Populations Living in the Vicinity of Vinyl Chloride-PVC Plants

| | . . . . . . Cases per Year of Exposure . . . . . . | |
Type of Effect	Linear Model	Log-Probit Model
All cancer	11	0.1-1.0
Liver angiosarcoma	5.5	0.05-0.5

Source: Reference (64-5) quoted in Reference (64)

Based on the linear model it was estimated that an incidence of 1 to 10 cases of liver angiosarcoma per year can be expected in the exposed population living in the vicinity of vinyl chloride and PVC plants. The calculation using the log-probit model predicted an incidence rate which is 10 to 100 times lower. The estimates for all cancers were about twice as great in both cases. The uncertainties in extrapolation process to low doses are reflected in this wide range of estimated effects.

The vinyl chloride-related cancer incidence probability calculations by Kuzmack and McGaughy (64-5) provide the best available quantitative estimate of the risk resulting from vinyl chloride exposure of a large segment of U.S. human population living in the vicinity of vinyl chloride-PVC plants. Recently published epidemiological studies indirectly support their conclusions. Brady, et al, (64-12) investigated the annual incidence rate for angiosarcoma of the liver among residents of New York State (excluding New York City). The study indicates that direct exposure to vinyl chloride, arsenic, and thorium dioxide was a significant factor in the etiology of this type of cancer (P = <0.02); and that it resulted in its increased incidence by a factor of 2 over the expected annual incidence for the U.S. (0.25 per million for New York State vs 0.14 per million for the U.S.). The important finding in this study was the diagnosis of five new cases of angiosarcoma of the liver in persons living in the vicinity of vinyl chloride polymerization and fabrication plants for 8 to 62 years prior to diagnosis of the disease.

The most recent report on this subject is a worldwide review of all cases of liver angiosarcoma in workers published by Spirtas and Kaminski in June, 1978 (64-13). The conclusions concerning the workers' age at diagnosis of the disease and the latency period, both of which appear to be increasing in recent years, are most important. It was reported in 1975 that the median age at diagnosis was 44 years and the latency period from first exposure to diagnosis averaged 17 years. Spirtas and Kaminski (64-13) reported 49 as the median age at diagnosis and a latency period of 21 years. It is probable that the initial cases may have had higher exposures of vinyl chloride and that the recent cases are due to more moderate exposures. It is also possible some variation is caused by statistical uncertainty in the age and latency parameter.

There are insufficient hard data available on the vinyl chloride exposure levels of persons living in the vicinity of vinyl chloride/PVC fabricating plants and on the amount of the vinyl chloride monomer released in time from various plastic products.

There are some initial data on vinyl chloride concentration in food packaged in PVC containers. The food oils require special attention; toxicologic data support this evidence.

Recent epidemiologic reports indicate that the median latency period for hemangiosarcoma occurrence in vinyl chloride-exposed workers is shifting to the right, and suggest that the recently diagnosed cases may have been due to lower exposures than the initial cases. This is an observation which, if confirmed, may have important consequences regarding the estimation of future risk for the population living in the vicinity of vinyl chloride/PVC plants, in addition to the workers.

Existing Guidelines and Standards: In the 1950s an upper limit of 500 ppm of VC at the workplace was recommended in the United States; for comparison, in the U.S.S.R, the upper limit was set at 400 ppm. Exposures in the U.S. were mostly below the time-weighted average (TWA) of 500 ppm; however, peak exposures as high as 4,000 ppm were recorded in some work areas (64-8). About 1960, Dow Chemical Company established a company standard for a limit of 50 ppm (TWA). They were successful in reducing exposures to workers to about 25 ppm vinyl chloride; however, excursions up to 500 ppm did occur. Dow Chemical also initiated continuous sampling and analysis using a multipoint remote sampler and gas chromatography.

In 1962, a Threshold Limit Value (TLV) of 500 ppm was set by the American Conference of Government Industrial Hygienists which was later adopted after its establishment by the Occupational Safety and Health Administration (Table 94).

Table 94: Regulations Concerning Vinyl Chloride

Year	Agency or Organization	Air Standard (ppm)	Other Action
1962	ACGIH	500 (TLV)	−
1971	OSHA	500 (TLV)	−
1974 (4/5)	OSHA	50 (Max. TLV)	Emergency temp. standard
1974	EPA	−	Banned as propellant in pesticide aerosols
1974	FDA	−	Banned as propellant in cosmetics and drug aerosols
1974	CPSC*	−	Banned as propellant in all aerosols for household use
1974 (10/4)	OSHA	1 (8 hr TWA)	5 ppm max. for 15 min.
1974	U.S. Coast Guard	−	Amended carriage on tank vessels
1975	EPA	−	Declared a hazardous pollutant (under Sec. 112, Clean Air Act), and proposed fugitive emission standard at the outlet not to exceed 10 ppm (acc. to BAT)
1976	EPA	−	Clarified proposed emission standard for various industrial processes including discharges in wastewater.

*Consumer Product Safety Commission.

Source: Reference (64)

Inhalation exposures dropped drastically after the carcinogenicity of vinyl chloride was reported (64-7). The Occupational Safety and Health Administration set an emergency temporary standard of 50 ppm (TWA) on April 5, 1974. A flurry of epidemiological studies was performed. Based on all of the information available at the time (64-15) a permanent standard of 1 ppm (TWA) with a maximum excursion of 5 ppm for a period of no longer than fifteen minutes in one day was promulgated for the workplace (64-14).

The U.S. EPA and other government agencies (Food and Drug Admin., Consum. Prod. Safety Comm.) have begun to investigate vinyl chloride inhalation exposures of humans in the general environment. Because of reports that forty-one pesticide spray products contained vinyl chloride as a propellant, there was published in 1974, a notice of intent to cancel registrations of all such products. Other aerosol products such as hair spray, also found to utilize vinyl chloride as a propellant, were banned from the market in the U.S. and some other countries shortly thereafter.

In 1975, the U.S. EPA declared vinyl chloride to be a hazardous substance under Sec. 112 of the Clean Air Act. Further, it proposed in 1975 and 1976 emission standards of total emissions with a limit of 10 ppm at the stack. Other government agencies have published new control measures during this time, or have new standards under consideration, e.g., FDA concerning packaging of food substances containing oil in PVC containers. Since 1975, when EPA published its intent to issue new standards for total emissions at the stack, the proposal was litigated in court action initiated by the Environmental Defense Fund and questioned by industry.

Summary of Proposed EPA Criteria: *Freshwater Aquatic Life* — No freshwater criterion can be derived for vinyl chloride using the Guidelines because no Final Chronic Value for either fish or invertebrate species or a good substitute for either value is available, and there are insufficient data to estimate a criterion using other procedures.

Saltwater Aquatic Life — No saltwater criterion can be derived for vinyl chloride using the Guidelines because no Final Chronic Value for either fish or invertebrate species or a good substitute for either value is available, and there are insufficient data to estimate a criterion using other procedures.

Human Health — For the maximum protection of human health from the potential carcinogenic effects of exposure to vinyl chlorides through ingestion of water and contaminated aquatic organisms, the ambient water concentration is zero. Concentrations of vinyl chloride estimated to result in additional lifetime cancer risks ranging from no additional risk to an additional risk of 1 in 100,000 are presented in the following section. The EPA is considering setting criteria at an interim target risk level in the range of 10^{-5}, 10^{-6}, or 10^{-7} with corresponding criteria of 517, 51.7, and 5.17 μg/l, respectively.

Basis for the Proposed Human Health Criteria: Vinyl chloride is a well-known human and animal carcinogen. Several occupational epidemiology studies in highly exposed workers have reported excess rates of liver angiosarcoma and tumors at other organ sites. Animal experiments using both inhalation and oral routes of exposure have also induced liver angiosarcoma.

The recommended water quality criterion is calculated using the tumor incidence data from chronic rate inhalation studies. The validity of these incidence rates for humans was established by evaluating the cancer incidence in workers after accounting for their exposure.

Under the Consent Decree in NRDC vs Train, criteria are to state "recommended maximum permissible concentrations (including where appropriate, zero) consistent with the protection of aquatic organisms, human health, and recreational activities." Vinyl chloride is suspected of being a human carcinogen. Because there is no recognized safe concentration for a human carcinogen, the recommended concentration of vinyl chloride in water for maximum protection of human health is zero.

Because attaining a zero concentration level may be infeasible in some cases and in order to assist the EPA and states in the possible future development of water quality regulations, the concentrations of vinyl chloride corresponding to several incremental lifetime cancer risk levels have been estimated. A cancer risk level provides an estimate of the additional incidence of cancer that may be expected in an exposed population. A risk of 10^{-5}, for example, indicates a probability of one additional case of cancer for every 100,000 people exposed, a risk of 10^{-6} indicates one additional case of cancer for every million people exposed, and so forth.

In the *Federal Register* notice of availability of draft ambient water quality criteria, EPA stated that it is considering setting criteria at an interim target risk level of 10^{-5}, 10^{-6} or 10^{-7} as shown in Table 95.

In Table 95 the risk levels and corresponding criteria are calculated by applying a modified "one-hit" extrapolation model to the animal bioassay and human epidemiological data presented in Summary of Pertinent Data. Since the extrapolation model is linear at low doses, the additional lifetime risk is directly proportional to the water concentration. Therefore, water concentrations corresponding to other risk levels can be derived by multiplying or dividing one of the risk levels and corresponding water concentrations shown in the table by factors such as 10, 100, 1,000, and so forth.

Table 95: Possible Alternative Criteria for Vinyl Chloride

	. Risk Levels and Corresponding Criteria .			
Exposure Assumptions (per day)	0	10^{-7}	10^{-6}	10^{-5}
	. . . . (μg/l)			
2 liters of drinking water and consumption of 18.7 g fish and shellfish*	0	5.17	51.7	517
Consumption of fish and shellfish only	0	260	2600	26,000

*Two percent of the vinyl chloride exposure results from the consumption of aquatic organisms which exhibit an average bioconcentration potential of 1.9 fold. The remaining 98% of vinyl chloride exposure results from drinking water.

Source: Reference (64)

Concentration levels were derived assuming a lifetime exposure to various amounts of vinyl chloride, (1) occurring from the consumption of both drinking water and aquatic life grown in waters containing the corresponding vinyl chloride concentrations and, (2) occurring solely from consumption of aquatic life grown in the waters containing the corresponding vinyl chloride concentrations.

Although total exposure information for vinyl chloride is discussed and an estimate of the contributions from other sources of exposure can be made, this data will not be factored into ambient water quality criteria formulation until additional analysis can be made. The criteria presented, therefore, assume an incremental risk from ambient water exposure only.

Summary of Pertinent Data — In a previous report on risks to vinyl chloride in the ambient air (64-5), the rat inhalation experiments of Maltoni and Lefemine (64-7) were combined with occupational epidemiology studies to estimate risks to inhaled vinyl chloride. The result was that a continuous exposure of 17 ppb of vinyl chloride results in a lifetime risk of 10^{-5}. On the assumptions that the same daily intake of vinyl chloride via 2 liters of drinking water produces the same risk, and that fish bioaccumulate vinyl chloride to a small degree (BCF = 1.9), the following calculation is used to find the water concentration giving a lifetime risk of 10^{-5}.

Intake of vinyl chloride via air is:

$$24 \text{ m}^3/\text{day} \times 17 \text{ ppb} \times (1 \ \mu g/m^3/0.387 \text{ ppb}) = 1.054 \times 10^3 \ \mu g/\text{day}.$$

If this intake comes from 2 liters of water and ingesting 18.7 g/day of fish and shellfish products, the ambient water concentration would have to be

$$(1.054 \text{ mg/kg/day})/[2 + 1.9(0.0187)] = 0.517 \text{ mg/l}.$$

References

(64-1)   Falk, H., et al, "Hepatic disease among workers at a vinyl chloride polymerization plant," *Jour. Am. Med. Assoc.*, 230, 59 (1974).

(64-2)   Maltoni, C., "Carcinogenicity of vinyl chloride: Current results. Experimental evidence." Proc. 6th Int. Symp. Biological Characterization of Human Tumors, Copenhagen, May 13-15, 1975.

See Vol. 3, *Biological characterization of human tumors,* New York, American Elsevier Publishing Co., Inc. (1976).

(64-3) U.S. EPA, *A scientific and technical assessment report on vinyl chloride and polyvinyl chloride,* Report No. EPA-600/6-75-004, Washington, D.C, Office of Res. and Dev. (1975).

(64-4) Filatova, V.S., and Gronsberg, E.S., "Sanitary hygienic working conditions in the production of polychlorvinylic tar and measures of improvement," *Gig. I. Sanit.,* 22, 38 (1957).

(64-5) Kuzmack, A.M. and McGaughy, R.E., *Quantitative Risk Assessment for Community Exposure to Vinyl Chloride,* Wash. D.C., U.S. Envir. Protect. Agency (1975).

(64-6) American Public Health Assoc., *Population Residing Near Plants Producing Vinyl Chloride* (1975).

(64-7) Maltoni, C. and Lefemine, G., "Carcinogenicity assays of vinyl chloride: current results, *Ann. N.Y. Acad. Sci.,* 246, 195 (1975).

(64-8) Ott, M.G., et al, "Vinyl chloride exposure in a controlled industrial environment: A long-term mortality experience in 595 employees," *Arch. Envir. Health,* 30, 333 (1975).

(64-9) Tabershaw, I.R. and Gaffey, W.R., "Mortality study of workers in the manufacture of vinyl chloride and its polymers," *Jour. Occup. Med.,* 16, (8), 509 (1974).

(64-10) Nicholson, W.J., et al, "Mortality experience of a cohort of vinyl chloride—polyvinyl chloride workers," *Ann. N.Y. Acad. Sci.,* 246, 225 (1975).

(64-11) Heath, C.W., Jr. and Falk, H., "Characteristics of cases of angiosarcoma of the liver among vinyl chloride workers in the United States, *Ann. N.Y. Acad. Sci.,* 246, 231 (1975).

(64-12) Brady, J., et al, "Angiosarcoma of the liver: An epidemiologic survey," *Jour. Nat. Cancer Inst.,* 59, 1383 (1975).

(64-13) Spirtas, R. and Kaminski, R., "Angiosarcoma of the liver in vinyl chloride/polyvinyl chloride workers, Update of the NIOSH Register, *Jour. Occup. Med.,* 20, 427 (1978).

(64-14) 39 *FR* 35890 (Oct. 4, 1974).

(64-15) National Inst. for Occup. Safety and Health, *Vinyl Halides: Carcinogenicity,* Current Intelligence Bulletin No. 28, Wash. D.C. (Sept. 21, 1978).

VINYLIDENE CHLORIDE

See "Dichloroethylenes" (27).

Z

ZINC (#65)

Zinc, symbol Zn, is an element in Group II of the Periodic Table. It has an atomic number of 30 and an atomic weight of 65.38.

Occurrence: Zinc is never found free in nature, but occurs as the sulfide, oxide, or carbonate. Because zinc is an element it can be expected to persist in the environment indefinitely in some form.

Physical Properties: Zinc is a bluish-white metal which dissolves readily in strong acids. It is fairly ductile and has a density in cast form of 7.1 g/cc. It has a melting point of 419.5°C and a boiling point of 906°C.

Chemical Properties: Zinc is divalent and also amphoteric. The metal is slowly oxidized in air, but moisture accelerates the rate of attack. Zinc reacts readily with mineral acids. It also reacts with alkali hydroxides forming alkali zincates, together with the evolution of hydrogen.

Uses: The principal uses of zinc include electroplating and the production of alloys.

Toxic Effects: In the aquatic environment zinc is acutely toxic to freshwater organisms at concentrations as low as 90 μg/l (65-1) and the lowest reported chronic effects lie between 26 and 51 μg/l (65-2). In marine waters, comparable values are 141 μg/l in acute tests (65-3) and 220 μg/l in chronic tests (65-4).

Water quality has been shown to affect zinc toxicity. The best studied of these is the protective effect exerted by water hardness, which has been incorporated into the freshwater criterion for the protection of aquatic life.

In humans, zinc ingestion has produced no clinical symptoms at daily intakes of 150 mg/day for as long as six months (65-5). Brown, et al (65-6) reported food poisoning from ingestion of a meal estimated to contain nearly 1,000 ppm of zinc and another case among people who had drunk punch containing zinc at a concentration of 2,200 ppm.

Current Levels of Exposure: It has been well established in several studies that the present intake of zinc via food for the adult U.S. population is from 10 to 20 mg. For the majority of the population the intake of zinc via drinking water will be only a few percent of the intake via food, but for some individuals the zinc concentration in tap water may cause an additional daily intake of 2 to 10 mg of zinc. The average exposure to zinc via ambient air will, even in the vicinity of zinc-emitting industries, be in the order of only a few tenths of a milligram. Smoking will contribute even less.

Special Groups at Risk: Since zinc may interfere with copper and other minerals, excessive intakes of zinc by people with a tendency to copper deficiency might cause reversible health effects. Patients treated for months or years with large oral doses of zinc salts, about ten times the intake via food, for curing of various diseases caused by zinc deficiency or to promote wound healing may constitute a group at special risk. Infants with copper deficiency or low intakes of copper may constitute another risk group. Occupational exposure to zinc oxide fumes may cause acute reversible reactions which may put persons subjected to such exposure at special risk.

Existing Guidelines and Standards: NIOSH (65-7) has recently reviewed the occupational hazards of exposure to zinc oxide and no changes were suggested regarding the existing standard for zinc oxide of 5 mg/m^3. ACGIH has an adopted threshold limit value (TLV) for zinc oxide of 5 mg/m^3. The TLV value has also been adopted in other countries. For zinc chloride a limit of 1 mg/m^3 has been adopted by ACGIH and OSHA also adopted a standard of 1 mg/m^3 for zinc chloride.

In addition, ACGIH has designated zinc stearate as a nuisance particulate with recommended limits of 10 mg/m^3 of total dust or 5 mg/m^3 of respirable dust.

Finally, ACGIH has set a TWA value of 0.05 mg/m^3 for zinc chromate with the notation that this is an industrial substance suspect of carcinogenic potential for man. This is, of course, simply a reflection of the chromium content of zinc chromate.

The present standard for drinking water, 5 mg/l, is based on organoleptic effects, i.e., some people will recognize the bitter taste caused by zinc present at such levels. The World Health Organization (WHO) has also proposed that the level should be 5 mg/l; however, the USSR has established a limit for zinc at 1 mg/l for other than health reasons (65-8).

There is no acceptable daily intake for zinc in food. Because zinc is an essential nutrient, there has been no reason to restrict the zinc levels in food.

In 1974, the National Academy of Sciences recommended that adults should have an intake of 15 mg of zinc per day, that pregnant women should have an intake of 20 mg/day and that preadolescent children should have 10 mg/day of zinc.

Summary of Proposed EPA Criteria: *Freshwater Aquatic Life* — For zinc, the criterion to protect freshwater aquatic life as derived using the Guidelines is:

$$e^{[0.67 \ln(\text{hardness}) + 0.67]}$$

as a 24-hour average and the concentration should not exceed

$$e^{[0.64 \ln(\text{hardness}) + 2.46]}$$

at any time.

Saltwater Aquatic Life — For saltwater aquatic life, no criterion for zinc can be derived using the Guidelines, and there are insufficient data to estimate a criterion using other procedures.

Human Health — For the prevention of adverse effects due to the organoleptic properties of zinc, the current standard for drinking water of 5 mg/l was adopted for ambient water criterion.

Basis for the Proposed Human Health Criteria: Zinc is an essential element and is not a carcinogenic agent. Studies on experimental animals and on human beings given zinc for therapeutic purposes together with observations of occupationally exposed persons show that large doses of zinc can be tolerated for long periods, provided that the copper status is normal.

Daily ingestion of about 150 mg of zinc as the sulfate has not resulted in adverse effects in most patients even after several months of treatment. A reduction of copper levels has been reported in patients with diseases such as sickle cell anemia and coeliac disease. A reduction of the dose of zinc and copper supplementation corrected the copper deficiency.

Laboratory animals have been shown to tolerate zinc concentration in the range of 100 to 300 mg/kg food and even higher for long periods when the intake of copper has been adequate. Copper-deficient animals have been shown to be more susceptible. In many animal experiments, zinc concentration in the diet of 1,000 to 2,000 mg/kg have been reported to be without effect. These concentrations should be compared to the average zinc content of human food, which is about 10 mg/kg.

The water quality criterion for zinc in water, based on available data on effects of ingested zinc would be about 10 mg/l for the adult U.S. population. Assuming a water intake of 2 liters per day, this exposure would not cause more than an additional intake of 20 mg which can be well tolerated. This concentration is above the present standard for drinking water which is 5 mg/l based on organoleptic effects.

There are some indications that infants and small children may have a high intake of water and an additional intake of 10 to 20 mg might have an influence on copper metabolism in children with low copper intakes or with copper deficiency due to e.g., intestinal diseases. However, due to insufficient amount of information available for this special group at risk, derivation of criterion lower than the current standard would be difficult to justify. Therefore, it is recommended that the current level be maintained for water quality criteria purposes (5 mg/l). As additional information becomes available, reconsiderations of appropriateness of the current standard should be performed.

References

(65-1) Rabe, F.W., and C.W. Sappington. *Biological productivity of the Couer D'Alene river as related to water quality.* Report on Project A-024-IDA. Water Resour. Res. Inst. Univ. Idaho. Moscow, Idaho. (1970)

(65-2) Spehar, R.L. "Cadmium and zinc toxicity to flagfish, *Jordanella floridae.*" *Jour. Fish. Res. Board Can. 33,* 1939. (1976).

(65-3) Calabrese, et al. "Survival and growth of bivalve larvae under heavy-metal stress." *Mar. Biol. 41,* 179. (1977).

(65-4) Reish, D.J., et al. "The effect of heavy metals on laboratory populations of two polychaetes with comparisons to the water quality conditions and standards in southern California marine waters." *Water Res. 10,* 299. (1976).

(65-5) Greaves, M.W., and A.W. Sillen, "Effects of long-continued ingestion of zinc sulfate in patients with venous leg ulceration." *Lancet.* (Oct. 31, 1970).

(65-6) Brown, M.A., et al. "Food poisoning involving zinc contamination." *Arch. Environ. Health. 8,* 657. (1964).

(65-7) Nat. Inst. for Occup. Safety and Health, *Criteria for a Recommended Standard: Occupational Exposure to Zinc Oxide,* NIOSH Doc. No. 76-104. (1976).

(65-8) National Academy of Sciences, *Drinking Water and Health,* Wash., D.C. (1977).

SUMMARY

An attempt has been made to summarize some of the major findings of the 65 Criteria Documents in one single table (Table 96).

Table 96: Summary of Some Criteria Document Findings

Pollutant	Proposed Allowable Limit in Water (μg/l)	Carcinogen or Suspect Carcinogen	Present or Absent in Cigarette Smoke
(1) Acenaphthene	20.0	No	Present
(2) Acrolein	6.5	No	Present
(3) Acrylonitrile	0.084*	Yes	Present
(4) Aldrin/dieldrin	4.5×10^{-5}*	Yes	Absent
(5) Antimony and compounds	145.0	No	Absent
(6) Arsenic and compounds	0.02*	Yes	Absent
(7) Asbestos	**, *	Yes	Absent***
(8) Benzene	15.0*	Yes	Absent
(9) Benzidine	0.00167*	Yes	Absent
(10) Beryllium and compounds	0.087*	Yes	Present
(11) Cadmium and compounds	10.0	Yes	Present
(12) Carbon tetrachloride	2.6*	Yes	Absent
(13) Chlordane	0.0012*	Yes	Absent
(14) Chlorobenzenes (except $C_6H_4Cl_2$)	20.0–0.5 (to Cl_5) 0.001 (HCB)*	HCB only	Absent
(15) Chlorinated ethanes	1.8–7.0*	Yes	Absent
(16) Chloroalkyl ethers (see 37)	11.5 (BCIE) 0.42 (BCEE)* 0.00002 (BCME)	Yes	Absent
(17) Chlorinated naphthalenes	0.08–3.9	No	Absent
(18) Chlorinated phenols (see 20, 28, 51)	3.0–263.0	No	Absent
(19) Chloroform	2.1*	Yes	Absent
(20) 2-Chlorophenol (see 18)	0.3	No	Absent
(21) Chromium and compounds	0.008 (Cr-VI)*	Yes	Absent
(22) Copper and compounds	1,000	No	Present
(23) Cyanides	200	No	Present
(24) DDT and metabolites	0.00098*	Yes	Absent
(25) Dichlorobenzenes (see 14)	230	No	Absent
(26) Dichlorobenzidine	0.0169*	Yes	Absent
(27) Dichloroethylenes	1.3*	Yes	Absent

(continued)

Table 96: (continued)

Pollutant	Proposed Allowable Limit in Water (μg/l)	Carcinogen or Suspect Carcinogen	Present or Absent in Cigarette Smoke
(28) 2,4-Dichlorophenol (see 18)	0.5	No	Absent
(29) Dichloropropane/propene	200.0/0.63	No	Absent
(30) 2,4-Dimethylphenol	†	Yes	Present
(31) Dinitrotoluenes	0.74*	Yes	Absent
(32) Diphenylhydrazines	0.40*	Yes	Absent
(33) Endosulfan	100	No	Absent
(34) Endrin	1.0	No	Absent
(35) Ethylbenzene	1,100	No	Present
(36) Fluoranthene	200	No	Present
(37) Haloethers (see 16)	(see 16)	(see 16)	Absent
(38) Halomethanes (see 12, 19)	2.0 (except fluorine compounds)	Yes	Absent
(39) Heptachlor	0.00023*	Yes	Absent
(40) Hexachlorobutadiene	0.77*	Yes	Absent
(41) Hexachlorocyclohexane (BHC)	0.00021*	Yes	Absent
(42) Hexachlorocyclopentadiene	1.0	No	Absent
(43) Isophorone	460	No	Absent
(44) Lead and compounds	50	No	Absent
(45) Mercury and compounds	0.2	No	Absent
(46) Naphthalene	143	No	Present
(47) Nickel and compounds	133	No	Present
(48) Nitrobenzene	30	No	Absent
(49) Nitrophenols	10-68.6	No	Absent
(50) Nitrosamines	0.01-0.11*	Yes	Present
(51) Pentachlorophenol (see 18)	140	No	Absent
(52) Phenol	3,400	No	Absent
(53) Phthalate esters	5,000 and up	No	Absent
(54) Polychlorobiphenyls (PCBs)	0.00026*	Yes	Absent
(55) Polynuclear aromatics	0.0097*	Yes	Present
(56) Selenium and compounds	10	No	Absent
(57) Silver and compounds	10	No	Absent
(58) Tetrachlorodibenzo-p-dioxin	4.6×10^{-7}*	Yes	Absent
(59) Tetrachloroethylene	2.0*	Yes	Absent
(60) Thallium and compounds	4.0	No	Present
(61) Toluene	12.4	No	Absent
(62) Toxaphene	0.00047*	Yes	Absent
(63) Trichloroethylene	21	Yes	Absent
(64) Vinyl chloride	517	Yes	Absent
(65) Zinc and compounds	5,000	No	Present

*Based on the probability of one additional case of cancer for every 100,000 (10^5) people exposed.

**300,000 fibers/liter.

***Asbestos exposure and cigarette smoking act synergistically to produce dramatic increases in lung cancer over that from exposure to either agent alone.

†Data insufficient to set a standard; contact should be minimized.

HAZARDOUS AND TOXIC EFFECTS
OF INDUSTRIAL CHEMICALS
1979

by Marshall Sittig

There is a continuing need to assess the status of potentially dangerous substances including those now available and those that may reach commercial availability in the future. This should be done with a predictive view to avoid or at least to ameliorate catastrophic episodes similar to those that have occurred with methyl mercury, polychlorinated biphenyls, vinyl chloride monomer, dioxin and a number of pesticides.

This handbook is intended to be a working guide for the industrial hygienist and other interested persons. Most of the individual chemical listings contain a number of literature references.

This book is intended to be a guide to these hazardous chemicals, to give first warning signals, and to serve as an introduction to the published literature and to government agencies offering detailed guidance.

Information (where available) under each chemical listing includes:

Description. Derivation, chemical structure and systematic chemical name.
Synonyms. Other chemical names, generic names and trademarks.
Potential Occupational Exposures.
Permissible Exposure Limits.
Routes of Entry.
Harmful Effects. Local, systemic.
Medical Surveillance.
Special Tests.
Personal Protective Methods.
Bibliography. References to articles in journals and government publications.

The book consists of about 250 individual monographs arranged alphabetically by the common name of each substance described. It is impossible to indicate here all of the chemical entries in this book. In order to give an indication of the vast scope of information dealt with here, the names of most entries in the beginning of the book are reproduced here.

Acetaldehyde	Bis(Chloromethyl) Ether	Coal Tar Products
Acetates	Bismuth & Compounds	Cobalt & Compounds
Acetic Acid	Boron & Compounds	Copper & Compounds
Acetic Anhydride	Boron Hydrides	Cotton Dust
Acetone (See Ketones)	Boron Trifluoride	Creosote
Acetonitrile	Brass	Cresol
Acetylaminofluorene	Bromine	Cyclohexanone
Acetylene	1,3-Butadiene	Diacetone Alcohol
Acridine	Butyl Alcohol	2,4-Diaminoanisole
Acrolein	Butylamine	4,4'-Diaminodiphenylmethane
Acrylamide	Cadmium & Compounds	Dibromochloropropane
Acrylonitrile	Calcium Cyanamide	1,2-Dibromoethane
Alkanes	Calcium Oxide	3,3'-Dichlorobenzidine
Allyl Alcohol	Carbaryl	1,2-Dichloroethane
Allyl Chloride	Carbon Dioxide	1,2-Dichloroethylene
Aluminum & Compounds	Carbon Disulfide	Dichloroethyl Ether
Aminodiphenyl	Carbon Monoxide	Diisobutyl Ketone
Ammonia	Carbon Tetrachloride	N,N-Dimethylacetamide
Amyl Alcohol	Carbonyls	4-Dimethylaminoazobenzene
Aniline	Cement Dust	N,N-Dimethylformamide
Antimony & Compounds	Cerium & Compounds	Dimethyl Sulfate
Arsenic	Chlorinated Benzenes	Dinitrobenzene
Arsine	Chlorinated Lime	Dinitro-o-Cresol
Asbestos	Chlorinated Naphthalenes	Dinitrophenol
Asphalt Fumes	Chlorine	Dinitrotoluene
Barium & Compounds	o-Chlorobenzylidene Malonitrile	Dioxane
Benzene	Chlorodiphenyls & Derivs.	Diphenyl
Benzidine & Salts	Chloroform	Epichlorohydrin
Benzoyl Peroxide	Chloromethyl Methyl Ether	Ethanolamines
Benzyl Chloride	Chloroprene	Ethyl Alcohol
Beryllium & Compounds	Chromium & Compounds	Ethylbenzene

plus 160 other chemicals

ISBN 0-8155-0731-3

460 pages

HAZARDOUS CHEMICAL SPILL CLEANUP 1979

Edited by J. S. Robinson

Pollution Technology Review No. 59

There is a delicate balance in nature involving a perfect blending of chemical, physical and biological elements. Once this balance is upset by a spillage of chemicals, it may take years to restore the original environment. Meanwhile, untold damage results. The deleterious effects, however, can be lessened if there is a rapid response reinforced by expertise in proper procedure. It is the intent of this book to provide the specific know-how needed to cope with chemical spillage quickly by correct containment, countermeasures, and cleanup.

After an introductory overview of legislation, Robinson offers practical advice and response techniques for different kinds of substances, including preferred methods of disposal and restoration. Managers in all fields with problems of potential spills should avail themselves of this information now.

The partial table of contents below lists chapter headings and **examples of some** subtitles.

INTRODUCTION
Upward Trend in Hazardous Spills
Legislative Background
Government Action—Recent Control Acts
National Contingency Plan
Spill Damage Restoration

1. PROCEDURE LEADING TO CLEANUP
Notification—Regional Research Centers
Information Sources—
   EPA; U.S. Coast Guard, Army; Transportation Emergency Assistance Plan, etc.
Identification and Assessment—
   On-Scene and Laboratory Responses
Classification Systems—
   Categorizing CHRIS (Chemical Hazard Resource Information System) Chemicals that Sink, Float, Disperse
Response Techniques for Various Classes
Cleanup in Industrial Areas

2. MECHANICAL CLEANUP METHODS
Dispersion and Dilution
Containment
Devices for Floating Hazardous Chemicals
Dredging—
   Equipment: Evaluation and Availability
Burial—
   Materials, Applicability, Controls

Barriers, Dikes and Trenches—
   Soil Surface Sealing, Encapsulation
Other Physical Methods—
   Solvent Extraction, Cryogens, Aerosols

3. CHEMICAL METHODS
Guidelines, Safety and Troubleshooting
Neutralization—
   Of Chemicals that Sink
   Of Representative CHRIS Chemicals
   Choice of Agents, Methods, Application
Precipitation—
   Of Sinking and CHRIS Chemicals
   Of Heavy Metals with Na Sulfide
Chelation—
   Treatable Spills
   Selecting Sequestrants, Precipitants
Redox Methods
Biodegradation
Portable Treatment Equipment Sources

4. SORBENTS, GELS AND FOAMS
Sorbents for Representative Chemicals
Activated Carbon & Ion Exchange Resins—
   "Teabags" and Other Packaging Concepts
   Flotation Methods
   Buoyant and Sinking Carbon Methods
   Deployment Techniques
Gels—
   For Sinking and Floating Chemicals
   Universal Gelling Agent for Land Spills
Foams—
   As a Response to Floating Spills
   High Expansion Rigid Urethane

5. MOBILE UNITS
Emergency Collection Bag System
Mudcat/Processing System—
   Freeing Pond Bottom of Simulated Matter
   Removal of Latex Paint
   Discussion of Field Results
Dynactor
In-Place Detoxifying of Spills in Soil
For Soluble Organics Spilled in Water—
   Design Criteria for Mobile System
Dispensing System for Multipurpose Gel
Unit for Activated Carbon Regeneration
Mobile Ozone Treatment System
Polyurethane Foam
Foamed Concrete Emergency Unit
Environmental Emergency Response Unit
Adapts
Remotely Controlled Countermeasures—
   Snail, Fire Cat, Foreign Devices

ISBN 0-8155-0767-4

406 pages